WQ 244

Heart Disease in Pregnancy

HEART DISEASE IN PREGNANCY

Edited by

Celia Oakley

Professor of Clinical Cardiology,
Hammersmith Hospital, London, UK

BMJ
Publishing
Group

First published in 1997
by the BMJ Publishing Group, BMA House, Tavistock Square,
London WC1H 9JR

British Library Cataloguing in Publication Data

A catalogue record for this book is available from the
British Library

ISBN 0-7279-1065-5

Typeset, printed and bound in Great Britain by
Latimer Trend and Company Ltd, Plymouth

Contents

Contributors

Muayad Al Zaibag
Section of Cardiology, Loma Linda University Medical Center, Loma Linda International Heart Institute, Loma Linda, California, USA

Mark H Anderson
Senior Registrar in Cardiology, St Mary's Hospital, London, UK

Anne H Child
Clinical Geneticist (Research) and Honorary Senior Lecturer, St George's Hospital, London, UK

Murdoch G Elder
Professor, Institute of Obstetrics and Gynaecology, Hammersmith Hospital, London, UK

Robert G Feldman
Senior Lecturer in Infectious Diseases and Bacteriology, Hammersmith Hospital, London, UK

Denis F Hawkins
Professor of Obstetric Therapeutics, Institute of Obstetrics and Gynaecology, Hammersmith Hospital, London, UK

Susan E Holder
Consultant Clinical Geneticist, The Kennedy Galton Centre, Northwick Park and St Mark's NHS Trust Hospital, Harrow, UK

J M B Hughes
Professor of Thoracic Medicine, Royal Postgraduate Medical School, Hammersmith Hospital, London, UK

Stewart Hunter
Paediatric Cardiologist, Freeman Hospital, Newcastle Upon Tyne, UK

Elizabeth A Letsky
Consultant Haematologist, Queen Charlotte's Hospital, London, UK

Petros Nihoyannopoulos
Senior Lecturer and Consultant Cardiologist, Division of Cardiology, Department of Medicine, Hammersmith Hospital, London, UK

Paulo Ribeiro
Associate Professor of Medicine, Section of Cardiology, Loma Linda
University Medical Center, Loma Linda International Heart Institute,
Loma Linda, California, USA

Stephen Robson
Professor of Obstetrics and Gynaecology, Royal Victoria Infirmary,
Newcastle Upon Tyne, UK

Claire Shovlin
Department of Genetics, Harvard Medical School, Boston,
Massachusetts, USA

Anita K Simonds
Consultant in Respiratory Medicine, Royal Brompton Hospital, London,
UK

Michael de Swiet
Consultant Physician, Queen Charlotte's Hospital, London, UK

Carole A Warnes
Consultant in Cardiovascular Diseases, Internal Medicine and Paediatric
Cardiology, Mayo Clinic, Rochester, Minnesota, USA

Julie Watts
Senior Registrar in Anaesthetics, Hammersmith Hospital, London, UK

David Zideman
Consultant Anaesthetist, Hammersmith Hospital, London, UK

Preface

This book is intended to help in the practical management of patients with cardiovascular problems in pregnancy and the puerperium.

The contributors were invited because of practical experience and expertise in their topics. Experience of heart disease in pregnancy is fragmented and diluted. The literature largely comprises case reports or reviews of anecdotal experience rather than the results of clinical trials, which are sparse even in the relatively common area of hypertension. Experts in the various cardiac disorders may not often see pregnant patients and personal experience of the many cardiac disorders in pregnancy tends to be small.

The Hammersmith experience stems from the setting up of an antenatal cardiac clinic 30 years ago with the late Geoffrey Dixon, a distinguished medical obstetrician and from a continuing team approach involving cardiologists, obstetricians, and anaesthetists. Because of the early development of open heart surgery at the hospital we have always had referrals of a rich mix of congenital and valvular heart disease in young women who are pregnant or wanting to become pregnant, related to our special interest in pregnancy complicating heart disease and heart disease complicating pregnancy. The Hammersmith Hospitals Trust includes Queen Charlotte's and has a large obstetric practice. Because the Royal Postgraduate Medical School is a multispecialty postgraduate institution, my colleagues in other specialties have many patients with non-cardiac disorders who develop cardiac complications and become pregnant or seek our advice. I am grateful to the many colleagues outside Hammersmith for their referrals, for their many telephone conversations about problem patients, and for the feedback which has greatly enriched our experience.

Acknowledgements

I owe much to my academic secretary of 18 years, Mrs Miriam Smith, without whose skill and patience there would have been no book. I am grateful also to my colleague, Dr Petros Nihoyannopoulos, for the echocardiographic material.

1: Overview

CELIA OAKLEY, MURDOCH G ELDER

Heart disease in pregnancy is an interdisciplinary subject which tends to be consigned to the perimeter of both cardiology and obstetrics. Cardiologists necessarily concentrate on coronary disease which is rare in pregnancy. Most pregnant women have normal hearts; they do not travel because they seek antenatal care from their general practitioner and local hospital. Experience is thereby diluted and individual cardiologists, obstetricians, and anaesthetists may see too few patients to gain confidence in their management.

The most common cause of maternal death is hypertension followed by pulmonary embolism and both of these plus peripartum cardiomyopathy can be considered as complications of the pregnancy. Heart disease is the third most common cause of maternal death and the most important non-obstetric cause.

Since the dramatic decline in the prevalence of rheumatic heart disease, which used to be found in up to 1% of young pregnant women, heart disease in pregnancy is perceived by some as a vanishing problem which involves either insignificant or obscure congenital or myocardial defects. Yet previously undetected mitral stenosis is not uncommon in young pregnant immigrants. It would be recognised immediately and promptly treated in their own countries but it now tends to be missed in the west because it has become rare. Abnormalities readily picked up by chest radiography and echocardiography are not diagnosed because neither investigation is made. Clinical competence is fast disappearing in favour of technology, but the chest radiograph is not requested because of the mistaken idea that a single radiograph is dangerous for the fetus and echocardiography requires at least a suspicion that there may be a cardiac cause for the breathlessness. The radiation dose from a chest radiograph is only half as much as the natural background radiation received in the course of a year and is about the same as that received during a flight to the USA.

Congenital heart disease is now both relatively and absolutely more common in pregnancy. Its increased prevalence in patients who are pregnant or seeking pregnancy is the result of the major improvement in the survival of children with congenital heart disease. During the same time paediatric and adult cardiology have become more separated and adult cardiologists

1

have often had inadequate exposure to congenital heart disease during their training.

Patients with simple defects do well but some more complex abnormalities may cause concern. Patients who have had holes closed or valves opened will sometimes have residual problems. Those who have survived heroic surgery during infancy for the palliation of complex defects need detailed assessment. Some of these patients face trouble in pregnancy. Aortic valve stenosis previously mild in childhood, may have become more severe but the patient has been lost to follow up until a pregnancy. Patients who have had non-restrictive ("big") ventricular septal defects closed and who have considered themselves cured may have been left with substantial but undiagnosed pulmonary hypertension. Ebstein's anomaly, Eisenmenger syndrome, or corrected transposition may be recognised for the first time at an antenatal clinic. Women with valved conduits, univentricular circulations, or interatrial (or arterial) switches for transposition all want to live normal lives and have families. A rich variety is seen. These patients seek advice about the risks of future pregnancy and want to know the genetic risks to a potential child.

Optimum management requires correct appraisal of the likely ability of the abnormal heart to make the necessary adaptations to the major haemodynamic and respiratory changes which take place during pregnancy, labour, and delivery. It is important to predict potential trouble in advance both for the mother and the baby and so reduce any likely adverse influences on the developing fetus, whose risks may be both environmental and genetic.

The use of drugs is avoided as much as possible during pregnancy but they may be necessary and their possible effects on the fetus need to be known. Rhythm disturbances may first develop or become more frequent during pregnancy and cause considerable concern over the best choice of management.

The increases in blood volume, stroke output, and heart rate (particularly if stroke volume cannot be increased) may not be well tolerated. The relaxation of smooth muscle which allows accommodation of the increased blood volume and the profound fall in systemic vascular resistance are beneficial to patients with regurgitant valve disease or left to right shunts, as the abnormal flows tend to diminish. Conversely when the left atrial pressure is raised it will rise further during pregnancy because of the increase in intrathoracic blood volume. This may lead to dyspnoea and pulmonary congestion in patients with mitral or aortic stenosis or in hypertrophic cardiomyopathy. Patients with impaired left ventricular function may benefit from a fall in afterload but this may be offset by the increase in preload. When stroke volume fails to rise the heart rate increases to maintain output and such reflex tachycardia betrays a lack of circulatory reserve. This may not matter when ventricular filling is rapid but may precipitate pulmonary oedema in patients with mitral stenosis or lead to myocardial ischaemia and failure in patients with aortic stenosis, hypertrophic cardiomyopathy, or pulmonary hypertension.

The fall in systemic vascular resistance causes right to left shunts to increase during pregnancy with resultant worsening of dyspnoea, fall in arterial oxygen saturation and rise in packed cell volume. Fetal perfusion suffers with risk of spontaneous abortion, prematurity, and dysmaturity. When the cyanosis is associated with pulmonary stenosis the mother may tolerate the pregnancy well albeit with the possible complications of venous thrombosis and paradoxical embolism, but if she has pulmonary hypertension (Eisenmenger syndrome) she faces mortal risk.

The highest maternal mortality due to heart disease occurs in patients with pulmonary hypertension whether solitary in the primary type or associated with bidirectional or reversed central shunt in the Eisenmenger syndrome. Maternal mortality may be as high as 50% in the Eisenmenger complex (with ventricular septal defect). This is the result of a highly sensitive "titre board" with finely balanced near-equal systemic and pulmonary vascular resistances upon which survival and well being depend. A fall in systemic resistance associated perhaps with a vagally induced systemic depressor reflex or increase in pulmonary vascular obstruction may result in virtually all of the right ventricular output bypassing the lungs. This can cause downward plummeting of arterial oxygen saturation followed by ventricular fibrillation. In patients with pulmonary hypertension unassociated with septal defects the stroke output may be relatively fixed, reflex tachycardia may lead to right ventricular ischaemia, and progressive congestion and failure are likely. Most deaths occur in the puerperium either suddenly or associated with a seemingly immutable increase in pulmonary vascular resistance which is unresponsive to all efforts to bring about vasodilatation.

In the peripartum and postpartum periods maternal heart failure may develop with seemingly explosive suddenness in women with peripartum cardiomyopathy. Patients may suffer myocardial infarction and the risk of thromboembolism is particularly high after caesarean section and in women with restricted cardiac outputs or cyanotic heart disease.

The choice of management of delivery, whether natural or caesarean under general or regional anaesthesia, is crucial to survival of both mother and baby in women with heart disease. The obstetric anaesthetist is an important member of the team looking after pregnant cardiac patients and there should be early discussion of the mode of delivery between cardiologist, obstetrician, and anaesthetist. While epidural analgesia or anaesthesia are well tolerated by patients with abundant circulatory reserve, vasodilatation can cause a redistribution of blood volume away from the thorax resulting in a fall in filling pressure and cardiac output which needs to be compensated by fluid loading. This has to be finely judged when systemic and pulmonary venous filling pressures are critical. If the stroke output cannot be raised the slight fall in blood pressure which usually accompanies epidural anaesthesia may become profound. In patients with right to left shunts vasodilatation leads to an increase in right to left shunting and to fetal as well as maternal hypoxaemia. In patients with stenotic lesions such as aortic stenosis or uncorrected coarctation, vasodilatation may lead to failure of perfusion distal to the circulatory obstruction.

In general, normal delivery has been favoured for women with heart disease. This dates from a time when the commonest maternal disease was mitral stenosis. Patients were kept in bed during the latter part of pregnancy and with the inferior vena cava compressed by the gravid uterus and intrapulmonary pressures thus minimised they came to term without the need for beta-blocking drugs to prevent tachycardia. The progress of labour was apparently expedited by the inotropic effects of digitalis upon the contracting uterus, and a little postpartum blood loss helped as well.

Good arguments can be made for more frequent use of caesarean delivery for certain cardiac patients. Heart disease tends to get worse, so the first pregnancy may be the only pregnancy and caesarean delivery has the advantage of minimal risk to the child. In addition to protecting the child, it safeguards patients with fragile circulatory reserve by eliminating maternal physical effort and expediting the birth process. In cyanosed women the effort of normal delivery causes increased right to left shunting and fetal hypoxaemia. Caesarean section gives babies who are usually premature and small for dates their best chance of survival. Caesarean delivery under epidural anaesthesia minimises aortic wall stress in women with the Marfan syndrome and it is of especial benefit if the baby is anticoagulated by maternal warfarin.

The clinical geneticist plays an increasing part as more becomes known about the inheritance of cardiovascular defects. The subject has become progressively more complex as knowledge has increased. In utero diagnosis by fetal echocardiography or fetal sampling or both is of growing importance.

Optimum management of pregnancy in women with heart disease is a team effort. Patients are best seen in joint antenatal cardiac clinics where their progress can be monitored and the delivery strategy planned.

2: Adaptation of the cardiovascular system to pregnancy

STEWART HUNTER, STEPHEN ROBSON

The human cardiovascular circulation is capable of coping with many adaptations and changes from fetal life through birth and into old age. After the neonatal period probably the most profound functional changes in the circulation occur during pregnancy. There are alterations in blood volume, cardiac output, arterial blood pressure, and vascular resistance. This chapter deals with the haemodynamic and structural adaptations during pregnancy and the implications for pathophysiological states.

Study of cardiovascular changes in pregnancy

The earliest studies of cardiac output used the inaccurate indirect Fick method. Following the development of cardiac catheterisation investigators changed to the direct Fick and dye dilution methods. Most such studies were cross sectional in design because of the inherent risks and were therefore of limited value because of the wide variation in cardiac output and stroke volume between individuals. Newer non-invasive techniques such as M mode echocardiography, impedance echocardiography, and Doppler ultrasound allowed serial measurements of cardiac indices such as cardiac output to be made without risk or discomfort for the patient. Of the available non-invasive techniques cross sectional echocardiography with Doppler ultrasound seems to be the most accurate and reproducible in pregnancy[1,2] while the impedance technique is probably the least accurate.[3]

Most serial studies of haemodynamic changes in pregnancy use postnatal measurements as baseline non-pregnant values. While most functional adaptations will have returned to non-pregnant values by six weeks postpartum this is not the case for stroke volume[4] and certain other structural changes.[5] Use of puerperal controls may therefore underestimate the size of changes induced by pregnancy. Longitudinal studies should recruit women before conception and three such detailed studies have included preconception haemodynamic measurements.[6-8]

The cardiovascular system is sensitive to posture, activity, and anxiety with resulting changes in catecholamine drive, heart rate, and cardiac output. Thus uniformity of standard resting conditions is important. For example, inferior caval obstruction by the gravid uterus in late pregnancy in supine patients leads to a reduction in venous return and therefore reduction in stroke volume and cardiac output.[9] All studies should therefore be made in the lateral position to avoid postural artefacts.

Changes in cardiac output, heart rate and stroke volume

The early direct Fick and dye dilution studies reviewed by Hytten and Leitch,[10] suggested an increase in cardiac output in early pregnancy. However, the studies included few measurements during the first trimester. The first investigation to study women from before conception was by Atkins et al.[6] They measured cardiac output by impedance cardiography and showed an increase from a non-pregnant mean of 6·5 l/min to 7·7 l/min at 12 weeks after conception. Robson et al measured cardiac output by cross sectional echocardiography and Doppler ultrasound at three sites within the heart (Figure 2.1).[8] In this study the mean non-pregnant output was 4·9 l/min rising to 6·6 l/min by 12 weeks, an increase of 35%. The increase was significant by five weeks after the last menstrual period and the rise in cardiac output was the result of increases in both heart rate and stroke volume.[7,8] During the menstrual cycle the maximum heart rate occurs on day 21 and thereafter a decrease of about five beats/min is noted.[11] If fertilisation occurs this fall is not seen and the heart rate continues to rise by 7 beats/min at four weeks and eight beats/min at 8 weeks. The earliest haemodynamic change associated with pregnancy therefore seems to be an increase in heart rate.

During the second trimester cardiac output increases further and maximum values are found at the end of the second trimester in most studies. In the study of Robson et al cardiac output reached a maximum of 7·1 l/min at 24 weeks' gestation (Figure 2.1), an increase of 45% over the preconception level.[8] Stroke volume contributes more than heart rate to the increase in cardiac output during the second trimester.[8,12-14]

The changes in cardiac output during the third trimester are less clear. The reduction in cardiac output reported by earlier investigators was possibly a postural artefact.[9] However, Ueland et al did show a fall in cardiac output in the lateral position using dye dilution studies from 7 l/min at 28 weeks to 5·7 l/min at 38–40 weeks.[12] There are also inconsistent results for M mode and Doppler studies in subjects in the lateral position; some patients show a further increase in cardiac output,[13-15] some show a decrease,[14,17] and most show no change.[8,9,14]

A further small increase in heart rate during the third trimester up to values of around 85 beats/min at term has been described by several authors.[8,13-15] The changes in stroke volume are inconsistent. Some investigators have reported a small decrease during the third trimester so

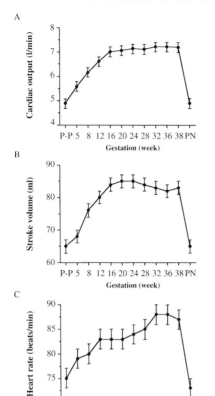

FIGURE 2.1—*Changes in cardiac output, stroke volume and heart rate during pregnancy measured by cross sectional and Doppler echocardiography in 13 women studied serially from before pregnancy (P-P) to 6 months after delivery (P-N). Figures are mean (SE) (derived from Robson et al[8]).*

that stroke volume at term is between 80 and 85 ml.[8,14,16,17] However, an increase has been reported by other investigators using both M mode and Doppler echocardiography.[13,15]

There are some haemodynamic data on normal pregnant women from cardiac catheterisation.[18,19] Clark *et al* studied a group of primigravid women at 36–38 weeks and recatheterised them 11–13 weeks after delivery to obtain non-pregnant control data.[19] These results are summarised in Table 2.1. In general terms the increases in cardiac output (43%) and heart rate (17%) noted at 36–38 weeks' gestation were in agreement with non-invasive data using ultrasound.[8,15,17] However, the non-pregnant output was lower than reported in most non-invasive studies. Indeed the mean value of 4·3 l/min is below most published normal ranges for resting cardiac output.[20]

Changes in total blood volume and preload

Preload is a term used to indicate how much stretch is applied to the myocardial fibres before contraction occurs. The amount of preload depends

TABLE 2.1—*Central (pulmonary artery catheterisation) haemodynamic measurements in 10 healthy primigravid women at term and at 11–13 weeks postpartum. Adapted from Clark et al.*[19]

Measurement	Postpartum Mean (SD)	At term Mean (SD)	Percentage change	p value
Cardiac output (l/min)	4·3 (0·9)	6·2 (1·0)	44	0·0003
Heart rate (beats/min)	71 (10)	83 (10)	17	0·015
Mean arterial pressure (mm Hg)	86·4 (7·5)	90·3 (5·8)	4·5	0·210
Systemic vascular resistance (dyne.cm.sec^{-5})	1530 (520)	1210 (266)	−21	0·100
Pulmonary vascular resistance (dyne.cm.sec^{-5})	119 (47)	78 (22)	−34	0·022
Central venous pressure (mm Hg)	3·7 (2·6)	3·6 (2·5)	−2·7	0·931
Pulmonary capillary wedge pressure (mm Hg)	6·3 (2·1)	7·5 (1·8)	19	0·187
Left ventricular stroke work index (g.m.m^{-2})	41 (8)	48 (6)	17	0·040

on the end diastolic volume of the ventricle. Studies using M mode and cross sectional echocardiography during pregnancy have shown increases in left and right sided chamber dimensions at end diastole.[7,8,13,21,22] The changes occur early in the first trimester and are fairly constant thereafter.[7,8] End diastolic dimensions measured by echocardiography correlate closely with end diastolic volume (measured by angiography) indicating that end diastolic volume is increased in pregnancy.

Total blood volume is made up of plasma volume and red cell mass. There have been two careful studies in the lateral position investigating changes in plasma volume in healthy primigravid women during pregnancy (Figure 2.2). Pirani *et al* measured plasma volume during pregnancy and 6–8 weeks after delivery and found that there was an increase of around 1250 ml from the non-pregnant mean value of 2600 ml.[23] Lind, in a group of women of mixed parity whom he studied before conception and during pregnancies, showed an increase of 57%, which was greater than the previous study because of the lower mean non-pregnant plasma volume (2297 ml).[24] These studies show that plasma volume increases mainly during the second trimester.

Plasma volume expansion is greater in multiparous women and substantial increases are seen in women with multiple pregnancies—the mean increase in twins being 1904 ml and in triplets 2400 ml.[25] There is also some evidence that plasma volume is related to fetal size.[26]

It might be expected that the changes in afterload and preload would affect the atrial contribution to ventricular filling. Transmitral Doppler flow velocities have been used to study left ventricular filling and there is evidence that the ratio between the peak early diastolic velocity and the

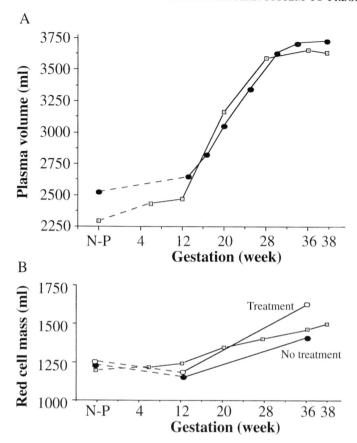

FIGURE 2.2—*Changes in plasma volume and red cell mass during pregnancy (N-P; not pregnant). The data on plasma volume were collected in the lateral position (reproduced from Pirani et al[23] —●— and Lind[24] —□—. Red cell mass data reproduced from Lind[24] —□— and Taylor and Lind[25] in women given iron and folic acid —○— and in women on no medication —●—.*

late atrial diastolic velocity (the E:A ratio) decreases in late pregnancy. Robson suggested that there is an increased contribution of atrial systole to ventricular filling in late pregnancy.[27] The E:A ratio is, however, not a particularly reproducible index of diastolic function.

The rate of change of left ventricular dimensions in diastole measured by echocardiography can be used to study volume loading of the left ventricle. The diastolic filling pressure during pregnancy seems not to change and the increase in peak rate of change of left ventricular dimension and posterior wall dimension may suggest a greater distensibility of the left ventricle.[26]

Femoral venous pressure has been reported to be raised in late pregnancy,[27] perhaps reflecting obstruction from the bulky gravid uterus, but there is no direct evidence that central venous pressure is increased.[19]

Plethysmography of the upper and lower limbs indicates that venous distensibility and capacitance are increased during pregnancy.[28,29] These changes are seen particularly during the second trimester and may be necessary to allow the increase in blood volume to be accommodated without increasing venous pressure. There are no data on intrathoracic and intrapericardial pressure during pregnancy.

Blood pressure and afterload

The errors and limitations of blood pressure measurement by standard mercury sphygmomanometry have been reviewed by de Swiet.[30] The sphygmomanometric reading of the systolic pressure is low compared with direct arterial pressure measurement. Diastolic pressure by sphygmomanometer is too high if the fourth Korotkoff sound is used and slightly less high if the fifth sound is used.[30] Comparisons between blood pressure studies during pregnancy are bedevilled by variations in posture and the method of measuring the blood pressure.[33] None the less, there seems to be a consistent change. Systolic pressure falls a little and diastolic pressure falls more, both reaching a nadir around 20 weeks with a progressive increase thereafter (Figure 2.3).[8,31,32] Most investigators have shown little difference between blood pressure at term and that in non-pregnant controls with the exception of Atkins et al[6] and Easterling et al[17] both of whom reported an increase in systolic pressure at term compared with postnatal values. The matter is complex as the effect of posture in pregnancy is difficult to assess. The blood pressure is said to be lower in the left lateral position than in the sitting or supine position.[6,34] However, around 1 in 10 of women in late pregnancy have a systolic pressure fall of 30 mm Hg or more between sitting and lying supine.

As cardiac output increases and blood pressure falls during the first half of pregnancy, systemic vascular resistance falls. Robson et al suggested that the systemic resistance was at its lowest at 20 weeks' gestation—34% below the preconception figures (Figure 2.3).[8] The percentage reduction was similar to the figures produced by Duvekot et al although the non-pregnant systemic vascular resistance in this latter group was higher.[34] Many workers have reported an increase in systemic vascular resistance of variable magnitude towards term. Cardiac catheterisation data have suggested that systemic vascular resistance is reduced by 21% at 36–38 weeks' gestation while pulmonary vascular resistance is reduced by 34%.

The great arteries (particularly the aorta) become more compliant during pregnancy. Hart et al showed that the ratio of aortic pressure to gross sectional area was significantly lower in later gestation and they concluded that the aorta was more compliant.[35] These changes may be related to histological changes in reticulin and elastin fibres in the aortic media during pregnancy.[36] Plasma viscosity is increased during pregnancy mainly because of increased fibrinogen concentration.[37] Whole blood viscosity falls during

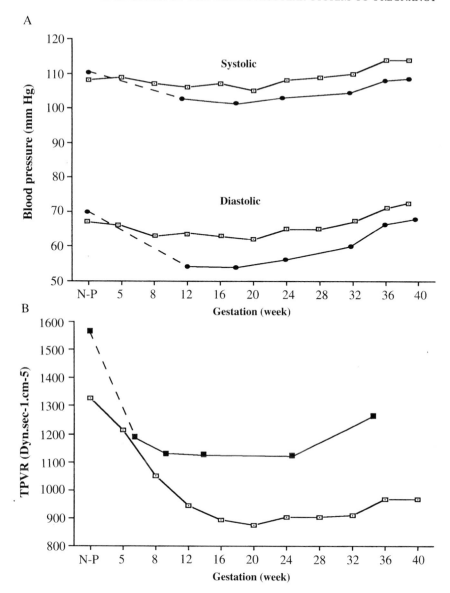

FIGURE 2.3—*Changes in blood pressure and total peripheral vascular resistance (TPVR) during pregnancy (N-P; not pregnant). Reproduced from Robson* et al[8] —□—, *MacGillivray* et al[31] —●—, *and Duvekot* et al[34] —■—).

the first 24 weeks and remains stable until 6–8 weeks from the end of pregnancy when it increases.[37]

There is therefore evidence that afterload is significantly reduced during the first half of pregnancy as a result of a reduction in vascular resistance and to some extent of a decrease in aortic compliance and blood viscosity. Later systemic and pulmonary vascular resistances rise together with blood viscosity although neither returns to non-pregnant levels.

Myocardial contractility

There have been numerous reported studies of ejection phase indices of left ventricular function using M mode echocardiography. The indices include fractional shortening, ejection fraction, and mean and peak rates of dimensional change of the left ventricular cavity (VCF or velocity of circumferential fibre shortening). It is debatable whether any of these is a genuine measurement of myocardial contractility as they are all to some extent affected by preload and afterload. None the less they are regularly used to assess myocardial function. Various studies have shown that ventricular performance is increased during the first two trimesters and falls towards term.[8,13,14,21,22]

Clark et al, using invasive methods, plotted left ventricular stroke work against capillary wedge pressure in normal women at term and found that ventricular function was normal.[19] Ventricular function curves are constructed to take account of preload change but are also influenced by afterload. The isolated perfused hearts of pregnant rats showed an increase in fractional shortening under fixed loading conditions.[38] The correlation between force and velocity was shifted upwards in pregnant rats suggesting that, at least in this species, contractility increases during pregnancy.

Structural changes in the heart

Left ventricular mass, which is calculated from M mode echo-cardiographic measurements of wall thickness, increases throughout pregnancy, reaching values 50% above those of the non-pregnant state.[8,13,21] Similar increases in wall thickness are seen in non-pregnant adults after only 12 weeks of exercise training.[39] Training seems to increase cardiac output and thus to increase end diastolic wall stress (which enlarges the internal diameter of the ventricle) and also systolic wall stress. As the wall thickness increases the systolic wall stress is normalised and this sequence of events probably operates during pregnancy.

All valve diameters and orifice areas measured by cross sectional or M mode echocardiography increase during pregnancy. This is true of all four valves[8,35,40] and probably accounts for the increased incidence of regurgitant velocities seen during pregnancy.[40,41]

Increased cardiac output and stroke volume in pregnancy are associated with changes in organ blood flow. There is an 80% increase in effective renal plasma flow between early pregnancy and 26 weeks when the levels are 400 ml/min greater than non-pregnant values.[42] Uterine blood flow rises from 60 ml/min during the first trimester to 180 ml/min at 28 weeks.[43] Mean values at term are 500 ml/min although there is wide individual variability.[44] Cutaneous vasodilatation leads to a substantial increase in peripheral blood flow. Blood flow in the hand is increased sevenfold and foot flow threefold.[45] Mean liver blood flow has been reported to rise during pregnancy by 75%.[46] However, this investigator reported high non-pregnant flows. Others have reported no significant change during pregnancy.[47,48] Cerebral blood flow is said to be unchanged in pregnancy.[49] Coronary and mammary blood flow are probably increased although there are no reliable data for either.

Haemodynamic changes during labour

Most of the early studies of cardiac output in labour were made with patients lying supine. The effects of posture and uterine contractions were studied by Ueland and Hansen.[50] They reported that cardiac output increased by 1·3 l/min in the supine position compared with 0·5 l/min in the lateral position. In the lateral position during contractions cardiac output increases throughout the first stage of labour by as much as 34%.[51] Initially this results from increased stroke volume but later both stroke volume and heart rate increase (Figure 2.4).[51-52] The cardiac output between contractions goes up by 12% during the first stage as a result of increase in stroke volume (Figure 2.4).[51] Ueland and Hansen, using dye dilution, reported further increases in cardiac output during the second stage of labour.[52]

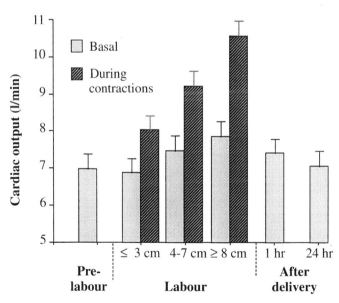

FIGURE 2.4—*Changes in cardiac output in 15 women during labour measured using cross sectional and Doppler echocardiography in the left lateral position. Figures are mean (SE), between contractions* ▤ *and during contractions* ▨. *Reproduced from Robson et al.*[51]

Epidural anaesthesia during labour removes the increase in heart rate during contractions[52] but does not effect the increase in stroke volume.[53]

It seems highly likely therefore that the increase in heart rate is a sympathetic response to pain and the increase in stroke volume is secondary to an increase in preload as blood is squeezed into the circulation from the choriodecidual space during a uterine contraction. Increases in central venous pressure of up to 5 mm Hg during contractions support this hypothesis.[54] When caudal anaesthesia is used there are smaller increases in cardiac output during the second stage of labour than are found with pudendal or paracervical anaesthesia.[52]

Blood pressure rises between contractions compared with values before labour, by a modest amount in the first stage and an increasing amount in the second stage.[54] During contractions there is a further increase with an even more pronounced difference between the first and second stage.[54] When pethidine is used for pain relief during labour both systolic and diastolic pressures increase during uterine contractions.[51,54]

The mechanism of cardiovascular changes in pregnancy

It is commonly believed that pregnancy is a state of volume loading (the so called "overfill" hypothesis) as indicated by increases in plasma and extracellular volume, glomerular filtration rate, and renal plasma flow. It is proposed that primary hypersecretion of aldosterone leads to sodium and water retention. Alternatively, the "underfill" hypothesis suggests that pregnancy is a state of reduced effective blood volume accompanied by secondary aldosteronism. According to this hypothesis arterial vasodilatation is the main circulatory change leading to underfilling of the circulation, a decrease in blood pressure, an increase in cardiac output secondary to reduction in afterload, stimulation of the renin-angiotensin-aldosterone axis, and release of vasopressin. Sodium and water are retained by the kidneys, leading to an enlargement of the extracellular and plasma compartments. There is evidence from both animal and human studies during early pregnancy to support the underfill hypothesis.[33,55]

The changes in vascular resistance are, however, mediated by mechanisms which are not clear. Oestrogens have an inconsistent effect on blood pressure but do increase cardiac output by increasing stroke volume and plasma volume.[56] Progesterone increases heart rate but it has little effect on blood pressure or cardiac output.[57] Prostacyclin and nitric oxide are vasodilators which are released by the endothelium in increased amounts in pregnancy but their contribution to vasodilatation is at present uncertain.[58,59]

Cardiac signs and symptoms during pregnancy

The changes in cardiac physiology during pregnancy produce symptoms and signs that may simulate disease. For instance Milne et al, found an increased incidence of breathlessness in the first trimester, which peaked at around 28–31 weeks.[60] This seemed not to correlate with any particular physiological variable, but fatigability and reduced exercise tolerance are common in normal pregnancy. Syncopal attacks or dizziness in late pregnancy, presumably as a result of mechanical compression of the inferior vena cava by the enlarged uterus, are caused by a decrease in venous return and a fall in cardiac output.[61] Overbreathing is a common feature in pregnancy and may result from compression of the basal parts of the lung by the enlarging uterus. The higher position of the diaphragm alters the electrical axis of the heart so that the apical impulse is displaced to the left. In addition there is often a right ventricular impulse palpable at the left sternal edge. Phonocardiography carried out during pregnancy by Cutforth and MacDonald showed a number of findings which are summarised in Figure 2.5.[62] A wide split first heart sound with a tendency to expiratory splitting of the second heart sound is seen in late pregnancy. Eighty-four percent of their patients had a further sound and 96% of pregnant women had systolic ejection flow murmurs. These are usually heard at the left sternal edge and are not particularly loud. They are thought to represent increased flow across the pulmonary artery and valve. Early diastolic murmurs indicating arterial valve regurgitation are not unknown in pregnancy and may reflect dilatation of annuli and increased flow across the arterial valves.

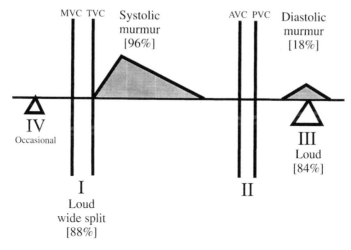

FIGURE 2.5—*Cardiac auscultatory findings during pregnancy. Abbreviations: MVC, mitral valve closure; TVC, tricuspid valve closure; AVC, aortic valve closure; PVC, pulmonary valve closure. (Adapted from Cutforth and Macdonald.*[62]*)*

Summary

It seems that the functional alterations in the cardiovascular system as a result of pregnancy are now well documented but the mechanisms which produce the changes remain unclear.

Cardiac output increases by up to 45% during pregnancy as a result of increases in both stroke volume and heart rate, maximum values being attained by mid-pregnancy and maintained thereafter in the lateral position until term. Arterial vasodilatation of the systemic vascular compartment occurs during the first trimester, leading to a fall in blood pressure and a reduction in afterload. There is an increase in blood volume and cardiac preload probably from stimulation of the renin-aldosterone axis and myocardial contractility does seem to be increased early in pregnancy. The mechanisms for these changes are uncertain but lead to an effective adaptation of the cardiovascular system to the demands of pregnancy.

This is particularly true of vasodilatation and a great deal of attention is currently being paid to the role of nitric oxide. In the non-pregnant subject the systemic vascular resistance seems to be under constant mediation by nitric oxide and there is some evidence to suggest that vascular synthesis of nitric oxide is increased in pregnancy. Understanding the mechanism of vasodilatation is of more than physiological interest because of its implications for the management of both pre-eclampsia and patients with pulmonary hypertension and pulmonary vascular disease.

References

1 Easterling TR, Carlson KL, Schmucker BC, Millard SP. Measurement of cardiac output in pregnancy by Doppler technique. *Am J Perinatol* 1990; **3**: 220–2.
2 Robson SC, Dunlop W, Moore M, Hunter S. Combined Doppler and echocardiographic measurement of cardiac output: theory and application in pregnancy. *Br J Obstet Gynaecol* 1987; **94**: 1014–27.
3 Secher NJ, Arnsbo P, Heslet Anderson L, Thompson A. Measurement of cardiac stroke volumes in various body positions in pregnancy and during caesarean section: a comparison between thermodilution and impedance cardiography. *Scand J Clin Lab Invest* 1979; **39**: 569–76.
4 Capeless EL, Clapp JF. When do cardiovascular parameters return to their preconception values? *Am J Obstet Gynecol* 1991; **165**: 883–6.
5 Robson SC, Hunter S, Moore M, Dunlop W. Haemodynamic changes during the puerperium: a Doppler and M mode echocardiographic study. *Br J Obstet Gynecol* 1987; **94**: 1028–39.
6 Atkins AJF, Watt JM, Milan P, Davies P, Selwyn Crawford J. A longitudinal study of cardiovascular dynamic changes throughout pregnancy. *Eur J Obstet Gynecol Reprod Biol* 1981; **12**: 215–24.
7 Capeless EL, Clapp JF. Cardiovascular changes in early phase of pregnancy. *Am J Obstet Gynecol* 1989; **161**: 1449–53.
8 Robson SC, Hunter S, Boys RJ, Dunlop W. Serial study of factors influencing changes in cardiac output during human pregnancy. *Am J Physiol* 1989; **256**: H1060–65.
9 Lees MM, Scott DB, Kerr MG, Taylor SH. The circulatory effects of recumbent postural change in late pregnancy. *Clin Sci* 1967; **32**: 453–65.
10 Hytten FE, Leitch I. Respiration. In: Hytten FE, Leitch I. *The physiology of human pregnancy.* 2nd ed. Oxford: Blackwell Scientific Publications, 1971: 111–31.
11 Kelleher C, Joyce C, Kelly G, Ferriss JB. Blood pressure alters during the normal menstrual cycle. *Br J Obstet Gynaecol* 1986; **93**: 523–6.
12 Ueland K, Novy MK, Peterson EN, Metcalfe J. Maternal cardiovascular dynamics. IV. The influence of gestational age on the maternal cardiovascular response to posture and exercise. *Am J Obstet Gynecol* 1969; **104**: 856–64.
13 Katz R, Karliner JS. Resnik R. Effects of a natural volume overload state (pregnancy) on left ventricular performance in normal human subjects. *Circulation* 1978; **58**: 434–41.

14 Mashini IS, Albazzaz SJ, Fadel HE, *et al.* Serial noninvasive evaluation of cardiovascular hemodynamics during pregnancy. *Am J Obstet Gynecol* 1987; **156**: 1208–13.
15 Mabie WC, DiSessa TG, Crocker LG, Sibai BM, Arheart KL. A longitudinal study of cardiac output in normal human pregnancy. *Am J Obstet Gynecol* 1994; **170**: 849–56.
16 Steegers EAP, van Lakwijk HPJM, Benaad T, *et al.* Atrial natiuretic peptide (ANP) in normal pregnancy: a longitudinal study. *Clinical and Experimental Hypertension in Pregnancy* 1990; **B9**: 273–92.
17 Easterling TR, Benedetti TJ, Schmucker BC, Millard SP. Maternal hemodynamics in normal and preeclamptic pregnancies: a longitudinal study. *Obstet Gynecol* 1990; **76**: 1061–9.
18 Wallenburg HCS. Hemodynamics in hypertensive pregnancy. In: Rubin PC, ed. *Hypertensions in pregnancy.* Amsterdam: Elsevier, 1988: 66–101.
19 Clark SL, Cotton DB, Lee W, *et al.* Central hemodynamic assessment of normal term pregnancy. *Am J Obstet Gynecol* 1989; **161**: 1439–42.
20 Wade OL, Bishop JM. Cardiac output and regional blood flow. Oxford: Blackwell, 1962: 1–44.
21 Laird-Meeter K, Van De Ley G, Bom TH, Wladimiroff JW. Cardiocirculatory adjustments during pregnancy—an echocardiographic study. *Clin Cardiol* 1979; **2**: 328–32.
22 Castillon G, Weissenburger J, Rouiffet M, Castillon V, Barat J. Etude echocardiographique des modifications hemodynamiques de la grossesse. *J Gynecol Obstet Biol Reprod* 1984; **13**: 499–505.
23 Pirani BBK, Campbell DM, MacGillivray I. Plasma volume in normal first pregnancy. *Journal of Obstetrics and Gynaecology of the British Commonwealth* 1973; **80**: 884–7.
24 Lind T. Hematologic system. In: Lind T. *Maternal physiology.* Washington: CREOG 25, 1985: 7–40.
25 Taylor DJ, Lind T. Red cell mass during and after normal pregnancy. *Br J Obstet Gynaecol* 1979; **86**: 364–70.
26 Rovinsky JJ, Jaffin H. Cardiovascular hemodynamics in pregnancy. I. Blood and plasma volumes in multiple pregnancy. *Am J Obstet Gynecol* 1965; **93**: 1–13.
27 Robson SC. *Haemodynamic changes during pregnancy.* Newcastle: University of Newcastle upon Tyne. MD Thesis, 1992.
28 McLennan CE. Antecubital and femoral venous pressure in normal and toxic pregnancy. *Am J Obstet Gynecol* 1943; **45**: 568–91.
29 Barwin BN, Roddie IC. Venous distensibility during pregnancy determined by graded venous congestion. *Am J Obstet Gynecol* 1976; **125**: 921–3.
30 de Swiet M. The cardiovascular system. In: Hytten FE, Chamberlain G, eds. *Clinical physiology in obstetrics.* Oxford: Blackwell Scientific Publications, 1991: 3–38.
31 MacGillivray I, Rose GA, Rowe B. Blood pressure survey in pregnancy. *Clin Sci* 1969; **37**: 395–407.
32 Schwarz R. Das Verhalten des Kreislaufs in der normalen Schwangerschaft. I. Der arterielle Blutdruck. *Archiv fur Gynäkologie* 1964; **199**: 549–70.
33 Eskes TKAB, Wyer A, Kramer N, Van Elteren P. Arterial blood pressure and posture during pregnancy. A prospective study. *Eur J Obstet Gynec Reprod Biol* 1974; **4**: 87–94.
34 Duvekot JJ, Cheriex EC, Pieters FAA, Menheere PPC, Peeters LLH. Early pregnancy changes in haemodynamics and volume homeostasis are consecutive adjustments triggered by a primary fall in systemic vascular tone. *Am J Obstet Gynecol* 1993; **169**: 1382–92.
35 Hart MV, Mortom MJ, Hosenpud JD, Metcalfe J. Aortic function during normal human pregnancy. *Am J Obstet Gynecol* 1986; **154**: 887–91.
36 Manalo-Estrella P, Barker AE. Histopathologic findings in human aortic media associated with pregnancy. *Archives of Pathology* 1967; **83**: 336–41.
37 Buchan PC. Maternal and fetal blood viscosity throughout normal pregnancy. *J Obstet Gynaecol* 1984; **4**: 143–50.
38 Buttrick SM, Schaibie TF, Malhotra A, Mattioli S, Schener J. Effect of pregnancy on cardiac function and myosin enzymology in the rat. *Am J Physiol* 1987; **252**: H846–50.
39 Lusiani L, Ronsisvalle G, Bonanome A, *et al.* Echocardiographic evaluation of the dimensions and systolic properties of the left ventricle in freshman athletes during physical training. *Eur Heart J* 1986; 7: 196–203.
40 Limacher MC, Ware A, O'Meara ME, Fernandez GC, Young JB. Tricuspid regurgitation during pregnancy: two dimensional and pulsed Doppler echocardiographic observations. *Am J Cardiol* 1985; **55**: 1059–62.

17

41 Robson SC, Richley D, Boys RJ, Hunter S. Incidence of Doppler regurgitant flow velocities during pregnancy. *Eur Heart J* 1992; **13**: 84–7.

42 Dunlop W. Serial changes in renal haemodynamics during normal pregnancy. *Br J Obstet Gynaecol* 1981; **88**: 109.

43 Assali NS, Rauramo L, Peltonen T. Measurement of uterine blood flow and uterine metabolism. VIII. Uterine and fetal blood flow and oxygen consumption in early human pregnancy. *Am J Obstet Gynecol* 1960; **79**: 86–98.

44 Assali NS, Douglas RA, Baird WW, Nicholson DB, Suyemoto R. Measurement of uterine blood flow and uterine metabolism. IV. Results in normal pregnancy. *Am J Obstet Gynecol* 1953; **66**: 248–53.

45 Ginsburg J, Duncan SLB. Peripheral blood flow in normal pregnancy. *Cardiovasc Res* 1967; **1**: 132–7.

46 Tindall VR. The liver in pregnancy. *Clin Obstet Gynecol* 1975; **2**: 441–62.

47 Robson SC, Mutch E, Boys RJ, Woodhouse KW. Apparent liver blood flow during pregnancy: a serial study using indocyanine green clearance. *Br J Obstet Gynaecol* 1990; **97**: 720–4.

48 Munnell EW, Taylor HC. Liver blood flow in pregnancy—hepatic vein catheterization. *J Clin Invest* 1947; **26**: 952–6.

49 McCall ML. Cerebral blood flow and metabolism in toxemias of pregnancy. *Surg Gynecol Obstet* 1949; **89**: 715–21.

50 Ueland K, Hansen JM. Maternal cardiovascular dynamics. II. Posture and uterine contractions. *Am J Obstet Gynecol* 1969; **103**: 1–7.

51 Robson SC, Dunlop W, Boys RJ, Hunter S. Cardiac output during labour. *BMJ* 1987; **296**: 1169–72.

52 Ueland K, Hansen JM. Maternal cardiovascular dynamics. III. Labour and delivery under local and caudal analgesia. *Am J Obstet Gynecol* 1969; **103**: 8–18.

53 Kjeldsen J. Haemodynamic investigations during labour and delivery. *Acta Obstet Gynecol Scand* 1979; **89(suppl)**: 77–195.

54 Lee W, Rokey R, Cotton DB, Miller JF. Maternal hemodynamic effects of uterine contractions by M-mode and pulsed Doppler echocardiography. *Am J Obstet Gynecol* 1989; **161**: 974–7.

55 Phippard AF, Horvarth JS, Glynn EM, *et al*. Circulatory adaptation to pregnancy—serial studies of haemodynamics, blood volume, renin and aldosterone in the baboon (Papio hamadryas). *J Hypertens* 1986; **4**: 773–9.

56 Walters WAW, Lim YL. Cardiovascular dynamics in women receiving oral contraceptive therapy. *Lancet* 1969; **ii**: 879–81.

57 Lumbers ER. Effects on sheep blood pressure of treatment with angiotensin, steroids and salt. *Clin Exp Pharm Physiol* 1990; **17**: 315–9.

58 Lewis PJ. Prostacyclin in pregnancy. *BMJ* 1980; **ii**: 1581–2.

59 Conrad KP, Joffe GM, Kruszyna H, *et al*. Identification of increased nitric oxide biosynthesis during pregnancy in rats. *FASEB J* 1993; **7**: 566–71.

60 Milne JA, Howie AD, Pack AL. Dyspnoea during normal pregnancy. *Br J Obstet Gynaecol* 1978; **85**: 260.

61 Kerr M. The mechanical effects of the gravid uterus in late pregnancy. *Journal of Obstetrics and Gynaecology of the British Commonwealth* 1965; **72**: 513–29.

62 Cutforth R, MacDonald MB. Heart sounds and murmurs in pregnancy. *Am Heart J* 1966; **71**: 741–7.

3: Haematological changes during pregnancy

ELIZABETH A LETSKY

There are substantial changes and wide variations in the circulating blood during pregnancy and the puerperium. It is not possible to assess the haematological status of pregnant women by criteria used for men and non-pregnant women.

There are dramatic changes in whole blood volume which affect the concentration of haemoglobin, red cell indices, and the metabolism of haematinics. In addition, the haemostatic mechanisms are profoundly altered compared with the non-pregnant state.

Blood volume

Plasma volume and total red cell mass are under separate control and bear no fixed relation to each other. Changes in pregnancy provide a dramatic illustration of this point.[1]

Healthy women in a normal first pregnancy increase their plasma volume from a non-pregnant level of about 2600 ml by about 1250 ml (50%). In subsequent pregnancies the increase is greater and may be about 1500 ml. Most of the rise takes place before 32–34 weeks' gestation, and thereafter there is relatively little change.

There is little doubt that the amount of increase in plasma volume is correlated with clinical performance and the birth weight of the baby. Women with multiple pregnancy have proportionately higher increments of plasma volume.[2,3] By contrast, women with poorly-growing fetuses, particularly multi-gravidae with a history of poor reproductive performance, have a correspondingly poor plasma volume response.[1]

There is less published information on red cell mass than plasma volume and the results are more variable. There is still disagreement as to how much the red cell mass increases in normal pregnancy. The extent of the increase is considerably influenced by iron medication. In iron replete pregnancies the Hb concentration is dependent largely on the plasma volume increase which is under separate control and directly reflects healthy reproduction. This has led to the erroneous association of high Hb concentrations instead of low plasma volume with poor outcome.[4,5]

If one accepts a figure of about 1400 ml for the quantity of red cells in the average healthy woman before pregnancy, then in round figures the rise during pregnancy in women not given iron medication is about 240 ml (18%) and in those given iron about 400 ml (30%). As with plasma volume, the extent of the increase is likely to be related to the size of the conceptus.[2,3]

Changes in blood volume at parturition and during the puerperium

Dramatic changes in maternal blood volume occur at delivery whether *per vaginam* or by caesarean section, as a result of the acute blood loss. If the blood loss at vaginal delivery is meticulously measured it proves to be slightly more than 500 ml during the delivery of one infant and almost 1000 ml when twins are delivered. Caesarean section is associated with an average loss of 1000 ml of blood if performed under general anaesthetic but there is anecdotal evidence that the blood loss is considerably less if it is done under epidural analgesia.[6]

The response of the mother to this acute blood loss differs from that of non-pregnant women, in whom rapid blood loss precipitates an immediate drop in blood volume compensated for by vasoconstriction. Within a few days the blood volume expands to near normal values because of an increase in plasma volume. This leads to a considerable fall in packed cell volume which is proportional to the amount of blood lost.

In the normal pregnant woman at term, the hypervolaemia modifies the response to blood loss considerably. The blood volume drops following the acute loss at delivery but remains relatively stable unless the blood loss exceeds 25% of the pre-delivery volume. There is no compensatory increase in blood volume and there is a gradual fall in plasma volume, primarily from diuresis. The red cell mass increase during pregnancy is not totally lost at delivery but slowly reduces as the remaining red cells come to the end of their lifespan. The overall result is that the packed cell volume gradually increases and the blood volume returns to non-pregnant levels.

In the first few days following delivery there are fluctuations in plasma volume and packed cell volume as a result of individual responses to dehydration, pregnancy hypervolaemia, and the rapidity of blood loss. The average blood loss which can be tolerated without causing a significant fall in haemoglobin concentration is around 1000 ml, but this depends in turn on a healthy increase in blood volume before delivery. Almost all the blood loss occurs within the first hour following delivery under normal circumstances. In the following 72 hours only about 80 ml are lost *per vaginam*. Patients with uterine atony, extended episiotomy, or lacerations will of course lose much more. If the packed cell volume or haemoglobin concentration at 5–7 days after delivery is significantly less than they were before delivery, either there was pathological blood loss at delivery, or there was a poor increase in blood volume during pregnancy, or both.

Benefits of hypervolaemia in pregnancy

The widely different response in plasma volume and red cell mass should have a rational basis and make biological sense.

The hypervolaemia *per se* combats the hazard of haemorrhage for the mother at delivery. It also protects the mother from hypotension in the last trimester when sequestration occurs in the lower extremities on standing, sitting, or lying supine.

The red cell mass should increase in line with the need for extra oxygen. By the end of pregnancy the requirement has been calculated to be around 15–16% more than the average non-pregnant requirement and is met adequately by an increase in red cell mass of 18–25%.

The role of the much greater increase in plasma volume becomes clear when the distribution of the raised cardiac output is defined. Most of the extra circulation is directed to the skin and kidneys. Both serve as organs of excretion during pregnancy. The basal metabolic rate increases by about 20% and the vastly increased blood flow in the skin allows for heat loss. There is also a decrease in viscosity which causes a decreased resistance to blood flow and a decrease in cardiac force required to maintain the circulation. This makes biological sense of what is often seen as a disproportionate increase in plasma volume.

Red cell production

There is evidence of a more rapid red cell production in pregnancy. There is a threefold increase in the concentration of erythropoietin in plasma by the second trimester and a considerable increase in the urine. Recent studies have confirmed the increase in erythropoietin concentration in normal pregnancy and have also shown that in the presence of anaemia or iron deficiency during pregnancy there is a further significant increase in the serum erythropoietin.[7–10] The concentration of other hormones such as placental lactogen is raised and may exert an effect on erythropoiesis, though this has never been shown in human pregnancy.

Together with the increase in erythropoiesis, there appears to be a reactivation of fetal haemoglobin production. Fetal haemoglobin (HbF) is largely replaced by adult haemoglobin (HbA) during the first year of life. The 1–2% of HbF which persists in the blood of normal adults is confined to a small number of red cells called F cells. There is a significant increase in F cells in all pregnancies. The number of F cells reaches a peak at 18–22 weeks and usually returns to normal by 8 weeks post partum.[11] Recent evidence indicates that the stimulus for maternal HbF synthesis is related to an increased rate of production of red cells.

Haemoglobin concentration

If the lowest normal haemoglobin in the healthy adult non-pregnant woman, living at sea level is accepted as 120 g/l, then it can be calculated from the plasma volume and red cell mass expansion in iron-sufficient subjects that the lowest haemoglobin in normal single pregnancy should be 106 g/l. In most published studies the mean minimum in pregnancy is between 110 and 120 g/l. This is in close agreement with the World Health Organisation figure of 110 g/l.[12] The lowest haemoglobin is observed at around 32 weeks' gestation when plasma volume expansion is maximal, after this time there is a rise of about 5 g/l. Clinical experience shows that many apparently healthy women are able to proceed through pregnancy with haemoglobins lower than 110 g/l without complications. On investigation, however, a fair proportion can be shown to be iron and folate deficient.

Mean cell volume (MCV)

Recently it has become clear that healthy iron-replete pregnancy is associated with a small physiological increase in red cell size, on average 4 fl, but in some women the increase may be as high as 20 fl.[13]

The increased drive to erythropoiesis resulting in a higher proportion of young large red cells masks the effect of iron deficiency on the MCV in pregnancy even when anaemia has become established. The MCV is a poor indicator of iron deficiency which develops during the course of pregnancy.[14] In a recent study (Ibidapo and Letsky, personal communication) of 160 patients attending the antenatal clinic at Queen Charlotte's Hospital the mean MCV remained in the normal range (90·7 fl) in the anaemic iron depleted patients (mean ferritin 0·9 µg/l) compared with the non-anaemic iron replete patients (mean MCV 90·6 fl). None of the values fell in the accepted microcytic range which indicates iron deficiency in the non-pregnant state.

Qualitative changes in the red cell

Maternal respiratory alkalosis enables the fetus to offload carbon dioxide but tends to increase maternal haemoglobin oxygen affinity. This is offset by a raised concentration of 2,3-diphosphoglycerate (2,3-DPG) in maternal red cells which pushes the oxygen dissociation curve to the right and thus facilitates oxygen release to the fetus and to maternal tissues. Oxygen transfer to the fetus is further helped by HbF which has a high affinity for oxygen and a low affinity for 2,3-DPG.[15]

However, the differential oxygen affinity across the placenta produced by HbA in the maternal circulation and the higher affinity HbF of the fetus is not essential to ensure adequate oxygen delivery for normal fetal development and growth.[16]

Iron metabolism

Requirements

In pregnancy the demand for iron is increased to meet the needs of the expanded red cell volume and the requirements of the developing fetus and placenta. By far the greatest single demand for iron is for the expansion of the red cell mass, which requires 570 mg. The fetus derives its iron from the maternal serum by active transport across the placenta mainly in the last four weeks of pregnancy. The iron transferred to the fetus is of the order of 200–370 mg. Moderate blood loss at delivery of 200–500 ml accounts for 100–250 mg iron, and breast feeding over six months results in the loss of another 100–180 mg. The increased need for iron is relatively small in early pregnancy and is greatest in the third trimester. Overall the requirement is 4 mg/day but this rises from 2·8 mg/day in the non-pregnant state to 6·6 mg/day in the last few weeks of pregnancy. This can be met only by mobilising iron stores in addition to achieving maximum absorption of dietary iron. It has been suggested that the main physiological role of iron stores is to satisfy the high iron requirements in late pregnancy.[17] Many women enter pregnancy with insufficient stores to cover the extra demands, particularly in the third trimester.

Absorption

The intestinal mucosal control of iron is complex and incompletely understood, but absorption is increased when there is erythroid hyperplasia, rapid iron turnover, and a high concentration of unsaturated transferrin—all of which are present in pregnant women. Absorption of dietary iron is enhanced and rates of up to 40% or higher may be attained in the latter half of pregnancy.[18,19] The amount of iron absorbed will depend on the rate of erythropoiesis, the status of the iron stores, the content of the diet, and whether or not iron supplements are being given.

Oral supplementation of 60–80 mg elemental iron per day from early pregnancy maintains the haemoglobin in the normal range in most subjects on a "western" diet, but does not maintain or restore the iron stores. The World Health Organisation recommends that supplements of 30–60 mg/day be given to those pregnant women with iron stores, and 120–240 mg to those women with none.[12]

Serum iron, transferrin, and total iron binding capacity

In health, the serum iron of adult non-pregnant women lies between 13 and 27 µmol/l (60–150 µg/dl), but it shows immense individual diurnal variability and fluctuates even from hour to hour. The total iron binding capacity (TIBC) in the non-pregnant state lies in the range 45–72 µmol/l (250–400 mg/dl). It is raised in association with iron deficiency and is low in chronic inflammatory states. The specific iron binding protein transferrin is between 1·2 and 2·0 g/l (120–200 µg/dl). Normally, in the non-anaemic individual, the TIBC is approximately one-third saturated with iron. Serum iron of less than 12 µmol/l (70 mg/dl) and a TIBC saturation of less than 15% indicate deficiency of iron during pregnancy.

Ferritin

Serum iron, even in combination with TIBC, is not a reliable indication of iron stores, because it fluctuates widely and is affected by recent ingestion of iron and other factors not directly involved with iron metabolism. The discovery that ferritin, a high molecular weight glycoprotein, circulates in the plasma of healthy adults in a range of 15–300 µg/l has considerably simplified the assessment of iron stores in pregnancy.[20] It is stable, is not affected by recent ingestion of iron and appears to reflect the iron stores accurately and quantitatively, particularly in the lower range associated with iron deficiency, which is so important in pregnancy.

Transferrin receptor (TfR)

Measurement of serum transferrin receptor provides a new allegedly reliable method for assessing cellular iron status.[21] Studies using sensitive immunological techniques have shown that transferrin receptor circulates in small amounts in the plasma of all individuals and that the concentration is proportional to the total body mass of TfR. The only notable exception is in patients with iron deficiency anaemia in whom the concentration of the receptor in serum is elevated some threefold. There is little or no change in serum receptor concentration during the early stages of storage iron depletion but as soon as *tissue* iron deficiency is established the serum TfR concentration increases directly proportional to the degree of iron deficiency. This measurement of iron status is particularly helpful in identifying iron deficiency in pregnancy.[22] It identifies the truly iron deficient women from those who have a low haemoglobin concentration from haemodilution or those who have low serum ferritin from storage iron mobilisation. In combination with serum ferritin TfR will give a complete picture of iron status—the serum ferritin reflecting iron stores and TfR the tissue iron status.[21]

Marrow iron

With the development of the new non-invasive tests of iron status described above, bone marrow examination will be reserved for the differential diagnosis of anaemia during pregnancy when the cause cannot be determined by any other means, and for the investigation of other haematological abnormalities which may arise de novo during the pregnancy.

Non-haematological effects of iron deficiency

Effect on the mother

Overt symptoms of iron deficiency are generally not prominent. Defects in oxygen-carrying capacity are compensated for but the health implications of iron deficiency have recently been examined in more detail. Of particular interest are effects produced by impairment of the function of iron-dependent tissue enzymes. These are not the ultimate manifestation of severe untreated iron deficiency, but develop hand in hand with the fall in haemoglobin concentration.

Tissue enzyme malfunction undoubtedly occurs even in the very first stages of iron deficiency. Treatment with oral or parenteral iron results in improved well being long before the haemoglobin starts to rise appreciably, suggesting a central nervous system effect.[23] Effects of iron deficiency on neuromuscular transmission may be responsible for the anecdotal reports of increased blood loss at delivery in anaemic women. The various effects of iron deficiency on cellular function may be responsible for the reported association between anaemia during pregnancy and preterm birth.[24,25]

Effect on fetus and newborn

The fetus derives its iron from maternal serum by active transport across the placenta in the last four weeks of pregnancy. Concentrations of ferritin in the cord blood are substantially higher than that in the mother's circulation at term whether she is iron deficient or not, and all fall within the normal adult range. However, babies born to iron deficient mothers have significantly lower cord ferritin levels than the others. This has an important bearing on iron stores and development of anaemia in the first year of life when iron intake is poor.[9,26,27]

Studies have also suggested that behavioural and developmental abnormalities in children with iron deficiency are related to changes in the concentration of chemical indicators in the brain.[28,29,30]

Even more far reaching effects of maternal iron deficiency during pregnancy have been suggested. A correlation has recently been shown between maternal iron deficiency anaemia, high placental weight, and an increased ratio of placental to birth weight. This suggests that maternal iron deficiency results in poor fetal growth compared with that of the placenta. High blood pressure in adult life has been linked to low birth weight and to birth weight that was lower than would be expected from the weight of the placenta. Prophylaxis of iron deficiency may therefore have important implications for the prevention of adult hypertension, which appears to have its origin in fetal life.[31]

Comment

There is still considerable controversy about whether all women need iron supplements during pregnancy. Many authors are not able to accept that the physiological requirements for iron in pregnancy are considerably higher than the usual intake of most healthy women with apparently good diets in industrial countries.[5,19] The arguments are complicated by the problems of applying strategies in countries at different stages of development. The greatest experience in prevention comes from those countries where iron deficiency is least common and least severe.

From what evidence is available it appears that a high proportion of women in reproductive years do lack storage iron. The reasons may be different in different populations. Over thousands of years the human race has changed its way of living and eating, from a society based on hunting and fishing to the present one with a lower intake of iron and a lower intake of meat and fish. Recent dietary changes in industrialised countries have made it difficult for women to build up iron stores so that iron balance can be maintained in pregnancy.

It has been suggested that women at risk of iron deficiency anaemia could be identified by estimating the serum ferritin concentration in the first trimester.[32] To explore this hypothesis, serum ferritin concentrations were estimated in 669 consecutive women who booked at 16 weeks gestation or earlier at Queen Charlotte's Hospital and who had haemoglobin concentrations of 110 g/l or above; 552 women (82·5%) had serum ferritin concentrations of 50 µg/l or below, and qualified for routine daily iron supplements. These women were drawn from a cosmopolitan, largely well-nourished population; 12% had serum ferritin concentrations of less than 12 µg/l and were already iron deficient in spite of having haemoglobin concentrations of 110 g/l or more. Only 51 (7·6%) had ferritin concentrations of 80 µg/l or above.[33]

In summary, negative iron balance throughout pregnancy, particularly in the latter half, may lead to iron deficiency anaemia in the third trimester. This hazard, together with the increasing evidence of non-haematological effects of iron deficiency on exercise tolerance, cerebral function, fetal, neonatal, and infant development leads to the conclusion that it is safer, more practical, and in the long term less expensive in terms of investigation, hospital admission, and treatment, to offer all women iron supplements from 16 weeks' gestation.[17]

Folate metabolism

Requirements for folate are increased in pregnancy to meet the needs of the growing fetus and the placenta, for uterine hypertrophy and the expanded maternal red cell mass. The placenta transports folate actively to the fetus even in the face of maternal deficiency but maternal folate metabolism is altered early in pregnancy like many other maternal functions, before fetal demands act directly.

Investigations of folate state

Plasma folate

After the haemoglobin concentration and plasma iron, folate must be one of the most studied substances in maternal blood, but there are comparatively few serial data available. It is generally agreed, however, that plasma folate concentration falls as pregnancy advances, so that, at term, it is about half the non-pregnant value.

Substantial day-to-day variations of plasma folate are possible and postprandial increases have been noted which limit the diagnostic value of an occasional sample taken at an antenatal clinic.

Red cell folate

The estimation of red cell folate may provide more useful information as it does not reflect daily or other short term variations in plasma folate concentrations. It is thought to give a better indication of overall amounts in tissues, but the turnover of red blood cells is slow and there is a delay before substantial reductions are evident in the folate concentration of the red cells in patients who are folate deficient.

A number of investigations of erythrocyte folate in pregnancy have shown a slight downward trend even though, as would be expected, the fall is not so pronounced as in plasma. There is evidence that patients who have low red cell folate at the beginning of pregnancy develop megaloblastic anaemia in the third trimester.

Excretion of formimino-glutamic acid (FIGLU)

A loading dose of histidine leads to increased FIGLU excretion in the urine when there is folate deficiency. As a test for folate deficiency in pregnancy it has little to recommend it, primarily because the metabolism of histidine is altered and this results in increased FIGLU excretion in normal early pregnancy.

Postpartum events

In the six weeks following delivery there is a tendency for all the folate indices to return to non-pregnant values. However, should any deficiency of folate have developed and remain untreated in pregnancy it may present clinically for the first time in the puerperium and its consequences may be detected for many months after delivery. Lactation is an added folate stress. Red cell folate concentrations in lactating mothers are significantly lower than those of their infants during the first year of life.

Interpretations of investigations during pregnancy

Outside pregnancy the hallmark of megaloblastic haemopoiesis is macrocytosis, first identified in routine laboratory investigations by a raised MCV. In pregnancy macrocytosis by non-pregnant standards is the norm and in any event may be masked by iron deficiency. Examination of the blood film may be more helpful. There may be occasional oval macrocytes in a sea of iron-deficient microcytic cells. Hypersegmentation of the neutrophil polymorph nucleus is significant because in normal pregnancy there is a shift to the left. If more than 5% of 100 neutrophils have five or more lobes, hypersegmentation is present, but hypersegmentation is observed in pure iron deficiency, uncomplicated by folate deficiency.

In the absence of any changes, megaloblastic haemopoiesis should be suspected when the expected response to adequate iron treatment is not achieved. Evidence of megaloblastic haemopoiesis may become apparent only after treatment with iron even though the rise in haemoglobin concentration appears adequate.

The diagnosis of folate deficiency in pregnancy has to be made entirely on morphological grounds and usually involves examination of a suitably prepared marrow aspirate. In current practice this investigation is not thought to be desirable or necessary. It is far better to provide routine supplements to cover the increased requirement.[13]

The fetus and folate deficiency

There is an increased risk of megaloblastic anaemia occurring in the neonate of a folate-deficient mother, especially if delivery is preterm.

The young infant's requirement for folate has been estimated at 20–50 µg/day (4–10 times the adult requirement on a weight basis). Serum and red cell folates are consistently higher in cord than in maternal blood, but the premature infant is in severe negative folate balance because of high growth rate and reduced intake. Earlier clinical investigations suggested an association between periconceptional folic acid deficiency and harelip, cleft palate and, most important of all, neural tube defects.[34]

To investigate the alleged association of maternal folate deficiency with neural tube defects, the Medical Research Council (MRC) ran a randomised double blind study of preconception together with early pregnancy folic acid supplements. This trial started in July 1983 at 33 centres in seven countries including over 1800 women, but was discontinued prematurely in April 1991 because the results were so clear cut.

Women with a history of neural tube defect given no folic acid supplements had a significantly higher recurrence rate (3·5% as opposed to 1%) than those women given folate.[35] The specific role of folic acid in the prevention of recurrence of neural tube defects was established. It has also been shown in a large randomised controlled trial that periconceptional supplement of 800 µg of folic acid prevented the first occurrence of neural tube defects.[36] What public health measures should be taken to ensure that the diet of a woman in her reproductive years contains adequate folic acid needs careful prospective planning.[37]

Prophylaxis of folate deficiency *during* uncomplicated pregnancy

The case for giving prophylactic folate supplements throughout pregnancy is a strong one and an example of excellent preventive medicine particularly in countries where overt megaloblastic anaemia is common.

The amount of folate needed to maintain the red cell folate concentration in a well nourished population is about 100 µg daily, but to meet the needs of all women, including those with poor dietary intake, the supplement needs to be of the order of 200–300 µg pteroylglutamic acid daily. This should be given in combination with iron supplements and there are several suitable combined preparations available.

The risk of adverse effects from folate supplements in a pregnant woman with B_{12} deficiency is small (see below). More important than this, there is not one report of subacute combined degeneration of the spinal cord occurring among the thousands of women who have received folate supplements during pregnancy. It is a hypothetical risk which should not detract from the vast benefit provided by routine use of folate supplements in pregnancy.[13,37]

Vitamin B_{12}

Muscle, red cell, and serum vitamin B_{12} concentrations fall during pregnancy. Non-pregnant serum concentrations of 205–1025 µg/l fall to 20–510 µg/l at term, lower concentrations being found in multiple pregnancy. Women who smoke tend to have lower serum B_{12} concentrations, which may account for the positive correlation between birth weight and serum concentrations in non-deficient mothers.[38]

Vitamin B_{12} absorption is unaltered in pregnancy. It is probable that tissue uptake is increased by the action of oestrogens, as oral contraceptives cause a fall in serum concentration of vitamin B_{12}. Cord blood vitamin B_{12} concentration is higher than that of maternal blood; the fall in serum concentration of vitamin B_{12} in the mother may be related to preferential transfer of absorbed B_{12} to the fetus at the expense of maintaining the maternal serum concentration, but the placenta does not transfer vitamin B_{12} with the same efficiency as it does folate. The vitamin B_{12} binding capacity of plasma increases in pregnancy, analogous to the rise in transferrin concentration. The rise is confined to the liver-derived transcobalamin II which is concerned with the transport of vitamin B_{12} rather than the leucocyte-derived transcobalamin I (the other vitamin B_{12} binding protein) the concentration of which is raised in the myeloproliferative conditions.

Pregnancy does not make a vast impact on maternal vitamin B_{12} stores: adult stores are of the order of 3000 µg or more, and vitamin B_{12} stores in the newborn are about 50 µg.[13]

Addisonian pernicious anaemia does not usually occur during the reproductive years and the vitamin B_{12} deficiency is associated with infertility. Pregnancy is likely only if the deficiency is remedied.

The recommended intake of vitamin B_{12} is 2·0 µg/day in the non-pregnant and 3·0 µg/day during pregnancy.[13] This will be met by almost any diet which contains animal products however deficient in other essential substances. Strict vegans who will not eat any animal-derived substances may have a deficient intake of vitamin B_{12} and their diet should be supplemented during pregnancy.[39]

Megaloblastic anaemia and pregnancy

The cause of megaloblastic anaemia in pregnancy is nearly always folate deficiency. Vitamin B_{12} is only rarely implicated. A survey of reports from the United Kingdom over the past two decades suggests an incidence of 0·2 to 5·0%, but a considerably greater number of women have megaloblastic changes in their marrow which are not suspected on examination of the peripheral blood alone.[20] The incidence of megaloblastic anaemia in other parts of the world is considerably greater and is thought to reflect the nutritional standards of the population. Several workers have pointed to the poor socio-economic status of their patients as the major aetiological factor contributing to the anaemia, which may be further exacerbated by seasonal changes in the availability of staple foodstuffs. Food folates are only partially available and the amount of folate supplied in the diet is difficult to quantify. In Great Britain analysis of daily folate intake in foodstuffs showed a range of 129–300 μg. The folate content of 24-hour food collections in various studies in Sweden and Canada was about 200 μg on average, with a range as large as 70 μg to 600 μg.

Foods that are rich in folate include broccoli, spinach, and brussel sprouts, but up to 90% of their folate content is lost within a few minutes, by boiling or steaming. These vegetables are unlikely to be eaten raw. Dietary folate deficiency megaloblastic anaemia occurs in about one third of all pregnant women in the world, despite the fact that folate is found in nearly all natural foods, because folate is rapidly destroyed by cooking, especially in foods such as beans and rice.[39] Asparagus, avocados, mushrooms, and bananas also have a fairly high folate content, which may delight social class I patients in the United Kingdom, but will not help the average working-class mother to improve her dietary intake.

The effects of dietary inadequacy may be further amplified by frequent childbirth and multiple pregnancy. Several reports have shown a markedly increased incidence of megaloblastic anaemia in multiple pregnancy.[13]

Other cellular components of the blood

White cells

Granulocytes

The total white cell count rises in pregnancy as a result of an increase in neutrophil polymorphonuclear leucocytes. There is a rise in the neutrophils from the 45th day of pregnancy to reach a peak at 30 weeks and plateau during the third trimester. There is a further neutrophilia at the onset of labour, the total leucocyte count rising as high as $40·0 \times 10^9/l$ in uncomplicated pregnancies. The count returns to non-pregnant levels by six days post partum. There is a tendency for the total leucocyte count to rise with increasing parity, but this is not significant. Normal pregnant women may have up to 3% myelocytes or metamyelocytes in their circulating blood.

The metabolic activity of granulocytes is increased during pregnancy. The leucocyte alkaline phosphatase score rises from the non-pregnant state to reach levels in the third trimester which are usually encountered only during the course of major infections in the non-pregnant. The activity returns to the non-pregnant level by six weeks post partum but breast feeding may prolong the elevation.

Hexose monophosphate activity, glucose oxidation and myeloperoxidase activity are also increased. The neutrophilia and the increase in metabolic activity appear to be the result of oestrogen stimulation.

Lymphocytes

The lymphocyte count does not alter during pregnancy and there is no change in the number of circulating T cells and B cells. However, factors in maternal serum suppress in vitro lymphocyte function, and cell-mediated immunity is profoundly depressed. The raised oestrogen concentrations in women taking oral contraceptives and in pregnancy may depress cellular immunity by increasing the concentration of glycoproteins which coat the lymphocyte surface, thus impairing responses to stimuli.

Other hormones associated with pregnancy, such as human chorionic gonadotrophin and prolactin, suppress lymphocyte function. In contrast there is no evidence of impairment in the production of immunoglobulins or of humoral immunity. The depression of cell-mediated immunity during pregnancy may be relevant to the survival of the fetus, but is associated with reduced resistance to viral infections. There are published reports of increased susceptibility to herpes,[40] influenza,[41] poliomyelitis,[42] rubella, and hepatitis.[43] Pneumococcal infections, particularly meningitis, are also more common and of greater severity in pregnancy according to one report from Nigeria.[44] Perhaps the most important result worldwide of altered immunity in pregnancy is the decreased resistance in immune women to malaria, particularly during the first pregnancy. The placenta is infected and this results in a high incidence of abortion, prematurity, and low birth weight.[45]

Platelets

Platelet counts decrease slightly but significantly during pregnancy and the decrease may be explained by haemodilution or by an increased consumption. Only a few studies of platelet function in pregnancy have been reported and no convincing evidence of any significant changes in function has been obtained. The platelets will be discussed in more detail in the section below which deals with haemostasis.

Haemostasis and fibrinolysis

The integrity and patency of the vascular tree is dependent upon a finely controlled interaction between the coagulation system and fibrinolysis. During pregnancy major changes occur in the components of the haemostatic system. Their significance and their relation to haemorrhage and thrombosis, which are major hazards for the pregnant woman can be appreciated only with a knowledge of the haemostatic mechanism in the healthy non-pregnant individual.

Haemostasis

Haemostasis in health has three primary functions:

- To confine the circulating blood to the vascular bed
- To maintain its fluidity
- To arrest bleeding from injured vessels.

All these aspects of haemostasis depend on a complex interaction between vasculature, platelets, coagulation factors, and fibrinolysis.

Vascular integrity—platelets—prostacyclin

The endothelial cell plays a vital part in the maintenance of vascular integrity and blood flow and also in the response to injury. Platelets do not adhere to the intact undamaged surface of a normal blood vessel and this phenomenon is not yet fully understood, although it is essential to maintain vascular integrity. Platelet adhesion occurs when the endothelial surface is damaged and when a vessel is severed or punctured so that sub-endothelial collagen components are exposed. The endothelial cell is a source of Von Willebrand's factor (VWF) which binds to both exposed collagen and glycoprotein receptors on the platelet surface, resulting in platelet adhesion.

Prostacyclin (PG1$_2$) is the principal prostanoid synthesised by blood vessels; it is a powerful vasodilator and a potent inhibitor of platelet aggregation. Moncada and Vane proposed that there is a balance between the production of prostacyclin by the vessel wall and the production of the vasoconstrictor and powerful aggregating agent thromboxane by platelets.[46]

There are several conditions in which production of prostacyclin is impaired, thereby upsetting the normal balance. Deficiency of prostacyclin production has been suggested in platelet consumption syndromes such as haemolytic uraemic syndrome and thrombotic thrombocytopenic purpura.[47] Prostacyclin production is also reduced in fetal and placental tissue from pre-eclamptic pregnancies,[48] and the current role of prostacyclin in the pathogenesis of pre-eclampsia is undergoing investigation.

Platelet production is thought to be regulated by humoral factors. The plasma and urine of thrombocytopenic animals and humans do contain megakaryocytopoietic and thrombopoietic activities that are lineage specific and distinct from known cytokines. These activities are referred to as megakaryocyte colony stimulating factor (meg-CSF) or thrombopoietin depending on their ability to effect proliferation (meg-CSF) or maturation (thrombopoietin). Recently meg-CSF/thrombopoietin-like protein in the plasma of irradiated pigs has been purified and cloned and the information used to isolate a human complementary DNA.[49] This protein has sequence homology with erythropoietin and has both meg-CSF and thrombopoietin-like activities. The availability of a recombinant protein affecting mega-karyocyte and platelet production makes a careful evaluation of its role in regulating thrombopoiesis and its potential to affect other haematopoietic activity possible.

Platelets produced in the bone marrow by the megakaryocytes have a lifespan of 9–12 days. At the end of their normal lifespan the effete cells are engulfed by cells of the reticulo-endothelium system and most damaged platelets are sequestered in the spleen.

There have been conflicting reports concerning the platelet count during normal pregnancy. The most recent studies, many surveying large populations with the use of automated counting equipment, suggest that if mean values for platelet concentration are analysed throughout pregnancy, there is a downward trend.[50,51]

Most investigators agree that low grade chronic intravascular coagulation within the utero-placental circulation is a part of the physiological response to pregnancy. This is partially compensated for and it is not surprising that the platelets should be involved, either showing evidence of increased turnover or in some cases a reduction in number.

A prospective study of 6715 consecutive deliveries over three years in healthy women delivered at a Canadian obstetric centre showed that 513 (7·6%) had mild thrombocytopenia at term.[51] Most of these (65%) were healthy women in whom thrombocytopenia was an incidental finding. The rest had a variety of medical and obstetric conditions ranging from diabetes, idiopathic thrombocytopenic purpura, and pregnancy induced hyper-tension. There was no direct morbidity or mortality resulting from thrombo-cytopenia in the mother or her infant.

Arrest of bleeding

An essential requirement of the haemostatic system is a rapid reaction to injury, the effect of which remains confined to the area of damage. This requires control mechanisms which stimulate coagulation after trauma but limit the extent of the response. The substances involved in the formation of the haemostatic plug normally circulate in the blood in an inert form until they are activated at the site of vascular injury or by some factor released into the circulation which triggers intravascular coagulation.

When a blood vessel is injured, the first event is the adherence of platelets to the collagen in the exposed subendothelium of the vessel wall. This triggers the release of adenosine diphosphate (ADP), serotonin, calcium, and secreted platelet proteins.[52] ADP increases the platelet plug by stimulating further aggregation of platelets at the site of injury. Serotonin promotes vasoconstriction and also stimulates further aggregation. The coagulation cascade is triggered and the action of thrombin leads to the formation of fibrin which in turn converts the loose platelet plug into a firm stable wound seal.

The end result of blood coagulation is the formation of an insoluble fibrin clot from the soluble precursor fibrinogen. This involves a complex interaction of clotting factors and a sequential activation of a series of proenzymes.[53]

When a blood vessel is injured, blood coagulation is initiated by activation of factor XII by collagen (intrinsic mechanism) and activation of factor VII by thromboplastin release (extrinsic mechanism) from the damaged tissue. Both intrinsic and extrinsic mechanisms are activated by components of the vessel wall and both are required for normal haemostasis. The two mechanisms are diagrammatically represented in Figure 3.1.

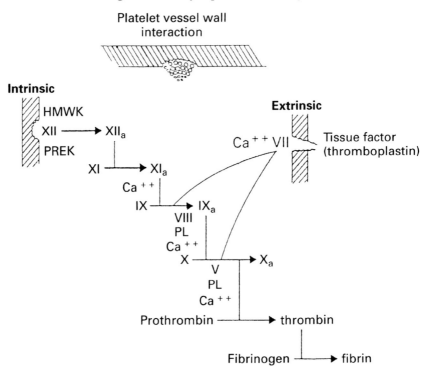

FIGURE 3.1—*Haemostatic/coagulation pathways.*

There is no strict division between the two pathways and interaction between activated factors in both pathways has been shown.[54] The system is a biochemical amplifier. Coagulation factors present in picogram amounts initiate a sequential series of enzyme conversions leading to the conversion of milligrams of fibrinogen to fibrin. The intrinsic and extrinsic systems share a common pathway, following the activation of factor X.

The naturally occurring anticoagulants

Mechanisms that limit and localise the clotting process at sites of trauma are critically important to protect against generalised thrombosis, and also to prevent spontaneous activation of those powerful procoagulant factors which circulate in normal plasma.

Recently investigation of healthy haemostasis has switched emphasis from the factors that promote clotting to those that prevent generalised and spontaneous activation of these factors. An account of the complex interactions and biochemistry of all of these factors is not appropriate here and only those of major importance in haemostasis and their relevance to pregnancy will be mentioned.

Antithrombin III

Antithrombin III (AtIII) is the main physiological inhibitor of thrombin and factor Xa and possibly the main inhibitor of factors IXa, XIa and XIIa. An inherited deficiency of AtIII is one of the few conditions in which there is a familial tendency to thrombosis.[55]

The activity in plasma which causes progressive destruction of thrombin was originally termed antithrombin III. It is now recognised that at least three proteins contribute towards this activity—two general proteinase inhibitors (α_1-antitrypsin and α_2-macroglobin) and α_2-globulin with more specific antithrombin activity, now known as antithrombin III (AtIII). Addition of a specific antibody to AtIII removes all the heparin cofactor activity from plasma and the evidence is overwhelming that these factors are identical. AtIII, therefore, is not only the major thrombin inhibitor in plasma but also the plasma protein through which heparin exerts its effect.[55,56] As AtIII is synthesised in the liver, its activity is low in cirrhosis and other chronic diseases of the liver as well as in protein-losing renal disease, disseminated intravascular coagulation (DIC), and hypercoagulable states.

During uncomplicated pregnancy there is no change in AtIII concentrations during the antenatal period,[57] but some lowering during delivery and then an increase one week post partum. The principle of laboratory measurement of biological activity of AtIII depends on its ability to neutralise thrombin or factor Xa.

Oral contraception and haemostasis

The commonest cause of a small reduction in plasma AtIII is the use of oral contraceptives (OC). In the past 20 years it has become obvious that there is a causal relation between OC steroids and venous thrombo-embolism, though this role in thrombopathogenesis has not been fully evaluated. The oestrogen content is important and since the introduction of low dose oestrogen pills the incidence of venous thromboembolism has fallen dramatically. A significant fall in AtIII concentration has been found in women taking combined OCs, regardless of the oestrogen content, but not in those taking progestogen-only pills.[58]

Accumulating evidence suggests that suppression of AtIII is only one of many interacting risk factors causing the association of venous thromboembolism with oestrogen-containing OCs.

Until recently, however, the only evidence for differences in the risk of thromboembolism between different types of combined OCs has been related to the oestrogen content. Those preparations containing 50 μg or more of ethinyl oestradiol were associated with greater risks than those containing less than 50 μg.[59] The low dose oestrogen containing pills have become the mainstay of contraceptive practice.

Since July 1995, several studies have shown an unexpected increased risk of thromboembolism related to different progestagens (gestodene and desogestrel) involved in two types of "third generation" combined OCs.

An increased risk for non-fatal venous thromboembolism associated with third generation combined OC (low dose oestrogen plus gestodene or desogestrel) compared with second generation OC (<35 μg oestrogen +levonogestrel) was found in a study based on 370 general practices in a cohort of 283 130 otherwise healthy women. The data were taken from the UK general practice research database.[60]

Probably the largest study to date describes the risk of venous thromboembolism with current use of combined OCs among 1143 patients and 2998 age-matched controls from 21 centres in Africa, Asia, Europe and Latin America.[61] Odds ratios associated with the use of combined OCs containing third generation progestagens were higher than for those observed with first generation progestagens (norethandrone type) and second (norgestrel group) generation.[61,62] In this study odds ratios were also increased in obese women and, an unexpected finding, in women with a history of hypertension in pregnancy.

The absolute risk of venous thromboembolism has been calculated to rise from 15/100 000 women/year with second generation OCs to 30/100 000/year in women using OCs containing desogestrel or gestodene. This is the first time that differences in incidence have been found between the newer low dose oestrogen OCs and linked to progesterone derivatives. To put this extra risk into perspective it should be noted that during pregnancy a woman's risk of thrombosis increases to about 60/100 000. However, the greatest risk to health comes from smoking while taking the pill, whatever type is used. Young women smokers who take OCs are 10 times more likely to develop myocardial infarction than those who do not smoke.[63] Venous thromboembolism remains rare among women in the reproductive years but we have to balance the risk of OCs of any sort against the possible benefits such as protection against myocardial infarction. Women with risk factors for venous thromboembolism (such as a personal or family history) should be screened for thrombophilia and it would be sensible not to start them on third generation OCs. It is hoped "that any disproportionate fear of litigation soon gives way to intelligent and well-informed collaborative decision-making".[64] As this chapter goes to press, active investigation and further epidemiological studies are under way. The US FDA has stated that it "considers it prudent to treat the data with caution before deciding on the policy implications".

Protein C-thrombomodulin—protein S—activated protein C cofactor

Protein C inactivates factors V and VIII in conjunction with its cofactors thrombomodulin and protein S. To exert its effect, protein C, a vitamin K dependent anticoagulant synthesised in the liver, must be activated by an endothelial cell cofactor termed thrombomodulin.

Many kindreds with a deficiency or a functional deficit of protein C resulting in recurrent thromboembolism have been described.[65] Purpura fulminans neonatalis is the homozygous expression of protein C deficiency with severe thrombosis and neonatal death.[66]

Protein S, also a vitamin K dependent glycoprotein, acts as a cofactor for activated protein C by promoting its binding to lipid and platelet surface, thus localising the reaction. Several families have been described with protein S deficiency and thromboembolic disease. Data on protein C and protein S concentrations in healthy pregnancy are sparse but a significant reduction in functional protein S concentration during pregnancy has been shown.[67,68,69]

Recently a cross sectional study of 91 normal pregnant women showed no change in antigenic or functional protein C but confirmed a significant fall in free protein S from first to second trimester.[70]

Activated protein C cofactor

A new cofactor in the protein C anticoagulant pathway

Deficiency of protein C, protein S, or AtIII is found in about 20% of patients with a history of thromboembolism under the age of 45 years. These deficiencies are especially common in those with a family history. Recently Dahlbäck et al identified a second cofactor for activated protein C in a family with thrombophilia.[71] The defect could be corrected by the addition of normal plasma. In a further study to establish the prevalence of activated protein C resistance in patients with venous thrombosis the defect was found in 33% of the patients studied.[72] Precipitating factors for thrombosis such as pregnancy and the use of oral contraceptives were identified in 60% of these patients. The defect was identified in the laboratory using a modified activated partial thromboplastin time (APTT) test. The results were expressed as activated protein C sensitivity ratios defined as APTT in the presence of activated protein C divided by APTT in the absence of activated protein C. An abnormal APTT ratio (<2·0) was detected in 64 of 301 (21%) consecutive young patients in The Netherlands on investigation of their first episode of thromboembolism.[73]

Dahlbäck and Hildebrand have recently identified the procoagulant factor V as the factor responsible for hereditary activated protein C resistance.[74] A single missense mutation in the factor V gene, which changes arginine to glutamine has been found in association with the vast majority of cases with an abnormal APTT ratio—the so-called factor V Leiden mutation. This defect is the most important cause of hereditary thrombophilia identified to date.

A recent retrospective study of thromboembolism associated with pregnancy and the use of OCs showed that 59% of 34 women during pregnancy and 30% of 28 women using OCs had activated protein C ratios of less than 2·0 indicating activated protein C resistance.[75]

Women who are carriers of factor V Leiden mutation and take OCs are at high risk of thromboembolism.[76]

Fibrinolysis

The fibrinolytic enzyme system has four components: plasminogen, plasmin, activators, and inhibitors.

Fibrin and fibrinogen are digested by plasmin, a proteolytic enzyme derived from an inactive plasma precursor, plasminogen. Plasminogen is a β-globulin and estimates of its molecular weight vary between 81 000 and 143 000. Synthesis, most probably in the liver, can take place fairly rapidly, and treatment with streptokinase results in an increase in the plasma plasminogen concentration from barely detectable levels to normal within 12–24 hours. Plasminogen is stable over a wide range of temperatures and pH in plasma and serum. It is a single polypeptide chain which, when converted to plasmin, becomes a two-chain molecule connected by a single disulphide bond.

Physiological fibrinolytic activity depends on plasminogen activators in the blood. Increased amounts are found in the plasma after strenuous exercise, emotional stress, surgical operations and other trauma. Plasminogen activator is difficult to assay because it is extremely labile and in vitro has a half-life of 15 minutes.

Naturally occurring activators are found in blood, tissue, and urine. Tissue activator can be extracted from most human organs with the exception of the placenta. Tissues especially rich in activator include the uterus, ovaries, prostate, heart, lungs, thyroid, adrenal glands, and lymph nodes. Activity in tissues is concentrated mainly around blood vessels, and veins have greater activity than arteries. Venous occlusion of the limbs stimulates fibrinolytic activity of the blood and this has been used as a test of a patient's potential to release activator from the vascular endothelium.[77]

Plasmin, the proteolytic enzyme derived from plasminogen, can digest many proteins including fibrinogen and fibrin. Normally the action of plasmin is confined to the digestion of fibrin because of the presence of plasmin inhibitors in the blood. Other proteins that can be digested by

38

plasmin include prothrombin, factors V and VIII, glucagon, adreno-corticotrophic hormone, and growth hormone.

There are two main inhibitors of the fibrinolytic system: antiactivators which inhibit plasminogen activation and antiplasmins which are inhibitors of formed plasmin. Antiactivators have been separated and identified in human serum and shown to develop during the process of spontaneous blood coagulation.

Several aliphatic-amino compounds are competitive inhibitors of plasminogen activation and include epsilon aminocaproic acid, tranexamic acid and aprotinin (Trasylol) which is prepared commercially from bovine lung.

Both plasma and serum exert a strong inhibitory action on plasmin. Platelets have antiplasmin activity which is probably of importance in stabilising platelet thrombi. Normally plasma anti plasmin concentration exceeds that of plasminogen and hence of potential plasmin, otherwise the stability of healthy vasculature would be destroyed.

Fibrin and fibrinogen degradation products (FDP)

When fibrinogen or fibrin is broken down by plasmin, FDP are formed (Figure 3.2). Plasmin first splits off fragment X with some smaller fragments A, B and C. Further digestion of fragment X (which is still slowly but completely clottable by thrombin) results in the formation of fragments Y and D, which will not clot as a result of the action of thrombin. Fragment Y is further broken down to fragments D and E, so-called "end split products". Fragments X and Y are termed "high-molecular-weight split products".

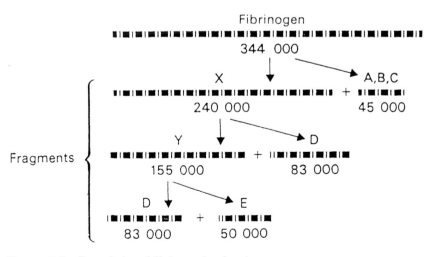

FIGURE 3.2—*Degradation of fibrinogen by plasmin.*

Serum can contain small amounts of fragment X, larger amounts of Y, D, and E, as well as complexes of fibrin monomers, fibrinogen, and fragments Y and X. All these components have antigenic determinants in common with fibrinogen, and will be recognised by antifibrinogen antisera.

In recent years the development of tests to measure specific fibrin–fibrinogen degradation products such as fibrinopeptide A and D-dimer using chromogenic assays has aided the laboratory investigation of fibrinolysis considerably.

Tests of haemostatic function

There are simple rapid screening tests which establish the competence of the haemostatic system. These tests can be done in any general haematological laboratory and do not require an expert coagulation unit. The easily available investigations are emphasized, the results of which help those in obstetric practice to come to a rapid decision about the nature of haemostatic failure in their patients.

All the tests referred to are performed on suitably prepared aliquots of specimens of whole blood acquired by venepuncture. In order to avoid testing artefacts it is essential that the blood is obtained by a quick, efficient, non-traumatic technique, with particular emphasis on the following points:

- *Thromboplastin contamination*: Thromboplastin released from damaged tissues may contaminate the specimen and alter the results. This is likely to occur if difficulty is encountered in finding the vein or if the vein is only partly canalised and the flow is slow, or if there is excessive squeezing of tissues and repeated attempts to obtain a specimen with the same needle. In such circumstances the specimen may clot in the tube in spite of the presence of anticoagulant or the coagulation times of the various tests are altered and do not reflect the true condition. Platelets may aggregate in clumps and give a falsely low count.
- *Heparin contamination*: Heparin prolongs the partial thromboplastin time and thrombin time out of proportion to the prothrombin time. As little as 0·05 units of heparin/ml prolongs the coagulation test times. It is customary, though not desirable, to take blood for coagulation tests from lines which have been washed through with fluids containing heparin to keep them patent. It is almost impossible to overcome the effect of the heparin on the blood passing through such a line, however much blood is taken and discarded before obtaining a sample for investigation. It is strongly recommended that blood be taken from another site not previously contaminated by heparin.
- *Fibrinolysis in vitro*: Any blood taken into a glass tube without anticoagulant will clot within a few minutes and natural fibrinolysis will continue in vitro. Unless the blood is taken into a fibrinolytic inhibitor such as epsilon aminocaproic acid, a falsely high concentration of FDPs is found which bears no relation to fibrinolysis in vivo. Similarly, leaving a tourniquet on too long before taking the specimen stimulates local fibrinolytic activity in vivo.

Screening tests for haemostatic function

Tests related to integrity of vasculature

- *Bleeding time*: The length of time a small skin wound continues to bleed depends largely on the number and function of platelets and their ability to form plugs at the site of injury. Ivy's method is recommended but the test is unpleasant for the patient and tedious if the bleeding is prolonged (normal range up to 7–10 minutes; 15–20 minutes is abnormal). It is not of value in assessing haemostatic failure in an obstetric emergency. Its use in coagulation laboratories is mainly in the investigation of bleeding disorders with a normal platelet count, such as thrombasthenia or Bernard Soulier syndrome. It is always prolonged in the presence of substantial thrombocytopenia. Details of platelet function tests can be found elsewhere.[78]

- *Platelet count*: The commonest platelet disorder is thrombocytopenia. It may be an isolated haemostatic defect or part of a generalised consumptive coagulopathy.

  Venous blood is taken into commercially provided containers containing the anticoagulant ethylenediamine-tetra-acetic acid (EDTA, sequestrene). These containers are also used when estimation of haemoglobin concentration, packed cell volume, and white cell count are required. Examination of the blood film by a competent haematology laboratory worker may also provide valuable information about the nature of the haemostatic disorders.

  The count is made electronically on a diluted whole blood specimen. The platelets are distinguished by size from other cells. The platelet count is a valuable rapid screening test in assessing acute obstetric haemostatic failure, particularly in helping the attendants to diagnose the presence and severity of disseminated intravascular coagulation.

Tests for coagulation mechanisms[78]   Blood for investigation should be taken into trisodium citrate; a measured standard amount of citrate is used so that the dilution factor is constant. It is essential that the exact amount of blood required for laboratory testing is delivered into the citrate-containing bottle. Variations in packed cell volume can introduce similar effects and may have to be allowed for by appropriate adjustment of the proportion of citrate. There are three simple, rapid tests of the integrity of the coagulation cascade:

- Activated partial thromboplastin time (APTT)—intrinsic system
- Prothrombin time (PT)—extrinsic system
- Thrombin time (TT)—final common pathway.

For the relation of these tests to the coagulation cascade see Figure 3.3.

- *Activated partial thromboplastin time (APTT)*: This test is also known as the partial thromboplastin time with kaolin (PTTK) and the kaolin cephalin clotting time (KCCT). If normal blood is allowed to clot in a glass tube with no additive the process takes from 4–11 minutes. The time-consuming reactions are those which lead to contact activation and those which cause aggregation and release of phospholipid from platelets. These reactions are accelerated or bypassed by pre-incubation of citrated plasma with kaolin to activate the contact factors and the addition of phospholipid to replace platelet activity.

The measurement of the clotting time of the citrated plasma after addition of calcium and phospholipid under these circumstances gives a crude assessment of the integrity of the intrinsic coagulation system. The normal range is between 35 and 45 seconds, but tests must always be compared with a known normal plasma. The time taken to complete this test in the laboratory is a distinct advantage over trying to perform bedside whole blood clotting tests which provide little information in an emergency. The APTT is not only quicker but much more informative. The whole blood clotting time is insensitive and can therefore be dangerously misleading.

- *Prothrombin time (PT)*: This test measures the clotting time of citrated plasma after the addition of an optimal concentration of tissue extract (thromboplastin) and recalcification.

  It was originally introduced by Quick as a measure of prothrombin, factor II, activity. It is now known to depend in addition on reactions between factors V, VII and X and thus is a measure of the overall efficiency of the extrinsic clotting system. Normal range is 10–14 seconds, but the values obtained in any laboratory depend on exactly how the test is undertaken and, in particular, on the source and type of thromboplastin used. The interpretation depends on meticulous quality control.

- *Thrombin time*: This test is a measure of the final common pathway of the extrinsic and intrinsic coagulation systems (Figure 3.3). Thrombin is added to a sample of citrated plasma and the time of fibrin clot to form is measured. The time taken is affected by the concentration and reaction of fibrin.

  Normal plasma has a thrombin clotting time of 15–19 seconds. The commonest causes of a prolonged thrombin time are the presence of fibrin degradation products, depletion of fibrinogen in disseminated intravascular coagulation, and the presence of heparin (see above).

Fibrinogen estimation (Clauss technique)[78] Diluted plasma is clotted with a strong thrombin solution. The plasma is diluted to yield a low concentration of inhibitors such as FDPs and heparin. The result is obtained from a previously prepared calibration curve using normal plasma. It should be remembered that in late pregnancy (after 30 weeks gestation) the normal non-pregnant range of fibrinogen (2·0 to 4·5 g/l) is increased to 4·0 to 6·0 g/l.

Detection of fibrinogen/fibrin degradation products (FDP) A suspension of latex particles is coated with specific antibodies to the purified FDP

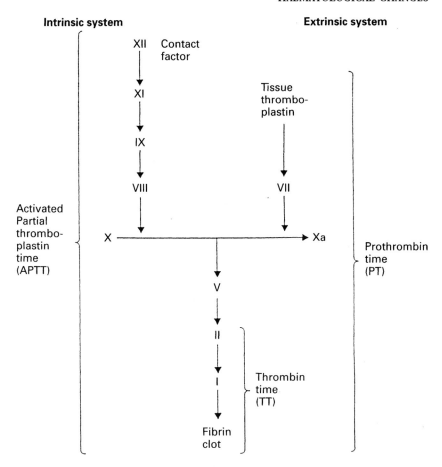

Intrinsic system

Extrinsic system

FIGURE 3.3—*In vitro screening tests of coagulation and their relation to systems involved.*

fragments D and E. The suspension is mixed with diluted patient's serum which has been taken into an antifibrinolytic agent to arrest in vitro fibrinolysis. Aggregation indicates the presence of FDPs. By testing serial dilutions of the sample a semi-quantitative assay can be performed.

Healthy subjects have FDP concentrations of less than 10 μg/ml. Concentrations between 10 and 40 μg/ml are seen in acute inflammatory disorders, in acute venous and arterial thrombosis, and after strenuous exercise or major surgery. High levels of FDPs are seen in association with severe acute DIC and following thrombolytic therapy with streptokinase.

In patients with acute or chronic haemostatic disorders these simple screening tests, together with a detailed clinical history, allow us to place them into categories or even to make a provisional diagnosis which indicates how to proceed further to confirm the diagnosis, for example, to platelet function tests or individual coagulation factor assays.

It is essential that these more exacting tests should be carried out in an expert, competent, and specialised laboratory and, because of the rapidity with which changes in coagulation factors take place in vitro, such units usually prefer to see the patient themselves rather than receiving blood samples taken at other centres, even if they are delivered by car or other rapid transport.

Coagulation and fibrinolysis during normal pregnancy

Coagulation system

Normal pregnancy is accompanied by major changes in the coagulation system. There are increases in the concentration of factors VII, VIII and X and a particularly pronounced increase in the concentration of plasma fibrinogen.[79-82] The increased quantity of fibrinogen in the plasma alters the negative surface charge of the red cells which, on standing, form aggregates in a pattern described as *rouleaux*, and these settle in a glass tube more quickly than single erythrocytes. The increase in fibrinogen is probably the chief cause of the accelerated erythrocyte sedimentation rate observed during pregnancy.

The effect of pregnancy on the coagulation factors can be detected from about the third month of gestation. The plasma fibrinogen concentration increases from non-pregnant levels of about 2·5–4·0 g/l to as high as 6·0g/l in late pregnancy and labour. If the increase in plasma volume is taken into consideration, the amount of fibrinogen in late pregnancy is at least double that of the non-pregnant state. This marked rise in fibrinogen results from increased synthesis. Factor VII in pregnancy may be increased as much as tenfold and an increase in this factor has also been observed in women taking oestrogen/progestagen contraceptives.

Factor VIII, antihaemophilic factor, is increased in late pregnancy, the coagulation activity being about twice that in the non-pregnant state. Some workers have found a parallel increase both in the biological activity of factor VIII (VIIIC) and in the factor VIII-related antigen (VWF) while others have found an increase in the ratio between the antigenic and coagulant activity. In uncomplicated pregnancies the ratio remains around 1·0 but it is raised in pregnancies complicated by severe pre-eclampsia or septic abortion because of a greater increase in VWF and reduction in factor VIIIC by thrombin activation.

Rises of factor IX (Christmas factor) concentrations during pregnancy have been reported by several authors, as have decreases in factor XI—with concentrations down to 60–70% of the non-pregnant value and a gradual fall in fibrin stabilising factor XIII reaching 50% of the normal non-pregnant value at term.

Increased concentrations of high molecular weight fibrin/fibrinogen complexes in the plasma have been found during normal pregnancy and confirmed by comparing the concentrations in normal pregnancy with those found in non-pregnant age-matched controls. An increase in the level of fibrinopeptide A and a thrombin-like influence on factor V activity has also been described. There appears to be an increased ability to neutralise heparin in late pregnancy as shown by the need for a moderately increased dose to achieve similar plasma levels in the third trimester in those women receiving prophylactic low-dosage unfractionated heparin[83] and low molecular weight heparin.[84]

These changes in the coagulation system in normal pregnancy are consistent with a continuing low grade process of coagulant activity. Under electron microscopy fibrin is seen to be deposited in the intervillous space of the placenta and in the walls of spiral arteries supplying the placenta.[85] As pregnancy advances, the elastic lamina and smooth muscle of these spiral arteries are replaced by a matrix containing fibrin. This allows an expansion of the lumen to accommodate an increasing blood flow and reduces the pressure of arterial blood flowing to the placenta. At placental separation during normal childbirth, a blood flow of 500–800 ml/min has to be staunched within seconds or serious blood loss will occur. Myometrial contraction plays a vital part in securing haemostasis by reducing the blood flow to the placental site. At separation of the placenta, rapid closure of the terminal part of the spiral arteries by the unique mechanism of myometrial contraction is facilitated by the structural changes described. The placental site is rapidly covered by a fibrin mesh following delivery; the amount of fibrinogen deposited represents 5 to 10% of the total circulating fibrinogen.

The increased levels of fibrinogen and coagulation factors during pregnancy are probably a compensatory response to local utilisation. The resulting hypercoagulability is advantageous to meet the sudden demand for haemostatic components at placental separation.

Fibrinolysis

Plasma fibrinolytic activity is reduced during pregnancy, remains low during labour and delivery and returns to normal within one hour of placental delivery. Fibrinolytic activity in the walls of veins is also reduced in late pregnancy.

The rapid return of systemic fibrinolytic activity to normal following delivery of the placenta and the fact that the placenta contains inhibitors which block fibrinolysis suggest that inhibition of fibrinolysis during pregnancy is mediated through the placenta.[86]

The identification of a placentally-derived circulating plasminogen activation inhibitor—PA1-2—supports this contention.[87] In addition, the activity of the fibrinolytic system in response to stimulation is significantly reduced during pregnancy.[77] This physiological impairment of fibrinolysis may contribute to the increased thrombotic risk in pregnancy.

As fibrinolysis is depressed during pregnancy, the level of FDP will not necessarily reflect the amount of local intravascular coagulation. The increase of FDP in the circulation in labour may originate from the uterus. FDP concentrations in uterine blood during caesarean section during labour are considerably higher than those during elective caesarean section.

Haemostatic problems associated with pregnancy

Pregnancy induces complex changes in the physiological systems concerned with haemostasis.[81,82,88,89] The alterations in the coagulation and fibrinolytic systems which take place during pregnancy, together with the increased blood volume and unique phenomenon of myometrial contraction, help to combat the hazard of haemorrhage during and after placental separation; however, they carry the risk of more rapid and increased response to coagulant stimuli. The tendency to venous stasis in the lower limbs may provide initiating conditions and the incidence of venous thrombosis, though low, is undoubtedly raised in pregnancy.

The local activation of the clotting system during parturition carries with it a risk not only of thromboembolism but of disseminated intravascular coagulation. Consumption of clotting factors and platelets leads to severe generalised—and in particular uterine—bleeding. Despite the advances in obstetric care and highly-developed blood transfusion services, haemorrhage is still a major factor in maternal mortality and morbidity.[90,91]

The most recent published report on Confidential Enquiries into Maternal Deaths in the UK highlights the hazard of pulmonary embolism, which has been second only to hypertension as a direct cause of maternal mortality in recent years.[91] Unexpectedly, the incidence of death from haemorrhage has increased in the last two triennia bringing haemorrhage into the first three leading direct causes of maternal mortality. Most of the reported deaths were not associated with DIC initially, which only appeared to develop after prolonged shock.

Fibrinolysis is stimulated by disseminated intravascular coagulation and the FDP resulting from the process interfere with the formation of firm fibrin clots; a vicious circle is thus established which results in further disastrous bleeding. The classic example of this complication is abruptio placentae. Tissue thromboplastin is released into the hypercoagulable maternal circulation from the placental site, and severe protracted post partum bleeding in cases of abruptio placentae is associated with high concentrations of FDPs and atony of the uterus. It is possible that high concentrations of FDP interfere not only with coagulation but also inhibit myometrial contraction.

A more subtle low grade process of intravascular coagulation is thought to occur in pre-eclampsia. Compared with findings in normal pregnancy the platelet count falls and serum FDP concentration rises around 24 weeks' gestation. The ratio of factor VIII-related antigen to factor VIII coagulant activity is considerably increased, and concentrations of soluble fibrin/fibrinogen complexes are high in patients with pre-eclampsia compared with those in normal pregnancy. Although administration of small doses of heparin substantially results in lowering of the FDP concentration and the return of the platelet count from thrombocytopenic levels to normal, there is no change in the clinical course of pre-eclampsia. Pilot studies have suggested that low dose aspirin may protect women at risk of developing pre-eclampsia and pregnancy associated hypertension; aspirin is thought to act by selectively inhibiting the production of thromboxane from arachidonic acid by the platelets, thereby enhancing the effect of prostacyclin generation from the endothelium. However, the results of the recently published Collaborative Low-dose Aspirin Study in Pregnancy do not support routine prophylactic or therapeutic adminis-tration of anti-platelet drugs to all women at increased risk of pre-eclampsia or intrauterine growth retardation.[92] This is discussed further in the section on "Use of anticoagulants in pregnancy".

Addendum

Developmental haemostasis and prenatal diagnosis of coagulation defects

Observations in the 1960s and 1970s on midterm miscarriages and preterm infants showed that clotting factors are present in fetal life and are independent of maternal blood concentrations. With the obstetric advances in ultrasound scanning and fetal blood sampling it has been possible to obtain serial measurements in utero of fetal concentration of platelets and of the important coagulation factors.[93]

Using these values, obstetric and laboratory techniques developed during the last decade have been successfully applied to the accurate prenatal diagnosis of congenital haematological disorders.[94,95,96] Fetal blood cannot be obtained easily before 18 weeks' gestation and if the findings indicate the need for termination of pregnancy this would mean a mid-trimester termination. However, a few conditions remain which cannot be diagnosed by any other method and this technique will continue to have value. In the past decade there has been an explosion of knowledge about human molecular genetics. There has been a change in emphasis in the analysis of human genetic disease from the clinical, cellular, and biochemical levels to the molecular level. Using recombinant DNA techniques, the new tools of molecular biology, it has been possible to study the structure of human genes directly, how their activity is controlled, and their role in protein synthesis.

The fetal tissue necessary for DNA analysis can be obtained much earlier in gestation and will therefore result in earlier termination of pregnancy if desired and indicated. The chromosomal site of many of the genes responsible for producing haemostatic factors are now known. Fetal sex may be established at a much earlier stage of pregnancy than was possible from amniotic fluid fibroblasts, by DNA analysis of chorionic biopsy material obtained at 8–10 weeks' gestation and also by the new more discriminating ultrasound. Cloning of the genes for factors VIII and IX has facilitated prenatal diagnosis in many but not all cases at risk of haemophilia. The identification of most haemophilia carriers as well as affected fetuses by analysis of DNA is now in routine practice.

For a review of the techniques involved and their application to clinical practice in this and many other conditions, the reader is referred to Weatherall's masterly monograph.[97]

With the help of this new discipline of molecular genetics the systems involved in the control of haemostasis continue to be unravelled. The discovery of new procoagulants, anticoagulants and fibrinolytic factors increase our understanding of their complex interactions and allow revisions of the model for physiological initiation, regulation, and control.[98]

References

1 Hytten F. Blood volume changes in normal pregnancy. In: Letsky EA, ed. *Haematological disorders in pregnancy*. Eastbourne: Saunders, 1985 (Clinics in Haematology 14).

2 Rovinsky JJ, Jaffin H. Cardiovascular hemodynamics in pregnancy. I. Blood and plasma volumes in multiple pregnancy. *Am J Obstet Gynecol* 1965; **93**: 1–15.

3 Fullerton WT, Hytten FE, Klopper AI, McKay E. A case of quadruplet pregnancy. *Journal of Obstetrics and Gynaecology of the British Commonwealth* 1965; **72**: 791–6.

4 Murphy JF, O'Riordan J, Newcombe RG, Coles EC, Pearson JF. Relation of haemoglobin levels in first and second trimesters to outcome of pregnancy. *Lancet* 1986; **i**: 992–5.

5 Steer P, Ash Alam M, Wadsworth J, Welch A. Relation between maternal haemoglobin concentration and birth weight in different ethnic groups. *BMJ* 1995; **310**: 489–91.

6 Combs CA, Murphy EL, Laros RK. Factors associated with hemorrhage in cesarean deliveries. *Obstet Gynecol* 1991; **77**: 77–82.

7 Beguin Y, Lipscei G, Oris R, Thoumsin H, Fillet G. Serum immunoreactive erythropoietin during pregnancy and in the early postpartum. *Br J Haematol* 1990; **76**: 545–9.

8 Riikonen S, Saijonmaa O, Jarvenpaa AL, Fyhrquist F. Serum concentrations of erythropoietin in healthy and anaemic pregnant women. *Scand J Clin Lab Invest* 1994; **54**: 653–7.

9 Milman N, Agger AO, Nielsen OJ. Iron status markers and serum erythropoietin in 120 mothers and newborn infants. Effect of iron supplementation in normal pregnancy. *Acta Obstet Gynecol Scand* 1994; **73**: 200–4.

10 Harstad TW, Mason RA, Cox SM. Serum erythropoietin quantitation in pregnancy using an enzyme-linked immunoassay. *Am J Perinatol* 1992; **9**: 233–5.

11 Popat N, Wood WG, Weatherall DJ, Turnbull AC. Pattern of maternal F-cell production during pregnancy. *Lancet* 1977; **ii**: 377–9.

12 World Health Organization. *Nutritional anaemias*. Geneva: WHO, 1972. (Technical Report Series No 503).

13 Chanarin I. Folate and cobalamin. In: Letsky EA, ed. *Haematological disorders in pregnancy*. London: Saunders, 1985. (Clinics in Haematology 14).

14 Thompson WG. Comparison of tests for diagnosis of iron depletion in pregnancy. *Am J Obstet Gynecol* 1988; **159**: 1132–4.

15 Oski FA. The unique fetal red cell and its function. *Pediatrics* 1973; **51**: 494.

16 Kaeda JS, Prasad K, Howard RJ, Mehta A, Vulliamy T, Luzzatto L. Management of pregnancy when maternal blood has a very high level of fetal haemoglobin. *Br J Haematol* 1994; **88**: 432–4.

17 Hallberg L. Prevention of iron deficiency. *Clin Haematol* 1994; 7: 805–14.

18 Hallberg L. Iron balance in pregnancy and lactation. In: Forget SJ, Zlotkin S, eds. *Nutritional anaemias*. New York: Raven Press, 1992.

19 Barrett JFR, Whittaker PG, Williams JG, Lind T. Absorption of non-haem iron from food during normal pregnancy. *BMJ* 1994; **309**: 79–82.

20 Jacobs A, Miller F, Worwood M, Beamish MR, Wardrop CA. Ferritin in serum of normal subjects and patients with iron deficiency and iron overload. *BMJ* 1972; **iv**: 206–8.

21 Cook JD. Iron deficiency anaemia. In: Clinical Haematology 7. London: Bailliere Tindall, 1994.

22 Carriaga MT, Skikne BS, Finley B, Cutler B, Cook JD. Serum transferrin receptor for the detection of iron deficiency in pregnancy. *Am J Clin Nutr* 1991; **54**: 1077–81.

23 Addy DP. Happiness is: iron. *BMJ* 1986; **292**: 969–70.

24 Allen LH. Iron-deficiency anemia increases risk of preterm delivery. *Nutr Rev* 1993; **51**: 49–52.

25 Scholl TO, Hediger ML, Fischer RL, Shearer JW. Anaemia vs. iron deficiency: increased risk of preterm delivery in a prospective study. *Am J Clin Nutr* 1992; **55**: 985–8.

26 Fenton V, Cavill I, Fisher J. Iron stores in pregnancy. *Br J Haematol* 1977; **37**: 145–9.

27 Milman N, Agger AO, Nielsen OJ. Iron supplementation during pregnancy. Effect on iron status markers, serum erythropoietin and human placental lactogen. A placebo controlled study in 207 Danish women. *Dan Med Bull* 1991; **38**: 471–6.

28 Oski FA. Iron deficiency—facts and fallacies. *Pediatr Clin N Am* 1985; **32**: 493.

29 Walter T. Effect of iron deficiency anaemia on cognitive skills in infancy and childhood. *Baillieres Clinical Haematology* 1994; 7: 815–27.

30 Idjradinata P, Pollitt E. Reversal of developmental delays in iron-deficient anaemic infants treated with iron. *Lancet* 1993; **341**: 1–4.

31 Godfrey KM, Redman CWG, Barker DJP, Osmond C. The effect of maternal anaemia and iron deficiency on the ratio of fetal weight to placental weight. *Br J Obstet Gynaecol* 1991; **98**: 886–91.

32 Bentley DP. Iron metabolism and anaemia in pregnancy. In Letsky EA, ed. *Haematological disorders in pregnancy.* Eastbourne: Saunders, 1985. (Clinics in Haematology 14).

33 Letsky EA. Anaemia in obstetrics. In: Studd J, ed. London: Churchill Livingstone, 1987. (Progress in Obstetrics and Gynaecology 6).

34 Smithells RW, Nevin NC, Seller MJ, *et al.* Further experience of vitamin supplementation for prevention of neural tube defect recurrences. *Lancet* 1983; **i**: 1027–31.

35 MRC Vitamin Study Research Group. Prevention of neural tube defects: results of the Medical Research Council vitamin study. *Lancet* 1991; **338**: 131–7.

36 Czeizel AE, Dudás I. Prevention of the first occurrence of neural-tube defects by periconceptional vitamin supplementation. *N Engl J Med* 1992; **327**: 1832–5.

37 Wald NJ, Bower C. Folic acid and the prevention of neural tube defects. *BMJ* 1995; **310**: 1019–20.

38 McGarry JM, Andrews J. Smoking in pregnancy and vitamin B_{12} metabolism. *BMJ* 1972; **ii**: 74–7.

39 Herbert V. Biology of disease—megaloblastic anaemias. *Lab Invest* 1985; **52**: 3–19.

40 Goyette RE, Donowho EM, Hieger LR, Plunkett GD. Fulminant herpes virus hominis hepatitis during pregnancy. *Obstet Gynecol* 1974; **43**: 191–6.

41 Greenberg M, Jacobziner H, Pakter J, Weisl BAG. Maternal mortality in the epidemic of Asian influenza, New York City 1957. *Am J Obstet Gynecol* 1958; **76**: 897.

42 Rindge ME. Poliomyelitis in pregnancy. *N Engl J Med* 1957; **256**: 281.

43 Anon. Nature's transplant. *Lancet* 1974; **i**: 345.

44 Lucas AO. Pneumococcal meningitis in pregnancy and the puerperium. *BMJ* 1964; **i**: 92.

45 MacGregor JD, Avery JG. Malaria transmission and fetal growth. *BMJ* 1974; **iii**: 433.

46 Moncada MD, Vane JR. Arachidonic acid metabolites and the interactions between platelets and blood-vessel walls. *N Engl J Med* 1979; **300**: 1142–7.

47 Lewis PJ, Boylan P, Friedman LA, Hensby CN, Downing I. Prostacyclin in pregnancy. *BMJ* 1980; **280**: 1581–2.

48 Lewis PJ. The role of prostacyclin in preeclampsia. *Br J Hosp Med* 1982; **28**: 393–5.

49 De Sauvage FJ, Hass PE, Spencer SD, *et al.* Stimulation of megakaryocytopoiesis and thrombopoiesis by the c-Mpl ligand. *Nature* 1994; **369**: 533–8.

50 O'Brien WF, Saba HI, Knuppel RA, Scerbo JC, Cohen GR. Alterations in platelet concentration and aggregation in normal pregnancy and pre-eclampsia. *Am J Obstet Gynecol* 1986; **155**: 486–90.

51 Burrows RF, Kelton JG. Thrombocytopenia at delivery: a prospective survey of 6715 deliveries. *Am J Obstet Gynecol* 1990; **162**: 731–4.

52 Niewiarowski S. Secreted platelet proteins. In: Bloom AL, Forbes CD, Thomas DP, Tuddenham EGD, eds. *Haemostasis and thrombosis.* 3rd ed. Edinburgh: Churchill Livingstone, 1994.

49

53 Forbes CD, Greer IA. Physiology of haemostasis and the effect of pregnancy. In: Greer IA, Turpie AGG, Forbes CD, eds. *Haemostasis and thrombosis in obstetrics and gynaecology.* London: Chapman & Hall, 1992.

54 Hathaway WE, Bonnar J. Hemostasis—general considerations. In: *Haemostatic disorders of the pregnant woman and newborn infant.* Chichester: John Wiley, 1987.

55 Lane DA, Olds RJ, Thein SL. Antithrombin and its deficiency. In: Bloom AL, Forbes CD, Thomas DP, Tuddenham EGD, eds. *Haemostasis and thrombosis.* 3rd ed. Edinburgh: Churchill Livingstone, 1994.

56 Barrowcliffe TW, Thomas DP. Heparin and low molecular weight heparin. In: Bloom AL, Forbes CD, Thomas DP, Tuddenham EGD, eds. *Haemostasis and thrombosis.* 3rd ed. Edinburgh: Churchill Livingstone, 1994.

57 Hellgren M, Blomback M. Blood coagulation and fibrinolysis in pregnancy, during delivery and in the puerperium. *Gynecol Obstet Invest* 1981; **12**: 141–54.

58 Conard J, Cazenave B, Samama M, Horellou MH, Zorn JR, Neau C. AtIII content and antithrombin activity in oestrogen-progestogen and progestogen-only treated women. *Thromb Res* 1980; **18**: 675–81.

59 Thorogood M. Oral contraceptives and cardiovascular disease: an epidemiologic overview. *Pharmacoepidemiology and Drug Safety* 1993; **2**: 3–16.

60 Jick H, Jick SS, Gurewich V, *et al.* Risk of idiopathic cardiovascular death and non-fatal venous thromboembolism in women using oral contraceptives with differing progestagen components. *Lancet* 1995; **346**: 1589–93.

61 World Health Organization Collaborative Study of Cardiovascular Disease and Steroid Hormone Contraception. Venous thromboembolic disease and combined oral contraceptives: results of international multicentre case-control study. *Lancet* 1995; **346**: 1575–82.

62 World Health Organization Collaborative Study of Cardiovascular Disease and Steroid Hormone Contraception. Effect of different progestogens in low oestrogen oral contraceptives on venous thromboembolic disease. *Lancet* 1995; **346**: 1582–8.

63 Lewis MA, Spitzer WO, Heinemann LAJ, *et al.* Third generation oral contraceptives and risk of myocardial infarction: an international case-control study. *BMJ* 1996; **312**: 88–90.

64 McPherson K. Third generation oral contraception and venous thromboembolism. *BMJ* 1996; **312**: 68–9.

65 Bertina RM, Briet E, Engesser L, Reitsma PH. Protein C deficiency and the risk of venous thrombosis. *N Engl J Med* 1988; **318**: 930–1.

66 Seligsohn U, Berger A, Abend M, *et al.* Homozygous protein C deficiency manifested by massive venous thrombosis in the newborn. *N Engl J Med* 1984; **310**: 559–62.

67 Malm J, Laurell M, Dahlbäck B. Changes in the plasma levels of vitamin K-dependent proteins C and S and of C4b-binding protein during pregnancy and oral contraception. *Br J Haematol* 1988; **68**: 437–43.

68 Comp PC, Thurnau GR, Welsh J, Esmon CT. Functional and immunologic protein S levels are decreased during pregnancy. *Blood* 1986; **68**: 881–8.

69 Warwick R, Hutton RA, Goff L, Letsky E, Heard M. Changes in protein C and free protein S during pregnancy and following hysterectomy. *J R Soc Med* 1989; **82**: 591–4.

70 Faught W, Garner P, Jones G, Ivey B. Changes in protein C and protein S levels in normal pregnancy. *Am J Obstet Gynecol* 1995; **172**: 147–50.

71 Dahlbäck B, Carlsson M, Svensson PJ. Familial thrombophilia due to a previously unrecognized mechanism characterized by poor anticoagulant response to activated protein C: prediction of a cofactor to activated protein C. *Proc Natl Acad Sci USA* 1993; **90**: 1004–8.

72 Svensson PJ, Dahlbäck B. Resistance to activated protein C as a basis for venous thrombosis. *N Engl J Med* 1994; **330**: 517–22.

73 Koster T, Rosendaal FR, de Ronde H, Briët E, Vandenbroucke JP, Bertina RM. Venous thrombosis due to poor anticoagulant response to activated protein C: Leiden Thrombophilia Study. *Lancet* 1993; **342**: 1503–6.

74 Dahlbäck B, Hildebrand B. Inherited resistance to activated protein C is corrected by anticoagulant cofactor activity found to be a property of factor V. *Proc Natl Acad Sci USA* 1994; **91**: 1396–1400.

75 Hellgren M, Svensson PJ, Dahlbäck B. Resistance to activated protein C as a basis for venous thromboembolism associated with pregnancy and oral contraceptives. *Am J Obstet Gynecol* 1995; **173**: 210–13.

76 Bloemenkamp KWM, Rosendaal FR, Helmerhorst FM, Büller HR, Vandenbroucke JP. Enhancement by factor V Leiden mutation of risk of deep-vein thrombosis associated

with oral contraceptives containing third-generation progestogen. *Lancet* 1995; **346**: 1593–6.

77 Ballegeer V, Mombarts P, Declerk PJ, *et al.* Fibrinolytic response to venous occlusion and fibrin fragment D-Dimer levels in normal and complicated pregnancy. *Thromb Haemost* 1987; **58**: 1030–2.

78 Dacie JV, Lewis SM. Investigation of haemostasis and a bleeding tendency. In: *Practical haematology.* 8th ed. Edinburgh: Churchill Livingstone, 1995.

79 Stirling Y, Woolf L, North WRS, Seghatchian MJ, Meade TW. Haemostasis in normal pregnancy. *Thromb Haemost* 1984; **52**: 176–82.

80 Letsky EA. *Coagulation problems during pregnancy.* Edinburgh: Churchill Livingstone, 1985. (Current Reviews in Obstetrics & Gynaecology 10).

81 Bonnar J. Physiology of coagulation in pregnancy. In: Hathway WE, Bonnar J, eds. *Hemostatic disorders of the pregnant woman and newborn infant.* Chichester: John Wiley and Sons, 1987.

82 Greer IA. Haemostasis and thrombosis in pregnancy. In: Bloom AL, Forbes CD, Thomas DP, Tuddenham EGD, eds. *Haemostasis and Thrombosis.* 3rd ed. Edinburgh: Churchill Livingstone, 1994.

83 Bonnar J. Long-term self-administered heparin therapy for prevention and treatment of thromboembolic complications in pregnancy. In: Kakkar VJ, Thomas DP, eds. *Heparin chemistry and clinical usage.* New York: Academic Press, 1976.

84 Sturridge F, Letsky EA, de Swiet M. The use of low molecular weight heparin for thromboprophylaxis. *Br J Obstet Gynaecol* 1994; **101**: 69–71.

85 Sheppard BL, Bonnar J. The ultrastructure of the arterial supply of the human placenta in early and late pregnancy. *Journal of Obstetrics and Gynaecology of the British Commonwealth* 1974; **81**: 497–511.

86 Wiman B, Csemiczky G, Marsk L, *et al.* The fast inhibitor of tissue plasminogen activator in plasma during pregnancy. *Thromb Haemost* 1984; **52**: 124–6.

87 Booth N, Reith A, Bennett B, *et al.* A plasminogen activator inhibitor (PA1-2) circulates in two molecular forms during pregnancy. *Thromb Haemost* 1988; **59**: 77–9.

88 Greer IA, Turpie AGG, Forbes CD. *Haemostasis and thrombosis in obstetrics and gynaecology.* London: Chapman & Hall Medical, 1992.

89 Letsky EA, de Swiet M. Maternal hemostasis: coagulation problems of pregnancy. In: Schafer AI, Loscalzo J, eds. *Thrombosis and hemorrhage.* Oxford: Blackwell Scientific Publications, 1994.

90 Letsky EA. Management of massive haemorrhage—the haematologist's role. In: Patel N, ed. *Maternal mortality—the way forward.* London: Royal College of Obstetricians and Gynaecologists, 1992.

91 Department of Health. *Report on confidential enquiries into maternal deaths in the United Kingdom 1991–93.* London: HMSO, 1996.

92 Collaborative Low-dose Aspirin Study in Pregnancy Collaborative Group CLASP: a randomised trial of low-dose aspirin for the prevention and treatment of pre-eclampsia among 9364 pregnant women. *Lancet* 1994; **343**: 619–29.

93 Mibashan R, Peake I, Nicolaides K. Prenatal diagnosis of hemostatic disorders. In: Alter BP, ed. *Perinatal hematology.* Edinburgh: Churchill Livingstone, 1990. (Methods in Haematology 21).

94 Nicolaides KH, Rodeck CH, Mibashan RS. Obstetric management and diagnosis of haematological disease in the fetus. In: Letsky EA, ed. *Haematological disorders in pregnancy.* London: WB Saunders, 1985. (Clinics in Haematology 14).

95 Forestier F, Daffos F, Kaplan C, Sole Y. The development of the coagulation system in the human fetus and the prenatal diagnosis and management of bleeding disorders with fetal blood sampling. In: Greer IA, Turpie AGG, Forbes CD, eds. *Haemostasis and thrombosis in obstetrics and gynaecology.* London: Chapman & Hall, 1992.

96 Letsky EA. Haematological disorders. In: Whittle M, Connor M, eds. *Prenatal diagnosis in obstetric practice.* 2nd ed. Oxford: Blackwell Scientific, 1995.

97 Weatherall DJ. *The new genetics and clinical practice.* 3rd ed. Oxford: Oxford University Press, 1990.

98 Tuddenham EGD, Cooper DN. *The molecular genetics of haemostasis and its inherited disorders.* Oxford: Oxford University Press, 1993.

4: Cardiovascular examination in pregnancy and the approach to diagnosis of cardiac disorder

PETROS NIHOYANNOPOULOS

Pregnancy is a physiological phenomenon during which there are major cardiovascular changes affecting the loading conditions of the heart. The mechanisms of the various cardiopulmonary adaptations during pregnancy are discussed in detail in chapter 2. Briefly, during the first trimester there is a steep increase in plasma volume which causes dilution and anaemia. The stroke volume and to a lesser extent the heart rate increase and the cardiac output increases progressively. This increase is around 40% to 50% above the pre-pregnancy level and is maintained throughout pregnancy. There is an accompanying decrease in vascular resistance, and diastolic and mean blood pressure. In cyanotic or potentially cyanotic congenital heart disease, the drop in peripheral vascular resistance encourages right to left shunting leading to increasing cyanosis, and a rise in haematocrit with increased risk of thrombosis and of paradoxical embolism.

While the normal heart tolerates the added load easily, abnormal hearts may not. When trouble occurs it usually begins early, often by the end of the first trimester. These considerations are of pivotal importance if the physician is to advise the woman correctly and not simply retreat with the easy option of advising against pregnancy or encouraging early termination.

Examination

History

Many disorders are apparent from the personal and family history, particularly cardiomyopathies, the Marfan syndrome, and congenital heart

52

disease. There may be previous knowledge of a cardiac murmur. The outcome of any previous pregnancies will be noted with particular attention to hypertension, pre-eclampsia, pulmonary oedema, or peripartum cardiomyopathy. Previous unsuccessful pregnancies ending in termination or stillbirth may signify maternal disease such as antiphospholipid antibody syndrome causing recurrent mid-trimester termination. Fetal abnormality may have been related to maternal medication such as anti-epileptic drugs or it may reflect a genetic disorder.

Systemic blood pressure

Pregnancy hypertension has been the largest cause of maternal death in England and Wales over the last 30 years, and continues to be so, and cerebrovascular accident is the commonest mode of death.[1] In systemic hypertension, the risks to the mother are largely related to the level of blood pressure and development of stroke or heart failure while the risk to the fetus is from failure of placental function. The ability of the placenta to exchange nutrients and gases with the fetus is dependent on blood flow. In systemic hypertension, blood flow to the placenta is reduced. When the blood pressure is above 170/110 mm Hg cerebral blood flow autoregulation is lost, the maternal risks are greatly increased and treatment should be prompt.

The blood pressure tends to fall in the first part of pregnancy but then gradually rises to equal or exceed pre-pregnancy levels in the last six weeks. Blood pressure should be measured with the woman seated or lying on her left side because if a woman lies supine the blood pressure may be misleadingly reduced. Even profound hypotension can occur in late pregnancy from mechanical obstruction of the inferior vena cava by the gravid uterus.

The measurement of blood pressure is confounded by non-standardised methodology. In the non-pregnant patient the 5th Korotkoff sound is usually noted, as it best corresponds to the intra-arterial measurement. In pregnancy the 4th Korotkoff sound has been recommended in the United States as more reproducible because audible sounds may continue down to zero.[2] Recently, de Swiet et al have made a compelling plea for recording diastolic pressure at the 5th Korotkoff sound as in the non-pregnant state. In a carefully conducted study they found that observers could always identify the 5th sound whereas inter-observer variation of the level of the 4th sound was much greater.[3]

Protein excretion increases during pregnancy from a maximum of 18 mg in 24 hours in the non-pregnant to over 300 mg total protein with albumin representing roughly 55% of this. A total protein excretion of over 300 mg is considered to be abnormal.[4] Women who develop pregnancy induced hypertension in the second trimester may show steadily worsening hypertension accompanied by the development of proteinuria, thrombocytopenia, and failing renal and hepatic function that defines pre-eclampsia. It is crucial to follow the blood pressure using a standardised method and to look for proteinuria particularly in women with a family history of hypertension or pre-eclampsia (Chapter 21).

Physical signs

Adaptive mechanisms bring a variation in the cardiovascular examination that may mimic heart disease. The palms flush, the extremities are warm, the soft tissues become more tense, the digital vessels throb, there may be capillary pulsation, and the pulse is full, bounding and often collapsing. The heart rate is slightly faster and there may be slight peripheral oedema.[5]

The jugular veins look distended from about the 20th week of pregnancy. The venous pressure may be raised with prominent a and v waves and brisk x and y descents because of hypervolaemia and vasodilatation. The increase in blood volume causes the heart to be mildly overloaded and may lead to an over-estimation of valve regurgitation. The increased intra-abdominal pressure caused by the gravid uterus indirectly leads to an increased intrathoracic pressure which in turn raises the jugular venous pressure but not the right ventricular filling pressure. This is important to differentiate from heart failure and avoid the potentially harmful administration of diuretics.

Normal pregnancy in a woman without heart disease is commonly accompanied by tachycardia, palpitations and increased numbers of premature atrial or ventricular beats, sometimes multiple. It is important to recognise these usually benign symptoms.

During pregnancy the apical impulse is slightly displaced to the left and is more abrupt and lively. It signifies an overfilled ventricle working against a low resistance as a result of peripheral vasodilatation. Pathological volume loaded conditions such as aortic or mitral regurgitation, or left to right shunting should be distinguished (Table 4.1).

The mitral closure sound may be slightly increased in intensity. A loud third sound confirms rapid ventricular filling and is found in up to 90% of pregnant women. There is no change in the character of the second heart sound during the first 30 weeks of pregnancy but later on pulmonary closure may be slightly increased with persistent expiratory splitting.[6]

A systolic aortic or pulmonary flow murmur is heard in 90% of pregnant women. A cervical venous hum best heard over the supraclavicular fossa, is common in children, and is also found in pregnancy. The mammary souffle, either systolic or continuous, is heard maximally at the second left or right intercostal space during late pregnancy in some women. This is easily differentiated from a persistent arterial duct by applying gentle pressure which makes the mammary souffle disappear.

TABLE 4.1—*Normal clinical findings that can mimic heart disease in pregnancy.*

- Raised jugular venous pressure
  (prominent a and v waves, brisk x and y descents)
- Volume loaded left ventricle
- Full, sharp and collapsing pulse
- Warm extremities
- Peripheral oedema
- Palpitations
- Tachycardia
- Premature atrial/ventricular beats
- Increased intensity of mitral closure sound
- Third heart sound
- Systolic murmur
- Continuous murmur from venous hum, mammary souffle

Special investigations

Electrocardiography

Electrocardiographic (ECG) changes can be related to a gradual change in the position of the heart. The ECG often shows a gradual shift of the QRS axis to the left in the frontal plane with a small Q wave, and inverted T wave in lead III as a result of rotation.

The heart rate may be increased by 10% to 15%. Re-entrant supra-ventricular tachycardia is a relatively common benign arrhythmia. Conversely, persistent sinus tachycardia, atrial flutter, atrial fibrillation, or ventricular tachycardia suggest underlying heart disease and should prompt further investigation. The appearance of ventricular tachycardia in late pregnancy or in the puerperium should arouse suspicion of peripartum cardiomyopathy.[7]

Chest radiograph

The most common normal finding in pregnancy is slight prominence of the pulmonary conus and simulation of left atrial enlargement in the lateral views.[8] These changes are predominantly the result of hyperlordosis and may in some instances suggest mitral stenosis.[9] Progressive elevation of the diaphragm leads to a more horizontal position of the heart and an increase in the cardiothoracic ratio. An increased intrathoracic blood volume and heavy breast shadows may raise suspicion of left to right shunting from an atrial septal defect, or pulmonary venous congestion caused by mitral stenosis.

A chest radiograph should be obtained in any pregnant patient with new onset of dyspnoea. Failure to do so has led to mistaken diagnosis of chest infection or adult respiratory distress syndrome and to missing mitral stenosis.[10] The general physician, intensive care consultant, or obstetrician do not resort to echocardiography unless they suspect heart disease. The chest x ray film may first suggest this in a distressed and breathless patient whose murmurs may be atypical or missed on account of tachycardia. With proper screening the risk to the fetus is minuscule.

Echocardiography

Modern echocardiography with its sophisticated Doppler and transoesophageal arsenal is well suited to the rapid diagnosis in pregnant women with known or suspected cardiac disorders. The performance and visual interpretation of echocardiographic studies can be achieved speedily and has a crucial impact on management. It is particularly important during pregnancy when the physical signs may be misleading with potential hazard to both mother and fetus.

Referral is often triggered by the detection of a systolic murmur by the obstetrician (Table 4.2). Occasionally, the distinction between normality and abnormality may be subtle and an expert interpretation should be sought before the final report. Doctors and technicians involved in the performance and interpretation of echocardiographic studies should be accredited by their national authority and fully acquainted with artifacts or variation of normal structures that are often seen in normal echocardiographic examinations. In most pregnancies echocardiography will reassure the mother-to-be who can then continue to enjoy her pregnancy.

TABLE 4.2—*Echocardiographic challenges during pregnancy.*

- Normal study
- Mitral stenosis
- Aortic stenosis
- Complex congenital heart disease
- Deterioration of ventricular function
- Assessment of prosthetic valves

Valve disease

More commonly echocardiography is requested for assessment of a patient with known valve disease. Because of the hyperkinetic circulation and increased stroke output, systolic velocities across native or prosthetic valves rise leading to an apparent "increase" in systolic gradients which should not be misinterpreted. Similarly, in regurgitant lesions, the physiological increase in volume which occurs during pregnancy may render a minor valvar leak more impressive. Multivalvar regurgitation (affecting all except the aortic valve) may be a normal finding on Doppler echocardiography during pregnancy and should not be reported if the regurgitation is slight and the valves look structurally normal.[11]

Despite the decline in rheumatic heart disease, one of the most common reasons for echocardiography is to assess the severity of mitral stenosis in a pregnant woman with pulmonary oedema. This may be difficult if tachycardia prevents accurate measurement of the pressure half time of mitral valve filling from the continuous Doppler display. Indeed, tachycardia is sometimes the cause of pulmonary oedema even when mitral stenosis is only moderate. If the tachycardia cannot be slowed by carotid massage[12] planimetry of the mitral orifice area at the tips of the leaflets is an alternative using a frame-by-frame method but this method is less accurate and it is better to reassess after administration of a beta-blocking drug.

A rarer echocardiographic task during pregnancy is assessment of the severity of aortic stenosis. The aortic valve can readily be described but the velocities and the derived pressure gradients across the valve are higher than in the non-pregnant state because of the increased stroke volume and may lead to over-assessment of severity.[13]

The reduced systemic resistance in pregnancy may precipitate effort induced syncope if stroke volume fails to increase. Even then, pregnancy can be continued with bed rest and beta-blockers in most patients until the baby is viable. Serial echocardiographic studies greatly help in decision-making in those difficult patients. Intervention is needed if left ventricular systolic function deteriorates or congestive heart failure develops. Balloon dilatation of the valve may provide temporary palliation. Otherwise aortic valve replacement should be preceded by caesarean delivery of the baby if viable.[14]

Congenital heart disease

The decreasing incidence of rheumatic heart disease and advances in medical and surgical treatment have resulted in an increase in both the relative and absolute incidence of congenital cardiac disorders seen in pregnancy.[15] Their assessment can be one of the most challenging tasks for the echocardiographer.

Patients with unoperated congenital heart defects are usually acyanotic and the defects include pulmonary stenosis, persistent ductus arteriosus, coarctation of the aorta, atrial and ventricular septal defects, aortic valve disease secondary to some form of bicuspid aortic valve, and Ebstein's anomaly. Pregnancy increases the risk of aortic dissection complicating coarctation and this should be considered if a patient develops chest pain. Interestingly, the incidence of toxaemia is lower in coarctation-related hypertension than in primary systemic hypertension.[16] Cyanotic patients with tetralogy of Fallot or the Eisenmenger syndrome rarely become pregnant. While patients with tetralogy of Fallot tolerate pregnancy well, patients with pulmonary hypertension do not.[14] Pulmonary vascular disease may deteriorate with possible fatal outcome and the decreased arterial oxygen content leads to poor fetal growth or spontaneous abortion.

The advantage of echocardiography is the ability to perform serial studies in the assessment of intracardiac flow disturbances and left and right ventricular function. Most patients with simple defects will see their pregnancy through with no complications and the role of echocardiography is simply documentative, but sometimes rare complex or potentially dangerous abnormalities are first recognised on antenatal echocardiographic screening. These include corrected transposition and coronary anomalies.

The second category of patients with congenital heart disease are those who have had previous surgery. If the operation was "corrective" pregnancy usually proceeds normally but is sometimes complicated by arrhythmia, usually benign, and endocarditis. Patients who have undergone palliative surgery may be at risk of heart failure or thromboembolism as well as infection and arrhythmia. Patients with Mustard or Senning repairs, Rastelli valve-bearing conduits, or Fontan univentricular circulations can have successful pregnancies (Chapter 6). Echocardiography and particularly transoesophageal imaging in these conditions permits detailed description of the surgical procedure and helps both in initial assessment of risk and in serial documentation of progress.

Cardiomyopathies

In women with cardiomyopathies echocardiography plays an important part in assessing left ventricular function. The cardiomyopathy may be diagnosed first during pregnancy. The left ventricle in hypertrophic cardiomyopathy seems to fill better during pregnancy and to accommodate the physiological increase in blood volume without undue rise in filling pressure in most cases. Pressure gradients may be high but this does not affect outcome. Coexisting mitral regurgitation can readily be detected.

When discovered during pregnancy, dilated cardiomyopathy may be regarded as peripartum because of its temporal relationship with pregnancy but when detected earlier in pregnancy the condition must have been pre-existing. Echocardiography shows a hypokinetic left ventricle which may or may not be dilated. In peripartum cardiomyopathy ventricular function may gradually improve within six months to a year of delivery. In an echocardiographic study of left ventricular function in 10 women with peripartum cardiomyopathy, the severity of left ventricular dysfunction did not predict outcome.[17] Over the first month following delivery, five of seven patients (71%) increased their ejection fraction and at four months left ventricular size and mass index decreased with further improvement in ejection fraction. Despite this improvement, the ejection fraction became normal in only 57% of women. Interestingly, two of these patients had subsequent normal pregnancies.[17] One of the patients with Eisenmenger VSD developed peripartum cardiomyopathy.[18] Echocardiography during pregnancy had shown excellent left and right ventricular function throughout. Repeat serial echocardiography after delivery showed sudden deterioration in ventricular function. Complete recovery of ventricular function occurred within two years with no advance in the pulmonary vascular disease (Figure 4.1).

14.11.86	23.7.87	18.5.90

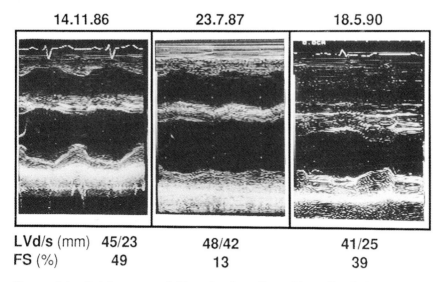

LVd/s (mm)	45/23	48/42	41/25
FS (%)	49	13	39

FIGURE 4.1—*Serial parasternal M mode echocardiographic studies during pregnancy (first panel), three months after delivery (middle panel) and three years later (third panel). The middle panel shows right ventricular hypertrophy and transient substantial left and right ventricular dysfunction. The fractional shortening dropped from 49% during pregnancy to 13% after delivery and subsequently recovered at 39%. Reproduced with permission.*[16]

Women with the Marfan syndrome are always a worry in pregnancy. The family history is important and also serial measurement of aortic root diameter in patients with either a family history of aortic rupture or evidence of aortic root widening (Chapter 12).

Transoesophageal echocardiography

Multiplane transducers have made transoesophageal echocardiography the ultimate echocardiographic method in the assessment of adults with complex congenital heart disease, thromboembolic episodes, and infective endocarditis, particularly in patients previously operated on or in patients with prosthetic valves. Transoesophageal echocardiography is safe during pregnancy.[19] Oxygen saturations should be monitored when midazolam is used for premedication, particularly in patients with chronic obstructive airways disease or in cyanotic patients because of the risks of hypoxia to the fetus. Antibiotic prophylaxis is not given as there is no evidence, even in high risk patients with prosthetic valves, that transoesophageal echocardiography has caused endocarditis.[19]

Some patients with severe mitral stenosis may require balloon valvotomy which is successful in suitable valves identified by echocardiography. The procedure can be monitored by transoesophageal echocardiography in the catheter laboratory to reduce the amount of radiation to the fetus.

Imaging the heart from the oesophagus using multiplane transducers has many advantages over precordial imaging in adults with complex congenital heart disease. One should adopt a sequential approach to the diagnosis of congenital heart lesions.The atrial situs (by defining the atrial appendages), the venous connection, and the detailed morphology of the atrial chambers and septum can easily be defined, in contrast to transthoracic windows when these posterior structures tend to be poorly imaged. The transoesophageal probe lies in contiguity with the posterior wall of the left atrium and is in an excellent position to image the morphology and sites of drainage of pulmonary veins and the venae cavae. Previous surgery may have been undertaken many years earlier and the details may not be available. Transoesophageal echocardiography therefore has a descriptive role as well as being diagnostic when possible sources of embolism, vegetation, or abscesses are being sought.

Assessment of the function of a Fontan circulation by transoesophageal imaging allows direct visualisation of atriopulmonary and cavopulmonary connections together with pulsed Doppler estimation of velocity profiles through the connections. Direct visualisation of Glenn or Blalock anastomoses, precise measurement of atrial shunting, and identification or exclusion of obstruction to pulmonary arterial or venous blood flow can all be achieved.

Patients who have undergone Senning or Mustard procedures can be difficult to assess by transthoracic imaging alone. From the transoesophageal approach, caval obstruction or obstruction within the mid-portion of the systemic venous atrium, the sites of baffle leakage, or obstruction to the drainage of individual pulmonary veins can easily be identified.

Stress testing

Coronary artery disease is rare during pregnancy but may be seen in women with familial hypercholesterolaemia, particularly the rare homozygotes, or in patients with lupus erythematosus and in the antiphospholipid syndrome.

Treadmill exercise testing is useful in the pre-pregnancy assessment of patients, particularly in symptom-free patients with aortic stenosis, looking for evidence of provocable subendocardial ischaemia or fall in blood pressure as an indication of probable risk. More formal measurement of cardiopulmonary exercise tolerance may be used before giving advice about fitness for pregnancy in other borderline patients.

Stress echocardiography either with exercise or dobutamine infusion may add to the diagnostic specificity of treadmill exercise testing in detecting the presence and extent of ischaemia in high risk patients with possible coronary artery disease.

Fetal echocardiography

Over the past 20 years fetal echocardiography has undergone major developments. The heart can usually be visualised at 16–18 weeks' gestation[20,21] and abnormalities can be detected as early as 18–20 weeks.[22,23] The single most valuable view is the four-chamber view centred on the atrio-ventricular junction. It gives the opportunity to assess the number and relative sizes of the ventricles and atria as well as the atrio-ventricular valves and is obtainable in 95% of pregnancies.[22–24] The following features should be sought: i) The heart should occupy no more than one third of the fetal thorax, ii) there should be two atria of equal size, iii) there should be two ventricles of equal size that contract equally briskly, iv) the two atrio-ventricular valves should meet the atrial and ventricular septa at the crux, v) the foramen ovale should be present, and vi) the ventricular septum must be intact (Table 4.3). Fetal echocardiography should be performed by operators with skills based on experience of pathology rather than just on the performance of a large number of "normal" scans. Transvaginal fetal echocardiography facilitates early visualisation of the fetal heart.

TABLE 4.3—*Routine checklist of fetal echocardiography.*

- Heart 1/3 of the fetal thorax
- Two atria of equal size
- Two ventricles of equal size contracting briskly
- Two equal size atrioventricular valves
- Patent foramen ovale
- Intact ventricular septum

Recognition of cardiovascular pathology is of great importance to adjust any medication appropriately and to plan the delivery and mode of anaesthesia. There are a few cardiac conditions such as the Eisenmenger syndrome or primary pulmonary hypertension that indicate the need for early interruption of pregnancy because of high maternal risk.

References

1 Turnbull A, *et al.* Report on confidential enquiries into maternal deaths in England and Wales 1982–1984. *Rep Health Soc Subj Lond* 1989; **34**: 1–166.
2 MacGillivray I, Rose G, Row B. Blood pressure survey in pregnancy. *Clin Sci* 1969; **37**: 395–9.
3 Shennon A, Gupta M, Halligan A, Taylor DJ, de Swiet M. Lack of reproducibility in pregnancy of Korotkoff phase IV as measured by mercury sphygmomanometry. *Lancet* 1996; **347**: 139–42.
4 Hughes EC. *Obstetrics-gynecological terminology.* Philadelphia: Davis, 1972: 422–3.
5 Wood P. *Diseases of the heart and circulation.* 2nd Edition. London: Eyre & Spottiswoode, 1956: 902–9.
6 Cutforth R, MacDonald CB. Heart sounds and murmurs in pregnancy. *Am Heart J* 1966; **71**: 741–7.
7 Perloff JK. *The cardiomyopathies.* Philadelphia: WB Saunders, 1988.
8 Szekely P, Snaith L. *Heart disease and pregnancy.* Edinburgh: Churchill Livingstone, 1974.

9 Turner AF. The chest radiograph in pregnancy. *Clin Obstet Gynecol* 1975; **18**: 65–74.

10 Morley CA, Lim BA. The risks of delay in diagnosis of breathlessness in pregnancy. *BMJ* 1995; **311**: 183–4.

11 Campos O, Andrade JL, Bocanegra J, *et al.* Physiological multivalvular regurgitation during pregnancy: a longitudinal Doppler echocardiographic study. *Int J Cardiol* 1993; **40**: 265–72.

12 Torrecilla EG, Garcia-Fernandez MA, Dan Roman DJ, Alberca MT, Delea JL. Usefulness of carotid sinus massage in the quantification of mitral stenosis in sinus rhythm by Doppler pressure half time. *Am J Cardiol* 1994; **73**: 817–21.

13 Burwash IG, Forbes AD, Sadahiro M, *et al.* Echocardiographic volume flow and stenoses severity measures with changing flow rate in aortic stenosis. *Am J Physiol* 1993; **265**: H1734–43.

14 Oakley CM. Pregnancy in heart disease. In: Jackson G. *Difficult cardiology.* London: Martin Dunitz, 1990: 1–18.

15 Perloff JK. Pregnancy and congenital heart disease. *J Am Coll Cardiol* 1991; **18**: 340–2.

16 Perloff JK. *Clinical recognition of congenital heart disease.* Philadelphia: WB Saunders, 1987.

17 Cole P, Cook F, Plappent T, Salzman D, Shilton M St J. Longitudinal changes in left ventricular architecture and function in peripartum cardiomyopathy. *Am J Cardiol* 1987; **60**: 871–6.

18 Oakley CM, Nihoyannopoulos P. Peripartum cardiomyopathy with recovery in a patient with coincidental Eisenmenger ventricular septal defect. *Br Heart J* 1992; **67**: 190–2.

19 Saltissi S, de Belder MA, Nihoyannopoulos P. Setting up a transoesophageal echocardiography service. *Br Heart J* 1994; **71(suppl)**: 15–9.

20 Allan LD, Tynan MJ, Cambell S, Wilkinson JL, Anderson RH. Echocardiographic and anatomical correlates in the fetus. *Br Heart J* 1980; **44**: 444–51.

21 Wyllie J, Wren C, Hunter S. Screening for fetal cardiac malformations. *Br Heart J* 1994; **71(suppl)**: 20–7.

22 Allan LD, Chita SK, Sharland GK, Fegg NLK, Anderson RH, Crawford DC. The accuracy of fetal echocardiography in the diagnosis of congenital heart disease. *Int J Cardiol* 1989; **25**:279–88.

23 Allan LD, Crawford DC, Chita SK, Tynan MJ. Prenatal screening for congenital heart disease. *BMJ* 1986; **292**: 1717–9.

24 Copel JA, Pila G, Green J, Hobbins JC, Kleinman CS. Fetal echocardiographic screening for congenital heart disease: the importance of the four chamber view. *Am J Obstet Gynecol* 1987; **57**: 48–55.

5: Acyanotic congenital heart disease

CELIA OAKLEY

Both the relative incidence and the absolute numbers of pregnant women with congenital heart disease has risen. This is because rheumatic heart disease in young adults is rare in the United Kingdom except in its immigrant population and because more children with complex congenital heart disease are surviving into the reproductive age following surgery in infancy and wanting to lead normal lives with job, car and family.[1-6]

Congenital heart disease is not infrequently discovered first during pregnancy, particularly now that structural heart disease can be differentiated with certainty from loud but innocent flow murmurs by recourse to echocardiography whenever there is clinical doubt.

Many congenital cardiac defects are compatible with survival to adult life. The most common is atrial septal defect. Ventricular septal defect and patent arterial duct are less common, having more often been detected and operated on in childhood. Pulmonary stenosis, ventricular septal defect with pulmonary stenosis or pulmonary hypertension, tetralogy of Fallot, corrected transposition, coarctation of the aorta, Ebstein's anomaly of the tricuspid valve, and aortic stenosis are all seen from time to time. Most of the simple acyanotic defects cause no trouble during pregnancy, but women with congenital heart disease are at risk if they have severe left ventricular outflow tract obstruction, pulmonary hypertension, cyanotic congenital heart disease, or restricted cardiac output (Table 5.1). Adults from medically unmonitored communities with previously unsuspected major cardiac defects may be seen first in pregnancy.

Most infants and children in the west are examined regularly and simple defects are usually corrected at a young age. Although only correction of a patent arterial duct can be regarded as a complete "cure" problems in later pregnancy are rare but arrhythmias may develop after closure of secundum atrial septal defect. Pulmonary vascular disease may progress after closure of non-restrictive ventricular septal defect and such patients are at risk as they may consider themselves normal and have been lost to follow up. Survivors of heroic but palliative surgery for complex congenital heart disease need to be considered for cardiovascular reserve, presence of pulmonary hypertension, arrhythmia, and conduction defects.

TABLE 5.1—*Congenital heart disease and pregnancy.*

Well tolerated

- Uncomplicated atrial septal defect
- Restrictive ventricular septal defect
- Small persistent ductus arteriosus
- Ebstein's anomaly
- Pulmonary stenosis
- Mild or moderate aortic stenosis
- Corrected transposition without other significant defects

Moderate risk

- Coarctation of the aorta
- Pulmonary stenosis with central right to left shunt
- Pulmonary hypertension with patent ductus, aortopulmonary defect, or ventricular septal defect

High maternal (and fetal) risk

- Pulmonary hypertension with reversed central shunt (the Eisenmenger syndrome)
- Severe aortic stenosis
- Marked cyanosis

Optimal management includes accurate diagnosis, correct prediction of the haemodynamic consequences of the pregnancy on the cardiac disorder and of the cardiac disorder on the baby's development, planned pregnancy after pre-conceptual counselling with explanation of the genetic risks, and fetal echocardiographic monitoring. This is best provided by a team made up of cardiologist (and echocardiographer), obstetrician, and obstetric anaesthetist.

Atrial septal defect

Secundum atrial septal defects in the region of the fossa ovalis and the rarer sinus venosus defects sited at the junction of the superior vena cava behave similarly and are considered together. Atrial septal defect (ASD) is by far the most common congenital cardiac defect to escape recognition until adult life. It is two or three times more common in women and it is not uncommon for it to be detected during pregnancy (Figure 5.1) when the pulmonary flow murmur becomes louder and echocardiography is undertaken (Figures 5.1 and 5.2). Most atrial septal defects are uncomplicated and asymptomatic during the reproductive years and no problems are encountered during pregnancy. Pulmonary vascular disease and arrhythmias are infrequent until later in life. Mitral regurgitation caused by a floppy anterior mitral leaflet is usually also a later development.

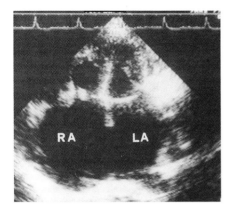

FIGURE 5.1—*Apical four chamber transthoracic echocardiographic view of a large secundum atrial septal defect. The caudal and ventral part of the septum is intact. The right heart chambers are dilated.*

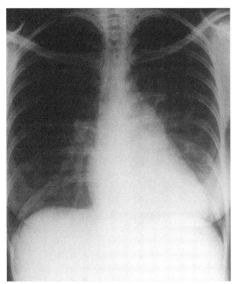
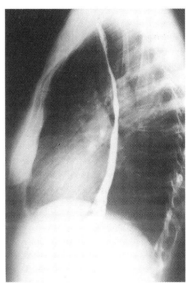

FIGURE 5.2—*Chest x ray picture of a patient with an uncomplicated secundum atrial septal defect who had a cardiac arrest after a modest postpartum haemorrhage.*

One of our patients, now in her late 80s, had nine children before her ASD was diagnosed when she was in her 50s. The defect was not closed despite a calculated shunt of 3·5:1 and she remains well.

A frailty of ASD which it is useful to know is poor tolerance of acute blood loss. If this occurs, systemic vasoconstriction coupled with a reduction in systemic venous return to the right atrium can cause massive diversion of blood (Figure 5.3) from left to right atrium. This occurred in a young woman who had a cardiac arrest following a postpartum haemorrhage. A casualty of late antenatal booking, she was successfully resuscitated and only subsequently found to have an ASD. A similar fall in blood pressure, sometimes with syncope, can occur in patients pregnant or not, who have atrial septal defects complicated by paroxysmal tachycardia. Verapamil can be used safely in pregnancy and may be successful in prophylaxis, but attacks of tachycardia are best converted by intravenous adenosine rather than verapamil (Chapter 19). The onset of atrial of flutter or fibrillation is uncommon but if it occurs it should be treated by DC cardioversion.

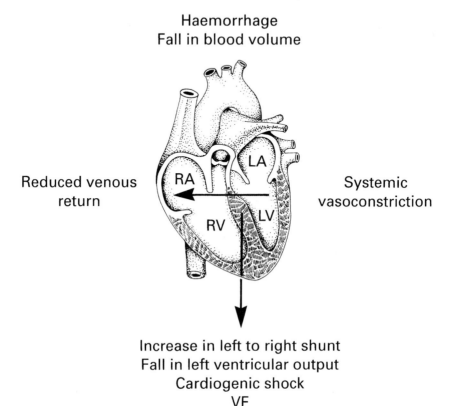

Haemorrhage
Fall in blood volume

Reduced venous return

Systemic vasoconstriction

Increase in left to right shunt
Fall in left ventricular output
Cardiogenic shock
VF

FIGURE 5.3—*Mechanism of sudden fall in left ventricular output after blood loss in atrial septal defect.*

Paradoxical embolism is a rare complication of ASD[7] but even patency of the foramen ovale has been found (by contrast echocardiography during the Valsalva manoeuvre) to be more commonly present in young patients with unexplained embolic stroke than in a control population.[8] A small right to left shunt can be shown by intravenous contrast echocardiography in most ASDs but the much larger flow of blood left to right probably checks entry of particulate matter into the systemic circulation. A strong association has, however, been found between aneurysm of the atrial septum and stroke. In a recent large study of 259 such aneurysms an interatrial shunt was detected in 61%, and 58% of the patients had a history of systemic embolism.[9]

Mitral regurgitation caused by prolapse of the anterior leaflet of the mitral valve is a complication which sometimes develops in older women with ASD and should be suspected in any patient with secundum ASD and an apical late or pansystolic murmur.[10] Mitral regurgitation increases left to right shunting and the venous pressure in the neck may suggest tricuspid regurgitation, but it is usually well tolerated.

A raised pulmonary vascular resistance is a relatively rare and late complication and the pulmonary artery pressure is rarely raised in young women with ASD. A pulmonary artery systolic pressure of over 50 mm Hg was found in only 7% of patients in the third decade.[11] Primary type pulmonary hypertension is sometimes associated with an anatomical secundum atrial septal defect in young women with undilated right heart chambers who have never developed a left to right shunt because they have retained a high pulmonary vascular resistance from birth. In these patients the physical signs, behaviour, and prognosis are similar to those of primary pulmonary hypertension. The atrial communication provides a vent for the right ventricle and allows maintenance of systemic output through right to left shunting though at the expense of reduced systemic arterial oxygen content. The risk of syncope and sudden death appears to be less and the prognosis somewhat better than in primary pulmonary hypertension without septal defect but pregnancy carries a high risk (Chapter 7). They are quite different from older patients who may develop pulmonary hypertension in association with a longstanding left to right shunt.

Patients with secundum ASD do not need antibiotic prophylaxis to cover dental treatment or complicated delivery unless the defect is complicated by a floppy mitral valve with mitral regurgitation.

Secundum atrial septal defect is sometimes inherited as an autosomal dominant condition but such families are rare and most cases are sporadic.

Atrioventricular canal defects (Endocardial cushion defects)

Atrioventricular canal defects whether partial or complete are usually diagnosed and treated surgically during infancy or childhood.

Partial atrioventricular defects with interatrial shunts and normal right ventricular pressures (ostium primum defects) are occasionally first diagnosed in young women and behave much like secundum atrial septal defects during pregnancy, unless mitral regurgitation is considerable and complicated by pulmonary hypertension, but they are at risk of infective endocarditis. A raised venous pressure with dominant V wave may reflect either mitral regurgitation or direct left ventriculo–right atrial shunting. Pregnancy is usually well tolerated but atrial arrhythmias occasionally develop and require treatment.

Atrioventricular canal defects are sometimes familial.

Pulmonary stenosis

Mild or moderate pulmonary stenosis is common and causes no trouble during pregnancy. No deaths have been reported and few complications.[12,13] Even severe pulmonary stenosis is usually tolerated although congestive features may appear from superimposition of gestational volume overload upon a hypertrophied and stiffened right ventricle. Percutaneous balloon valvuloplasty with maximum uterine shielding may be considered for the rare patient with severe or symptomatic pulmonary stenosis who is seen first only during pregnancy. These patients will usually have a supra-systemic pressure in the right ventricle. The procedure carries little risk of serious complication although hypotension, arrhythmias, and transient right bundle branch block have been reported. Mild pulmonary regurgitation may follow but is unimportant. Balloon valvuloplasty should be delayed until after organogenesis is complete and if possible until the second trimester. It is the procedure of choice for the treatment of pulmonary stenosis and is now usually carried out in childhood. Only rarely will it be necessary during pregnancy in patients whose severe pulmonary stenosis has not previously been detected.

Infundibular stenosis either isolated or, as sometimes, associated with a restrictive ventricular septal defect is similarly well tolerated but much rarer.

Persistent ductus arteriosus

Narrow arterial ducts with only small shunts and normal pulmonary artery pressure give rise to no haemodynamic difficulties during pregnancy. Women with bigger ducts with larger shunts may develop congestive heart failure and should be closed before pregnancy is contemplated. Uncorrected widely patent ducts with pulmonary hypertension may be complicated by the development of a pulmonary artery aneurysm (of which persistent ductus is the commonest single cause).[14]

Dissecting aneurysm of the main pulmonary artery may develop with spontaneous rupture during pregnancy or postpartum.[14-16] Cystic medial necrosis and atheroma are usually found and both are related to severe pulmonary hypertension. Both systemic and pulmonary arterial dissections seem to have an increased incidence in pregnancy[17] perhaps as a result of increased uptake of water by connective tissue mucopolysaccharides.[18]

Most ducts cause a typical machinery murmur and the continuous flow is well shown on continuous wave Doppler. We have seen a number of women with harsh systolic left infraclavicular murmurs which sounded organic but were too high for a ventricular septal defect and too long for mild pulmonary stenosis. These were shown on echocardiographic Doppler to be caused by small patent ducts but the diastolic flow was inaudible (even after the diagnosis was known). These small ducts do not of course require to be closed. There is no haemodynamic threat and the only hazard is the small one from infection.

Ventricular septal defect

Small ventricular septal defects are noisy and the loud pansystolic murmur at the lower left sternal edge will usually have been discovered earlier. Some may have been non-restrictive in infancy but become smaller through differential growth or partial closure, or both, by adherence of the septal leaflet of the tricuspid valve. Defects in the muscular septum may give rise to early non-pansystolic murmurs because the defect is closed by muscular contraction during systole. They are heard best towards the apex. Such small defects are not seen on imaging but are readily identified by colour flow Doppler. The only risk is from infective endocarditis and prophylaxis is needed for dental work or complicated delivery.

Some small ventricular septal defects may be identified first in pregnancy when murmurs tend to become louder with increased blood flow across pressure drops and also because of good antenatal care and referral of women with systolic murmurs for echocardiographic examination. Many of these murmurs may previously have been dismissed as innocent (and the defects are indeed benign unless complicated by infection) and missed even on echocardiography until the advent of colour flow.

Patients with unoperated non-restrictive defects and "obligatory" pulmonary hypertension who are still acyanotic and shunting left to right and who have no symptoms are occasionally encountered particularly in our immigrant community. They are usually quite well and may give no history of infantile heart failure or failure to thrive. Such patients may tolerate pregnancy without difficulty. Accelerated progression of pulmonary vascular disease is a hazard though not inevitable. Heart failure is not a risk as the shunt is usually only small so the heart was not volume loaded before pregnancy. Provided the patient remains acyanotic fetal growth is normal. Acute blood loss or vasodilatation during delivery can lead to shunt reversal. This is avoided by generous volume replacement and avoidance of systemic vasodilators. Vasoconstricting oxytocic agents are well tolerated.

A symptom-free acyanotic immigrant Asian patient with a non-restrictive ventricular septal defect, obligatory pulmonary hypertension, near Eisenmenger complex, and small persistent left to right shunt was first seen when 24 weeks pregnant. She developed postpartum cyanosis and low output failure after tolerating the pregnancy well and delivering a well grown baby.[19] She was found to have reduced left and right ventricular function as a result of peripartum cardiomyopathy. This eventually improved but only after about two years, during which she remained cyanosed, hypotensive, and in failure. Now she is again without symptoms or cyanosis, with a small heart and normal left and right ventricular function. She has been sterilised. Peripartum cardiomyopathy may complicate structural heart disease (Chapter 16).

The risk in pregnancy after closure of a ventricular septal defect does not differ from that in patients without heart disease unless there is residual pulmonary hypertension. Infants and children who have large non-restrictive ventricular septal defects closed (or less often large aorto-pulmonary communications) may be left with pulmonary hypertension. Sometimes this is progressive, sometimes stable in the years following surgery. Such patients need to be considered individually. Some patients with stable pulmonary hypertension and no symptoms may go through several pregnancies without trouble. Others behave more as patients with primary-type pulmonary hypertension with progression of right ventricular decompensation and a high chance of not surviving.[20] The risk of pregnancy should be considered to be high if the pulmonary artery pressure is close to systemic, particularly if there are associated symptoms of shortness of breath and fatigue.

The functions of the left and right ventricles should receive close attention. Impairment is occasionally seen, particularly in patients whose defects were closed early in surgical experience. The right ventricle is most vulnerable to failure of myocardial protection, and impaired function combined with residual pulmonary hypertension may seriously compromise cardiovascular reserve. Preconceptual cardiopulmonary exercise testing is indicated when there is doubt, to assess exercise tolerance and functional reserve.

The patient should rest as much as possible and be seen frequently for evaluation of right ventricular function both clinically and by echo-cardiography. Admission to hospital is needed for any patient with significant pulmonary vascular disease with a view to delivery by caesarean section under general anaesthetic. The puerperium is the time of greatest risk even in patients who seem to have tolerated pregnancy and delivery well. Consideration should be given to administering nitric oxide or nebulised prostacycline prenatally to try to prevent the postnatal rise in pulmonary vascular resistance which sometimes occurs.

Patients who have undergone pulmonary artery banding in infancy without closure of the defect are seen occasionally. One such patient with multiple defects in whom further surgery had been repeatedly postponed had an uneventful pregnancy. Her pulmonary vascular resistance was normal (Figure 5.4).

The risk of occurrence of ventricular septal defects in the offspring of women with the condition is high, and defects are found in nearly a quarter of live born children.[21]

Aortic stenosis

Severe valve stenosis is seldom encountered during pregnancy and there are few published reports.[22-28] Congenital aortic valve stenosis is common but is about five times as prevalent in male as in female subjects.

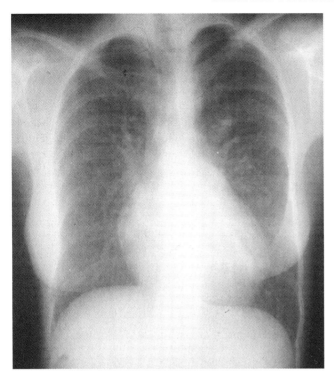

FIGURE 5.4—*Chest* x *ray picture of a young woman with multiple ventricular septal defects who had undergone pulmonary artery banding in infancy and came to clinic at 22 weeks' gestation (see text).*

Pregnancy in women with severe left ventricular outflow tract obstruction is risky. The increase in blood volume and stroke volume leads to an increase in left ventricular pressure and pressure gradient across the obstruction. The increase in left ventricular work demands augmentation of coronary blood flow. Women who were free of symptoms before pregnancy may develop angina, left ventricular failure, pulmonary oedema, or sudden death. Individual experience is small. A widely quoted 1978 review of 23 heterogeneous cases from the literature disclosed a maternal mortality of 17% and a perinatal mortality of 32% but such figures are uninformative and can be misleading when considering an individual patient.[16] Aortic stenosis can be hazardous in pregnancy but the risk is dependent on the severity of the obstruction. Patients with mild or moderate stenosis do well and pregnancy need not be discouraged. Indeed such women should plan to complete their families before their valves deteriorate and the stenosis worsens.

Left ventricular outflow tract obstruction may be valvular, supra-valvular, or caused by discrete membranous or the tunnel type of subvalvular aortic stenosis. Outflow tract gradients associated with hypertrophic cardio-myopathy are considered in chapter 15. Rheumatic aortic valve stenosis is rare in pregnancy (Chapter 8) and is then invariably associated with mitral stenosis, usually in older women.

Supravalvar stenosis is rare and often associated with other arterial stenoses. Discrete subvalvar stenosis may be a problem because of severe hypertrophy, previous surgery leaving residual obstruction, mitral regurgitation, left ventricular dysfunction, and associated anomalies such as coarctation.

Congenital aortic valve stenosis is usually the result of some variety of bicuspid aortic valve with varying degrees of valve thickening and commissural fusion. There is often some narrowing of the aortic root, asymmetry of the sinuses of Valsalva and an eccentric orifice. Regurgitation is usually absent or mild. Other left sided lesions such as coarctation of the aorta and patent ductus are associated in about 20%. Patients may have had open aortic valvotomy or balloon valvotomy in childhood. The earlier the procedure was needed the more severe the stenosis was likely to have been and the greater the deformity of the valve. Left ventricular systolic function is usually good but rarely this may be impaired. This is sometimes the result of endocardial fibroelastosis which, if seen in combination with mild or moderate aortic stenosis, poses a rather different problem. The danger is now left ventricular function rather than outflow tract obstruction, but a low Doppler aortic valve velocity in the presence of reduced left ventricular function may reflect severe valve stenosis needing urgent relief.

Echocardiography shows a thickened aortic valve which domes in systole (Figure 5.5) and on cross sectional views may show only two commissures usually with a third "rudimentary" raphe and with the non-coronary sinus occupying a greater aortic circumference than the right and left coronary sinuses, but appearances vary. The rudimentary raphe represents a fused commissure. Sometimes the valve is truly bicuspid with only two sinuses. Associated aortic regurgitation may be present particularly if a rudimentary third commissure is only partially fused. The coronary ostia are usually normally placed except in truly bicuspid valves when two equal sized sinuses of Valsalva are placed anteriorly and posteriorly, the right coronary ostium anteriorly and the left coronary ostium facing it posteriorly.

An exercise test is useful in deciding fitness for pregnancy in a patient without symptoms who has moderately severe aortic valve stenosis (aortic valve peak velocity <4·5 m/sec), good ECG (normal or with only voltage changes of left ventricular hypertrophy) and excellent left ventricular function. If she can exercise up to or near her target heart rate with a rise in or at least maintenance of her blood pressure, without symptoms of angina or the development of ST segment depression or T wave inversion, she will almost certainly go through pregnancy without trouble. Failure of the blood pressure to rise or an actual fall indicates inability to increase stroke volume, or a baroreceptor depressor reflex. ST segment depression suggests the development of subendocardial ischaemia and pregnancy is contraindicated. Such exercise tests need to be medically supervised both for safety and for maximum information (Table 5.2).

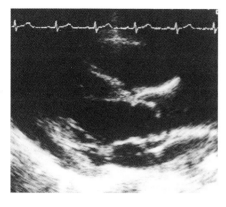

FIGURE 5.5—*Transthoracic long axis echocardiogram from a patient with congenital aortic valve stenosis with a bicuspid valve shown doming in systole. There is post-stenotic dilatation of the ascending aorta.*

TABLE 5.2—*Aortic stenosis and pregnancy.*

Fit for pregnancy

- Normal exercise tolerance

- Normal electrocardiogram or voltage increase only

- Negative exercise test: normal blood pressure rise
  achievement of target heart rate
  absence of inducible ST-T wave changes

- Good left ventricular function

- Peak aortic velocity on echocardiography <4·5 m/sec

Symptom-free patients with aortic valve stenosis who have repolarisation changes on the ECG, a positive exercise test, or impaired left ventricular function on echocardiography should be advised against pregnancy until after the aortic stenosis has been relieved. According to the condition of the valve, which varies in its intrinsic anatomy and with the age of the patient, balloon aortic valvotomy[25-30] or aortic valve replacement[31] may be advised. Balloon aortic valvotomy is of limited efficacy in these structurally deformed valves and its indications in pregnancy are restricted to high risk otherwise surgical patients.[29,30] It may relieve the stenosis sufficiently to allow the pregnancy to proceed[24,26,27] but carries a risk of causing severe aortic regurgitation requiring surgery, embolism, aortic rupture, and haemopericardium. Open aortic valvotomy, which was the only option short of valve replacement before the balloon technique, was likewise only palliative because the deformity permits only incomplete relief of stenosis with choice of slightly wider opening if some regurgitation is preferred. Even dividing the commissural fusion leaves appreciable stenosis if the aortic root is small. The rudimentary raphe can be opened only a little, otherwise the leaflets prolapse causing severe regurgitation. The results of balloon valvuloplasty are therefore unpredictable. In older women or in patients who have had a previous balloon procedure aortic valve replacement may be needed (Chapter 10).

73

Patients with severe aortic valve stenosis may not be seen until they are already pregnant and if the pregnancy is advanced or termination refused they require careful supervision through the pregnancy as do women whose fitness for pregnancy was considered marginal but who went ahead with it anyway. Patients who are expected to do well should also be seen regularly and checked for development of symptoms of dyspnoea, angina, light headedness, or syncope with ECG and echocardiography repeated particularly if there is any cause for concern.

Symptoms which develop during pregnancy in patients with aortic stenosis are sometimes hard to assess. One such patient aged 40 in a second pregnancy was referred urgently because of two syncopal attacks. She had severe aortic stenosis with a peak gradient of 100 mm Hg, good left ventricular function and a normal ECG. Neither of the syncopal attacks had occurred in relation to exertion. On both occasions she had fainted while sitting as teller at a check-out counter. She was given a small dose of metoprolol to prevent tachycardia and the pregnancy continued to term without trouble. Only exertional or immediately post exertional syncope or faintness should be attributed to aortic stenosis and pregnant patients with aortic stenosis are not immune from syncope caused by uterocaval compression.

If the pregnancy is proceeding well, serial echocardiographic Doppler velocities show an increase in the peak velocity of flow across the valve. This indicates a normal rise in stroke volume. Failure of this velocity to rise suggests no change or a fall in stroke volume (Table 5.3). New repolarisation changes in the ECG indicate subendocardial ischaemia in a patient who may have developed angina. Patients who become dyspnoeic or start to have anginal pain should be admitted to hospital for rest and given a beta-blocker such as metoprolol to slow the heart rate and improve the time available for diastolic coronary blood flow. This is usually followed by relief of symptoms and improvement in the ECG.

TABLE 5.3—*Aortic stenosis and pregnancy.*

Signs of trouble

Onset of:

- Tachycardia
- New dyspnoea
- Angina
- Electrocardiographic deterioration
- Fall in peak aortic velocity
- Deterioration in left ventricular function
- Pulmonary congestion or oedema
- Congestive failure

Every effort should be made to bring the pregnancy to term. If the mother's condition is still giving cause for alarm, the baby should be delivered by caesarean section under general anaesthesia *before* proceeding with aortic valve surgery. This is usually followed by immediate improvement in the mother's condition which may even allow surgery to be delayed for a week or two, although the patient should be kept in hospital until this is carried out. The pregnant patient with severe aortic stenosis is extremely intolerant of changes in left ventricular pre-load. A fall caused by haemorrhage or regional anaesthesia can lead to cardiogenic shock and a rise may precipitate pulmonary oedema. Careful monitoring is needed.

If maternal difficulties develop and the valve looks suitable an emergency balloon valvotomy may relieve the stenosis sufficiently for the pregnancy to continue to term or until the fetus has a good chance of survival. If this is done the risk of creating severe aortic regurgitation needing immediate or early valve replacement needs to be considered and discussed. Severe aortic regurgitation of sudden onset is not well tolerated in patients with previous severe aortic stenosis because the hypertrophied left ventricle is relatively indistensible leading to an abrupt rise in its diastolic pressure with subendocardial ischaemia, premature mitral valve closure, fall in stroke volume, tachycardia, and reduction of coronary blood flow.

The risk of open heart surgery to the fetus remains high particularly if the mother's condition is poor.[31,32] The fetus may die during induction of anaesthesia if this increases haemodynamic instability with swings in blood pressure, heart rate, and output or it may die during cardiopulmonary bypass despite modern technological improvements with membrane oxygenators and pulsatile flow especially if this is prolonged. Cardio-pulmonary bypass for valve replacement during pregnancy after the fetus is viable not only jeopardises the fetus unnecessarily but also increases the hazard to the mother because of tissue oedema, high diaphragms, and poor operating conditions for the surgeon.

Patients who respond well to rest and beta-blockers need to be kept in hospital but then can often be brought safely to term or to the stage of fetal viability without the need to deal with the aortic stenosis during the pregnancy. Delivery by caesarean section can be carried out and followed by a planned valve procedure.

Discrete subvalvar aortic stenosis, either the so-called membranous form or the tunnel variety, is much rarer than valve stenosis but the haemodynamic effects and assessment are similar. Membranous subaortic stenosis is to some extent dynamic, often with misleadingly brisk arterial pulses, but the ECG may show more marked hypertrophy than seems warranted by the apparent severity of the stenosis. In this respect it has some similarities with hypertrophic cardiomyopathy with outflow gradient but the subvalvar diaphragm is usually readily seen on echocardiography. Absence of an ejection click, silent aortic closure and usually a soft early diastolic murmur differentiate it clinically from valve stenosis. The aortic valve is seen on the echocardiograph to be slightly thickened but it does not dome during systole. Typically it fails to open fully during ejection because of the narrow jet of blood passing through the subvalvar obstruction and there is usually some regurgitation.

Subvalvar aortic stenosis can be alleviated by balloon dilatation during pregnancy but a definitive operation is still needed and there is some risk of tearing an aortic cusp as well as the anterior leaflet of the mitral valve from which the membranous part of the obstruction is an extension.[30]

Women with a history of discrete subaortic stenosis operated on in childhood may have residual abnormalities which include some outflow tract stenosis, aortic or mitral regurgitation or both, and left ventricular dysfunction. Patients with mainly regurgitant residual valve lesions may do well as did one young woman despite quite severe residual aortic and mitral regurgitation. Individual assessment is needed.

Supravalvar aortic stenosis either with or without the Williams–Beuren syndrome is rarely seen in pregnancy.[33,34] Peripheral pulmonary artery branch stenoses may be associated, as well as peripheral arterial dysplasia.[34] When the gradient across the supravalvar stenosis is small and other serious vascular stenoses are absent the prognosis is good.

Coarctation of the aorta

Coarctation of the aorta should be corrected in infancy or childhood. It is three times more common in men but may be first recognised during pregnancy when raised blood pressure is found. Uncorrected coarctation causes premature death. Earlier accounts described experience of pregnancy in patients with uncorrected coarctation from a time before early surgical treatment was common.[35] Most patients with uncorrected uncomplicated coarctation now do well and the outcome is successful but there are risks of aortic dissection or rupture of an intracranial berry aneurysm, of infective endocarditis, and of heart failure.[36] These are the complications that caused a mortality of 17% in the first reports but of less than 3% in recent ones.[36,37,38]

In coarctation of the aorta circulation to the distal segment is conducted almost entirely through collateral channels. Mild coarctations are rare. Surgical correction can be performed without interrupting the pregnancy because clamping of the aorta does not affect flow to the lower segment, but the additional risk of the clamp causing a dissection rarely justifies surgery at this time. Heart failure or uncontrollable hypertension are both uncommon but might be reasons for considering correction of the coarctation during pregnancy. The nature of the coarcted segment in the adult does not usually lend itself to successful balloon dilatation Left ventricular failure is not anticipated unless there is endocardial fibro-elastosis, a bicuspid valve with aortic stenosis, or a floppy mitral valve with regurgitation. Bicuspid aortic valve is present in at least a third of patients with coarctation but severe stenosis is uncommon in this age group. Abnormalities of the mitral valve may coexist as well as other deformities of the left side of the heart in a "left heart syndrome" but all are rarely encountered in pregnancy.

Pregnancy may be complicated by aortic dissection and rupture. This has been reported more often during pregnancy than in the postpartum period. Apart from pregnancy the dissection most commonly occurs in the low pressure but abnormal distal segment. Dissection of the aorta is a disaster which may occur during pregnancy in apparently healthy women and this risk is increased in women with coarctation during pregnancy and particularly during labour. Rupture or dissection of the proximal segment may occur or cerebral haemorrhage from rupture of a cerebral berry aneurysm.[38] This is presumably because of an unavoidable rise in systolic blood pressure with large swings in blood pressure and wide pulse pressure at this time. Vaginal delivery is usual unless prolonged labour is anticipated but it is important for the second stage to be curtailed to minimise arterial stress. If there is any doubt on obstetric grounds caesarean section is preferable.

Fetal development is normal indicating adequate maintenance of utero-placental blood flow through the collateral circulation. Pre-eclamptic toxaemia and malignant hypertension or papilloedema are rare.

A bicuspid aortic valve increases the risk of endocarditis. When this occurs it is nearly always on the bicuspid valve rather than on the coarctation. A higher incidence of congenital heart disease has been reported in the infants of mothers with uncorrected coarctation compared with mothers with corrected coarctation.[21] This is unexplained.

Drug treatment of hypertension is unsatisfactory in patients with uncorrected coarctation. Untreated, the resting blood pressure tends to fall slightly in pregnancy as in normal women, but considerable rises in systolic pressure and pulse pressure occur on exercise with attendant risks. Blood pressure lowering agents such as hydralazine, methyldopa, labetalol, or metoprolol may be used to temper this, but over-enthusiastic blood pressure reduction will diminish placental perfusion and be detrimental to fetal growth. Pregnant patients with uncorrected coarctation should avoid strenuous exercise to minimise stress on the arterial wall because surges in blood pressure and pulse pressure with exercise are not wholly prevented by blood pressure lowering drugs. Although both native coarctation[39,40] and re-coarctation[41] have been treated by percutaneous balloon angioplasty, initial tears may be created[42] and late development of aneurysms has been reported.[43] These risks are likely to be higher in pregnancy and the procedure should be avoided at this time.

Although surgical repair of coarctation has a favourable effect on prognosis by correcting hypertension or by making it possible to treat the hypertension more effectively, long term risks remain. These relate to the development of progressive aortic stenosis or regurgitation, left ventricular failure especially if there is associated mild endocardial fibro-elastosis, premature coronary artery disease, and endocarditis. Other long term complications relate to re-coarctation, dissection, or other problems such as aneurysm or pseudo aneurysm of the aorta, or to do with the repair.

Restenosis is common following correction during infancy and may require further surgery in childhood. Babies operated on at under one year of age are at higher risk of restenosis than those treated after the first year.[44] Early corrective surgery improves long term survival by reducing the otherwise high incidence of persistent hypertension requiring drug treatment as well as the later complications of hypertension, particularly cerebral berry aneurysm and coronary artery disease.[45,46] Late problems after repair include the development of aneurysms, particularly after the patch graft operation which is needed when end-to-end anastomosis is technically difficult because of a long hypoplastic segment.[46] An aneurysmal bulge may develop opposite the patch which may progress to aneurysm,[46] or rarely to pseudo-aneurysm perhaps as a result of previous infection.[47] These may not cause symptoms but are at risk of rupture.[48]

These possible late complications are uncommon but should be considered in any woman with a history of repaired coarctation who wishes to become pregnant. The integrity of the repair should be assessed by measuring the blood pressure in both arms and in the feet by Doppler technique, and by checking for brachio-femoral pulse delay and for a murmur over the site of the coarctation on the back or from periscapular collaterals. An aortic ejection click or murmur may indicate a bicuspid stenosed or regurgitant valve. The ECG in patients with coarctation may show right bundle branch block more often than in the normal population, but left ventricular hypertrophy or repolarisation changes suggest significant hypertension (perhaps only on exercise), aortic valve disease, or endocardial fibro-elastosis. Echocardiographic study is important to assess the coarctation site and adjacent aorta as well as the aortic valve. A transoesophageal study provides good detail of the coarcted segment and with multiplane ultrasound most of the aortic arch can now be visualised as well as the distal segment. If a patient with coarctation or repaired coarctation is referred during pregnancy with a suspected local complication the investigation of choice after conventional study is a transoesophageal echocardiograph. It is quick and avoids irradiation.

Corrected transposition

Corrected transposition (atrioventricular discordance with ventriculo-arterial discordance) is usually accompanied by other defects, particularly ventricular septal defect and subpulmonary and pulmonary valve stenosis or an Ebstein-like malformation of the left sided tricuspid valve with or without regurgitation. Sometimes it is recognised for the first time during pregnancy (or because of acquired coronary artery disease later on). Without other substantive defects it may well be missed altogether but commonly the patient is referred because of a "mitral" regurgitant murmur or with an ejection systolic murmur caused by subpulmonary stenosis with or without an associated ventricular septal defect.

One young woman was referred with suspected pulmonary hypertension because of a loud "pulmonary" closure sound and abnormal ECG. The loud second sound was produced by aortic valve closure (left sided and anterior). If the pulmonary stenosis is severe and there is a VSD large enough (or an associated atrial communication) the patient is cyanosed but if the pulmonary stenosis is mild the patient is likely to be symptom-free and pink. The diagnosis may be suspected from the ECG which usually shows Q waves in the right chest leads and RS waves in the left sided leads. If an x ray film has been taken it may show the characteristic smoothly curving profile of the left sided ascending aorta with absent aortic knob and narrow mediastinum.

Dysfunction of the systemic (morphologic right) ventricle tends to develop as patients with corrected transposition get older and particularly if there is associated atrioventricular valve regurgitation.

A review of 18 patients aged between 16 and 61 years at first presentation and without associated defects showed that three were referred because of abnormal ECGs, four with complete heart block (thought to be congenital in three), two with an abnormal routine chest radiograph, five with systolic murmurs from mild left sided atrioventricular valve regurgitation, three on account of paroxysmal supraventricular arrhythmia and one with a systolic murmur and questionable cyanosis from a left superior vena cava draining into the left atrium.[49] Fourteen of the 18 were well and free of symptoms. Four more patients developed heart block during follow up and needed pacemakers. Three of the nine women had uneventful pregnancies and the nine produced seven children, none of whom had congenital heart disease.

The prevalence of such symptom-free patients in the general population, leading normal lives, going through pregnancies, getting later complications

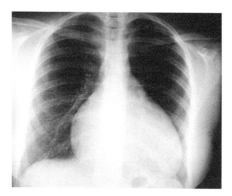

FIGURE 5.6—*Chest* x *ray picture of a young woman with acyanotic Ebstein's anomaly who presented with an embolic stroke presumed to have been caused by paradoxical embolism. Transthoracic and transoesophageal echocardiography showed no evidence of intra-atrial thrombus and there was no history of arrhythmia.*

(or not), but not entering the statistics, is unknown. That it is uncommon is suggested by the frequency of heart block in patients with diagnosed corrected transposition but its rarity in pacing clinics. Coronary artery disease is common in the general population but corrected transpositions are rare.

Heart block may develop at any time in life and may complicate pregnancy but patients with corrected transposition and without serious accompanying defects tolerate pregnancy without incident. Patients with accompanying defects need to be considered individually on the basis of their circulatory reserve. The accompanying congenital defects determine prognosis in the first three or four decades but acquired problems from left atrioventricular valve regurgitation and failure of the right ventricle usually occur later. Patients with corrected transposition and without other serious defects can be reassured about pregnancy but are at risk of heart block and endocarditis.

Ebstein's anomaly of the tricuspid valve

Ebstein's anomaly is associated with caudal displacement of the septal or posterior or both leaflets of the tricuspid valve together with an often sail-like abnormality of a normally attached anterior leaflet. An interatrial communication, either patent foramen ovale or septal defect, is commonly associated but not invariable.

Patients with Ebstein's anomaly often reach childbearing age. They are usually acyanotic and tolerate pregnancy well but may be bothered by atrioventricular tachycardia caused by right-sided pre-excitation.[50-51] This carries a risk of sudden death (with which this anomaly is classically associated) if atrial flutter develops. This can lead to one to one antidromic conduction down the accessory pathway and be followed by syncope or ventricular fibrillation. Paradoxical embolism can occur even in the asymptomatic patient (Figure 5.6) or late development of cyanosis ("cyanosis tardive") with reduction in the prospect of a successful pregnancy (Chapter 6).

References

1 Whittemore R, Hobbins JC, Engle MA. Pregnancy and its outcome in women with and without surgical treatment of congenital heart disease. *Am J Cardiol* 1982; **50**: 641–51.
2 Elkayam U, Gleicher N. Cardiac problems in pregnancy. I. Maternal aspects: the approach to the pregnant patient with heart disease. *JAMA* 1984; **251**: 2838–9.
3 Shime J, Mocarski EJM, Hastings D, Webb GD, McLaughlin PR. Congenital heart disease in pregnancy: short- and long-term implications. *Am J Obstet Gynecol* 1987; **156**: 313–22.
4 McFaul PB, Dornan JC, Lamki H, Boyle D. Pregnancy complicated by maternal heart disease: a review of 519 women. *Br J Obstet Gynaecol* 1988; **95**: 861–7.
5 Pitkin RM, Perloff JK, Koos BJ, Beall MH. Pregnancy and congenital heart disease. *Ann Intern Med* 1990; **112**: 445–54.

6 Oakley CM. Cardiovascular disease in pregnancy. *Can J Cardiol* 1990; **6(suppl B)**: 33B–44B.

7 Harvey JR, Teague SM, Anderson JL, Voyles WF, Thadani V. Clinically silent atrial septal defects with evidence for cerebral embolisation. *Ann Intern Med* 1986; **105**: 695–7.

8 Lynch J, Schuchard GH, Gross CM, Wann LS. Prevalence of right to left atrial shunting in a healthy population: detection by valsalva manoeuvre contrast echocardiography. *Am J Cardiol* 1984; **53**: 1478–80.

9 Marazanof M, Roudaut R, Cohen A, *et al*. Atrial septal aneurysm. Morphological characteristics in a large population: pathological associations. A French multicentre study on 259 patients investigated by transoesophageal echocardiography. *Int J Cardiol* 1995; **52**: 59–65.

10 Davies MJ. Mitral valve in secundum atrial septal defect. *Br Heart J* 1981; **46**: 126.

11 Markman P, Howitt G, Wade EG. Atrial septal defect in the middle aged and elderly. *Q J Med* 1965; **34**: 409–26.

12 Perloff JK, Koos BJ, Phil D, Beall MH. Pregnancy and congenital heart disease. *Ann Intern Med* 1990; **112**: 445–54.

13 Presibitero P, Prever SB, Brusca A. Interventional cardiology in pregnancy. *Eur Heart J* 1996; **17**: 182–8.

14 Green NJ, Rollason TP. Pulmonary artery rupture in pregnancy complicating patent ductus arteriosus. *Br Heart J* 1992; **68**: 616–18.

15 D'Arbela PG, Mugerwa JW, Patel AK, Somers K. Aneurysm of pulmonary artery with persistent ductus arteriosus and pulmonary infundibular stenosis. Fatal dissection and rupture in pregnancy. *Br Heart J* 1970; **32**: 124–6.

16 Hankins GDV, Brekken AL, Davis LM. Maternal death secondary to a dissecting aneurysm of the pulmonary artery. *Obstet Gynecol* 1985; **65(suppl)**: 45–8.

17 Guthrie W, MacLean H. Dissecting aneurysms of arteries other than the aorta. *J Pathol* 1972; **108**: 210–35.

18 Robertson EG. Oedema in normal pregnancy. *J Reprod Fertil* 1969; **9(suppl)**: 27–36.

19 Oakley CM, Nihoyannopoulos P. Peripartum cardiomyopathy with recovery in a patient with coincidental Eisenmenger ventricular septal defect. *Br Heart J* 1992; **67**: 190–2.

20 Jackson GM, Dildy GA, Varner MW, Clark SL. Severe pulmonary hypertension in pregnancy following successful repair of ventricular septal defect in childhood. *Obstet Gynecol* 1993; **82(suppl)**: 680–2.

21 Wooley CF, Sparks EH. Congenital heart disease, inheritable cardiovascular disease and pregnancy. *Prog Cardiovasc Dis* 1992; **35**: 41–60.

22 Lao TT, Sermer M, MaGee L, Farine D, Colman JM. Congenital aortic stenosis and pregnancy—A reappraisal. *Am J Obstet Gynecol* 1993; **169**: 540–5.

23 Rose BJ, Holbrook RH Jr, Wyner J, Cohen S, Ueland K. Efficacy of Doppler echocardiography in the evaluation of aortic stenosis during pregnancy. *Obstet Gynecol* 1987; **69**: 431–2.

24 Easterling TR, Chadwick HS, Otto CM, Benedetti TJ. Aortic stenosis in pregnancy. *Obstet Gynecol* 1988; **72**: 113–18.

25 Angel JL, Chapman C, Knuppel RA, *et al*. Percutaneous balloon valvuloplasty in pregnancy. *Obstet Gynecol* 1988; **3**: 438–40.

26 McIvor RA. Percutaneous balloon aortic valvuloplasty during pregnancy. *Int J Cardiol* 1991; **32**: 1–4.

27 Banning AP, Pearson JF, Hall RJC. Role of balloon dilatation of the aortic valve in pregnant patients with severe aortic stenosis. *Br Heart J* 1993; **70**: 544–5.

28 Sholler GF, Keane JF, Perry SB, Sanders SP, Lock JE. Balloon dilatation of congenital aortic valve stenosis: results and influence of technical and morphologic features on outcome. *Circulation* 1988; **78**: 351–60.

29 Rosenfeld HM, Landzberg MJ, Perry SB, Colan SD, Keane JF, Lock JE. Balloon aortic valvuloplasty in the young adult with congenital aortic stenosis. *Am J Cardiol* 1994; **73**: 1112–17.

30 Rocchini AR, Beckman RH, Ben-Shacher G, Benson L, Schwartz D, Kan G. Balloon aortic valvuloplasty: results of the valvuloplasty and angioplasty of congenital anomalies registry. *Am J Cardiol* 1990; **65**: 784–9.

31 Becker RM. Intracardiac surgery in pregnant women. *Ann Thorac Surg* 1983; **36**: 453–8.

32 Bernal JM, Miralles PJ. Cardiac surgery with cardiopulmonary bypass during pregnancy. *Obstet Gynecol Surv* 1986; **41**: 1–6.

81

33 von Son JAM, Danielson GK, Puga FJ, *et al.* Supravalvular aortic stenosis: long term results of surgical treatment. *J Thorac Cardiovasc Surg* 1994; **107**: 103–15.

34 Wessel A, Pankau R, Kececioglu D, Ruschewski W, Bursch JH. Three decades of follow-up of aortic and pulmonary vascular lesions in the Williams–Beuren syndrome. *Am J Med Genet* 1994; **52**: 297–301.

35 Goodwin JF. Pregnancy and coarctation of the aorta. *Lancet* 1958; **i**: 16.

36 Deal K, Woolley CF. Coarctation of the aorta and pregnancy. *Ann Intern Med* 1973; **78**: 706–10.

37 Clark SL. Cardiac disease in pregnancy. *Obstet Gynecol Clin North Am* 1991; **18**: 237–56.

38 Koller M, Rothlin M, Senning A. Coarctation of the aorta: review of 362 operated patients; long-term follow-up and assessment of prognostic variables. *Eur Heart J* 1987; **8**: 670–9.

39 Cooper RS, Ritter SB, Golinko RJ. Balloon dilatation angioplasty: non-surgical management of coarctation of the aorta. *Circulation* 1984; **70**: 903–7.

40 Allen HD, Marx GR, Ovitt TW, Goldberg SJ. Balloon dilatation angioplasty for coarctation of the aorta. *Am J Cardiol* 1986; **57**: 828–32.

41 Saul JP, Kearne JF, Fellows KT, Lock JE. Balloon dilatation angioplasty of postoperative aortic obstruction. *Am J Cardiol* 1987; **59**: 943–8.

42 Cooper RS, Ritter SB, Rothe WB, Chan CK, Griepp R, Golinko RJ. Angioplasty for coarctation of the aorta: long term results. *Circulation* 1987; **75**: 600–4.

43 Schuster SR, Gross RE. Surgery for coarctation of the aorta: a review of 500 cases. *J Thorac Cardiovasc Surg* 1962; **43**: 54–70.

44 Bobby JJ, Emami JM, Farmer RDT, Newman CGH. Operative survival and 40 year follow-up of surgical repair of aortic coarctation. *Br Heart J* 1991; **65**: 271–6.

45 Maron BJ, Humphries JO, Rowe RD, Mellits ED. Prognosis of surgically corrected coarctation of the aorta: a 20 year postoperative appraisal. *Circulation* 1973; **47**: 119–26.

46 Bergdahl L, Ljungqvist A. Long-term results after repair of coarctation of the aorta by patch grafting. *J Thorac Cardiovasc Surg* 1980; **80**: 177–81.

47 Kirsh MM, Perry B, Spooner E. Management of pseudoaneurysm following patch grafting for coarctation of the aorta. *J Thorac Cardiovasc Surg* 1977; **74**: 636–9.

48 Forfang K, Rostad H, Sorland S, Levorstad K. Late sudden death after surgical correction of coarctation of the aorta. *Acta Med Scand* 1979; **206**: 375–9.

49 Presbitero P, Somerville J, Rabajoli F, Stone S, Conte MR. Corrected transposition of the great arteries without associated defects in adult patients: clinical profile and follow up. *Br Heart J* 1995; **74**: 57–9.

50 Waickman LA, Storton DJ, Varmer MW, Ehmke DA, Goplerud CP. Ebstein's anomaly in pregnancy. *Am J Cardiol* 1984; **53**: 357–8.

51 Connolly HM, Warnes CA. Ebstein's anomaly: outcome of pregnancy. *J Am Coll Cardiol* 1994; **23**: 1194–8.

6: Cyanotic congenital heart disease

CAROLE A WARNES

When cyanosis accompanies congenital heart disease, the underlying anomaly is commonly complex. Many patients with congenital heart disease undergo successful repair in infancy or childhood, but some lesions associated with increased pulmonary vascular resistance (Eisenmenger syndrome) are not amenable to surgical repair. In addition, a number of patients with compensated anomalies survive to adulthood without surgical intervention. These include patients with Ebstein's anomaly and mild tetralogy of Fallot. Sometimes the lesion was unrecognised in childhood but as more blood was shunted from the right to the left circulation, the patient became progressively cyanosed. Sometimes surgery was refused by the patient or their family.

Cyanotic congenital heart disease can be divided into those lesions associated with low pulmonary blood flow and those associated with high pulmonary blood flow. In both circumstances, cyanosis poses risks for both the mother and the fetus.

Maternal risks

Patients with right to left shunts usually have erythrocytosis, and the more severe the hypoxia, the more elevated are the haemoglobin and packed cell volume. During pregnancy, as there is increased platelet adhesiveness and decreased fibrinolysis, there is an increased risk of thrombotic complications for the cyanotic mother. Over zealous treatment with diuretics should therefore be avoided because of the risk of haemoconcentration and abnormal renal function. A recent study by Presbitero et al evaluated pregnancy outcomes in 44 cyanotic patients who had 96 pregnancies.[1] In this series, patients with the Eisenmenger syndrome were excluded because it was considered that elevated pulmonary vascular resistance is a greater hazard than the presence of cyanosis. Two patients in this series had thrombotic complications (pulmonary and cerebral); their haemoglobin concentrations were 170 and 180 g/l. Cardiovascular complications occurred in 14 patients (32%). Eight patients developed heart failure, three requiring hospital admission at 32–36 weeks of gestation.

Peripartum bacterial endocarditis occurred in two patients (4·5%), both with palliated tetralogy of Fallot.

If cyanotic patients develop thrombophlebitis or deep venous thrombosis, they are at risk not only of pulmonary, but also paradoxical embolism. There must therefore be meticulous attention to leg care during pregnancy, and this is particularly important during labour and the puerperium. These risks can be minimised by arranging coordinated care with cardiologists, obstetricians, and anaesthetists throughout pregnancy and during labour and delivery. Patients should be adequately hydrated during labour. Elastic support stockings should be used, and patients mobilised early. Anticoagulation should not be used routinely in cyanotic patients as they are also at risk of bleeding. This is because they are usually deficient in the clotting factors produced in the liver, and the platelet count may be low and platelet function abnormal. It is possible, however, that the use of low dose aspirin after the first trimester is safe without increasing the risk of bleeding and perhaps may help to reduce thrombotic complications. It does not have an adverse effect on the fetus. Prophylactic doses of heparin may be used during the period of greatest risk while the patient is in hospital and are safe.

Fetal risk

Cyanosis also poses a substantial risk to the fetus, and results in increased fetal loss, prematurity, and small birth weight. Neill and Swanson reported that with increasing cyanosis, as reflected in the maternal haemoglobin, the incidence of spontaneous abortion increased, and the handicap to fetal growth was more pronounced.[2] In their series, no infant survived if the maternal haemoglobin was greater than 180 g/l, and most babies were lost in the first trimester. Whittemore estimated maternal hypoxia using the packed cell volume and showed that infants born to mothers with a packed cell volume greater than 0·44 were all below the 50th percentile of birth weight for gestational age.[3] The recent study by Presbitero et al also demonstrated that with increasing maternal hypoxia, as reflected by the mother's haemoglobin, the percent of live born infants fell, and when the mother's haemoglobin exceeded 200 g/l, only 8% of children were live born (Table 6.1).[1] Similarly, when the maternal oxygen saturation was ≤85%, only 2/17 pregnancies (12%) resulted in live born infants. In total, 41 of the 96 pregnancies (43%) produced a live birth. Twenty-six of these babies reached term, and 15 were premature. There were 49 spontaneous abortions and 6 stillbirths, again reflecting the high risk cyanotic congenital heart disease poses for the fetus. Congenital heart disease was found in two of 41 live infants (4·9%).

Tetralogy of Fallot

Tetralogy of Fallot consists of a ventricular septal defect immediately beneath the aortic valve and an overriding aorta which lies over the

TABLE 6.1—*Fetal outcome in cyanotic congenital heart disease and its relation with maternal cyanosis.*

	No of pregnancies	No of live births	Percentage born alive
*Haemoglobin, g/l**			
≤160	28	20	71
170–190	40	18	45
≥200	26	2	8
Arterial oxygen saturation (%)†			
≤85	17	2	12
85–89	22	10	45
≥90	13	12	92

Reproduced from Presbitero *et al* with permission;[1] *Haemoglobin concentration unknown in two pregnancies; †arterial oxygen saturation unknown in 44 pregnancies.

ventricular septal defect. Pulmonary outflow tract obstruction usually occurs at infundibular level and often with associated pulmonary valve stenosis, and this causes secondary right ventricular hypertrophy. Because of the right ventricular outflow tract obstruction, there is a right to left shunt through the ventricular septal defect and blue blood enters the aorta. Patients with mild tetralogy of Fallot may survive into adulthood without substantial symptoms but usually the pulmonary stenosis progresses, increasing the right to left shunt and the severity of cyanosis.

Because of the fall in peripheral vascular resistance which occurs during a normal pregnancy, there may be an increase in the right to left shunt with subsequent increase in the cyanosis. Thus, even mothers with mild cyanosis may notice a deterioration during pregnancy. Labour and delivery is a particularly hazardous time, as the blood loss associated with delivery may induce hypotension and again exaggerate the right to left shunt.

Right and left heart failure may occur during pregnancy, particularly when there is associated aortic regurgitation.[4] Aortic regurgitation tends to be progressive in unoperated patients with tetralogy of Fallot because the aortic valve leaflets have no support and prolapse into the defect. In addition, the aorta itself is usually larger than normal because it is carrying increased blood flow. Further problems may occur during pregnancy with the onset of atrial arrhythmias which are more common in the third and fourth decade.[5] Rarely, pulmonary stenosis has been surgically palliated during pregnancy.[6] Presbitero *et al* reported the outcome of 21 patients with 46 pregnancies who had either tetralogy of Fallot or pulmonary atresia with aortopulmonary collaterals.[1] There were 15 live births (33%), and 9 babies were premature. There were 26 abortions and 5 stillbirths. Eight of the mothers experienced cardiovascular complications, including two with peripartum bacterial endocarditis.

The risk of a congenital heart defect in the offspring of a parent with tetralogy has been reported to be 2·5% to 8·3%.[7–10] In the largest series reported so far of 127 parents (62 women, 65 men), congenital heart defects occurred in 3 (1·2%) of the 253 children.[11] One of these children had tetralogy of Fallot, one had ventricular septal defect, and the other had truncus arteriosus. The reasons for these discrepancies in risks depends on many factors, including ascertainment bias, environmental factors, and how vigorously congenital heart disease in the offspring is sought (for example, physical examination compared with echocardiography).

Following successful surgical repair of tetralogy of Fallot, the outcome is considerably improved.[12] Singh et al reported 40 pregnancies in 27 patients with surgically repaired tetralogy of Fallot.[8] There were no serious complications in any of the pregnancies, and the incidence of miscarriage was no higher than that in the general population. Of 31 pregnancies about which detailed information was available, 30 resulted in normal infants, the one abnormal infant having pulmonary atresia.

Each patient should be assessed before conception with careful history-taking to determine functional status, exercise capacity, and the presence or absence of other lesions. Echocardiography should be done to delineate the haemodynamics and find out whether or not there is any right ventricular outflow tract obstruction, pulmonary regurgitation, or right ventricular dysfunction. Any residual defects, such as ventricular septal defect or aortic regurgitation, should also be discovered, in addition to assessment of left ventricular function. If necessary, exercise testing should be done to assess functional capacity. Provided there are no major residual defects, it is likely that pregnancy and delivery will be uncomplicated.

Pulmonary atresia

Pulmonary atresia represents an extreme form of Fallot's tetralogy in which there is congenital absence of the pulmonary valve and main pulmonary artery, and the lungs receive their blood supply from arteries arising from the descending aorta. Patients rarely survive to adulthood without surgical intervention, or more commonly following a palliative shunt. Little information is available about the outcome of pregnancy in women with pulmonary atresia. Connolly et al reported 14 patients with complex pulmonary atresia who had 24 pregnancies resulting in 10 live births (including one twin pregnancy).[13] There was one neonatal death from abruptio placentae at 27 weeks. Six pregnancies were terminated in women with unoperated pulmonary atresia.

Six patients had successful pregnancies; two unoperated patients had three deliveries (including twins—four births), two palliated patients had three deliveries, and two patients had two successful and two unsuccessful pregnancies after complete repair. One pregnancy was complicated by high right ventricular pressure from conduit obstruction, and one unoperated patient had congestive heart failure requiring admission to hospital in the last month of pregnancy. No pregnancy-related maternal deaths occurred. The mean maternal haemoglobin in patients with successful pregnancies was 149 (SD 13) g/l compared with 183 (SD 21) g/l in patients who terminated pregnancy (p = 0·01) and 164 (SD 22) g/l in patients with unsuccessful pregnancies. None of the offspring had congenital heart disease. Thus, pregnancy in patients with complex pulmonary atresia can be accomplished successfully, but there is an increased risk of fetal loss even without maternal hypoxia (miscarriage rate 50%).

Assessment of pulmonary pressures and degree of cyanosis is necessary before pregnancy is contemplated, and for those patients following radical repair, ventricular and conduit function must also be evaluated.

Ebstein's anomaly

This malformation consists of an inferior displacement of the tricuspid valve with resulting tricuspid regurgitation and enlargement of the right heart chambers. At least 50% of patients with Ebstein's anomaly have either an atrial septal defect or a patent foramen ovale and may therefore be cyanosed. While Ebstein's anomaly is an uncommon congenital malformation, many patients survive to adulthood without surgical intervention, but their functional status varies widely depending on the degree of tricuspid regurgitation and right ventricular dysfunction. Several small series have reported the outcome of pregnancy in women with Ebstein's anomaly.[14,15] The largest series was reported by Connolly et al who reported the outcome of 44 women with Ebstein's anomaly who had pregnancies (Figure 6.1).[16] Forty-four women had 111 pregnancies, resulting in 85 live births (76%). The pregnancy outcomes are shown in Figure 6.2. Eighteen women were cyanotic at the time of pregnancy (16 had documented interatrial communication; two did not have an atrial septal defect or patent foramen ovale). The 18 cyanotic women had 52 pregnancies resulting in 39 live births (75%). Among the 39 live births were 12 preterm infants born to six cyanotic women (31%). The outcome of pregnancy of the cyanotic patients compared to the acyanotic women is shown in Table 6.2.

The mean birth weight of infants born to cyanotic women was significantly lower than that of infants born to acyanotic women (2530–3140 g, p<0·001). This difference persisted when premature infants were excluded from analysis. In this study, the miscarriage and fetal loss rates were only slightly increased at 18% (19/104), compared with the expected rate of 10–15%.[17] Although arrhythmias are a common complication in patients with Ebstein's anomaly, particularly as accessory conduction pathways are often associated, none of the patients in this series had significant arrhythmias during pregnancy. Of the 83 offspring, five had congenital heart disease, an incidence of 6%. Two had aortic valve abnormalities, one had pulmonary atresia with intact ventricular septum, and two had ventricular septal defects that closed spontaneously.

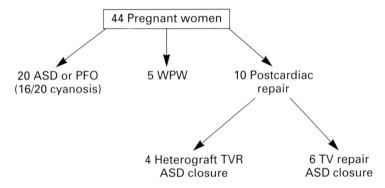

FIGURE 6.1—*Characteristics of 44 women with Ebstein's anomaly who had pregnancies. Twenty had an interatrial communication (either atrial septal defect [ASD] or patent foramen ovale [PFO]) at the time of pregnancy; 16 were cyanotic. Five women had one or more accessory pathways (Wolff–Parkinson–White [WPW]). Ten women had pregnancies after successful cardiac repair; all had ASD closure and reduction atrioplasty; six had tricuspid valve (TV) repair; and the remaining four had tricuspid valve replacement (TVR) with a heterograft prosthesis. Reproduced from Connolly et al with permission.*[16]

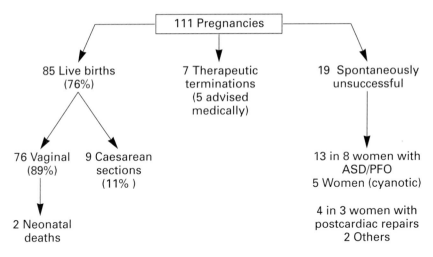

FIGURE 6.2—*Of 111 pregnancies in women with Ebstein's anomaly, 85 (76%) resulted in live births. Of these, 76 children (89%) were born by vaginal delivery, and nine (11%) by caesarean section (C-section). Of the 19 spontaneously unsuccessful pregnancies, 13 occurred in women with atrial septal defect (ASD) or patent foramen ovale (PFO); five of the eight women with ASD or PFO were cyanotic. Four unsuccessful pregnancies occurred in three women after successful cardiac repair and two occurred in women who had no ASD or PFO and had not had cardiac repair. Reproduced from Connolly et al with permission.*[16]

As Ebstein's anomaly may encompass a wide spectrum of anatomical and functional severity, it is recommended that all patients have a thorough evaluation before they become pregnant, with particular reference to

TABLE 6.2—*Outcome of pregnancy in Ebstein's anomaly: cyanotic compared with acyanotic women. Figures are number (%).*

	Cyanotic (n = 18)	Acyanotic (n = 26)	p Value
Preterm delivery	3 (17)	8 (31)	0·627
Miscarriage	4 (22)	4 (15)	0·928
Preterm + miscarriage	3 (17)	2 (8)	0·733
Total	10 (56)	14 (54)	0·844

Reproduced from Connolly *et al* with permission.[16]

ventricular size and function. Many cyanotic patients with Ebstein's anomaly may be amenable to surgical repair with a good functional result.[18] As the Connolly study showed, pregnancy is well tolerated after tricuspid valve repair or replacement, and the risk of paradoxical embolism is obviated after closure of the atrial septal defect. Therefore, while there is an increased risk of fetal loss, prematurity, and a low birth weight infant, in most cases one can be optimistic about the outcome of pregnancy.

Single ventricle/tricuspid atresia

Patients with a morphological single ventricle (univentricular atrioventricular connection) may have atresia of one or other atrioventricular valve (commonly tricuspid atresia). There may be two atrioventricular valves entering the main ventricular chamber (double inlet left ventricle), or there may be one large atrioventricular valve entering the main ventricular chamber (commonly morphologically right ventricle). Few patients survive to reproductive age without surgery, although some cases have been reported.[19] Most commonly, patients survive because of previous palliative surgery in the form of a shunt or following definitive repair. The presence of pulmonary hypertension is a major determinant of maternal risk. Some of these patients survive to adulthood with pulmonary vascular disease, but the majority have pulmonary stenosis. If there is modest pulmonary stenosis and good ventricular function associated with a moderate degree of cyanosis, pregnancy may be possible, but is associated with an increased risk, both for the mother and the fetus. There are only a few isolated reports in the literature regarding pregnancy and single ventricle. Stiller *et al* reported a patient with double inlet left ventricle and significant pulmonary stenosis with a systolic gradient of 89 mm Hg.[20] She delivered a healthy infant at 30 weeks' gestation weighing 2353 g. Leibbrandt *et al* reported a 29 year old woman with single ventricle and transposed great arteries who had only mild stenosis, but who tolerated two pregnancies.[21] Collins *et al* reported a 23 year old woman with tricuspid atresia and a previous Blalock–Taussig shunt who delivered a low birth weight infant but survived the pregnancy.[22] Two years later, however, she became pregnant again, had a stroke and subsequently aborted a two month fetus. Finally, in another

89

pregnancy, she had two pulmonary emboli, refused termination, and at 24 weeks delivered a premature infant which did not survive. Following delivery she had another pulmonary embolus but survived.

The important determinants of maternal and fetal survival is therefore ventricular function and degree of cyanosis. The pulmonary artery pressure must be assessed before pregnancy. For those with moderate pulmonary stenosis, pregnancy may be tolerated with an increased risk and particular caution to avoid hypotension during pregnancy and labour.

The definitive repair for both tricuspid atresia and single ventricle is the Fontan operation or one of its modifications.[23,24] This operation is designed to separate the systemic and pulmonary venous returns and to reduce the volume load on the left ventricle. This is accomplished by a right atrial to pulmonary artery anastomosis or a modification to divert caval blood to the pulmonary circuit. For those women who have had a successful Fontan operation, pregnancy may be successfully accomplished provided there are no significant residual lesions.[25] There is, however, an increased risk of fetal loss.

One multicentre study reported 28 pregnancies in 11 mothers following the Fontan operation.[25] Of these 11 women, seven had the Fontan operation for tricuspid atresia; two for single ventricle, and two had complex anomalies. There were 12 (43%) live births; one had two term pregnancies. There were nine (32%) first trimester miscarriages, five elective abortions, and two women currently pregnant. The gestational age of the infants averaged 36·2 weeks and their mean weight was 2331 g (range 1050–3575). One infant had an atrial septal defect. None of the mothers experienced any cardiac complications.

Each case must be assessed before pregnancy, including evaluation of functional capacity and echocardiography to assess residual lesions and ventricular function. For those patients with considerable right atrial enlargement, there is an increased risk of atrial arrhythmias, thrombus formation within the right atrium, and thromboembolism. This may be particularly true if spontaneous echo contrast is noted. Marked leg oedema tends to develop during pregnancy after the Fontan operation.

Transposition of the great vessels

In this anomaly, the aorta arises from the morphological right ventricle, and the pulmonary artery from the morphological left ventricle, with a communication between the two circulations in the form of either an atrial septal defect, a ventricular septal defect, or a patent ductus arteriosus. These patients do not survive to adulthood without surgical intervention, but with the development of reparative operations, most infants now survive to reach childbearing age. The most common type of repair seen in women of childbearing age is the Mustard operation, which was introduced in the 1960s.[26] The Mustard atrial baffle repair directs pulmonary venous return to the right ventricle and the transposed aorta, and the systemic venous blood is directed to the mitral valve and left ventricle and hence out to the pulmonary artery. This allows the blood to go in the appropriate direction but through the incorrect ventricle, so the right ventricle is left to support the systemic circulation.

There have been several reports of successful pregnancy after a Mustard procedure.[27,28] Lynch-Salamon et al reported three women who had Mustard operations in childhood and each had a successful pregnancy.[27] Two of the pregnancies were complicated by failure of the systemic ventricle, and one by preterm labour.

Clarkson et al reviewed nine women with 15 pregnancies following Mustard procedures.[29] They were symptom free before pregnancy and remained so during each pregnancy. There were 12 live births, two spontaneous abortions, and one intrauterine death. None of the live born infants had evidence of congenital heart disease. As anticipated, right ventricular volumes increased during pregnancy, as is the case in normal individuals, but none had overt failure. The authors concluded that in this group with good functional capacity, pregnancy was well tolerated. While many patients do well for two or three decades after the Mustard procedure, the degree of right ventricular dysfunction is variable, and this needs to be carefully assessed at the time of pregnancy counselling. Echocardiography should be done to assess the degree of right ventricular dilatation, dysfunction, and the degree of tricuspid regurgitation. Associated residual lesions should also be looked for, and if necessary, exercise testing should be done to assess the functional capacity. The good outcome of pregnancy in the cohorts reported should not always be extrapolated to women who show evidence of right ventricular impairment before pregnancy.

The Rastelli procedure is a type of surgical repair for patients with transposition and pulmonary stenosis, and many patients who have had this operation also survive to childbearing age.[30] The procedure involves placing a conduit between the right ventricle and the pulmonary artery to relieve the pulmonary stenosis and closing the ventricular septal defect in such a way as to divert the blood from the left ventricle into the aorta. Provided ventricular function is adequate and there are no residual lesions (such as subaortic stenosis or conduit obstruction), a pregnancy may be tolerated after this procedure.

Corrected transposition with ventricular septal defect and pulmonary stenosis

Congenitally corrected transposition (atrioventricular discordance with ventriculoarterial discordance) is commonly associated with ventricular septal defect, pulmonary stenosis, and left atrioventricular valve regurgitation. A common additional problem is congenital complete heart block. When ventricular septal defect exists with pulmonary stenosis, right to left shunting can occur, causing cyanosis. Few data are available about pregnancy in this condition. Presbitero et al reported five patients with ten pregnancies, producing six live births (60%).[1] There were four spontaneous abortions, and two babies were premature. Comparing the outcome of these pregnancies, however, with those with single ventricle or tricuspid atresia or both, and with those with tetralogy of Fallot or pulmonary atresia, the outcome was considerably better (60% versus 31% and 33%, respectively). Since the morphological right ventricle is supporting the systemic circulation in this condition, the volume load of pregnancy may induce ventricular failure. Therefore functional capacity as well as ventricular function and degree of cyanosis must be evaluated at prepregnancy counselling.

The Eisenmenger syndrome

The Eisenmenger syndrome is associated with high pulmonary vascular resistance and a reversed or bidirectional shunt, either at ventricular, aortopulmonary, or atrial level.[31] The degree of pulmonary vascular obstructive disease, therefore, determines the degree of cyanosis. Many patients with Eisenmenger syndrome survive to reproductive age but often get increasing symptoms in the third decade. Pulmonary vascular disease in pregnancy poses significant risks because it limits the right ventricular output through the lungs, and the systemic vasodilatation which occurs favours right to left shunting and therefore exaggerates the degree of cyanosis. Thus, even a minor fall in blood pressure, such as vasovagal faint or minor blood loss, can precipitate sudden death. Clinical experience with the Eisenmenger syndrome in a single institution is limited, and a number of published cases are unsatisfactorily or incompletely documented. Gleicher et al reviewed 44 well documented published cases of the Eisenmenger syndrome and these women had 70 pregnancies.[32] Fifty-two percent of these women died in connection with one of their pregnancies. There was no difference in maternal mortality between the first, second, and third pregnancies, suggesting that if a woman has one successful pregnancy, this should not be taken as a positive prediction for further pregnancies. A particularly high incidence of maternal death was associated with hypovolaemia, thromboembolic phenomena, and pre-eclampsia. Thirty-four percent of all vaginal deliveries, three out of four caesarean sections, and only one out of 14 pregnancy interruptions (the only one by hysterotomy) resulted in maternal death. The number having caesarean section was small and it may be that they were a high risk group already in a haemodynamically compromised state. Only 25·6% of all pregnancies reached term, and 54·9% of all deliveries occurred prematurely. Perinatal mortality was 28·3% and was strongly associated with prematurity. The conclusion from this study was that the prognosis for any woman with Eisenmenger syndrome and pregnancy was extremely grave and that elective abortion was considerably safer than any kind of delivery. Labour and delivery may be a particularly precarious time. Even if the mother has a successful delivery, death often occurs in the next few days from either deteriorating haemodynamics or pulmonary infarction.[34-36] Sudden death has been described up to 22 days after delivery.[37] Thus, women with the Eisenmenger syndrome should be advised strongly against pregnancy.

If a patient becomes pregnant against medical advice, she should be advised to have the pregnancy terminated. A first trimester dilatation and curettage appears to be the procedure of choice for interruption of pregnancy.[32] If she insists on continuing the pregnancy, the following management strategy may be considered:

(1) Careful and coordinated follow-up between the cardiologist and obstetrician with frequent observation to detect early haemodynamic deterioration. A coordinated approach is also essential with the anaesthetist at the time of labour and delivery.

(2) Bed rest is encouraged to reduce the cardiac demands. Rest should be undertaken in the lateral position to avoid fetal compression of the inferior vena cava and so maintain venous return. Complete bed rest should be considered with admission to hospital in the third trimester.

(3) Oxygen delivered by face mask may be administered during episodes of dyspnoea,[37] though there is little evidence that it improves either the maternal or fetal outcome.[38,39]

(4) Fetal wellbeing must be carefully monitored with estriol estimations and fetal ultrasound to evaluate growth.

(5) Congestive heart failure, if it occurs, can be treated with digoxin and diuretics, but diuretics must be used with caution to avoid haemoconcentration.

(6) Controversy exists regarding the use of heparin during pregnancy, and there is no consensus established.[32,40] While there is certainly a hypercoagulable state during pregnancy, these patients are also paradoxically at increased risk of bleeding because of the inherent haemostatic diathesis secondary to their cyanotic heart disease. Prophylactic doses of heparin should be used during the period of bed rest in hospital when the risk is highest, but no case comparison exists and the literature is anecdotal. The largest personal series, recently published, reported a strategy of heparin anticoagulation before delivery by caesarean section under general anaesthesia with coumarin anticoagulation started postpartum.

(7) Vaginal delivery appears to have been chosen more often than elective section.[32] Blood loss with caesarean section is greater than with vaginal delivery. While a normal patient may tolerate blood loss of 500–1000 ml without difficulty, a patient with the Eisenmenger syndrome may not be able to adjust her pulmonary circulation to a sudden fall in peripheral resistance[32] so that blood lost should be replaced immediately volume for volume.

(8) Labour and delivery should take place in an intensive care unit next to an operating room. Cardiac monitoring should be continuous with intravenous lines and intra-arterial lines and frequent measurements of arterial blood gases. A Swan–Ganz catheter may be helpful and permit rapid detection of changes in shunt flow and facilitate haemodynamic assessment,[36,38] but there may be complications in implanting this device,[41] and changes in shunt flow can be monitored by pulse oximetry.

(9) Epidural anaesthesia appears to be safe, provided there is no hypotension. Any fall in blood pressure should immediately be counteracted by the administration of norepinephrine, and loss of blood by transfusion.[39]

(10) Vaginal delivery should be performed. The second stage of delivery should be kept short, assisted by elective forceps or a vacuum extractor.

(11) The patient should be kept in bed and monitored continuously for at least the first day after delivery and then gradually activated. Thromboguards may be helpful in preventing venous stasis and thrombosis in the legs.

(12) The patient should stay in hospital for up to 14 days after delivery because of the continued risk of sudden death.

Editorial comment

Management of labour and delivery in the Eisenmenger syndrome is controversial because individual experience is small. Our own (unpublished) experience is in concert with the Brazilian experience.[33] We favour elective caesarean section under general anaesthesia for reasons given in chapter 26 and always use prophylactic heparin.

References

1 Presbitero P, Somerville J, Stone S, Aruta E, Spiegelhalter D, Rabajoli F. Pregnancy in cyanotic congenital heart disease. Outcome of mother and fetus. *Circulation* 1994; **89**: 2673–6.

2 Neill CA, Swanson S. Outcome of pregnancy in congenital heart disease. *Circulation* 1961; **24**:1003 (abstr).

3 Whittemore R. Congenital heart disease: its impact on pregnancy. *Hosp Pract* 1983; **18**: 65–74.

4 Higgins CB, Mulder DG. Tetralogy of Fallot in the adult. *Am J Cardiol* 1972; **29**: 837–46.

5 Meyer EC, Tulsky AS, Sigmann P, Silber EN. Pregnancy in the presence of tetralogy of Fallot. *Am J Cardiol* 1964; **14**: 874–9.

6 Baker JL, Russell CS, Grainger RG, Taylor DG, Thornton JA, Verel D. Closed pulmonary valvotomy in the management of Fallot's tetralogy complicated by pregnancy. *J Obstet Gynecol* 1963; **70**: 154–7.

7 Dennis NR, Warren J. Risks to the offspring of patients with uncommon congenital heart defects. *J Med Genet* 1981; **18**: 8–16.

8 Singh H, Bolton PJ, Oakley CM. Pregnancy after surgical correction of tetralogy of Fallot. *BMJ* 1982; **285**: 168–70.

9 Ando M, Takao A, Mori K. Genetic and environmental factors in congenital heart disease. In: Inouye E, Nishimura H, eds. *Gene-environment interaction in common diseases*. Baltimore: University Park Press, 1977: 71–88.

10 Nora JJ, Nora AH. Recurrence risks in children having one parent with congenital heart disease. *Circulation* 1976; **53**: 701–2.

11 Zellers MT, Driscoll DJ, Michels VV. Prevalence of significant congenital heart defects in children of parents with Fallot's tetralogy. *Am J Cardiol* 1990; **65**: 523–6.

12 Gersony WM, Batthany S, Bowman FO, Malm JR. Late follow-up of patients evaluated hemodynamically after total correction of tetralogy of Fallot. *J Thorac Cardiovasc Surg* 1973; **66**: 209–13.

13 Connolly HM, Warnes CA. Outcome of pregnancy in women with complex pulmonary atresia. *J Am Coll Cardiol* 1995: 377A.

14 Waickman LA, Skorton DJ, Varner MW, Ehmke DA, Goplerud CP. Ebstein's anomaly in pregnancy. *Am J Cardiol* 1984; **53**: 357–8.

15 Donnelly JE, Brown JM, Radford DJ. Pregnancy outcome and Ebstein's anomaly. *Br Heart J* 1991; **66**: 368–71.

16 Connolly HM, Warnes CA. Ebstein's anomaly: outcome of pregnancy. *J Am Coll Cardiol* 1994; **23**: 1194–8.

17 Beischer NA, MacKay EV. *Obstetrics and the newborn*. 2nd ed. Sydney: WB Saunders, 1986; 406–20.

18 Danielson GK, Driscoll DJ, Mair DD, Warnes CA, Oliver WC. Operative treatment of Ebstein's anomaly. *J Thorac Cardiovasc Surg* 1992; **104**: 1195–202.

19 Ammash NM, Warnes CA. Long-term survival in unoperated single ventricle. *J Am Coll Cardiol* 1995: 378A.

20 Stiller RJ, Vintzileos AM, Nochimson DJ, Clement D, Campbell WA, Leach CN. Single ventricle in pregnancy. Case report and review of the literature. *Obstet Gynecol* 1984; **64**: 18S–20S.

21 Leibbrandt G, Münch U, Gander M. Two successful pregnancies in a patient with single ventricle and transposition of the great arteries. *Int J Cardiol* 1982; **1**: 257–62.

22 Collins ML, Leal J, Thompson NJ. Tricuspid atresia and pregnancy. *Obstet Gynecol* 1977; **50(I suppl)**: 72S–3S.

23 Fontan F, Baudet E. Surgical repair of tricuspid atresia. *Thorax* 1971; **26**: 240–8.

24 Kreutzer G, Galindez E, Bono H, de Palma C, Laura JP. An operation for the correction of tricuspid atresia. *J Thorac Cardiovasc Surg* 1973; **66**: 613–21.

25 Canobbio M, Mair D. Pregnancy outcome following Fontan operation. *Circulation* 1993; **88**: I–290.

26 Mustard WT. Successful two-staged correction of transposition of the great vessels. *Surgery* 1964; **55**: 469–72.

27 Lynch-Salamon DI, Maze SS, Combs CA. Pregnancy after Mustard repair for transposition of the great arteries. *Obstet Gynecol* 1993; **82(Part II suppl)** : 676–9.

28 Warnes CA, Somerville J. Transposition of the great arteries: results in adolescents and adults late after the Mustard procedure. *Br Heart J* 1987; **58**: 148–55.

29 Clarkson PM, Wilson NJ, Neutze JM, North RA, Calder AL, Barratt-Boyes BG. Outcome of pregnancy after the Mustard operation for transposition of the great arteries with intact ventricular septum. *J Am Coll Cardiol* 1994; **24**: 190–3.

30 Rastelli GC, McGoon DC, Wallace RB. Anatomic correction of transposition of the great arteries with ventricular septal defect and subpulmonary stenosis. *J Thorac Cardiovasc Surg* 1969; **58**: 545–51.

31 Wood P. The Eisenmenger syndrome. *BMJ* 1958; **2**: 701–9.

32 Gleicher N, Midwall J, Hochberger D, Jaffin H. Eisenmenger's syndrome and pregnancy. *Obstet Gynecol Surv* 1975; **34**: 721–41.

33 Avila WS, Grinberg M, Snitcowsky R, *et al*. Maternal and fetal outcome in pregnant women with Eisenmenger's syndrome. *Eur Heart J* 1995; **16**: 460–4.

34 Lieber S, Dewilde PH, Huyghens L, Traey E, Gepts E. Eisenmenger's syndrome and pregnancy. *Acta Cardiol* 1985; **40**: 421–4.

35 Heytens L, Alexander JP. Maternal and neonatal death associated with Eisenmenger's syndrome. *Acta Anaesth Belg* 1986; **37**: 45–51.

36 Arias F. Maternal death in a patient with Eisenmenger's syndrome. *Obstet Gynecol* 1977; **50(suppl)**: 76S–80S.

37 Neilson G, Gatea EG, Blunt A. Eisenmenger's syndrome and pregnancy. *Med J Aust* 1971; **1**: 431–4.

38 Midwall J, Jaffin H, Herman MV, Kupersmith J. Shunt flow and pulmonary hemodynamics during labor and delivery in the Eisenmenger syndrome. *Am J Cardiol* 1978; **42**: 299–303.
39 Bitsch M, Johansen C, Wennevold A, Osler M. Eisenmenger's syndrome and pregnancy. *Eur J Obstet Gynecol Reprod Biol* 1988; **28**: 69–74.
40 Pitts JA, Crosby WM, Basta LL. Eisenmenger syndrome in pregnancy. Does heparin prophylaxis improve the maternal mortality rate? *Am Heart J* 1977; **93**: 321–6.
41 Devitt JH, Noble WH, Byrick RJ. A Swan–Ganz catheter related complication in a patient with Eisenmenger's syndrome. *Anesthesiology* 1982; **57**: 335–7.

7: Pulmonary hypertension

CELIA OAKLEY

Whatever its cause pulmonary hypertension is associated with high maternal risk during pregnancy. If the abnormally raised pulmonary vascular resistance is maintained blood flow through the lungs may fail to rise with resultant fall in systemic blood pressure, increased right to left shunting or right ventricular failure.

Pulmonary hypertension is termed primary when no cause can be found. It is a rare disease seen most commonly in women and is usually fatal.[1-5] It has an incidence of only about 1 in 500 000/year and only about 100 deaths/year from this cause are registered with the Office for Population Censuses and Surveys (OPCS) in the United Kingdom. Most series give an average survival of three years[1-5] from the time of diagnosis but diagnosis tends to be late and the duration of the disease is variable, ranging from weeks or months to 30 or 40 years.[5-7] In a study from the Mayo Clinic only 24 of 120 patients were alive after five years.[3] Young women in their childbearing years are most commonly affected. Few cardiac centres will see more than one or two new patients a year unless they have a special interest. Experience of the disease in pregnancy is therefore small.

Aetiology

A growing literature on an association between amphetamine like anorexigens[8-10] particularly fenfluramine[11-14] and primary pulmonary hypertension is consistent with previous observations of an "epidemic" of primary pulmonary hypertension after introduction of aminorex fumarate in the 1960s[19] and with use of dexfenfluramine[17,18] more recently. These agents are less commonly prescribed in the UK where the disease is far less common than in France and Belgium where 20% of 73 patients with primary pulmonary hypertension described from a specialist centre had taken fenfluramines.[20] Genetic susceptibility may be a factor. Familial cases unassociated with appetite suppressants have been reported.[21] Most cases in the UK are not associated with their use.[19] Other causative factors may play a role including HIV infection[22,23] and cirrhosis[24,25] but these two account for only a small proportion of cases.

Primary pulmonary hypertension (PPH) in typical form is easily diagnosed after clinical examination with ECG (Figure 7.4) and chest radiograph (Figure 7.5). Echocardiography (Figures 7.6 and 7.7), a perfusion lung scan (Figure 7.8) and pulmonary arteriography (Figures 7.1 and 7.2) complete the diagnostic studies[26] but it is important to exclude underlying conditions. Structural heart disease, particularly mitral valve disease and congenital septal defects if not detected clinically, are shown on echocardiography, and collagen vascular diseases, interstitial lung disease, chronic hypoventilation in muscular dystrophies or the Pickwickian syndrome by an autoimmune screen, lung function tests, and arterial blood gases.

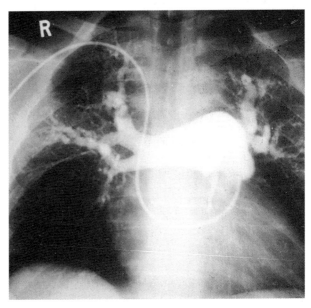

FIGURE 7.1—*Pulmonary arteriogram from a patient with chronic pulmonary hypertension apparently dating from an unsuccessful first pregnancy some years earlier. There was no history or evidence to suggest autoimmune disease. A coagulopathy was not detected and the pulmonary hypertension was considered to be thromboembolic in origin. Both lower lobe pulmonary arteries were completely blocked and the arteriogram also shows obstruction of sub-branches to the upper lobes. The main pulmonary artery is seen to be grossly dilated and the pulmonary artery pressure was at systemic level. This patient subsequently survived a pregnancy (undertaken against advice).*

Chronic thromboembolic pulmonary hypertension[27–29] and postarteritic pulmonary hypertension,[30] (Chapter 13) with or without a Takayasu syndrome affecting the systemic arteries, are even rarer than primary pulmonary hypertension. Pulmonary arteriography shows major arterial obstructions and perfusion lung scans show segmental or lobar gaps in perfusion. In this age group chronic thromboembolic pulmonary hypertension is usually associated with an inherited coagulopathy and a family and personal history of venous thrombosis and pulmonary embolism. Continued anticoagulant treatment is essential.

Pulmonary hypertension may also persist or advance after repair of ventricular septal defect in childhood (Table 7.1).[31]

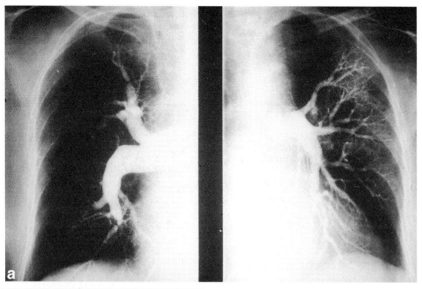

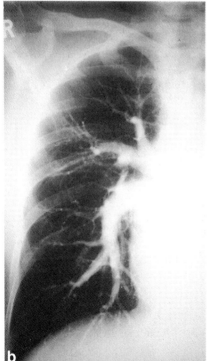

FIGURE 7.2—(a) *Right (on the left) and left pulmonary arteriograms from a woman with chronic pulmonary hypertension of presumed thromboembolic origin. The central pulmonary arteries are dilated and peripheral filling is poor especially to the right lung as a result of multiple peripheral "webs" and blocks in segmental pulmonary artery branches. The pulmonary artery pressure was at systemic level. This arteriogram is shown for comparison with the normal right pulmonary arteriogram. (b) From a patient with severe primary pulmonary hypertension.*

Primary type pulmonary hypertension may complicate many auto-immune diseases,[32] systemic lupus (SLE),[33,34] mixed connective tissue disease (MCTD),[35] systemic sclerosis,[36] Sjögren's syndrome,[37] and rheumatoid arthritis.[38] As many as 14% of SLE patients screened by

TABLE 7.1—*Classification of pulmonary hypertension.*

- **Pulmonary hypertension** (Unassociated with cardiac or pulmonary parenchymal disease)

  Primary pulmonary hypertension
  Primary-type pulmonary hypertension in:
     Systemic lupus erythematosus
     Mixed connective tissue disease
     Rheumatoid arthritis
     Sjörgen's syndrome
  Residual after repair of congenital cardiac septal defects in childhood

- **Postarteritic pulmonary hypertension** affecting the larger pulmonary arteries (with or without Takayasu syndrome)

- **Thromboembolic pulmonary hypertension** with inherited coagulopathy

echocardiographic Doppler have pulmonary hypertension.[34] Because of its high incidence, pulmonary hypertension should be excluded in any patient with collagen vascular disease, particularly lupus, before reassuring the patient that she is fit for pregnancy (Chapter 13). Neither the pathology nor the clinical course differ from those of primary pulmonary hypertension unassociated with these disorders.

Pathology and pathophysiology

The pathology and pathophysiology of primary pulmonary hypertension have been reviewed recently by Rubin.[39] By the time patients with primary pulmonary hypertension are diagnosed most of the lung vessels show irreversible changes (Figure 7.3) and only a few pulmonary arteries are capable of responding to a vasodilator.

Table 7.2 shows the pathology of primary pulmonary hypertension under four headings. The first two are often combined in the same patient. Pulmonary veno-occlusive disease tends to be a distinct entity but some patients with a plexiform arteriopathy also show veno-occlusive changes.

TABLE 7.2—*Vascular lesions causing pulmonary hypertension.*

- Thrombotic arteriopathy
- Plexiform arteriopathy
- Pulmonary veno-occlusive disease
- Pulmonary capillary haemangiomatosis

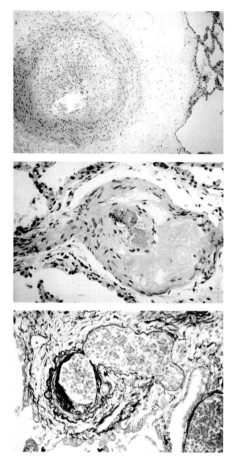

FIGURE 7.3—(a) Proliferative changes with increased cellularity and intimal thickening, (b) a nearly completely occluded small pulmonary artery, and (c) a typical plexiform lesion in postmortem sections from a patient with primary pulmonary hypertension.

Primary pulmonary hypertension and pregnancy

Primary pulmonary hypertension is associated with high maternal risk and mortality,[40-43] 15 out of 37 patients with PPH died during pregnancy or in the early postpartum period in one series.[40] Mild or early cases are rarely recognised.

This high mortality is to be expected from the haemodynamics. Right ventricular stroke volume is seriously compromised by the throttle imposed by the small resistance vessels in the lung. Cardiac output is dependent on heart rate and blood pressure on systemic vascular resistance. The right ventricle is much less well vascularised than the left ventricle as it is normally an undemanding low pressure chamber and receives both systolic and diastolic coronary flow. When the right ventricular pressure rises systolic coronary blood flow ceases and it then becomes like the left ventricle, dependent on diastolic coronary blood flow. Tachycardia increases the ischaemia already imposed by high pressure.

Diagnosis

The predominant symptoms are usually progressive dyspnoea and excessive fatigue, and some patients are first seen on account of effort-associated syncope. Anginal chest pain may result from right ventricular ischaemia.[30]

Haemoptysis can be troublesome in patients with PPH and occasionally is a first symptom. It can be caused by rupture of thin-walled plexiform vascular dilatations in the lung and exacerbated by warfarin treatment but it is not usually a major problem and warfarin should be continued. It can also result from pulmonary thromboembolism and be prevented by long-term warfarin treatment.

The physical signs are often subtle though there is usually a pulmonary ejection click and loud pulmonary closure sound as well as a dominant venous A wave in the neck and there may be an early diastolic murmur of pulmonary regurgitation. Patients with more advanced disease may also have an inspiratory tricuspid regurgitant murmur and prominent jugular V wave.

Pregnancy may precipitate anginal chest pain, hypotension, syncope, and right ventricular failure. The systemic arterial oxygen content may be normal or it may be reduced either as a result of shunting across a patent foramen ovale or because of mismatching in the lungs and, in advanced cases, the increased venous admixture caused by the low oxygen saturation of venous blood returning to the heart. Moreover, the disease itself may advance during pregnancy as there is some suggestion that it is under hormonal influence.[44,45]

Such is the risk as well as the potentially deleterious effect on the disease that pregnancy is permanently contraindicated. Patients should be told this early on. Medical treatment may alleviate but does not cure the disease so tubal ligation is advised. Oestrogen-containing oral contraceptives may accelerate the rate of progression of the disease.[44,45]

Unfortunately patients are sometimes first diagnosed during pregnancy. These include those with a long history of dyspnoea of unrecognised cause as well as some patients with recent onset or deterioration of previously mild disease. Syncope is a common presenting symptom. The condition is often missed because it is not considered, dyspnoea being disregarded because of the pregnancy and even syncope explained away. The ECG although abnormal, may also be overlooked or pulmonary embolism suspected (Figure 7.4). A chest x ray (Figure 7.5) and perfusion lung scan may have been omitted on account of the pregnancy, and echocardiography although diagnostic is sought only if there is suspicion of cardiac abnormality. It shows the dominant right ventricle and dilated main pulmonary arteries (Figure 7.6). The relation between right and left ventricular systolic and diastolic pressures can be assessed from movement of the ventricular septum and the right ventricular pressure can be estimated from the tricuspid regurgitant velocity (Figure 7.7). Lung scans (Figure 7.8) and cardiac catheterisation are unnecessary if the patient insists on continuing the pregnancy.

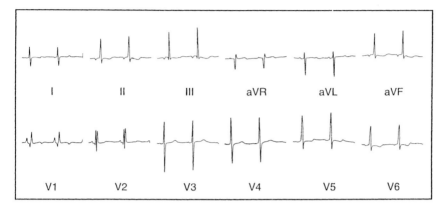

FIGURE 7.4—*Typical electrocardiogram in primary pulmonary hypertension showing sinus rhythm with right atrial P waves (V1), an inferior axis and evidence of right ventricular pressure overload. The changes are perhaps not dramatic but indicate severe disease—the pulmonary artery pressure was at systemic level in this patient who has since undergone successful heart–lung transplantation. Right ventricular hypertrophy is much more pronounced in patients who have had pulmonary hypertension since childhood.*

Termination should be advised in any patient with PPH who has become pregnant. If the patient refuses termination close supervision of her management and progress are necessary. Maximum rest is desirable because of the limited cardiac output and the risk of right ventricular failure, exercise-induced fall in blood pressure causing syncope, or increase in right to left shunting either within the lung or across a foramen ovale with consequent hypoxaemia. Early admission to hospital is advisable for rest and monitoring both of mother and fetus.

Management in pregnancy

Anticoagulant treatment with warfarin should be continued during pregnancy despite a small risk to the fetus but the international normalised ratio need not be higher than 2·0. Anticoagulants are needed because the thrombotic arteriopathy is thought to be due to thrombosis in situ on an abnormal or denuded endothelium and because of the risk of venous thromboembolism as a result of the low output and the hypercoagulable state induced by pregnancy. Pulse oximetry should be used to detect any fall in systemic oxygen saturation. A calcium channel blocker such as nifedipine or diltiazem should be given to try to induce some pulmonary

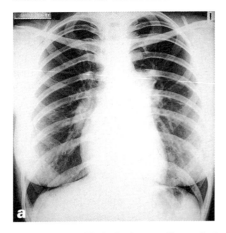
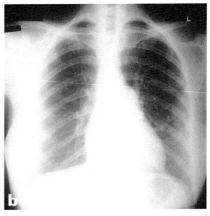

FIGURE 7.5—*Typical chest radiograph in primary pulmonary hypertension. (a) A prominent dilated main pulmonary artery and a dilated right atrium and clear lung fields with increased transradiency because of diminished pulmonary capillary volume. The peripheral pulmonary artery branches are narrowed ("pruned") rather abruptly distal to the heavy hilar branches. In (b) the abnormalities are much less florid but the dilated main pulmonary artery is clearly seen. This x ray film was passed as normal in a young woman whose severe primary pulmonary hypertension was diagnosed the following year when she developed right ventricular failure in pregnancy.*

vasodilatation. Not everyone responds favourably with a fall in pulmonary vascular resistance and a rise in right ventricular stroke volume. Like any other vasodilators used in pulmonary hypertension, these agents can cause a fall in oxygen saturation as a result of increased "shunting" within the lung, and systemic hypotension if the cardiac output fails to increase, and this includes continuous infusion of prostacyclin which does not confer any advantage. Oxygen should be used through nasal cannulae to minimise hypoxaemia and also because of its pulmonary vasodilating effect. Nitric oxide inhalation may lower calculated pulmonary vascular resistance but as with prostacycline, patients with advanced disease fail to benefit because of sometimes profound drops in systemic arterial saturation (Table 7.3).

Despite every therapeutic effort, symptomatic deterioration is usually progressive particularly in the second and third trimester, with extreme dyspnoea, almost equally disabling fatigue, right ventricular failure, and often chest pain as a result of right ventricular ischaemia. Most deaths are peripartum and are precipitated by hypotension especially after blood loss, sudden arrhythmia, pulmonary embolism, or right ventricular failure.[41] Premature labour is common and fetal wastage is high.

Management of delivery

Slowing of fetal growth or maternal deterioration may bring a need for early delivery. Elective caesarean section is preferable to vaginal delivery

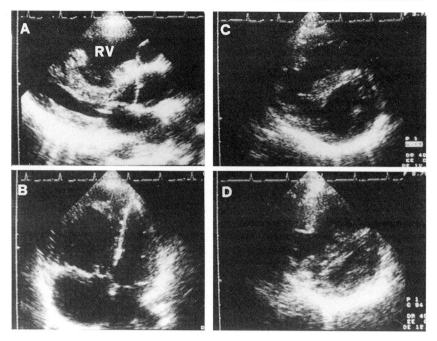

FIGURE 7.6—*Echocardiograms from a patient with severe primary pulmonary hypertension. The parasternal long axis view (A) shows a prominent dilated right ventricle (RV) which is displacing the ventricular septum posteriorly. The dilatation of the right heart chamber is shown also on the apical four chamber view (B). The short axis views show squashing of the left ventricle by the displaced septum in systole (D) indicating that the right ventricular pressure is suprasystemic. The septum assumes a more normal but still rather flat appearance in diastole (C).*

because it is much quicker and spares the mother the physical exertion, thereby protecting the fetus from hypoxaemia.

Although epidural analgesia is popular with anaesthetists for delivery of patients with heart disease, general anaesthesia is preferable for anyone with a fixed low cardiac output in whom vasodilatation may precipitate a drop in blood pressure or increase right to left shunting and hypoxaemia. It provides rest with reduced metabolic demand, maximum oxygenation, and minimal interference with the forces conserving a fragile circulatory reserve. Vasodilatation and shifts in the distribution of the blood volume can be minimised. The anaesthetist should avoid agents with a negative inotropic effect. Hydration should be generous and any blood loss immediately corrected because maintenance of cardiac output is dependent on a high right ventricular filling pressure.

Epidural anaesthesia is worse. The patient is awake and worried. The opiate infusion usually given is a venodilator and reduces venous return. The epidural agent is a systemic vasodilator. The combination tends to redistribute blood out of the thorax and into the periphery. If there is then

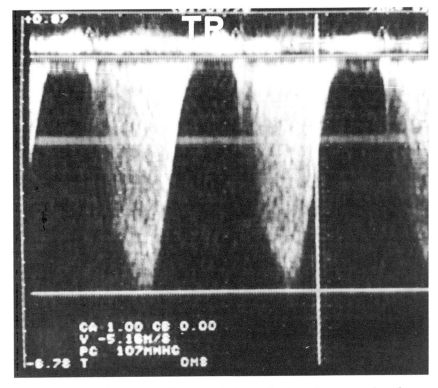

FIGURE 7.7—*Continuous wave Doppler velocity profiles from the same patient show a peak tricuspid regurgitant (TR) velocity of 5·0 m/sec corresponding to an instantaneous peak gradient of 107 mm Hg and a right ventricular pressure of about 115 mm Hg.*

any uncorrected blood loss the blood pressure may plummet and cardiac arrest follow.

Management postpartum

After delivery patients should be returned to the ICU with continued monitoring of venous and arterial blood pressure and arterial saturation, followed by slow mobilisation and resumption of anticoagulant treatment. Swan–Ganz catheterisation and an intra-arterial line are not usually necessary because the systemic blood pressure and the central venous pressure are the best guidelines.

Right ventricular failure may resolve dramatically after delivery. In one patient first recognised late in pregnancy and referred to us at term in profound right ventricular failure, haemodynamic stability was restored after successful delivery by caesarean section under general anaesthesia. Five years later she remains stable in New York Heart Association class II. She is not in right ventricular failure, she still has severe pulmonary hypertension which, however, is no worse.

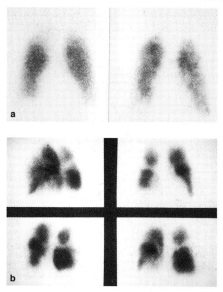

FIGURE 7.8—(a) *Ventilation (on the left) and perfusion lung scans from a patient with advanced primary pulmonary hypertension. The perfusion scan shows a rather mottled fluffy appearance throughout the lungs and contrasts sharply with the stark holes in perfusion seen in a patient with postarteritic pulmonary hypertension and multiple branch stenoses* (b) *(four views).*

TABLE 7.3—*Treatment of primary pulmonary hypertension.*

High dose calcium channel blocking agents: nifedipine or diltiazem

Anticoagulation with warfarin

Antiplatelet agents—aspirin or dipyridamole

Prostacyclin (epoprostenol)—by continuous intravenous infusion

Nitric oxide inhalation—10 to 40 parts/million in air intermittently

Oxygen inhalation—by nasal cannulae 60% continuously

Atrial septostomy—to maintain systemic output (at the expense of arterial oxygen desaturation)

Heart–lung transplantation

Pulmonary veno-occlusive disease and pulmonary capillary haemangiomatosis are both exceptionally rare but the hazard of pregnancy is the same.

Residual pulmonary hypertension after repair of congenital cardiac defects in childhood

An increasing number of children who have undergone successful surgery for congenital heart disease now live to become adults. Many are no longer

107

being followed up because they have moved, their cardiologist has retired, or they have lost touch. They and their doctors may believe that follow up is no longer necessary or that they are "cured" because they are murmur-free. Particularly after closure of non-restrictive ventricular septal defect pulmonary hypertension may persist but be asymptomatic until pregnancy which may precipitate right ventricular failure. Thorough cardiac evaluation is necessary for any woman with a history of repaired congenital heart disease who seeks advice about pregnancy or who is already pregnant (Chapter 5).[31]

Postarteritic pulmonary hypertension

Postarteritic pulmonary hypertension may be associated with renovascular hypertension, aortic regurgitation, systolic hypertension caused by non-expansile conducting arteries or acquired aortic coarctations, or seemingly occur on its own. Each patient is different and needs full evaluation. The haemodynamic hazard from pulmonary hypertension in pregnancy depends on the severity of the right ventricular outflow obstruction and on whether cardiac output can be increased, as well as on the coexistence of abnormalities in the systemic circulation.

Postarteritic pulmonary hypertension affecting the major pulmonary artery branches may accompany a large vessel systemic arteritis in the Takayasu syndrome.[46-48] It may coexist with systemic lupus erythematosus or relapsing polychondritis (Chapter 13) or occur apparently on its own. A patchy pulmonary arteritis may attract occlusive thrombus or be followed by arterial strictures identified clinically by murmurs heard over the lungs. Haemoptysis from systemic bronchial collateral vessels can be a presenting feature or complicate pregnancy. Haemoptysis is more common and apt to be larger and more dangerous in large vessel pulmonary hypertension than in primary type pulmonary hypertension because segments of lung denuded of a pulmonary arterial supply depend on enlarged bronchial vessels which run submucosally to anastomose with pulmonary artery radicals. The inflammatory arteritis appears to be self-terminating and pulmonary hypertension of this type may not be relentlessly progressive. Because patients may present with constitutional features or haemoptysis the pulmonary hypertension may be recognised when it is mild or moderate and pregnancy is not invariably contraindicated.

Advice about the safety of pregnancy needs to be individually based on the severity of the right ventricular obstruction, cardiovascular reserve, and the presence or absence of other complications caused by the systemic arteritis. These patients can be stable for many years and deterioration of the disease does not seem to occur during pregnancy. One patient who presented with haemoptysis in pregnancy has now been followed for more than 25 years and is well despite a pulmonary artery pressure at systemic level, pulmonary regurgitation and systemic hypertension. Another who was referred with dyspnoea and murmurs over both lungs has completed two pregnancies and two others remain well with burned out disease after successful pregnancies.

One patient who was first seen at the age of 19 on account of systemic hypertension caused by renal artery stenosis and treated successfully by angioplasty was subsequently referred with dyspnoea at age 23, and was found to have moderately severe pulmonary hypertension with large vessel disease. Although she had previously been strongly counselled against pregnancy we advised her that pregnancy should be safe though it was likely that she would become more breathless during it. She has since had two successful pregnancies without developing right ventricular failure or perceptible deterioration but has had a number of worrying haemoptyses treated by embolisation of the bronchial collateral supply to the right upper lobe of her lung, to which the pulmonary artery branch was completely occluded. She also has occlusion of the left carotid and left subclavian arteries at their origins from the aortic arch but has had no evidence of active disease since she was first seen.

Chronic thromboembolic pulmonary hypertension

Chronic thromboembolic pulmonary hypertension is much rarer than acute pulmonary embolism which, if not quickly fatal, usually resolves completely. Most patients with chronic thromboembolic pulmonary hypertension have a coagulopathy. This may be an inherited abnormality of haemostatic factors such as antithrombin III, protein S, or protein C deficiency so a family history of thrombosis and embolism should be sought. Parents should also be checked for the presence of antiphospholipid antibodies or malignancy, particularly adenocarcinoma or chorion carcinoma which may embolise to the lungs. Chronic thromboembolic pulmonary hypertension affecting the major or first segmental pulmonary artery branches may be treated successfully by surgical thrombectomy. This must be followed by lifelong anticoagulant treatment. The safety of pregnancy needs to be judged on an individual basis as these are rare and individually disparate patients.

Pulmonary hypertension whatever its origin is associated with substantial morbidity and mortality, particularly when it complicates pregnancy. Although it always causes considerable dyspnoea on exertion, diagnosis tends to be late and there are few therapeutic options. Earlier diagnosis may come from heightened awareness and as treatment has recently been shown to be effective in a few patients this could be of value. Nevertheless, the prospects for safe and successful pregnancy remain poor for the majority.

References

1 Rich S, *et al.* Primary pulmonary hypertension: a national prospective study. *Ann Intern Med* 1987; **107**: 216–23.

2 Suarez LD, Sciandro EE, Llera JJ, *et al.* Long term follow-up in primary pulmonary hypertension. *Br Heart J* 1979; **41**: 702–8.
3 Fuster V, *et al.* Primary pulmonary hypertension: natural history and the importance of thrombosis. *Circulation* 1984; **70**: 580–7.
4 Oakley CM. Primary pulmonary hypertension: case series from the United Kingdom. *Chest* 1994; **105(suppl)**: 29S–32S.
5 Rozkovec A, Montanes P, Oakley CM. Factors that influence the outcome of primary pulmonary hypertension. *Br Heart J* 1986; **55**: 449–58.
6 Charters AD, Baker WD. Primary pulmonary hypertension of unusually long duration. *Br Heart J* 1970; **32**: 130–3.
7 Trell E. Benign, idiopathic pulmonary hypertension. Two further cases of unusually long duration. *Acta Med Scand* 1973; **193**: 137–43.
8 Malmquist J, Trell E, Torp A, Lindstrom C. A case of drug-induced (?) pulmonary hypertension. *Acta Med Scand* 1970; **188**: 265–72.
9 Cameron J, Wagh L, Loadsman T, White P, Radford DJ. Possible association of pulmonary hypertension with an anorectic drug. *Med J Aust* 1984; **140**: 595–7.
10 Nall KC, Rubin LJ, Lipkind S, Sennesh JD. Reversible pulmonary hypertension associated with anorexigen use. *Am J Med* 1991; **91**: 97–9.
11 Douglas JG, Munro JF, Kitchen AH, Muir AL, Proudfoot AT. Pulmonary hypertension and fenfluramine. *BMJ* 1981; **223**: 881–3.
12 Gaul G, Blazek G, Deutsch E, Heeger H. Ein fall von chronischer Pulmonar Hypertonie nach Fenfluramineinnahme. *Wien Klin Wochenschr* 1982; **22**: 618–21.
13 McMurray J, Bloomfield P, Miller HC. Irreversible pulmonary hypertension after treatment with fenfluramine. *BMJ* 1986; **292**: 239–40.
14 Pouwels HMM, Smeets JLRM, Cheriex EC, Wouters EFM. Pulmonary hypertension and fenfluramine. *Eur Respir J* 1990; **3**: 606–7.
15 Follath F, Buckart F, Schweizer W. Drug-induced pulmonary hypertension. *BMJ* 1971; **i**: 265–6.
16 Kay JM, Smith P, Heath D. Aminorex and the pulmonary circulation. *Thorax* 1971; **26**: 262–70.
17 Atanassoff PG, Weiss BK, Schmid ER, Tornic M. Pulmonary hypertension and dexfenfluramine. *Lancet* 1992; **i**: 436.
18 Roche N, Labrune S, Braun JM, Huchon GJ. Pulmonary hypertension and dexfenfluramine. *Lancet* 1992; **i**: 436–7.
19 Thomas SHL, Butt AY, Corris PA, *et al.* Appetite suppressants and primary pulmonary hypertension in the United Kingdom. *Br Heart J* 1995; **74**: 660–3.
20 Brenot F, Herve P, Petipretz P, Parent F, Duroux P, Simmoneau G. Primary pulmonary hypertension and fenfluramine use. *Br Heart J* 1993; **70**: 537–41.
21 Langleben D. Familial pulmonary hypertension. *Chest* 1994; **105(suppl)**: 13S–16S.
22 Legou B, Piette AM, Bouchet PE, *et al.* Pulmonary hypertension and HIV infection. *Am J Med* 1990; **89**: 122.
23 Mette SA, Palevsky HI, Pietra GG. Primary pulmonary hypertension in association with human immuno-deficiency virus infection: a possible viral aetiology for the forms of hypertensive arteriopathy. *Am Rev Resp Dis* 1992; **145**: 1196–1200.
24 Hadengue A, Benhayoun MK, Lebrec D, *et al.* Pulmonary hypertension complicating portal hypertension: prevalence and relation to splanchnic haemodynamics. *Gastroenterology* 1991; **100**: 520–8.
25 McDonnell PJ, Toye PA, Hutchins GM. Primary pulmonary hypertension and cirrhosis: are they related? *Am Rev Respir Dis* 1983; **127**: 437–41.
26 Oakley CM. Investigation and diagnosis of pulmonary hypertension in adults. In: Morice AH, ed. *Clinical pulmonary hypertension.* London: Portland Press Ltd, 1995: 81–113.
27 Rich S, Levitsky S, Brundage BH. Pulmonary hypertension from chronic pulmonary thromboembolism. *Ann Intern Med* 1988; **108**: 425–34.
28 Moser KM, Auger WR, Fedullo PE. Chronic major vessel thromboembolic pulmonary hypertension. *Circulation* 1990; **81**: 1735–43.
29 Durant JR, Cortes EM. Occlusive pulmonary vascular disease associated with haemoglobin SC disease. *Am Heart J* 1966; **71**: 100–6.
30 Lande A, Bard R. Takayasu's arteritis: an unrecognized cause of pulmonary hypertension. *Angiography* 1976; **27**: 114–21.
31 Jackson GM, Dildy GA, Varner MW, Clark SL. Severe pulmonary hypertension in pregnancy following successful repair of ventricular septal defect in childhood. *Obstet Gynecol* 1993; **82(suppl 21)**: 680–2.

32 Kasukawa R, Nishimaki T, Takagi T, Miyawaki S, Yokohari R, Tsunematsu T. Pulmonary hypertension in connective tissue disease. Clinical analysis of sixty patients in multi-institutional study. *Clin Rheumatol* 1990; **9**: 56–62.

33 Santini D, Fox D, Kloner RA, *et al.* Pulmonary hypertension in systemic lupus erythematosus: haemodynamics and effects of vasodilator therapy. *Clin Cardiol* 1980; **3**: 406–11.

34 Simonson JS, Nelson BS, Petri M, Hellmann DB. Pulmonary hypertension in systemic lupus erythematosus. *J Rheumatol* 1989; **16**: 918–25.

35 Kobayash H, Sano T, Fi K, *et al.* Mixed connective tissue disease with fatal pulmonary hypertension. *Acta Patholofica Jpn* 1982; **32**: 1121–9.

36 Morgan JM, Griffiths M, du Bois RM, Evans TW. Hypoxic pulmonary vasoconstriction in systemic sclerosis and primary pulmonary hypertension. *Chest* 1991; **99**: 551–6.

37 Hedgpeth MT, Boulware DW. Pulmonary hypertension in primary Sjögren's syndrome. *Ann Rheum Dis* 1988; **47**: 251–3.

38 Asherson RA, Morgan SH, Hackett D. Rheumatoid arthritis and pulmonary hypertension. *J Rheumatol* 1984; **12**: 154–9.

39 Rubin LJ. Pathology and pathophysiology of primary pulmonary hypertension. *Am J Cardiol* 1995; **75**: 51A–4A.

40 Elkayam U, Gleicher N. Primary pulmonary hypertension in pregnancy. In: Elkayam U, Gleicher N, eds. *Cardiac problems in pregnancy: diagnosis and management of maternal and fetal disease.* New York: Alan R Liss, 1982: 153–60.

41 Nelson DM, Main E, Crafford W, *et al.* Peripartum heart failure due to primary pulmonary hypertension. *Obstet Gynecol* 1983; **62**: 599–635.

42 Dawkins KD, Burke CM, Billingham ME, *et al.* Primary pulmonary hypertension and pregnancy. *Chest* 1986; **89**: 383–8.

43 Takenchi T, Nishii O, Okamura T, *et al.* Primary pulmonary hypertension in pregnancy. *Int J Gynaecol Obstet* 1988; **26**: 145–50.

44 Oakley CM, Somerville J. Oral contraceptives and progressive pulmonary vascular disease. *Lancet* 1968; **i**: 890–3.

45 Kleiger RE, Boer M, Ingham RE, *et al.* Pulmonary hypertension in patients using oral contraceptives: a report of six cases. *Chest* 1976; **69**: 143–7.

46 Ishikawa K, Matsuura S. Occlusive thromboaortopathy (Takayasu's disease) and pregnancy: clinical course and management of 33 pregnancies and deliveries. *Am J Cardiol* 1982; **50**: 1293–1300.

47 Wong VCW, Wang RYE, Tse TF. Pregnancy and Takayasu's arteritis. *Am J Med* 1983; **75**: 597.

48 Winn HN, Setaro JF, Mazor M, *et al.* Severe Takayasu's arteritis in pregnancy: the role of central haemodynamic monitoring. *Am J Obstet Gynecol* 1988; **159**: 1135–6.

8: Rheumatic heart disease

PAULO RIBEIRO, MUAYAD AL ZAIBAG

The incidence of rheumatic heart disease is dwindling in the western world and in many areas the disease has virtually disappeared.[1-5] We practise in a tertiary care referral centre on the west coast of the United States and have seen only two pregnant patients with rheumatic heart disease during the past three years, despite recent reports of the resurgence of pockets of rheumatic fever in this country. In contrast, in the 1980s, during our practice in Saudi Arabia where rheumatic heart disease is still prevalent, mitral stenosis was the most common cardiac lesion in pregnant patients with heart disease.[6,7] In developing countries rheumatic heart disease is the main cause of morbidity and mortality during pregnancy. Mitral stenosis is responsible for most of the complications in pregnant patients with rheumatic heart disease (Figure 8.1).[7-10] In this chapter we discuss the interaction between pregnancy and rheumatic heart disease and their management.

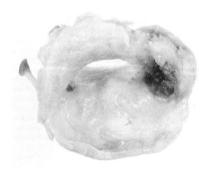

FIGURE 8.1—*Severe rheumatic stenosis of a surgically excised mitral valve. Note the small valve orifice area, which causes a decrease in cardiac output and increase in left atrial pressure and is responsible for the symptoms in pregnant patients.*

Acute rheumatic fever in pregnancy

During our practice in Saudi Arabia where 40% of pregnant patients in the antenatal heart disease clinic had rheumatic heart disease, we never diagnosed a case of rheumatic fever during pregnancy, which supports Roess' report that rheumatic fever during pregnancy is rare.[11] During the 1950s and 1960s acute rheumatic fever with carditis in pregnancy was associated with both fetal and maternal mortality.[11-14] Castleden *et al*[13] reported that all nine pregnant patients with acute rheumatic fever had died of heart failure, and subsequent studies corroborated its grave prognosis during pregnancy. Chorea gravidarum, described by Lewis and Parsons, can lead to miscarriage with both fetal and maternal death.[15] The treatment of acute rheumatic fever in pregnancy includes high doses of steroids. All patients in developing countries with rheumatic disease should have antibiotic prophylaxis for acute rheumatic fever until the age of 30 and throughout pregnancy.

Rheumatic mitral stenosis in pregnancy

Mitral valve stenosis is the most common valvular lesion resulting from rheumatic fever. The rheumatic process evolves over a period of one or two decades leading to mitral commissural fusion. The disease may extend to the chordae, causing thickening, shortening, and fusion with leaflet fibrosis and retraction (Figure 8.1).

In pregnant patients mitral stenosis is responsible for most of the morbidity and mortality of rheumatic heart disease. Heart failure develops during the third trimester and early puerperium in 75% of pregnant patients with rheumatic mitral stenosis. This finding is corroborated by the maternal death rate which reaches a peak during the third trimester of pregnancy.[16–18]

Pathophysiology

Diastolic blood flow through the mitral valve is slowed and consequently left atrial pressure rises (Figure 8.2).[16,19–21] This can lead to lung congestion and eventually to pulmonary oedema with the onset of clinical symptoms in women who were previously symptom free. There may be secondary pulmonary hypertension with dilatation and hypertrophy of the right ventricle. Eventually the right ventricle may fail and tricuspid regurgitation, right heart failure, ankle oedema, and varicose veins then develop.[22]

During pregnancy there is a 30–50% increase in cardiac output and intravascular blood volume.[16,17,24–32] A peak is reached by the 20–24th week of pregnancy. The increase in cardiac output is the result of an increase in stroke volume and of resting heart rate by an average of 10 beats/minute. A rise in heart rate is deleterious in pregnant patients with mitral stenosis as the decrease in diastolic filling time raises left atrial pressure further and failure to maintain stroke volume causes a further reflex rise in heart rate (Figure 8.2). Cardiac output fails to rise appropriately with exercise and the pregnant patient complains of shortness of breath on mild exercise or even at rest. The onset of atrial fibrillation in pregnant patients with mitral stenosis causes rapid uncontrolled ventricular contractions, loss of atrial contractions, and further increase in left atrial pressure. The result is acute pulmonary oedema and a further fall in cardiac output.

113

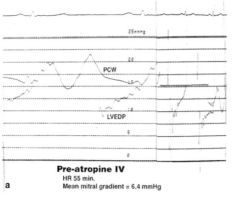

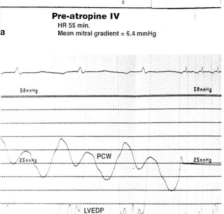

FIGURE 8.2—*Severe rheumatic mitral valve stenosis. This haemodynamic study shows a considerable increase in left atrial pressure from 15 mm Hg at a heart rate of 55 beats/minute to a mean pressure of 25 mm Hg after atropine at 102 beats/minute. There is a substantial increase in mitral valve gradient. This simulates the haemodynamics during pregnancy, during which the resting tachycardia considerably increases left atrial pressure and leads to symptoms and pulmonary oedema, particularly during the second and third trimester.*

The onset of pulmonary hypertension as a result of raised left atrial pressure causes a further decrease in cardiac output but is in a way protective to the lungs as only a few pregnant patients with mitral valve stenosis complicated by pulmonary hypertension have severe symptoms of breathlessness.[22]

As a result of the decrease in cardiac output pregnant patients complain of excessive fatigue and the low output also jeopardises fetal perfusion. The development of severe pulmonary hypertension may increase the pregnancy related mortality of 5% to more than 30%.[22] During labour and delivery there may be a 10–65% increase in cardiac output.[24] Studies by Clark *et al* showed that postpartum volume shifts as a result of relief of inferior vena cava compression, and also secondary to placental and uterine contraction, may cause pulmonary oedema.[23] This increase in intravascular volume may be balanced by an immediate blood loss of 500 ml with vaginal delivery and 1000 ml with caesarean section.[16,17,22,28-32] Tachycardia reaches its peak 5–15 minutes postpartum, causing a further decrease in diastolic filling time which contributes to the observed 10 mm Hg increase in left atrial pressure. This period is the most dangerous for patients with severe mitral stenosis. Heart rate can be controlled by short acting intravenous beta-blockers[33-35] and invasive haemodynamic monitoring may be indicated in patients with severe mitral stenosis during this period.[9,36]

Diagnosis

The clinical diagnosis of mitral stenosis during the second and third trimester of pregnancy should be made easier by the increase in intravascular volume and heart rate and consequent decreased left ventricle filling time. The mitral rumble becomes louder and the A2 mitral valve opening interval further decreases.[23] Doppler echocardiographic examination is the most important investigation to estimate mitral valve area and pulmonary artery pressure but tachycardia over 75 beats/minute tends to result in over-estimation of mitral valve area. Carotid sinus massage or short-acting beta-blockade with intravenous esmolol enables more accurate measurement of pressure half-time.[37] We consider mitral stenosis severe when the area is $<1 \cdot 1$ cm^2. Patients with mild stenosis have a mitral valve area of $>1 \cdot 5$ cm^2 and moderate mitral stenosis between $1 \cdot 1-1 \cdot 5$ cm^2. With mild and moderate stenosis the patient should have an uneventful pregnancy unless atrial fibrillation develops. The development of pulmonary hypertension further increases pregnancy morbidity and warrants serial Doppler studies particularly during the second and third trimester of pregnancy.

Management

We manage most pregnant patients with severe rheumatic mitral valve stenosis medically. In our experience beta-blockers are the cornerstone of treatment[33-35]; left atrial pressure rises as the length of the left ventricular diastolic filling period shortens. In a prospective study of 25 consecutive pregnant patients with severe mitral valve stenosis, 92% had marked clinical improvement after the heart rate was reduced from a mean of 86 to 78 beats/minute.[34] The dose is titrated according to the patient's symptoms and heart rate. We had two patients who had poor compliance with beta-blockers and developed pulmonary oedema requiring urgent mitral valvotomy. During treatment with beta-blockers we monitored fetal heart rate which ranged between 130–150 beats/minute. All infants were delivered at term and no side effects from beta-blockers were observed.[33]

Diuretics complement beta-blockers during the third trimester and peripartum period in some patients. We never use them during the first trimester. Diuretics need to be used judiciously as a decreased intravascular volume may jeopardise placental blood flow during this period. Loop diuretics are useful in the immediate postpartum period in patients who develop pulmonary oedema secondary to the sudden increase in intravascular volume or with the onset of atrial fibrillation. In these patients we control the ventricular rate with an intravenous beta-blocker complemented with diuretic therapy. Cardioversion may be necessary in patients who have developed pulmonary oedema and fast atrial fibrillation.

We had one patient in the eighth month of pregnancy who despite adequate beta-blockers and diuretics died of pulmonary oedema before we could intervene.

Systemic emboli may occur in 1–1·5% of patients with severe rheumatic heart disease. This figure comes from a survey of 1048 consecutive pregnancies in patients with rheumatic heart disease, 90% of whom had mitral stenosis. They had been observed by Szekely et al over a 28 year period.[7] The incidence of atrial fibrillation in this large population was between 6·5% and 8·4%. Anticoagulation is needed in patients who are in atrial fibrillation. The risks of warfarin in pregnancy must be taken into consideration. Heparin can be given during the first trimester of pregnancy and peripartum period and coumarin anticoagulation during the second and third trimester and peripartum period. The thromboembolic risk is not as high in these patients as in those with mechanical valve prostheses so the use of heparin is justified during the period of risk of embryopathy in the first trimester.

For those patients who are not controlled by medical treatment or are poorly compliant, balloon valvotomy or surgical intervention are indicated.[38–41] We reported balloon valvotomy for pregnant patients with severe pliable rheumatic mitral valve stenosis using the Inoue technique with total abdominal and pelvic shielding (Figure 8.3a and 8.3b).[39,40] The mean mitral valve area increased from 0·8 to 1·9 cm^2 with no complications (Figure 8.4a and 8.4b). Pregnancy was uneventful in all patients and normal babies were delivered. Several authors have reported similar findings using both the Inoue and the double balloon technique. Successful use of the double balloon technique in 38 pregnant women was reported from Tunisia where rheumatic fever is still endemic.[41] The technique was employed in 454 patients of whom 70% were women. Pregnancy proceeded uneventfully after the procedure and 38 normal babies were delivered. We believe that the Inoue technique is superior in pregnant patients as it is technically less demanding and faster. Consequently, balloon valvotomies done with the Inoue technique cause less radiation exposure to the fetus. Balloon valvotomy can be aided by transoesophageal echocardiography to reduce radiation time.

In third world countries, surgical closed mitral valvotomies are done with excellent results.[42,43] The operation requires expertise and practice that is no longer widely available in the western world, as the incidence of mitral stenosis is dwindling. Although open surgical valvotomy also provides excellent results, extracorporeal circulation causes a higher fetal mortality.[43]

During delivery epidural analgesia may be indicated in the active phase of labour. Caesarean section has been recommended in patients with severe mitral stenosis to avoid the haemodynamic changes of normal delivery, but the anaesthesia can itself cause a substantial increase in heart rate and lead to pulmonary oedema. Heart rate needs to be controlled with an intravenous beta-blocking drug such as esmolol. Vaginal delivery is usually to be preferred in these patients.

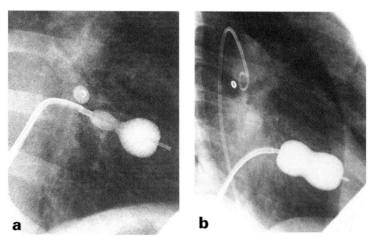

FIGURE 8.3a AND 8.3b—*(a) Inoue balloon valvotomy during pregnancy showing the initial inflation of the balloon and (b) full inflation during successful valvotomy.*

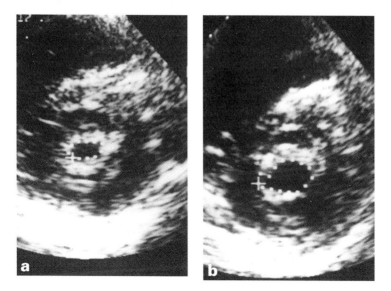

FIGURE 8.4a AND 8.4b—*Echocardiographic study with parasternal short axis view of the mitral valve before balloon valvotomy and after balloon valvotomy in a pregnant patient with severe symptomatic mitral stenosis. Note the increase in valve area from 0·86 cm² to 1·9 cm² after successful balloon valvotomy and commissural splitting. The patient lost her symptoms after the intervention and delivered a healthy baby. (Reproduced with permission from* Am Heart J *1992;* **124***: 1562–7)*

Rheumatic mitral regurgitation in pregnancy

In our experience patients with moderate and severe rheumatic mitral regurgitation do well through pregnancy, and pulmonary oedema rarely develops. Despite severe regurgitation both clinically and by echocardio-

117

graphic Doppler criteria the left atrial pressure is usually well below pulmonary oedema levels. This can be explained by stretching and dilatation of the left atrial cavity and the decrease in systemic resistance observed during the second and third trimester further unloads the left ventricle.[16,17,21] Vasodilators may help to prevent left ventricular systolic functional deterioration and dilatation, though proof is lacking.

Rheumatic aortic stenosis in pregnancy

Rheumatic aortic stenosis during pregnancy is uncommon and is nearly always associated with mitral valve stenosis. The pathology is characteristic and distinct from congenital aortic valve stenosis. The leaflets show variable commissural fusion (Figure 8.5) and this may have important therapeutic implications as balloon valvotomy can split the fused commissures.[44,45]

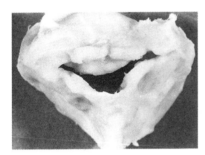

FIGURE 8.5—*Excised aortic valve showing rheumatic stenosis. There is severe commissural fusion indicating that during pregnancy it would have been feasible to do balloon valvotomy to achieve commissural splitting.*

Pathophysiology

We studied 10 rheumatic valves excised from patients with severe rheumatic aortic stenosis. Commissural fusion was the hallmark of the disease (Figure 8.5). The leaflets were thick and fibrotic with little or no calcification and there was a degree of retraction accounting for central aortic regurgitation. In pregnant patients with severe aortic stenosis increase in cardiac output can occur only if the heart rate increases if stroke volume is fixed. When the aortic stenosis is more severe, stroke volume and aortic systolic gradient decline. Mean left atrial and pulmonary artery pressures increase. Pulmonary hypertension and right heart failure eventually ensue.[8,9,10,20,46]

Diagnosis

Diagnosis of the presence and severity of rheumatic aortic stenosis in pregnant patients is established by echocardiographic Doppler studies; the aetiology of the aortic valve stenosis can rapidly be established because the mitral valve invariably also shows features of rheumatic valve disease. The outflow velocity increases particularly in the second and third trimester of

118

pregnancy if the left ventricle is able to increase stroke volume and cardiac output, particularly in those patients with combined aortic stenosis and regurgitation. This increased flow across the valve may lead to overesti-mation of the degree of stenosis. In patients with pure severe aortic valve stenosis, the stroke volume cannot be increased. In patients with critical aortic stenosis (valve area <0·6 cm^2) the aortic gradient may actually fall as a result of decreased stroke volume. Therefore, aortic valve area calculations from echocardiographic Doppler studies are less important than serial observations of Doppler velocity and left ventricular function.[47]

Management

In our experience coexistent rheumatic mitral stenosis usually dominates the clinical picture during pregnancy and is somewhat protective to pregnant patients with severe aortic stenosis by decreasing cardiac output. Patients with severe aortic stenosis usually do well provided mitral stenosis is treated with appropriate drugs—beta-blockers and diuretics. For those patients who suddenly deteriorate and develop congestive heart failure the onset of atrial fibrillation is usually the underlying cause. Atrial contraction is important in pregnant patients with aortic stenosis as it maintains optimal left ventricular filling without a rise in mean left atrial pressure. Emergency cardioversion or medical therapy with diuretics and quinidine may be indicated, particularly for those who develop acute pulmonary oedema.

Arias and Pineda,[44] reported a maternal mortality of 17% in pregnant patients with aortic stenosis and 31% fetal mortality. Several reports have shown that termination of pregnancy is also risky for the patient with aortic stenosis.[46] Surgical replacement of the valve may be an alternative in pregnant patients with heart failure refractory to medical treatment, though fetal mortality is high.[46] We have carried out balloon valvotomy with abdominal and pelvic shielding with good immediate outcome.[45] If valve replacement is required it should if possible be delayed until the fetus has been delivered.[21] Balloon valvotomy may permit this.

For those pregnant patients with severe aortic stenosis who are symptom-free or respond to medical treatment, vaginal delivery is permissible. Epidural anaesthesia in pregnant patients with severe aortic stenosis is not recommended as the sympathetic blockade and reduction in peripheral vascular resistance may reduce the blood pressure and be hazardous.

Rheumatic aortic regurgitation in pregnancy

We followed up several pregnant patients with severe rheumatic aortic regurgitation. Before becoming pregnant, patients were symptom-free and showed the classic physical signs of severe aortic regurgitation. Echocardio-graphic Doppler studies showed a dilated left ventricular cavity with preserved fractional shortening in most patients. The mitral valve is not usually affected. This is in contrast to patients with rheumatic aortic stenosis

119

who invariably have coexisting mitral stenosis. Few patients who had left ventricular systolic dysfunction were still free of symptoms. During pregnancy and labour patients continued to do well without the need for drugs, even when there was severe aortic regurgitation with diastolic pressures as low as 30 mm Hg. In pregnancy there is a decrease in systemic vascular resistance and a decline in blood pressure together with a 30–50% increase in cardiac output.[16,17] The maximum decrease in systemic resistance during the second and third trimester of pregnancy occurs at a time when the increase in intravascular volume and heart rate has peaked. The decreased systemic resistance is the result of circulating prostaglandins and the low resistance circuit in the pregnant uterus.[16,17,19,28] The reduction in systemic resistance may explain why pregnant patients with considerable aortic regurgitation tolerate pregnancy well. The beneficial role of vasodilators in patients with severe aortic regurgitation has been shown outside pregnancy and warrants investigation in pregnancy. They may have a role in preventing further left ventricular dilatation.

Tricuspid stenosis in pregnancy

Pathological studies have shown that patients with rheumatic tricuspid valve disease all have mitral valve disease.[49,50] In pregnancy mitral valve disease invariably dominates the clinical picture. We studied 43 patients with echocardiographic features of tricuspid stenosis, 4% of patients with rheumatic heart disease in Saudi Arabia.[51] The rheumatic process leads to pure tricuspid valve regurgitation in more than half the cases. Pure tricuspid stenosis is rare and was observed in only six of the 194 cases in Hank's study.[49]

Pathophysiology

The area of the normal tricuspid valve orifice is 7 cm^2 so the degree of commissural fusion must be severe to cause haemodynamically relevant tricuspid stenosis, particularly in pregnancy when the tricuspid annulus dilates further.[52-55] In our haemodynamic studies the mean right atrial pressure was normal at rest in patients with severe tricuspid valve stenosis (Figures 8.6 and 8.7).[56] The main haemodynamic disturbance in tricuspid stenosis is a low cardiac output and a diastolic tricuspid gradient.[56] In pregnant patients the increase in cardiac output and heart rate, which reaches a peak during the second trimester, causes a rise in right atrial pressure, a decrease in the tricuspid diastolic filling time, and an increase in the tricuspid diastolic gradient.[19,56] We studied this phenomenon by amplifying the tricuspid valve gradient both with atropine and fluid challenge, simulating conditions observed during pregnancy, in 42 patients with tricuspid stenosis.[56] Pregnant patients with tricuspid stenosis developed tiredness and shortness of breath with mild exercise as the cardiac output can rise only twofold on exercise.[53]

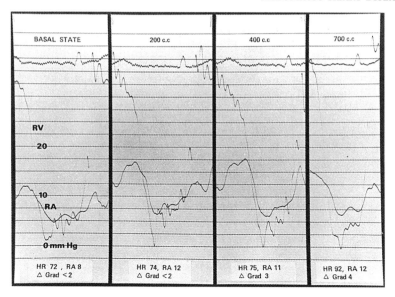

BASAL STATE	200 c.c	400 c.c	700 c.c
HR 72 , RA 8 △ Grad < 2	HR 74, RA 12 △ Grad < 2	HR 75, RA 11 △ Grad 3	HR 92, RA 12 △ Grad 4

FIGURE 8.6—*Haemodynamic studies showing the effects of heart rate and volume increase on the right atrial pressure and tricuspid valve gradient. With infusion of saline and atropine the tricuspid valve gradient increases markedly, simulating the increase in resting heart rate and intravascular volume which occur in pregnancy. The tricuspid gradient was detected only after provocation with fluid challenge and atropine.*

In patients with haemodynamically severe tricuspid regurgitation right atrial mean pressure increases and the cardiac output decreases.[58,59] Most patients with tricuspid valve disease have predominant regurgitation and the valve shows echocardiographic features of rheumatic heart disease. In pregnancy the increase in intravascular volume further increases mean right atrial and V wave pressure.[16,19] The increase in resting heart rate in pregnancy does not translate into an appropriate increase in cardiac output, as right ventricular stroke volume fails to increase and symptoms of right heart failure, liver congestion, and varicose veins ensue.

Diagnosis and management

In pregnancy, the clinical diagnosis of tricuspid valve disease is confirmed by echocardiography (Figure 8.8). The echocardiographic features include diastolic doming of all three leaflets.[51] We showed that 57% of patients with 2-dimensional echocardiographic features of tricuspid stenosis have haemodynamically relevant stenosis.[51] As the 2-dimensional echocardiographic features of tricuspid stenosis are not a precise indicator of haemodynamically important stenosis, combined Doppler studies with calculation of tricuspid valve gradient and valve area are indicated (Figure 8.9).[51,56] The severity of tricuspid regurgitation is estimated by colour Doppler flow studies. Functional tricuspid regurgitation occurs commonly in normal pregnancy.[52,59,60]

121

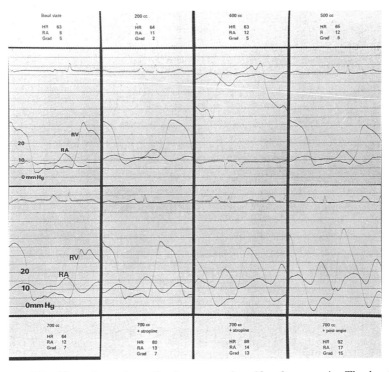

Basal state	200 cc.	400 cc	500 cc
HR 63	HR 64	HR 63	HR 65
RA 8	RA 11	RA 12	R 12
Grad 5	Grad 2	Grad 5	Grad 5

700 cc	700 cc + atropine	700 cc + atropine	700 cc + post angio
HR 64	HR 80	HR 89	HR 92
RA 12	RA 13	RA 14	RA 17
Grad 7	Grad 7	Grad 13	Grad 15

FIGURE 8.7—*Haemodynamic studies in severe tricuspid valve stenosis. The baseline tricuspid diastolic gradient increases markedly during saline infusion and rises further after atropine, simulating the haemodynamics in pregnancy, particularly during the second and third trimesters. (Reproduced with permission from* Am J Cardiol *1988; 61: 1307–11)*

In pregnant patients with tricuspid stenosis the symptoms are primarily the result of reduced cardiac output both at rest and on exercise.[53,54,55] The increase in heart rate of about 10–20 beats/minute at term further decreases diastolic filling time and increases the right atrial pressure. There seems to be little role for medical treatment in patients with symptomatic tricuspid stenosis. Beta-blockers control the heart rate, but at the expense of a further decrease in cardiac output. Digoxin does not control heart rate in pregnant patients in sinus rhythm. Diuretics may improve symptoms of right heart failure in patients with severe tricuspid regurgitation but may reduce uterine blood flow and placental perfusion. Diuretics should therefore be used judiciously, particularly during the first trimester.[16] Fetal side effects such as neonatal thrombocytopenia, hyponatraemia, and jaundice have been reported with thiazide diuretics.[61,62]

In pregnant patients with symptomatic concomitant mitral valve disease and severe tricuspid stenosis (Figure 8.10), surgical intervention or balloon tricuspid valvotomy should be considered.[63] We previously described a technique for tricuspid balloon valvotomy.[57] This should include total abdominal and pelvic shielding in pregnant patients.[63,64] Valvotomy resulted

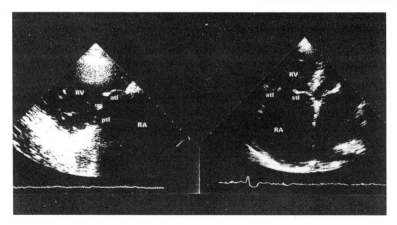

FIGURE 8.8—*During pregnancy the diagnosis of rheumatic tricuspid stenosis is made by echocardiography, using both the right ventricle inflow view and the apical four chamber view. This study shows doming and thickening of all three leaflets. RV = right ventricle; atl = anterior tricuspid leaflet; RA = right atrium; stl = septal tricuspid leaflet; ptl = posterior tricuspid leaflet. (Reproduced with permission from* Am J Cardiol 1988; **61**: 1307–11)

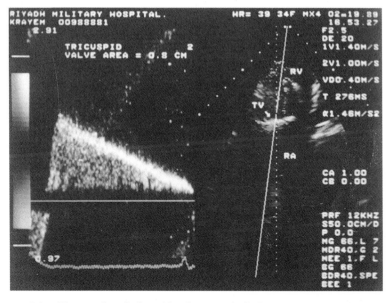

FIGURE 8.9—*The severity of tricuspid valve stenosis during pregnancy can be estimated by Doppler valve area calculation as seen in this patient. RV = right ventricle; TV = tricuspid valve; RA = right atrium.*

in an immediate and long term improvement in symptoms and an increase in tricuspid valve area with a decrease in tricuspid gradient. The tricuspid valve areas achieved were comparable to those achieved by surgical valvotomy and were maintained at three year follow up.[64]

123

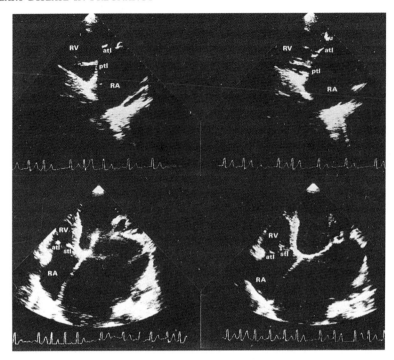

FIGURE 8.10—*Echocardiogram during pregnancy showing severe mitral and tricuspid valve stenosis in a patient with a giant left atrium. The Doppler calculations of valve area complement the echocardiographic studies. RV = right ventricle; RA = right atrium; atl = anterior tricuspid leaflet; ptl = posterior tricuspid leaflet; stl = septal tricuspid leaflet.*

Left ventricular function in pregnant patients with rheumatic heart disease

The most common sequelae of rheumatic heart disease involve the cardiac valves. As the acute process involves all areas of the heart—acute pancarditis—it can also impair right and left ventricular function.[43,65] The long standing volume overload of rheumatic mitral and aortic regurgitation can further jeopardise left ventricular function during pregnancy and lead to progressive left ventricular dilatation. These patients should therefore be followed by serial longitudinal echocardiographic studies.

Mitral valve involvement occurs in 65%–90% of patients with rheumatic heart disease.[7] Left ventricular dysfunction is observed in up to 40% of patients with rheumatic mitral stenosis and further complicates the management of pregnant patients with rheumatic heart disease.[65–67] Pregnant patients tolerate mild and moderate abnormalities in left ventricular function well, whereas when severe left ventricular dysfunction is combined with severe mitral valve disease medical treatment is complex. Beta-blockers may be given to control heart rate, combined with vasodilators to unload the ventricle. Termination of pregnancy should be considered in those patients who do not respond to treatment. Alternatively, relief of the mitral stenosis by balloon valvotomy or surgical valvotomy followed by vasodilator treatment may be successful in certain high risk pregnancies. In patients with mitral and aortic regurgitation vasodilators may constitute the cornerstone of treatment to prevent deterioration of left ventricular systolic function. Clinical studies are warranted to investigate the role and safety of vasodilators in pregnant patients with left ventricular dysfunction.

Acknowledgements

We thank Sally Angell for secretarial assistance and the medical illustration department at Loma Linda University Medical Center for the figures.

References

1 Bland EF. Declining severity of rheumatic fever. *N Engl J Med* 1960; **262**: 597–9.
2 Gordis L. The virtual disappearance of rheumatic fever in the U.S. Lessons in the rise and fall of disease. *Circulation* 1985; **72**: 1155–9.
3 Pope RM. Rheumatic fever in the 1980s. *Bull Rheum Dis* 1989; **38**: 1–8.
4 Bland EF. Declining severity of rheumatic fever: a comparative study of the past four decades. *N Engl J Med* 1960; **262**: 557–62.
5 Agarwal BL. Rheumatic heart disease unabated in developing countries. *Lancet* 1981; **ii**: 910–11.
6 WHO Study Group. Rheumatic fever and rheumatic heart disease. *WHO Technical Reports in Science* 1989; **764**: 21–5.
7 Szekely P, Turner R, Snaith L. Pregnancy and the changing pattern of rheumatic heart disease. *Br Heart J* 1973; **35**: 1293–303.
8 Ueland K. Rheumatic heart disease and pregnancy. In: Elkayan U, Gleicher N, eds. *Cardiac problems in pregnancy: diagnosis and management of maternal and fetal disease.* 2nd ed. New York: Alan R Liss, 1990: 99–107.
9 Elkayam U. Pregnancy and cardiovascular disease. In: Braunwald E, ed. *Heart disease.* Philadelphia: WB Saunders, 1984: 1790–1806.
10 McFaul PB, Dorman JC, Lamki H. Pregnancy complicated by maternal heart disease. A review of 519 women. *Br J Obstet Gynecol* 1988; **95**: 861–8.
11 Roess TJ. Acute rheumatic fever with carditis in pregnancy. Report of one case and review of the literature. *N Engl J Med* 1958; **258**: 605–7.
12 Ueland K, Metcalfe J. Acute rheumatic fever in pregnancy. *Am J Obstet Gynecol* 1966; **95**: 586–7.
13 Castleden LIM, Hamilton-Paterson JL, Rosser EI. Acute rheumatism in pregnancy. *Journal of Obstetrics and Gynaecology of the British Empire* 1951; **58**: 253–8.
14 Drury MI, O'Driscoll MK, Hanratty TD, Barry AP. Rheumatic heart disease complicating pregnancy. *BMJ* 1954; **1**: 70–3.
15 Lewis BV, Parsons M. Chorea gravidarum. *Lancet* 1966; **1**: 284–6.
16 Perloff JK. Pregnancy and cardiovascular disease. In: Braunwald E, ed. *Heart disease.* 2nd ed. Philadelphia: WB Saunders, 1984: 1763–81.
17 Ueland K, Metcalfe J. Circulatory changes in pregnancy. *Clin Gynecol* 1975; **18**: 41–50.
18 Zaibag MA, Halim MA. Mitral valve stenosis. In: Zaibag MA and Duran CMG, ed. *Valvular heart disease.* New York: Marcel Dekker, 1994; **6**: 209–47.
19 Ueland K. Cardiovascular physiology of the normal pregnancy. In: Gleicher N, Elkayam U, Galbraith RM, *et al*, eds. *Principles of medical therapy in pregnancy* New York: Plenum, 1985: 643.
20 Elkayam U, Gleicher N. Hemodynamics and cardiac function during normal pregnancy and the peurperium. In: Elkayam U, Gleicher N, eds. *Cardiac problems in pregnancy: diagnosis and management of maternal and fetal disease.* 2nd ed. New York: Alan R Liss, 1990: 5.
21 Oakley CM. Cardiovascular disease in pregnancy. *Can J Cardiol* 1990; **6(suppl B)**: 30B–9.
22 Sinnenberg RJ. Pulmonary hypertension in pregnancy. *South Med J* 1980; **73**: 1529–32.

23 Clark S, Phelan JP, Greenpoon J, Aldahl D, Horenstein J. Labor and delivery in the presence of mitral stenosis: central hemodynamic observation. *Am J Obstet Gynecol* 1985; **152**: 984–8.

24 Robson SC, Hunter S, Boys RJ, *et al.* Serial study of factors influencing changes in cardiac output during human pregnancy. *Am J Physiol* 1989; **256**: H1060–5.

25 Longo LD. Maternal blood volume and cardiac output during pregnancy. A hypothesis of endocrinologic control. *Am J Physiol* 1983; **245**: R720–9.

26 Ueland K, Hansen JM. Maternal cardiovascular dynamics: II. Posture and uterine contractions. *Am J Obstet Gynecol* 1969; **103**: 1–7.

27 Metcalfe J, Ueland K. Maternal cardiovascular adjustment to pregnancy. *Prog Cardiovasc Dis* 1974; **16**: 363–74.

28 Lees MM, Taylor SH, Scott DB, Kerr MG. A study of cardiac output at rest and throughout pregnancy. *Journal of Obstetrics and Gynaecology of the British Commonwealth* 1967; **74**: 319–28.

29 Artal R. Cardiopulmonary responses to exercise in pregnancy. In: Elkayam U, Gleicher N, eds. *Cardiac problems in pregnancy: diagnosis and management of maternal and fetal disease.* 2nd ed. New York: Alan R Liss, 1990: 25.

30 Robson SC, Dunlop W, Boys RJ, *et al.* Cardiac output during labour. *BMJ* 1987; **295**: 1169–72.

31 Ueland, K. Rheumatic heart disease and pregnancy. In: Elkayam U, Gleicher N, eds. *Cardiac problems in pregnancy: diagnosis and management of maternal and fetal disease.* 2nd ed. New York: Alan R Liss, 1990: 99.

32 Walters WAW, MacGregor WG, Hillo M. Cardiac output at rest and during pregnancy and the puerperium. *Clin Sci* 1966; **30**: 1–11.

33 Al-Kasab S, Sabag T, Al-Zaibag M, Bitar I, Halim MA, Abdullah MA. Beta-adrenergic receptor blockade in the management of pregnant women with mitral stenosis. *Am J Obstet Gynecol* 1990; **163**: 37–40.

34 Frishman WH, Chesner M. Use of beta-adrenergic blocking agents in pregnancy. In: Elkayam U, Gleicher N, eds. *Cardiac problems in pregnancy: diagnosis and management of maternal and fetal disease.* 2nd ed. New York: Alan R Liss, 1990: 351–5.

35 Narasimtian C, Joseph G, Singh TC. Propranolol for pulmonary oedema in mitral stenosis. *Int J Cardiol* 1994; **44**: 178–9.

36 Elkayam U, Gleicher N. Diagnostic approaches to maternal heart disease. In: Elkayam U, Gleicher N, eds. *Cardiac problems in pregnancy: diagnosis and management of maternal and fetal disease.* 2nd ed. New York: Alan R Liss, 1990: 41.

37 Torrecilla EG, Garcia-Fernandez MA, San Roman DJ, Alberca MT, Delca JL. Usefulness of carotid sinus massage in the quantification of mitral stenosis in sinus rhythm by Doppler pressure halftime. *Am J Cardiol* 1994; **73**: 817–21.

38 Esteves CA, Ramos AL, Braga SC, Harrison JK, Sousa JE. Effectiveness of percutaneous balloon valvotomy during pregnancy. *Am J Cardiol* 1991; **68**: 930–4.

39 Ribeiro PA, Fawzy ME, Awad M, Dunn B, Duran CG. Balloon valvotomy for pregnant patients with severe pliable mitral stenosis using the Inoue technique with total abdominal and pelvic shielding. *Am Heart J* 1992; **124**: 1558–62.

40 Ribeiro PA, Al Zaibag M. Mitral balloon valvotomy in pregnancy. *Journal of Heart Valve Disease* 1992; **2**: 206–8.

41 Ben Farhat M, Betbout F, Gamra H, *et al.* Results of percutaneous double-balloon mitral commissurotomy in one medical centre in Tunisia. *Am J Cardiol* 1995; **76**: 1266–70.

42 Goon MS, Ramam S, Sinnathuray JA. Closed mitral valvotomy in pregnancy. A Malaysian experience. *Obstet Gynecol* 1987; **27**: 173–7.

43 Becker R. Intracardiac surgery in pregnant women. *Ann Thorac Surg* 1983; **36**: 453–8.

44 Arias F, Pineda J. Aortic stenosis in pregnancy. *J Reprod Med* 1978; **20**: 229–320.

45 Ribeiro P, Zaibag MA, Rajendran V. Double balloon aortic valvotomy for rheumatic aortic stenosis. *Eur Heart J* 1989; **10**: 417–23.

46 Bernac JM, Miralles PJ. Cardiac surgery with cardiac pulmonary bypass during pregnancy. *Obstet Gynecol* 1989; **41**: 1–6.

47 Burwash IG, Forbes AD, Sadahiro M, *et al.* Echocardiographic volume flow and stenosis severity measures with changing flow rates in aortic stenosis. *Am J Physiol* 1993; **265**: H1734–43.

48 Angel JL, Chapman C, Knappel RA, *et al.* Percutaneous balloon aortic valvuloplasty in pregnancy. *Obstet Gynecol* 1988; **72**: 438–40.

126

49 Hank AJ, Freeman DP, Ackerman DM, Danielson GK, Edwards WD. Surgical pathology of the tricuspid valve: a study of 363 cases spanning 25 years. *Mayo Clin Proc* 1988; **63**: 851–63.
50 Virmani R. The tricuspid valve. *Mayo Clin Proc* 1983; **63**: 943–6.
51 Ribeiro PA, Zaibag MA, Sawyer, W. A prospective study comparing the hemodynamic with the cross-sectional echocardiographic diagnosis of rheumatic tricuspid stenosis. *Eur Heart J* 1989; **10**: 120–6.
52 Limacher MC, Ware JA, O'Meara ME, Fernandez GC, Young JB. Tricuspid regurgitation during pregnancy: two-dimensional and pulsed Doppler echocardiographic observations. *Am J Cardiol* 1985; **55**: 1059–62.
53 Kitchen A, Turner R. Diagnosis and treatment of tricuspid stenosis. *Br Heart J* 1964; **26**: 354–79.
54 Gibson R, Wood P. The diagnosis of tricuspid stenosis. *Br Heart J* 1955; **17**: 552–9.
55 Killip T, Lunas DS. Tricuspid stenosis: physiologic criteria for diagnosis and hemodynamic abnormalities. *Circulation* 1957; **16**: 3–13.
56 Ribeiro PA, Al Zaibag M, Al Kasab S, *et al*. Provocation and amplification of the transvalvular pressure gradient of rheumatic tricuspid stenosis. *Am J Cardiol* 1988; **61**: 1307–12.
57 Ribeiro PA, Al Zaibag M, Al Kasab S, *et al*. Percutaneous double balloon valvotomy for rheumatic tricuspid stenosis. *Am J Cardiol* 1988; **61**: 660–2.
58 Sepulveda G, Lukas DS. The diagnosis of tricuspid insufficiency. Clinical features in 60 cases with associated mitral valve disease. *Circulation* 1955; **11**: 552–63.
59 Limacher MC, Ware JA, O'Meara ME, *et al*. Tricuspid regurgitation during pregnancy: two-dimensional and pulsed Doppler echocardiographic observations. *Am J Cardiol* 1985; **55**: 1059–62.
60 Campos O, Martinez E, Andrade JL, *et al*. Detection of right-sided valve regurgitation during normal pregnancy by Doppler echocardiography. *J Am Coll Cardiol* 1990; **15**: 139A.
61 Dicke JM. Cardiovascular drugs in pregnancy. In: Gleicher N, Elkayam U, Galbraith RM, *et al*, eds. *Principles of medical therapy in pregnancy*. New York: Plenum, 1985: 646–55.
62 Elkayam U, Gleicher N. Cardiac problems in pregnancy. I. Maternal aspects: the approach to the pregnant patient with heart disease. *JAMA* 1984; **251**: 2838–9.
63 Al Zaibag M, Ribeiro PA, Al Kasab S. Percutaneous balloon valvotomy for tricuspid stenosis. *Br Heart J* 1987; **57**: 51–3.
64 Ribeiro PA, Zaibag M, Idris M. Percutaneous double balloon tricuspid valvotomy: three year follow-up study. *Eur Heart J* 1990; **11**: 1109–12.
65. Hildner F, Javier R, Cohen L, *et al*. Myocardial dysfunction associated with valvular heart disease. *Am J Cardiol* 1972; **30**: 319–26.
66 Mohan JC, Khalilullah M, Arora R. Left ventricular intrinsic contractibility in pure rheumatic mitral stenosis. *Am J Cardiol* 1989; **64**: 240–6.
67 Gash AK, Carabello BA, Cepin D, Spann JF. Left ventricular ejection performance and systolic muscle function in patients with mitral stenosis. *Circulation* 1983; **67**: 148–52.

127

9: Mitral valve prolapse

CELIA OAKLEY

The term "mitral valve prolapse" describes abnormal protrusion of one or both mitral leaflets into the left atrium during ventricular systole with or without mitral regurgitation.[1] Since the first clinical description in the early 1960s the condition has generated huge interest and has become one of the most common cardiac diagnoses. It is frequently diagnosed in young women of child bearing age.[2,3]

Mitral valve prolapse is termed primary when it occurs in the absence of other systemic or cardiac diseases and secondary when associated with a connective tissue disorder or other cardiac abnormality (Table 9.1). Numerous synonyms are in use (Table 9.2).

TABLE 9.1—*Mitral valve prolapse.*

- **Primary mitral valve prolapse**

"Echo-only" prolapse	Normal valve
Floppy mitral valve	Sometimes familial
The mitral valve prolapse syndrome	Occurs in only a small proportion of patients with prolapse
Wear and tear prolapse	Occurs in middle or later age

- **Secondary mitral valve prolapse**

  Associated with hereditary connective tissue disorders:
  Marfan syndrome
  Ehlers–Danlos syndrome type IV
  Osteogenesis imperfecta
  Pseudoxanthoma elasticum

  Associated with structural heart disease:
  Atrial septal defect (secundum)
  Hypertrophic cardiomyopathy
  Rheumatic carditis
  Post-infective

The early understanding of mitral valve prolapse came from linking the physical signs of non-ejection click or clicks and late systolic murmur with phonocardiography and angiocardiography.[4] Later studies largely ignored auscultatory features and depended on M mode echocardiography before more rigorous criteria using cross sectional echocardiography were evolved. Prolapse began to be over-diagnosed particularly in young women without abnormal auscultatory signs in whom slight bowing of the mitral valve leaflets to the atrial side of the annulus during systole can be a normal

128

TABLE 9.2—*Mitral valve prolapse—synonyms.*

- Barlow's syndrome
- Click-murmur syndrome
- Floppy mitral valve
- Billowing mitral leaflet
- Mitral leaflet prolapse

finding. This led to a reported prevalence even as high as 17% in females in their 20s and in up to one third of underweight young women but in only 1% of middle-aged women.[5] Such surveys suggested that silent prolapse diagnosed by echocardiography in young women was a normal phenomenon which disappeared with increasing age and girth. It was an "echo-only" diagnosis.

True mitral valve prolapse is associated with myxomatous transformation[6] and redundancy of part or all of the leaflets which are elongated and their chordae lengthened, resulting either in localised protrusion of part of a leaflet or generalised billowing into the left atrium.[7,8] Mitral annular dilatation is usually associated.

"Echo-only" prolapse

There is no evidence to suggest that structurally normal mitral valves that bow slightly towards the left atrium in systole are abnormal. Such bowing is prevalent in the young and underweight, varies with posture, is poorly reproducible, unaccompanied by thickening or folding of the leaflets and is seen also in conditions which reduce left ventricular volume such as primary pulmonary hypertension, constrictive pericarditis and transposition of the great arteries. This "echo only" prolapse is not abnormal, not a risk, and tends to disappear during pregnancy when left ventricular volume and stroke output increase. These young women may have a variable isolated click but this too tends to disappear during pregnancy. They should be strongly reassured.

Primary mitral valve prolapse

Primary mitral valve prolapse is inherited as an autosomal dominant condition in families with asthenic build but no other features of Marfan syndrome (Table 9.3).[9–11] Some of these families may have mutations in the fibrillin gene but most patients do not have a family history of the condition.

Even extreme billowing as a result of elongation and redundancy of both leaflets may still allow coaptation of the leaflet edges so that there is little or no regurgitation. This is in contrast to abnormality affecting only a part

129

TABLE 9.3—*Physical features often found in familial mitral valve prolapse.*

- Asthenic habitus
- Straight back syndrome
- Pectus excavatum
- High arched palate
- Hypermobility
- Unilateral hypomastia

of a leaflet, which is commoner in older patients with degenerative "wear and tear" type myxomatous degeneration. This often affects only one scollop of the posterior leaflet and causes severe mitral regurgitation.

Pathology

The term myxomatous (mucoid) degeneration describes disruption of normal valvular architecture, fragmentation of valvular collagen, and mucopolysaccharide accumulation but without inflammatory changes. Electron microscopy shows disruption of collagen fibrils and considerable increase in the ground substance. With increasing bulk of the myxoid stroma the leaflets become thickened and redundant with a tendency to endothelial disruption and fibrin deposition. These become sites for platelet aggregation, thrombus formation, and the development of infective endocarditis if bacteraemia occurs. Involvement of the mitral annulus and chordae can lead to annular dilatation and to chordal lengthening and rupture. Development of a flail leaflet causes severe regurgitation. Similar changes may be seen in the aortic and tricuspid valves in a few patients but haemodynamically relevant disturbance of their function is rare.[6-8]

Secondary mitral valve prolapse

Secondary mitral valve prolapse may develop in association with other disorders of the mitral valve such as acute rheumatic carditis, following mitral valvotomy and with hypertrophic cardiomyopathy as well as in the inherited connective tissue disorders, Marfan syndrome,[12] Ehlers–Danlos syndrome,[13] and pseudoxanthoma elasticum[14] (Chapter 12).

Symptoms

Most patients with mitral valve prolapse are free of symptoms and are found when a late systolic murmur sometimes preceded by one or more clicks leads to echocardiography.

TABLE 9.4—*Possible mechanisms of syncope and pre-syncope in the mitral valve prolapse syndrome.*

- Tachyarrhythmias
- Orthostatic phenomena leading to decreased intrathoracic blood volume and causing increased mitral valve prolapse
- Tachycardia
- Hypotension
- Arrhythmias (often exercise-provoked ventricular ectopic beats)
- Low stroke volume
- Sympathetic abnormality
- Parasympathetic abnormality
- Baroflex abnormality

A number of non-specific symptoms have been attributed to mitral valve prolapse such as chest pain, dizziness, syncope, fatigue, and shortness of breath, but these cannot result from the slight haemodynamic abnormality and are absent in most patients.[1,2,15] The term "mitral valve prolapse syndrome" has been given to a minority of patients with true mitral valve prolapse but non-attributable symptoms, some of whom may have an autonomic disorder with overactivity both of the adrenergic and vagal systems (Table 9.4).[3] Unfortunately mitral valve prolapse also became a convenient diagnostic label to give to young women with unexplained symptoms but normal hearts in whom prolapse was sought by clinicians and found as an "echo-only" phenomenon by helpful technicians (Table 9.1).

Specific symptoms are the result of arrhythmias[16] or in a minority of progressive mitral regurgitation.[17] Palpitation has a definite association even when regurgitation is mild and may be caused either by supraventricular or ventricular ectopic beats. The latter characteristically increase with exercise. Sudden death has been attributed to arrhythmia associated with mitral valve prolapse but must be exceedingly rare.[18] In general the syndrome is benign.

Diagnosis

Diagnosis is based on physical examination[4] and echocardiography.[19] A family history of the condition may be obtained. The auscultatory signs are easily recognisable: a variable late systolic click with or without a late systolic murmur. Increase in regurgitation is associated with earlier onset of the murmur and clicks if present. The murmur becomes pansystolic when regurgitation becomes more severe although retaining a characteristic late accentuation.

These auscultatory features are sensitive to changes in left ventricular volume which is most easily induced by changes in posture. The systolic click is earlier and the murmur longer with upright posture or tachycardia. It becomes later or may even disappear transiently on squatting. Diminution or loss of the auscultatory features in pregnancy fits in with these observations.[20]

Abnormalities in the arterial pulse and cardiac impulse are found only in patients with billowing valves with greatly increased excursion. The jerky ill-sustained arterial pulse and left ventricular impulse are explained by sudden cessation of forward ejection because systolic increase in left ventricular volume coincides with displacement of the mitral leaflets into the left atrium. These features too are lessened during pregnancy.[20]

Most patients have normal electrocardiograms but non-specific ST segment changes and T wave inversion are sometimes seen in the inferior and lateral leads.[21] The chest x ray is usually normal. A long lean thoracic cage is usual and tends to obscure increases in left ventricular size in patients with mitral regurgitation.[22]

Cross sectional echocardiography allows prolapse to be identified in multiple views. Bowing of the leaflets in young women can be recognised as a normal variant and diagnosis of abnormality needs association of prolapse with redundancy, elongation, thickening, folding, or hooding of the leaflets. In others it may be difficult or impossible to decide between normality and abnormality. There is a range. Redundancy is well shown on short axis views with deformity of the usual mitral "smile" by puckering of the outline and repeated changing of the shape of the orifice as it opens and closes as well as from one cycle to the next, rather like a sea anemone. The mitral regurgitant jet is often hard to quantify because it is non-central and slanted, swirling around the posterior wall of the left atrium when prolapse is mainly of the anterior leaflet and striking the atrial septum in mainly posterior prolapse. Even when mitral regurgitation is severe, a jet spurting into the cavity and hitting the posterior wall of the left atrium is rarely seen and thus the severity of the regurgitation may be underestimated. Recognition of a volume loaded left ventricle is therefore an important adjunct to the assessment which is greatly aided also by transoesophageal imaging plus Doppler.

Effects on pregnancy

Mitral regurgitation resulting from prolapse is well tolerated in pregnancy both because the prolapse tends to lessen when cardiac volume increases and because regurgitation is reduced by systemic vasodilatation. Even women with considerable mitral regurgitation have no problems in pregnancy. Most patients can be confidently reassured that they can expect to have an uncomplicated pregnancy and to deliver normally at term.[23] Patients with the mitral prolapse syndrome also do well and may lose some of their symptoms during pregnancy (Table 9.4).[14]

When mitral valve prolapse is associated with Marfan syndrome the risks of pregnancy are those of Marfan syndrome (Chapter 12).

132

Women with prolapsing valves and mitral regurgitation are at risk of infective endocarditis which can lead to sudden increase in severity (Chapter 11).[24,25] It is the commonest cardiac disorder underlying infective endocarditis in women and second only to bicuspid aortic valve in men. This is because of the high velocity jet and the presence of endothelial breaks which attract platelet aggregates. These may cause transient ischaemic attacks.[26]

Most patients require no medication. Only those with symptomatic cardiac arrhythmias should be prescribed a beta-blocker during pregnancy. Patients who have had a transient ischaemic attack should take low dose aspirin but stop this before term.

Antibiotic prophylaxis is not needed for routine vaginal delivery in patients with structural heart disease but should be given for complicated delivery and to cover dental or surgical procedures in women with prolapse who have a mitral regurgitant murmur. Antibiotic prophylaxis is not needed for patients who have only isolated clicks or no abnormal physical signs (Chapter 11).

Summary

Mitral valve prolapse is common in young women but not nearly as common as the early literature suggested. Only anatomical abnormality that has been defined echocardiographically should qualify for the diagnosis. Signs of mitral prolapse tend to become less or disappear with increased cardiac volume during pregnancy. Most patients have normal pregnancies. Complications are rare. No special precautions are necessary except for antibiotic prophylaxis in selected cases. The genetic risk should be explained in patients with familial primary prolapse or an associated connective tissue disorder. Cardiological follow up is needed only rarely for patients without significant mitral regurgitation.

References

1 Oakley CM. Mitral valve prolapse. In: Acar J, Bodnar E, eds. *Textbook of acquired heart valve disease. Vol 1*. London: ICR Publishers UK, 1995: 433–53.
2 Oakley CM. Mitral valve prolapse. *Q J Med* 1985; **219**: 317–20.
3 Boudoulas H, Kobilbash AJ Jr, Baker P, *et al*. Mitral valve prolapse and the mitral valve prolapse syndrome. A diagnosis classification and pathogenesis of symptoms. *Am Heart J* 1989; **118**: 796–818.
4 Barlow JB, Pocock WA, Marchand P, Denny M. The significant late systolic murmurs. *Am Heart J* 1963; **66**: 443–52.
5 Devereux RB, Brown WT, Lutas EM, Kramer-Fox R, Laragh JH. Association of mitral valve prolapse with low body weight and low blood pressure. *Lancet* 1982; **ii**: 792–5.
6 Pomerance A. Ballooning deformity (mucoid degeneration) of atrioventricular valves. *Br Heart J* 1969; **31**: 343–51.
7 Davies MJ, Moore BP, Braimbridge MW. Floppy mitral valve: study of incidence, pathology, and complications in surgical necropsy, and forensic material. *Br Heart J* 1978; **40**: 468–81.

133

8 Olsen EGJ, Al-Raufair HK. The floppy mitral valve: study on pathogenesis. *Br Heart J* 1980; **44**: 674–83.
9 Read RC, Thal AP, Wendy VE. Symptomatic valvular myxomatous transformation (the floppy valve syndrome): a possible forme fruste of the Marfan syndrome. *Circulation* 1965; **32**: 897–910.
10 Chen WW, Chan FL, Wong PH, Chow JS. Familial occurrence of mitral valve prolapse. Is this related to the straight back syndrome? *Br Heart J* 1983; **50**: 97–110.
11 Beighton P. Mitral valve prolapse and a Marfanoid habitus. *BMJ* 1982; **284**: 920.
12 Pyeritz RE, Wappel MA. Mitral valve dysfunction in Marfan syndrome. *Am J Med* 1983; **74**: 797–807.
13 Jaffe AS, Geltman EM, Rodney GE, Uitto J. Mitral valve prolapse. A consistent manifestation of type IV Ehlers–Danlos syndrome. The pathogenetic role of the abnormal production of type III collagen. *Circulation* 1981; **64**: 121–5.
14 Lebwohl MG, Distefano D, Prioleau PG, *et al.* Pseudoxanthoma elasticum and mitral valve prolapse. *N Engl J Med* 1982; **307**: 228–31.
15 Chesler E, Gornick CC. Maladies attributed to myxomatous mitral valve. *Circulation* 1991; **83**: 328–32.
16 Winkle RA, Lopes MG, Fitzgerald J, Goodman D, Schroeder J, Harrison DC. Arrhythmias in patients with mitral valve prolapse. *Circulation* 1975; **52**: 73–81.
17 Cohn LH, Disesa VJ, Couper GS, *et al.* Mitral valve repair for myxomatous degeneration and prolapse of the mitral valve. *J Thorac Cardiovasc Surg* 1983; **86**: 323–37.
18 Shappell SD, Marshall CE, Brown RE, Bruce TA. Sudden death and the familial occurrence of mid-systolic click, late systolic murmur syndrome. *Circulation* 1973; **48**: 1128–34.
19 Alpert MA, Carney RJ, Flaker GC, *et al.* Sensitivity and specificity of two-dimensional echocardiographic signs of mitral valve prolapse. *Am J Cardiol* 1984; **54**: 792–6.
20 Haas JH. The effect of pregnancy on the mid-systolic click and murmur of the prolapsing posterior leaflet of the mitral valve. *Am Heart J* 1976; **92**: 407–8.
21 Pocock WA, Barlow JB. Etiology and electrocardiographic features of the billowing posterior mitral leaflet syndrome. *Am J Med* 1971; **51**: 731–9.
22 Bon Tempo CP, Ronan JA, de Leon AC Jr, Twigg HL. Radiographic appearance of the thorax in systolic click-late systolic murmur syndrome. *Am J Cardiol* 1975; **36**: 27–36.
23 Rayburn WF, Fontana ME. Mitral valve prolapse and pregnancy. *Am J Obstet Gynecol* 1981; **141**: 9–11.
24 Macmahon SW, Hickey AJ, Wilcken DEL, *et al.* Risk of infective endocarditis in mitral valve prolapse with and without systolic murmurs. *Am J Cardiol* 1987; **59**: 105–8.
25 Danchin N, Briancon S, Mathieu P, *et al.* Mitral valve prolapse as a risk factor for infective endocarditis. *Lancet* 1989; **i**: 743–5.
26 Barletta GA, Gagliardi R, Benvenuti L, Fantini F. Cerebral ischaemic attacks as a complication of aortic and mitral valve prolapse. *Stroke* 1985; **16**: 219–23.

134

10: Artificial heart valves

CELIA OAKLEY

Some controversy still persists concerning the choice of valvular prosthesis for young women who may wish to have a family.[1,2] Bioprostheses offer a normal outlook for mother and fetus[3-6] as anticoagulants are not needed if sinus rhythm is maintained, but they lack durability in the young and deteriorate at an accelerated rate during pregnancy.[6-9] Mechanical prostheses are reliable but continued anticoagulant treatment is essential.

Women who are likely to need a heart valve prosthesis should be encouraged to have their children early before the valve disease deteriorates further. Although most women with artificial valves have more than adequate cardiovascular reserve for pregnancy there is concern about the hazard to the fetus from oral anticoagulants and about maternal safety from thromboembolism if she is transferred from an oral anticoagulant to heparin.

The hypercoagulable state induced by pregnancy increases dependence on anticoagulant prophylaxis of thromboembolism and the need for meticulous control.[10-12] Oral anticoagulants cross the placenta and carry a risk of fetal malformation (chondrodysplasia punctata) if used during the first trimester and a continuing risk of fetal cerebral haemorrhage throughout.[13-16] Although heparin has been described as the anticoagulant of choice[17] there is growing doubt about its safety and efficacy for long term use in patients with artificial valves during pregnancy.[6,8,18-21]

Bioprostheses

Accelerated deterioration of bioprostheses during pregnancy has turned us away from their use in young women. Both bioprostheses manufactured from porcine aortic valve and from bovine pericardium have shown limited durability because of progressive calcification of the porcine and mechanical wear of the pericardial valve. Planned obsolescence of bioprostheses chosen to provide time for one or more safe pregnancies is often readily accepted by the potential parents but they should also understand that re-replacement will be needed only a few years after the first operation at a time when the badly wanted children are still small and dependent and that re-operation carries an appreciable risk. The current 30 day mortality is still over 10% but is individually unpredictable.[22] It is highest for patients in New York Heart Association functional class IV with impaired left ventricular function, prosthetic valve endocarditis, or in emergency but it is probably still at least 5% when carried out electively in an otherwise fit young woman. The patient must also survive repetition of the relatively high risk first postoperative year when paravalvular leaks may develop and embolism and prosthetic valve endocarditis are most likely.

Most women who have undergone valve replacement for rheumatic valve disease are still in sinus rhythm when they have their children but they will eventually go into atrial fibrillation. They will then require anticoagulant treatment anyway. Bioprostheses are not free of thromboembolic risk and for patients with mitral bioprostheses the incidence is similar in patients not taking anticoagulants to that in patients with mechanical prosthetic valves taking anticoagulants.[23] Increased risk of thromboembolism may be indicated by spontaneous echocardiographic contrast "smoke" within the left atrium.[24] Infection, especially respiratory infection, may be a trigger factor for thromboembolism. Prompt treatment and elimination of smoking are important.[25]

Mechanical prostheses

Uncertainty is still expressed concerning the risks of pregnancy in women with mechanical prosthetic valves as well as about the choice of anticoagulants. This is because of lack of good data. Properly controlled trials have never been conducted because of small numbers, the many variables of prosthetic site, size, number, type, and thrombogenicity as well as the difficulty of organising the close monitoring required for later recall of both anticoagulant dose and effect throughout pregnancy.

Heparin

Heparin was thought to be ideal because it does not reach the fetus but its safety and efficacy when given long term for the prevention of arterial thromboembolism has never been shown. Its powerful effects combined with short duration of action and narrow therapeutic index make it difficult to maintain an antithrombotic effect without haemorrhage complications.[26,27] Recommendations differ about the route, dose and duration of treatment.[1,28–33] A change to heparin has been advocated for the first trimester, for the entire pregnancy, or even before conception, and advice from the United States has included fertility testing of couples contemplating pregnancy, to minimise the time on heparin. Intravenous administration using a heparin lock has been proposed so as to avoid painful subcutaneous injections and inevitable bruising but this route provides a portal of entry for bacteria and seems unwise (staphylococcal endocarditis has been described).[34] A much higher dose is needed to prevent prosthetic valve thrombosis or embolism than to prevent venous thromboembolism. The usual test is the activated partial thromboplastin time (APTT). A target APTT of 1·5 suggested in 1989 is clearly insufficient.[28] More recently a minimum of 2·0 was suggested, measured half-way between 12 hourly injections.[1] The heparin requirement goes up during pregnancy and the half-life of heparin clearance increases with the dose. The consequence of this is that as dosage increases toward the therapeutic range even a small increment may bring about considerable prolongation of the APTT with risk of bleeding.[1,36] Sub-anticoagulant doses are ineffective.[8,19,35] Stringent monitoring is required because of the narrow window of safety. Heparin treatment is arduous for the patient. Regular blood counts are required to detect thrombocytopenia which brings a paradoxical risk of thrombosis because it is caused by platelet aggregation.[26] Heparin induces osteopenia when used long term.[37] This complication has been reported most often in pregnant women perhaps because they have been the group most often subjected to long term treatment and also because of the pregnant woman's high calcium turnover. Other side effects include urticaria, bronchospasm, and anaphylaxis.[38,39]

Low molecular weight heparins have so far been licensed only for the prevention of venous thromboembolism. With molecular weights down to about 3000 daltons, they still do not cross the placenta. Thrombocytopenia is thought to be less common with these fractionated heparins.

Oral anticoagulants

Early reports of oral anticoagulants during pregnancy were largely anecdotal but collected together into a much quoted review in which experience with warfarin and heparin was compared in patients with various conditions, not all requiring long term treatment. Their use was associated with similar fetal loss, prematurity and stillbirth rates although about two-thirds of the pregnancies were successful (Table 10.1). The conclusion of Hall et al was that heparin did not appear to be a clearly superior alternative to coumarin derivatives.[40]

The risk of fetal damage has probably been exaggerated in reports from the US because of higher dosage there than in Europe.[41,42] A higher prevalence of major bleeding complications has been reported in non-pregnant patients with prosthetic valves in the US compared with Europe because the US was slow to adopt the International Normalised Ratio (INR). Thromboplastins used there have lower responsiveness than European thromboplastins and give rise to less prolongation of the prothrombin time for the same warfarin dose. With International Sensitivity Indices (ISI) ranging between 1·7 and 2·8 prothrombin time ratios in the US of between 2·7 and 5·2 are equivalent to INRs between 5·0 and 10·0. Overdosing of American women with prosthetic valves during pregnancy may have resulted in unduly high rates of fetal complications. Moreover it has been shown that INRs controlled to between 2·5 and 3·3 according to valve site (aortic or mitral) and type (first, second, or third generation prostheses) reduce the risk of bleeding complications without increasing the thromboembolic risk in non-pregnant patients.[43,44]

TABLE 10.1—*Fetal and neonatal complications following maternal anticoagulant treatment in pregnancy.*[40] *Figures are number (%) of patients.*

	Coumarin Drugs (n = 418)	Heparin (n = 135)
Live born with problems:	57 (14)	30 (22)
Embryopathy	16 (4)	0
CNS defects	6 (1)	0
Premature (fatalities)	4 (1)	10 (7)
Spontaneous abortions	36 (9)	2 (1)
Still births	32 (8)	17 (13)
Premature (healthy)	8 (2)	19 (14)
Live born without problems	293 (70)	86 (64)

From Hall *et al.*[40] (Reproduced with permission).

The fetus is in any case unavoidably overdosed compared with its mother because the fetal liver produces small amounts of vitamin K dependent clotting factors and the molecules of maternal procoagulants are too large to cross the placental barrier. The risk to the fetus is dose-dependent and the maternal dose requirement varies widely but has not been taken into consideration when computing fetal risk. Women who require only a small dose of warfarin for anticoagulant control have less risk of fetal damage than those needing a bigger dose. The risk of embryopathy appears to be under 5% for all degrees of severity of deformity and all maternal dosages of warfarin. The risk of coumarin induced fetal damage may be lower than this in women who require a low dose. Conversely the risk of both embryopathy and fetal haemorrhage later in pregnancy is higher in women with a high dose requirement.

An increased rate of miscarriage reported with warfarin anticoagulation compared with healthy women may be caused partly by bleeding, partly by damage to the fetuses, partly by the condition for which the patient is being treated, and partly the result of a self-fulfilling prophecy. Spontaneous abortion in early pregnancy may only rarely be recorded in the notes at annual follow-up cardiological visits unless it is thought to have been drug induced.

Reported experience

Personal series of patients with prosthetic valves and pregnancy began to be collected in the late 1970s and 1980s from countries with a high incidence of rheumatic heart disease in the young, bringing a need for valve replacement but where good anticoagulant control might be difficult to achieve. Only four thromboembolic events (1·9%) were recorded by Salazar's group in Mexico among 212 patients receiving oral anticoagulant treatment during the second and third trimesters.[8,19] This suggested that warfarin treatment provides good protection from thromboembolism during pregnancy. The same group found that a fixed dose of 5000 units of heparin subcutaneously 12 hourly was ineffective. Three patients had massive prosthetic valve thrombosis, two of them in the first trimester and one immediately postpartum, with two deaths. None of the women developed prosthetic valve thrombosis while on oral anticoagulants. Thrombosis of mechanical prostheses has been noted in other reports of women receiving subcutaneous or intravenous heparin.[35,45-48]

Ben Ismail et al reported on the course of 71 pregnancies in 51 Tunisian women with cardiac valve prostheses.[49] They found that heparin was less effective than oral anticoagulants and that transfer to heparin in the first trimester was therefore not justified. They did not encounter any teratogenic effects. Wang et al encountered five thromboembolic events in 10 patients after substitution of subcutaneous heparin for warfarin in the first trimester.[50] Larrea et al found a lower incidence of fetal complications in women who had changed to intravenous heparin in the first trimester than in those taking warfarin throughout, but at the expense of a higher maternal mortality.[51]

Like Hall et al,[40] both Salazar et al[8] and Ayan et al[52] found that fetal wastage was as high in women taking heparin as in those on coumarins and Lee et al[53] reported a miscarriage rate of 50% with the use of adjusted doses of subcutaneous heparin aimed to achieve an APTT of 1·5 (which is less than that now recommended[1]). The weighty recommendation to give adjusted doses of subcutaneous heparin throughout pregnancy was not justified by the information then available nor has it been ratified by subsequent experience.[54]

In a report from India of 47 pregnancies in 37 patients with mechanical prostheses, oral anticoagulants had been continued throughout pregnancy apart from transfer to heparin before labour.[55] No embryopathies occurred. Valve thrombosis developed in two patients, but was successfully treated surgically. Among 49 patients with 60 mechanical valves receiving warfarin Sareli et al in South Africa reported no thromboembolic complications or deaths even though only 39% of INRs were within or greater than the target range.[56]

In two recent surveys from Europe the outcomes with different regimens of warfarin and heparin were compared from information obtained retrospectively by questionnaires addressed to centres of excellence in which the quality of anticoagulant control was likely to have been high, though the dose requirement and levels of anticoagulation achieved throughout pregnancy could not be fully assessed. In our own study 13 mechanical valve thromboses (four of them fatal) were reported during 124 pregnancies.[6] Ten of these occurred while patients were on heparin and one in a woman with an aortic prosthesis who refused anticoagulant treatment. Excluding spontaneous abortions (because they were unlikely to have been fully reported or the information might have been selectively acquired because of bias), 91% of women with bioprostheses and 85% of women with mechanical valves had healthy babies. This difference was not significant but there were more premature births (p = <0·05) in the women with mechanical valves (Tables 10.2 and 10.3). Pregnancy was more likely to be successful in women taking heparin followed by warfarin than in women taking heparin throughout (p = <0·05). Pregnancies in women taking warfarin throughout came in between (Table 10.4). Maternal complications or death were, however, more likely to occur while on heparin. No deaths occurred in women with bioprostheses. In a French study 10 valve thromboses were reported among 108 women with mechanical valves.[20,21] Six of the patients were on heparin, two were unsatisfactorily controlled on an oral anticoagulant and two were not taking their oral anticoagulant at the time. Even on an intention to treat basis the thromboembolic risk was calculated to be 4·5 times higher for women on heparin than for women taking an oral anticoagulant.

TABLE 10.2—*Outcome of pregnancy in women with mechanical valves.*

Outcome	No (%)
Pregnancies	124
Healthy babies:	105 (85)
Full term	75 (60)
Premature	30 (25)
Stillbirths	9 (7)
Neonatal deaths	3 (2)
CNS abnormalities	1
Embryopathies	0
Therapeutic abortions	3 (2)
Not delivered (maternal death)	2
Ectopic pregnancy	1

From: Sbarouni and Oakley[6] (reproduced with permission).

TABLE 10.3—*Outcome of pregnancy: comparison between mechanical valves and bioprostheses. Figures are number (%) of patients.*

	Bioprostheses (n = 57)	Mechanical (n = 124)
Healthy babies:	52 (91)	105 (85)
Full term	48 (84)	75 (60)
Premature	4 (7)*	30 (25)*
Stillbirths	2 (4)	9 (7)
Therapeutic terminations	3 (5)	3 (2)

*p<0·05
From: Sbarouni and Oakley[6] (reproduced with permission).

The only fetal embryopathy among my patients was in a woman (seen since our study) with a mitral bioprosthesis, sinus rhythm, and a previous

TABLE 10.4—*Outcome of pregnancy according to different anticoagulant regimens. Figures are number (%) of patients.*

	No anticoagulant (49B)	Heparin for first trimester (64M + 2B)	Warfarin throughout (31M + 5B)	Heparin throughout (29M + 1B)
Healthy babies:	44 (91)	61 (92)†	30 (83)	22 (73)†
Full term	41 (84)	42 (64)	23 (64)	17 (57)
Premature	3 (6)*	19 (29)*	7 (19)	5 (17)
Stillbirths	2 (4)	1 (1·5)‡	4 (11)‡	4 (13)‡
Neonatal deaths	0	1 (1·5)	2 (3)	0
Therapeutic termination	3 (6)	0	1 (3)	2 (7)

*, †, ‡; p<0·05. B = bioprostheses; M = mechanical valves.
From: Sbarouni and Oakley[6] (reproduced with permission).

embolus who required 16 mg of warfarin daily. The baby had multiple malformations and died. The woman needed re-replacement with a mechanical valve shortly after the pregnancy.

Advice to patients

When discussing the fetal risks with a patient with a mechanical valve who wishes to become pregnant, her dose requirement should be taken into consideration. For most patients warfarin treatment should not be interrupted during pregnancy. The quoted embryopathy risk of 3 to 4% does not take dose into account. Cotrufo found no cases of embryopathy in a small series of 20 women requiring less than 5 mg per day treated throughout pregnancy.[57] Rare patients require high doses of 15 mg to 20 mg a day. They probably run a much higher risk both of fetal embryopathy and of fetal intra-cerebral bleeding throughout the pregnancy. For a woman who needs such a dose transfer to heparin for the first trimester may seem attractive but the maternal risk of so doing needs to be discussed. This includes disabling stroke as well as death. Moreover, if she resumes warfarin an enhanced risk of fetal haemorrhage attributable to the high dose will prevail throughout the pregnancy. It is impossible to put a figure on this as there are no data relating fetal outcome to maternal warfarin dose.

Management of delivery

It has been conventional to advise conversion to heparin for the last two weeks of pregnancy. For this to be given most effectively and safely the practice in the United Kingdom has been to give intravenous heparin in hospital where its effect can be closely monitored and where early detection of maternal or fetal complications can be expected. This imposes a period of risk (as well as increased cost) while waiting for natural labour to start. If the birth is to be induced, two weeks off warfarin are needed to allow fetal coagulation to return to normal. Elective caesarean section at 38 weeks not only provides a safer birth route for these precious babies but it also minimises the length of time that the mother is unprotected by warfarin.[57] Fresh frozen plasma should be given before surgery to counteract the warfarin effect (not vitamin K) and warfarin restarted as soon as possible postoperatively, with heparin prophylaxis in between.

Prosthetic valve thrombosis

Most women with prosthetic heart valves have more than adequate cardiovascular reserve and tolerate pregnancy well. Certainly this is true of patients in class I or II before the pregnancy (where there is doubt exercise tolerance should be tested before conception). The development of unexpected dyspnoea should hint at the possibility of prosthetic valve thrombosis. This is not always associated with embolism. It is detected clinically by muffling of the normally clear prosthetic clicks and the development of systolic and diastolic murmurs. Confirmation comes from echocardiography which shows either immobilisation or reduced excursions of the occluder or poppet or of one or both leaflets of a bileaflet valve. Fortunately valves tend to stick in a half open, half closed position which is not immediately fatal so the development of thrombosis is always associated with new regurgitation as well as stenosis. Both are detected and measured by echo Doppler with colour flow revealing the site and mechanism of regurgitation and continuous wave the extent of the stenosis.

Thrombolytic treatment is the choice for thrombosis of a tricuspid prosthesis and has increasingly been shown to be possible for left sided valves although with a risk of systemic embolism.[58] Thrombolytic treatment is not necessarily incompatible with continuation of the pregnancy although retroplacental haemorrhage may result in loss of the fetus. These risks have to be weighed against the risk of emergency cardiac surgery for both mother and fetus.

Summary

The use of heparin is associated with more prosthetic valve thrombosis and higher maternal mortality than warfarin. The risk of warfarin embryopathy is low, no cases occurring in some series despite continuing oral anticoagulants during the first trimester (Table 10.5). The highest incidence was reported from a centre which used clinical geneticists to detect mild cases which might otherwise have been missed.

Anticoagulant control during pregnancy should be meticulous with increased frequency of testing of INR. An INR of 2·5 is sufficient for a patient with a third generation bileaflet aortic prosthesis and 2·7 for patients with mitral prostheses.[43] In non-pregnant patients these lower levels have

TABLE 10.5—*Advantages and disadvantages of heparin and of warfarin anticoagulant treatment during pregnancy.*

Warfarin		Heparin	
Advantages	Disadvantages	Advantages	Disadvantages
Low maternal risk	Overdoses fetus	Does not reach fetus	Parenteral

Safe and effective	3% to 4% Risk of embryopathy (maximal 6th to 9th week)		Bad pharmacokinetics
			  Short action
			  Narrow therapeutic
			    index

	Risk of fetal loss
	  Termination
	  Prematurity
	  Stillbirth
			How to monitor?
			  Which test?
			  Which target?
			  How often?

			Maternal hazards
			  Valve thrombosis
			  Haemorrhage
			  Osteopenia
			  Thrombocytopaenia

			Risk of fetal loss
			  Termination
			  Prematurity
			  Stillbirth
			  (retroplacental
			  haemorrhage)

been shown to diminish the risk of bleeding complications while not incurring an increase in thromboembolism.[59] Low dose aspirin may be added but should be stopped at least a week before anticipated delivery because of possible premature closure of the arterial duct through prostaglandin inhibition. Patients with bioprosthetic valves should have regular echocardiographic monitoring during and after pregnancy to detect early deterioration before the development of haemodynamic problems.

The first successful pregnancy and delivery in a patient with a prosthetic heart valve was reported in 1966 in a patient with a Starr Edwards mitral prosthesis.[60] Thirty years later the anticoagulant management of pregnancy in women with mechanical prostheses remains unsettled despite accumulating experience showing that safe and effective heparin anticoagulation is impractical long term and cannot be achieved. Both warfarin and heparin carry hazards during pregnancy but whereas warfarin brings a small risk to the fetus, heparin compromises the mother (whose safety must be paramount). Experience with mechanical valves in pregnancy has been reduced in North America and in Europe by selection of bioprostheses in young women as well as by cautioning against pregnancy in women who already have mechanical heart valves. Neither is right. Bioprostheses deteriorate especially fast in pregnancy and need re-replacement at uncertain risk. Women with mechanical valves eager to comply with advice need not face added risk to themselves and have a high chance of a successful outcome on oral anticoagulant treatment.[61]

References

1 Ginsberg JS, Barron WM. Pregnancy and prosthetic heart valves. *Lancet* 1994; **344**: 1170–2.
2 Oakley CM. Pregnancy and prosthetic heart valves. *Lancet* 1994; **344**: 1643–4.
3 Oakley CM, Doherty P. Pregnancy in patients after valve replacement. *Br Heart J* 1976; **38**: 1140–6.
4 Denbow CE, Matadial L, Sivapragasam S, Spencer H. Pregnancy in patients after homograft cardiac valve replacement. *Chest* 1983; **83**: 540–1.
5 Nunez L, Larrea JL, Aguado MG, Reque JA, Matorras R, Minguez JA. Pregnancy in 20 patients with bioprosthetic valve replacement. *Chest* 1983; **84**: 26–8.
6 Sbarouni E, Oakley CM. Outcome of pregnancy in women with valve prostheses. *Br Heart J* 1994; **71**: 196–201.
7 Bortolloti U, Milano A, Mazzucco A, *et al*. Pregnancy in patients with a porcine valve prosthesis. *Am J Cardiol* 1982; **50**: 1051–4.
8 Salazar E, Zajarias A, Gutiarraz N, Iturbe I. The problem of cardiac valve prostheses: anticoagulants and pregnancy. *Circulation* 1984; **70**: 169–77.
9 Badduke ER, Jamieson RE, Miyashima RT, *et al*. Pregnancy and childbearing in a population with biologic valvular prostheses. *J Thorac Cardiovasc Surg* 1991; **102**: 179–86.
10 Todd ME, Thompson JH Jr, Bowie ETJ, Owen LA. Changes in blood coagulation during pregnancy. *Mayo Clin Proc* 1965; **40**: 370–83.
11 Shaper AG. The hypercoagulable states. *Ann Intern Med* 1985; **102**: 814–28.
12 Renzulli A, De Luca L, Caruso A, Verde R, Galzerano D, Cotrufo M. Acute thrombosis of prosthetic valves: a multivariate analysis of the risk factors for a life threatening event. *Eur J Cardiothorac Surg* 1992; **6**: 412–21.
13 Bloomfield DK. Fetal deaths and malformations associated with the use of coumarin derivatives in pregnancy. A critical review. *Am J Obstet Gynecol* 1990; **107**: 883–6.
14 Fillmore SJ, DeVitt E. Effects of coumarin compounds on the fetus. *Ann Intern Med* 1970; **73**: 731–4.
15 Holzgreve W, Carey JF, Gallus AS. Warfarin induced fetal abnormalities. *Lancet* 1976; **ii**: 914–15.
16 Chong MKB, Harvey D, de Swiet MD. Follow up study of children whose mothers were treated with warfarin during pregnancy. *Br J Obstet Gynaecol* 1984; **91**: 1070–3.
17 Rutherford JD, Hauder MR. Therapeutics and management during pregnancy. In: Douglas P, ed. *Heart disease in women*. Philadelphia: FA Davies, 1989: 113–25.
18 Ben Ismail M, Fekih M, Taktak M, *et al*. Prostheses valvularies cardiaques et grossesse. *Arch Mal Coeur Vaiss* 1979; **2**: 192–4.
19 Iturbe-Alessio I, Delcarmen Fonesca M, Mutchinik D, Santos MA, Zajarias A, Salazar E. Risks of anticoagulant therapy in pregnancy: women with artificial heart valves. *N Engl J Med* 1986; **27**: 1390–3.
20 Hanania G, Thomas D, Michel PL, Garbarz E, Age C, Acar J. Pregnancy in patients with valvular prostheses: Retrospective Cooperative Study in France (155 cases). *Eur Heart J* 1994; **87**: 429–37.
21 Hanania G, Thomas D, Michel PL, Garbarz E, Age C, Acar J. Pregnancy in patients with valvular prostheses: Retrospective Cooperative Study in France (155 cases). *Eur Heart J* 1994; **15**: 1651–8.
22 Taylor KM. *Report of the United Kingdom Heart Valve Registry 1993*. London: HMSO, 1995.
23 Edmunds LH Jr. Thrombotic and bleeding complications of prosthetic heart valves. *Ann Thorac Surg* 1987; **44**: 430–45.
24 Daniel WG, Nellessen U, Schroder E, Nonnast-Daniel B, Nikutta P, Lichtler PR. Left atrial spontaneous echo contrast in mitral valve disease: an indicator for increased thromboembolic risk. *J Am Coll Cardiol* 1988; **11**: 1204–11.
25 Butchart EG, Moreno de la Santa P, Rooney SJ, Lewis PA. The role of risk factors and trigger factors in cerebrovascular events after mitral valve replacement. *J Card Surg* 1994; **9(suppl)**: 228–36.

26 Routledge P, Shett HGM. Pharmacology of anticoagulants. In: Butchart EG, Bodnar E, eds. *Thrombosis, embolism and bleeding.* London: ICR Publishers, 1992: 263–76.

27 Whitfield LR, Lele AS, Levy G. Effect of pregnancy on the relationship between concentration and anticoagulation action of heparin. *Clin Pharmacol Ther* 1983; **34**: 23–8.

28 Ginsberg JS, Hirsh J. Anticoagulants during pregnancy. *Ann Rev Med* 1989; **40**: 79–86.

29 Ginsberg JS, Kowalchuk G, Hirsch K, Brill-Edwards P, Burrow R. Heparin therapy during pregnancy. *Ann Intern Med* 1989; **149**: 2233–6.

30 Ginsberg JS, Hirsh J. Use of anticoagulants during pregnancy. *Chest* 1989; **95**: 156S–160S.

31 Hirsh J. Heparin oral anticoagulant drugs. *N Engl J Med* 1991; **324**: 1865–75.

32 Brill-Edwards P, Ginsberg JS, Johnston M, Hirsh J. Establishing a therapeutic range for heparin therapy. *Ann Intern Med* 1993; **119**: 104–9.

33 Hirsh J, Poller L, Deykin D, Lerne M, Dalen JE. Optimal therapeutic range of oral anticoagulants. *Chest* 1989; **95**: 55–115.

34 Bigardi GE, Barrett S, Foale R, Spyrou N. Pregnancy and prosthetic heart valves. *Lancet* 1994; **344**: 1644.

35 Bennett GG, Oakley CM. Pregnancy in a patient with mitral valve prosthesis. *Lancet* 1968; **i**: 616–19.

36 Howell R, Fidler J, Letsky E, de Swiet M. The risks of antenatal subcutaneous prophylaxis: a controlled trial. *Br J Obstet Gynaecol* 1983; **90**: 1124–8.

37 De Swiet M, Dorrington M, Fidler J. Prolonged heparin therapy in pregnancy causes bone demineralization. *Br J Obstet Gynaecol* 1983; **90**: 1129–34.

38 Oakley CM. Anticoagulants in pregnancy. *Br Heart J* 1995; **74**: 107–11.

39 Oakley CM. Clinical perspectives: anticoagulation and pregnancy. *Eur Heart J* 1995; **16**: 1317–19.

40 Hall JG, Pauli RM, Wilson KM. Maternal and fetal sequelae of anticoagulation during pregnancy. *Am J Med* 1980; **68**: 122–40.

41 Hirsh J, Cade JF, O'Sullivan EF. Clinical experience with anticoagulant therapy during pregnancy. *BMJ* 1970; **i**: 270–3.

42 Hirsh J. Is the dose of warfarin prescribed by American physicians unnecessarily high? *Arch Intern Med* 1987; **147**: 769–71.

43 Butchart EG. Prosthesis-specific and patient-specific anticoagulation. In: Butchart EG, Bodnar E, eds. *Thrombosis, embolism, and bleeding.* London: ICR Publishers, 1992: 293–317. (Current issues in heart valve disease)

44 Butchart EG, Lewis PA, Kulatilike ENP, Breckenridge IM. Anticoagulation variability between centres: implications for comparative prosthetic valve assessment. *Eur J Cardiothorac Surg* 1988; **2**: 72–81.

45 Donzeau GP, Ng Yen, Touchot B. Acute thrombosis of a St Jude Medical Aortic prosthesis in a pregnant woman. *J Thorac Cardiovasc Surg* 1985; **33**: 248–9.

46 Shemin RJ, Phillippe M, Djau V. Acute thrombosis of a composite ascending aortic conduit containing a Bjork–Shiley valve during pregnancy. Successful emergency caesarian section and operative repair. *Clin Cardiol* 1986; **9**: 299–301.

47 Gonzalez-Santos JM, Vallejo JL, Rico MJ. Thrombosis of a mechanical valve prosthesis late in pregnancy. *Thorac Cardiovasc Surg* 1986; **34**: 335–7.

48 Tapanainen J, Ikaheimo M, Jouppila P, *et al.* Thrombosis in a mechanical aortic valve prosthesis during subcutaneous heparin therapy in pregnancy. A case report. *Eur J Obstet Gynecol Reprod Biol* 1990; **36**: 175–7.

49 Ben Ismail M, Abid F, Trabelsi S, Taktak M, Fekih M. Cardiac valve prostheses, anticoagulation and pregnancy. *Br Heart J* 1986; **55**: 101–5.

50 Wang RYC, Lee PK, Chow JF, Chen WWC. Efficacy of low dose subcutaneously administered heparin in treatment of pregnant women with artificial heart valves. *Med J Aust* 1983; **2**: 126–7.

51 Larrea JL, Nunez L, Reque JA, *et al.* Pregnancy and mechanical valve prostheses a high risk situation for the mother and the fetus. *Ann Thorac Surg* 1983; **36**: 459–63.

52 Ayan A, Yapar EG, Yuce K, *et al.* Pregnancy and its complications after cardiac valve replacement. *Int J Gynaecol Obstet* 1991; **35**: 117–22.

53 Lee PK, Wang RYC, Cho JSF, Cheung K, Wong VCW, Chan TK. Combined use of warfarin and adjusted heparin during pregnancy in patients with artificial valves. *J Am Coll Cardiol* 1986; **8**: 221–4.

54 Chesebro JH, Adam PC, Fuster V. Antithrombotic therapy in patients with valvular heart disease and prosthetic heart valves. *J Am Coll Cardiol* 1986; **8(suppl B)**: 41B–56B.

55 Pavunkumar P, Venugopal P, Kaul U, *et al.* Pregnancy in patients with prosthetic cardiac valve. A 10 year experience. *Scand J Thorac Cardiovasc Surg* 1988; **22**: 19–22.

56 Sareli P, England MJ, Berk MR, *et al.* Maternal and fetal sequelae of anticoagulation during pregnancy in patients with mechanical heart valve prostheses. *J Am Coll Cardiol* 1989; **63**: 1462–5.

57 Cotrufo M, de Luca TSL, Calabro R, Mastrogiovanni G, Lama D. Coumarin anticoagulation during pregnancy in patients with mechanical heart valve prostheses. *Eur J Cardiothorac Surg* 1991; **5**: 300–5.

58 Birdi I, Angelini GD, Bryan AJ. Thrombolytic therapy for left sided prosthetic heart valve thrombosis. *J Heart Valve Disease* 1995; **4**: 154–9.

59 Gohlke-Barwolf C, Acar J, Oakley C, *et al.* Study Group of the Working Group on Valvular Heart Disease of the European Society of Cardiology: guidelines for prevention of thromboembolic events in valvular heart disease. *Eur Heart J* 1995; **16**: 1320–30.

60 DiSaia PJ. Pregnancy and delivery of a patient with a Starr–Edwards mitral valve prosthesis: report of a case. *Obstet Gynecol* 1966; **28**: 469–72.

61 Elkayam U, Gleicher N. Anticoagulation in pregnant women with artificial heart valves. *N Engl J Med* 1987; **316**: 1664.

11: Infective endocarditis

CELIA OAKLEY

Infective endocarditis is a rare complication of pregnancy but when it is encountered it presents some particularly difficult problems in management. Moreover, the diagnosis may be missed because it is not considered and because interpretation of murmurs may be difficult. The typical systolic flow murmur and third heart sound in pregnancy together with a mammary souffle may either falsely suggest or alternatively obscure the diagnosis. The increase in stroke volume, cardiac output, blood volume, and heart rate that occur during pregnancy can precipitate heart failure caused by fever and new valve lesions. Antibiotics must be chosen to save the life of the mother but also to try to avoid damage to the fetus. The need for surgical treatment in pregnancy must be judged against the risk of losing the infant.

Although there is evidence of increased susceptibility to virus infections during pregnancy, associated with diminished cellular immunity, it is uncertain whether the risk of bacterial infection is increased or whether the incidence of infective endocarditis is higher in women with susceptible heart disease in pregnancy than outside it. Twenty years ago Nazarian *et al* estimated the incidence of infective endocarditis in pregnancy as one in 8000.[1] Nearly forty years ago Crockett *et al* found one case in every 200 pregnant women with rheumatic heart disease but that was when rheumatic heart disease was found in 1% of pregnant women.[2] The prevalence of endocarditis in pregnancy has dropped and now largely comprises women with congenital defects except in parts of the world where rheumatic fever is still common.

Infective endocarditis is a microbial infection of the endothelial lining of the heart or of the vascular endothelium, characterised by fever, positive blood cultures, vegetations on valves or congenital defects, embolism, and immunological phenomena. Except for some patients with tricuspid endocarditis virtually all patients with endocarditis have a heart murmur and endocarditis should be suspected in any such patients with unexplained fever. The other phenomena develop only later when the infection has taken hold, but embolism to any site can be the first feature.

The pathognomonic lesion of infective endocarditis is the vegetation. Damaged endothelium provides the nidus for infection and is particularly likely to be caused by high velocity jets as occur with flow from a high to a low pressure chamber. High pressure streams are associated with low pressure sinks with bacterial deposition. Endothelial breeches are thrombogenic. These are particularly a feature of floppy mitral valves. Bacteria are rapidly covered in platelet fibrin aggregates—the vegetations—which develop downstream to the jet, on the atrial surface of the mitral valve, on the right ventricular side of a ventricular septal defect, distal to a coarctation, or on the venous end of an arteriovenous fistula. Within the cardiac vegetation microorganisms are protected from host defence mechanisms by a dense covering of fibrin within which they multiply rapidly until they reach maximal density after which they become metabolically relatively inactive and are no longer easily killed by antibiotics.

Despite the poignancy of a classic illness with a high mortality which threatens both the mother and the unborn baby, infective endocarditis in pregnancy is the same disease requiring the same alert and often interventional management as it does outside pregnancy. Infective endocarditis complicating pregnancy or the puerperium has no special characteristics since the virtual disappearance of endocarditis complicating puerperal sepsis and criminal abortion in the West.[3-6] Sadly these are still found to be the commonest causes of isolated right sided endocarditis in India.[7]

The modern classification of infective endocarditis is usually into native valve and prosthetic valve endocarditis rather than into acute and subacute although the virulent pyogenic organisms such as *Staphylococcus aureus* and *Streptococcus pneumoniae* tend to produce a more aggressive and rapidly destructive invasive process than infections by streptococci of the viridans group.

With the reduction in rheumatic and syphilitic heart disease, the most common underlying conditions in young women are mitral valve prolapse and congenital heart disease.[8] A history of a known cardiac abnormality or murmur is usually present except in especially virulent diseases.[9] Endocarditis on previously normal tricuspid valves is usually staphylococcal and occurs particularly in intravenous drug abusers but can also complicate pelvic sepsis or skin infection in women with no history of drug abuse.[10] Infection on prosthetic valves accounts for about a third of all cases seen in regional centres nowadays but for a much smaller proportion in the young. The success of surgeons in palliating complex congenital cardiac malformations in infancy contributes to an increasing number of infections in young women with surgically created shunts or valve bearing conduits, and uncorrected common defects particularly aortic stenosis and ventricular septal defect are vulnerable.[11]

Any organism capable of causing endocarditis in the non-pregnant state may cause it in pregnancy but because endocarditis is a rare disease (about 1500 cases a year in the UK), pregnancy complicated by endocarditis with unusual organisms is more likely to be reported.[3,5,6] The range of organisms is probably similar to endocarditis in the non-pregnant state though organisms cultured from the vagina and postpartum uterus have been reported to cause infective endocarditis after obstetric and gynaecological procedures[3] including complicated delivery,[7] criminal abortion, curettage, and pelvic inflammation. One reviewer estimated that obstetric and gynaecological procedures may have been the source of infection in about 20% of women with enterococcal endocarditis.[3]

The reported mortality of women with infective endocarditis during pregnancy has been much the same as in the non-pregnant state. With antibiotic treatment this otherwise fatal infection should always be curable but the mortality remains between 10% and 30% in different series usually because of delayed diagnosis and failure to ask for surgical treatment.[12,13]

Infective endocarditis may present with fever, a murmur, embolism, or fulminant cardiac failure. Most often it presents with protean symptoms which could be caused by almost any other infection including tuberculosis, meningitis or encephalitis, glomerulonephritis, or acute rheumatic fever. In the fulminant acute form it can present with stroke, myocardial infarction, limb embolism, lung or cerebral abscess, or with severe congestive heart failure.

Fever is almost invariable and in its absence the diagnosis is unlikely unless antibiotics have been given. Previous antibiotics are the usual reason for negative blood cultures in patients with a clinical diagnosis of infective endocarditis.[14] Echocardiography has greatly increased the accuracy of diagnosis and has been included in the Duke criteria[15] for the diagnosis of infective endocarditis which now supersede the classic von Reyn criteria.[16] The Duke modification includes major and minor signs (as in the Duckett and Jones criteria for the diagnosis of acute rheumatic fever) and performs well.[17]

Fever, echocardiographic evidence of vegetations, and persistently positive blood cultures with a pathogenic organism are the major basis for a diagnosis of infective endocarditis. Transoesophageal echocardiography should always be used if transthoracic imaging is technically difficult or unhelpful because of the much finer detail provided by this view.[18] It is essential also in patients with suspected prosthetic valve endocarditis or possible abscess in any patient who has failed to respond to appropriate antibiotic treatment or for whom surgery is contemplated (Figure 11.1).

Once a clinical diagnosis has been made or is seriously suspected, treatment should begin as soon as three successive blood cultures have been sent to the laboratory.[19,20] This should be during the course of an hour or so. Start of antibiotic treatment should not wait on receipt of news from the microbiology department. Classic signs such as petechiae, vasculitic rash, Osler's nodes, splinter haemorrhages, and Roth's spots are usually absent in early cases. Splenomegaly usually takes about six weeks to develop as does clubbing of the fingers. These are late signs. Red cells are not found in the urine of uncomplicated cases and when present they indicate infarction or glomerulonephritis. In the latter case proteinuria and casts will also be found.

The main complications of infective endocarditis are the results of valve destruction, embolism, and an often profound immunological response

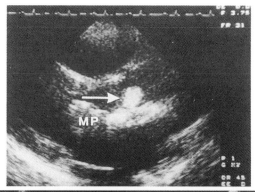

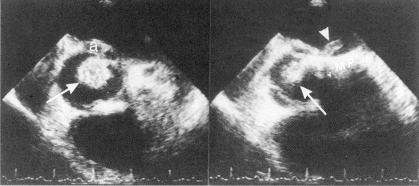

FIGURE 11.1—*Echocardiogram of a 22 year old woman with prosthetic valve endocarditis following a mitral valve replacement for endocarditis. Although the large vegetation on the aortic valve (arrows) was well seen on transthoracic views (parasternal view—top) the posterior aortic root abscess (a) and the vegetations on the mitral valve prosthesis (arrowhead) were seen only on the transoesophageal study shown below.*

with a focal crescentic glomerulonephritis. The risk of embolism is highest early in the course of the disease and diminishes with treatment. Large fluffy vegetations found on the first echocardiographic study, with or without previous embolism, may be an indication for surgery and in such cases a conservative approach to the infected valve may be possible.[21]

In pregnancy penicillin, rifampicin, and fusidic acid are safe but gentamicin can cause fetal deafness. If needed the dose should be kept low and it should not be given for more than two weeks. The use of antibiotics in pregnancy is considered in chapter 22.

The indications for surgery are the same as in the non-pregnant state and are primarily haemodynamic to save life in the face of heart failure resulting from acute valve destruction, particularly when the infecting organism is a virulent one such as a coagulase positive staphylococcus. It may be tempting to delay surgical intervention until after delivery of the baby but this should not be considered when the indications for surgery are urgent. If the baby is viable it should be delivered before the cardiac surgery.

Prophylactic antibiotics

Prevention of infective endocarditis remains a hope rather than an expectation. Pregnant women get free dental treatment under the National Health Service in England and most patients with susceptible heart disease are given antibiotic prophylaxis cards to show to their doctor and dentist. These give specific recommendations for prophylaxis in accordance with the guidelines of the British Society for Antibiotic Chemotherapy Working Party.[22] The new American guidelines are similar.[23] The indications for antibiotic prophylaxis during pregnancy are the same as in the non-pregnant state to cover any procedures or conditions likely to be associated with bacteraemia in any woman with susceptible heart disease. Prophylaxis for anticipated normal delivery is discretionary but should be given to patients with a history of previous infective endocarditis and to patients with prosthetic valves.

The incidence of bacteraemia following normal delivery has been estimated as between 0 and 5%[24,25] and the occurrence of infective endocarditis complicating normal delivery in women with heart disease unprotected by prophylactic antibiotics is negligible.[26,27] No proven case occurred among more than 2000 normal deliveries of cardiac patients in one survey.[26] In most cases of infective endocarditis the cause and portal of entry of the preceding bacteraemia remains unknown. Despite the low risk of infection some obstetricians choose to cover an anticipated normal delivery in a susceptible patient because complications are unpredictable.[26,27]

The recommended UK regimen for operative delivery is 1 g of amoxycillin (or ampicillin) intravenously or intramuscularly, plus 120 mg of gentamicin at the time of induction of anaesthesia, and 500 g amoxycillin orally six hours later. For patients allergic to penicillin or who have had penicillin more than once in the previous month vancomycin 1 g should be given by slow intravenous infusion over 100 minutes followed by gentamicin 120 mg intravenously at the time of induction or 15 minutes before the surgical procedure. Teicoplanin 400 mg intravenously (+ gentamicin) can be given instead of vancomycin.[22]

If antibiotics are given to cover anticipated normal delivery the time of possible bacteraemia is less predictable and may be more prolonged. Amoxycillin 3 g can be given orally as it provides more prolonged bactericidal blood levels but may cause nausea. Parenteral dosing may be better but needs to be repeated.

If cardiac surgery is required antibiotic cover should be with flucloxacillin and gentamicin for 48 hours or with a single dose of ceftriaxone 1 g.[27]

References

1 Nazarian M, McCullough GH, Fielder DL. Bacterial endocarditis in pregnancy. *J Thorac Cardiovasc Surg* 1976; **86**: 880–3.

2 Crockett EJ, Batchelor TM, Corbeil J. Pregnancy and subacute bacterial endocarditis. *Obstet Gynecol* 1960; **16**: 43–95.
3 Lein JN, Stander RW. Subacute bacterial endocarditis following obstetric and gynecologic procedures. *Obstet Gynecol* 1959; **13**: 568–73.
4 Hanson GC, Phillips J. A fatal case of subacute bacterial endocarditis in pregnancy. *Journal of Obstetrics and Gynaecology of the British Commonwealth* 1965; **72**: 781–4.
5. Anand CM, MacKay AD, Evans JI. Haemophilus aphrophilus endocarditis in pregnancy. *J Clin Pathol* 1976; **29**: 812–14.
6 Holshouser CA, Ansbacher R, McNitt T, Steele R. Bacterial endocarditis due to listeria monocytogenes in a pregnant diabetic. *Obstet Gynecol* 1978; **51(suppl)**: 9S–10S.
7 Grover A, Anand IS, Varma J, *et al.* Profile of right-sided endocarditis: An Indian experience. *Int J Cardiol* 1991; **33**: 83–8.
8 Danchin N, Volrai P, Briancon S, *et al.* Mitral valve prolapse as a risk factor for infective endocarditis. *Lancet* 1989; **i**: 743–6.
9 Holt S, Hicks DA, Charges RG, Coulshed N. Acute staphylococcal endocarditis in pregnancy. *Practitioner* 1978; **220**: 619–22.
10 Clifford CP, Eykyn SJ, Oakley CM. Staphylococcal tricuspid valve endocarditis in patients with structurally normal hearts and no evidence of narcotic abuse. *Q J Med* 1994; **87**: 755–7.
11 Gersony WM, Hayes CJ, Driscoll DJ, *et al.* Bacterial endocarditis in patients with aortic stenosis, pulmonary stenosis or ventricular septal defect. *Circulation* 1993; **87(suppl 1)**: 121–6.
12 McKinsey DS, Ratts TE, Binos AL. Underlying cardiac lesions in adults with infective endocarditis. The changing spectrum. *Am J Med* 1987; **82**: 681–8.
13 Verheul HA, van den Brink RBA, van Vreeland T, Moulijn AC, Duren DR, Dunning AJ. Effects of changes in management of active infective endocarditis on outcome in a 25 year period. *Am J Cardiol* 1993; **72**: 682–7.
14 Oakley CM. The medical treatment of culture-negative infective endocarditis. *Eur Heart J* 1995; **16(suppl B)**: 90–3.
15 Durack DT, Bright DK, Lukes AS. Duke Endocarditis Service: New criteria for diagnosis of infective endocarditis: utilization of specific echocardiographic findings. *Am J Med* 1994; **96**: 200–9.
16 von Reyn CF, Levy BS, Arbeit RD, Friedland G, Crumpacker CS. Infective endocarditis: An analysis based on strict case definitions. *Ann Intern Med* 1981; **94**: 505–17.
17 Bayer AS, Ward JI, Ginzton LE, Shapiro SM. Evaluation of new clinical criteria for the diagnosis of infective endocarditis. *Am J Med* 1994; **96**: 211–19.
18 Lowry RW, Zoghbi WA, Baker WB, Wray RA, Quinones MA. Clinical impact of transoesophageal echocardiography in the diagnosis and management of infective endocarditis. *Am J Cardiol* 1994; **73**: 1089–91.
19 Working Party of the British Society for Antimicrobial Chemotherapy. Antibiotic treatment of streptococcal and staphylococcal endocarditis. *Lancet* 1985; **2**: 815–17.
20 Oakley CM. Endocarditis. In: Jackson G, ed. *Difficult concepts in cardiology.* London: Martin Dunitz, 1994: 337–56.
21 Hendren WG, Morris AS, Rosenkranz ER, *et al.* Mitral valve repair for bacterial endocarditis. *J Thorac Cardiovasc Surg* 1992; **103**: 124–9.
22 Working Party of the British Society for Antimicrobial Chemotherapy. Antibiotic prophylaxis and infective endocarditis. *Lancet* 1992; **i**: 1292–3.
23 Wilson WR, Karchmer AW, Dajani AS, *et al.* Antibiotic treatment of adults with infective endocarditis due to streptococci, enterococci, staphylococci and HACEK micro-organisms. *JAMA* 1995; **274**: 1706–13.
24 Redlead PD, Fadell EJ. Bacteraemia during parturition. *JAMA* 1959; **160**: 1284–5.
25 Baker TH, Hubbell R. Reappraisal of asymptomatic peurperal bacteremia. *Am J Obstet Gynecol* 1967; **97**: 575–6.
26 Sugrue D, Blake S, Troy P, MacDonald D. Antibiotic prophylaxis against infective endocarditis after normal delivery—is it necessary? *Br Heart J* 1980; **44**: 499–502.
27 Hall JC, Christiansen K, Carter MJ, *et al.* Antibiotic prophylaxis in cardiac operations. *Ann Thorac Surg* 1993; **56**: 916–22.

12: Management of pregnancy in Marfan syndrome, Ehlers–Danlos syndrome, and other heritable connective tissue disorders

ANNE H CHILD

The major heritable disorders of connective tissue that cause problems in obstetric management include Marfan syndrome, Ehlers–Danlos syndrome, osteogenesis imperfecta, achondroplasia, and other short-stature syndromes.[1] Although individually rare, together they form an important group, requiring cooperative management by several specialists during pregnancy. Improved medical and surgical management permits affected female patients to reach child bearing age, but good advice should begin during family or individual counselling sessions, well before child bearing starts. The genetic risk, the possibilities of prenatal diagnosis and the obstetric risk to women should also be discussed later with the prospective parents, and if pregnancy is contraindicated, the alternatives of childlessness, adoption, or ovum donation should be discussed.

Pregnancy in patients with Marfan syndrome

Marfan syndrome is the most serious dominantly inherited fibrillin deficiency disorder, affecting all systems, but mainly eyes, heart, and skeleton. Signs of classical involvement in two out of three main systems constitute the diagnostic criteria,[2] and there is a family history of affected relatives in about 75% of cases. In 25% of patients the syndrome arises as a spontaneous mutation in either ovum or sperm. If unaffected parents have such a child, then the risk of recurrence in a subsequent pregnancy is the population incidence (one in 5000) and is negligible. To date there is no report of two unaffected parents having more than one affected child.

153

If one parent has Marfan syndrome then there is a 50/50 chance in each pregnancy that the child will inherit the single dominant gene. This expresses itself in most instances with the same degree of severity as in the affected parent's family. On average, one in ten children will be severely affected, requiring surgery for eye, heart, or skeletal problems in early life. The overall risk of producing a severely affected child is therefore one in twenty (one in two multiplied by one in ten). However, the risk is greater than one in ten in a severely affected family. The parents must accept that the baby may be like any of the affected family members. Each child, of either sex, has a 50/50 chance of inheriting the gene. Those who do *not* inherit the gene, cannot pass it on.

Marfan syndrome does not skip generations. Mildly affected people must be examined by an experienced clinician to determine whether they are carrying the gene or not. DNA from blood or skin fibroblast culture may be tested to confirm the presence of a mutation in the gene. At present, 80% of mutations in the fibrillin gene (FBN1) on chromosome 15q 21.3 can be detected using heteroduplex screening.[3]

Gene testing

Provided parents would consider termination, prenatal diagnosis of Marfan syndrome in the first fourteen weeks is possible, in two situations. In the first, the affected parent's family contains at least two people with Marfan syndrome in two generations, and study of blood samples from affected and unaffected members demonstrates linkage to the chromosome 15 gene.[4] These tests should be arranged well before planning a pregnancy, as they may take 6 to 9 months to be analysed. Testing may be arranged by referral to the patient's nearest genetic counselling unit. If the family demonstrates linkage to FBN1, during pregnancy the fetal blood sample may then be analysed for carrier status.

In the second situation, the affected parent has been shown to have a mutation in the FBN1 gene. Chorionic villus sample at 11 weeks may be studied directly or grown, and fibroblast RNA/DNA analysed for the same mutation. If parents simply wish to learn whether their infant is affected, testing should occur in the newborn period using cord blood sample. This avoids the 1% risk of miscarriage incurred during fetal sampling by any method.

Maternal health

Before pregnancy, a woman with Marfan syndrome should be assessed fully for cardiological problems. Women with minimal cardiac involvement (aortic root diameter less than 4·0 cm, and no significant aortic or mitral regurgitation) should be told of a 1% risk of aortic dissection, or other serious cardiac complications such as endocarditis or congestive cardiac failure during pregnancy.[5] Family history must be taken into account, as three pregnant women at our hospital dissected when the aortic root diameter was less than 5 cm. Two came from families in which dissection at a low aortic root diameter was a feature. One of these patients died, although her infant was delivered by emergency caesarean section, and is unaffected. The other was operated on to replace the ascending aortic root and valve, as her dissection occurred three months after delivery. Her child appears to be unaffected.

Patients with substantial cardiac complications, including those who have had aortic root or mitral valve replacement, or women with an aortic root diameter of more than 4 cm, are usually advised against pregnancy because of the high risk of dissection. If such a woman decides to go ahead with pregnancy, she must be considered at high risk of further cardiac complications. We have three patients who have had successful pregnancies after mitral valve replacement.

Other options

In a recent survey of reproductive decisions by 102 adult women with Marfan syndrome in the UK, 10% had decided not to have children because of the one in two risk that each child would be affected.[6] Five had adopted children, and three had tried unsuccessfully to adopt. If the parent is mildly affected, a letter from the genetic counsellor or medical practitioner stating that a normal life expectancy is expected or at least that 20 years can most likely be given to raising an adopted child, may persuade the adoption panel to allow adoption to proceed. Adoption of a foreign child, in which case parental medical health may not be considered such an important determinant, has also been successful for a few women.

If the husband has Marfan syndrome, then artificial insemination by donor may be considered the genetic solution. The infant is then 50% genetically the offspring of the couple, and 100% the environmental child of the couple. If the mother is affected, then ovum donation would virtually eliminate the genetic risk. For affected mothers with serious heart disease, a further possibility is to find a surrogate mother. The cost and availability of these methods varies, depending on the particular country and city in which the couple live. In vitro fertilisation with pre-implantation diagnosis is now a real possibility, if the couple are willing to accept the rather low 40% average success rate (live birth) after three attempts.

Cardiovascular complications

Cardiovascular changes during normal pregnancy include thinning of the aortic wall, and increased cardiac workload due to increased blood volume to supply the placenta, and increased heart rate and cardiac output. For this reason, a careful cardiological assessment of the mother with Marfan syndrome should be made before pregnancy, including echocardiogram and electrocardiogram looking carefully for aortic root diameter, valvar insufficiency, and left ventricular enlargement and diminished contractility.

Each pregnancy should be supervised jointly by a cardiologist and an obstetrician who are knowledgeable about the possible complications in women with Marfan syndrome. These include aortic dissection, aortic rupture, increasing aortic and mitral regurgitation, congestive cardiac failure, and need to prescribe beta-blocker drugs or bed rest or both if aortic root enlargement is shown and possible early delivery to reduce the cardiac stress. The risk period extends to six months postpartum, and beyond if the infant is breast fed. Echocardiograms each trimester, and at three and six months postpartum should be carefully compared to look for signs of aortic dilatation. Dissection can occur without dilatation. Severe chest or abdominal pain should be treated as possible aortic dissection and immediate ultrasound assessment of the entire aorta should be made. Cardiac surgery may be indicated, and the infant may need to be delivered by caesarean section if the pregnancy has advanced far enough.[7]

Labour and delivery should be managed so that minimal cardiovascular stress develops.[8] Delivery should be by the least stressful route, and normally this means an uninduced labour, with vaginal delivery. The woman may be allowed to labour on her side or in a semi-erect position to minimise stress on the aorta. Caesarean delivery is, however, the safest mode for women with aortic root diameters of more than 4·5 cm.

Beta-blocker drugs, if given before pregnancy, need not be stopped. No adverse effects on the fetus have been reported. If a woman has had cardiac surgery before becoming pregnant and is taking warfarin, it has been thought that this should be changed to an alternative anticoagulant regimen such as heparin or aspirin for the first trimester, to avoid fetal damage from warfarin,[9,10] and again at term to avoid postpartum haemorrhage.[11] However, the more recent view is that coumarin anticoagulants should be continued through pregnancy, because the risk of embryopathy is low, except for those rare women who require high doses (see chapter on artificial valves, and chapter on anticoagulants).

Aortic dissection during pregnancy

The dissected aorta poses the greatest challenge to the surgeon. There is general agreement that acute dissections of the ascending aorta are surgical emergencies; repair with a composite graft is the procedure of choice.[12] An acute dissection with origin beyond the left subclavian artery should be managed medically by reduction of blood pressure and dP/dt (change in pressure/change in time) until the clinical condition stabilises. Dissection of the descending aorta does not usually need surgery, and can be followed by MRI at regular intervals. However, progressive dilatation to 50 mm, recurrent pain, or signs consistent with fresh dissection, and organ or limb ischaemia, are all indications for repair. Crawford *et al*[13] pioneered the staged approach to aortic surgery, and performed the first successful replacement of the entire aorta in a patient with Marfan syndrome.[14]

156

About 500 families are known to us in the UK. Over the past ten years, eight women have developed dissections during pregnancy or in the six months after delivery. Of these, one died suddenly three weeks before term, the infant was delivered by emergency caesarean section, survived, and seems unaffected. The other women survived, and have ultrasound assessment of the entire aorta every six months. Each patient is on beta-blocker drugs to protect the aortic wall from high pressure. Three have had further dissections requiring aortic root replacement, and two of these required subsequent abdominal and then thoracic aneurysm replacement. One died soon after operation. The other has had two episodes of endocarditis necessitating hospital admission and prolonged intravenous antibiotic therapy.

Anaesthesia

Anaesthetic management of caesarean section, followed by repair of aortic dissection, must take account of fetal and maternal risks.[7] The goal should be to minimise fetal exposure to depressant drugs while ensuring a well-controlled haemodynamic environment for the mother. Sodium thiopentone for induction at a dose of 4 mg/kg causes minimal fetal depression. To counter expected increases in heart rate or blood pressure at induction, labetolol may be given before induction. Fentanyl for analgesia limits fetal exposure to opioids. Epidural and spinal anaesthesia should be undertaken only after consideration of the possibility of dural ectasia;[15] arachnoid cysts might result in considerable dilution. Emergency surgery, using hypothermic extracorporal circulation, when the fetus is premature, may lead to fetal death.[7]

Maternal non-cardiovascular complications

Women with predominantly skeletal manifestations may find that their joint pains worsen, or, more often, improve as a result of the hormonal effects of pregnancy. Generally, joints become slightly more lax, and so symptoms such as low back pain may worsen. Patients with moderately severe untreated scoliosis should probably have repeated lung function studies done, and the risk of pulmonary symptoms during pregnancy, from increased cardiac output, and increased pressure on the diaphragm should be discussed with their physician. Some patients report that their eyesight changes slightly during pregnancy, and they may need an altered prescription for spectacles part way through pregnancy. For those who have had dislocated lens or retinal detachment, the risk of further such complications is not significantly increased, but this should be discussed with their ophthalmologist before pregnancy.

Outcome of pregnancy

Miscarriage under 20 weeks of pregnancy may be slightly more common, particularly if this is a familial tendency in female members affected.[5] This does not appear to be the result of cervical incompetence, as is seen in other connective tissue disorders such as Ehlers–Danlos syndrome. Premature rupture of fetal membranes does not seem to be a problem, but it is advisable not to take long journeys far from the intended centre of delivery in the last month of pregnancy. Excessive vaginal haemorrhage at the time of delivery is a problem in a small number of women who also tend to bruise easily, and therefore cross-matched blood for transfusion should be available. In those who show signs of poor wound healing (thin, stretched scars on knees or elsewhere, or stretch marks which extend from the lumbar region to the upper back, over the shoulders, or on the thighs), if stitching is required, then buttressing, and leaving the stitches in longer than one would for a normal woman, are recommended. In such cases, the antibiotic cover, which should be provided routinely for delivery and three days postpartum, should be extended until sutures are removed. Babies with Marfan syndrome tend to be long and thin, with aged, wise-looking faces, high palate and long fingers, and may have low birth weight due to lack of subcutaneous fat. They may be hypotonic and have difficulty feeding. This improves with age. Each infant should have a neonatal echocardiogram as there is a 1% chance of congenital structural heart disease.[16] Ophthalmological examination for dislocated lenses should also be made soon after birth.

Future pregnancies

Each woman with Marfan syndrome should be assessed cardiologically before starting a further pregnancy. In our experience, the couples who have an unaffected infant, frequently go on to plan a second pregnancy. Those who have an affected infant often decide not to have further family. The wish to have children is a strong biological urge in some couples, but may not be as strong in others. For this reason, only the couples themselves, having taken expert advice from medical advisors, and after discussing the problem with their support team, including religious advisor, parents, brothers and sisters, and close friends, are capable of making the decision to have a child. Whatever the decision of the couple, the medical profession is always prepared to support the decision fully by providing the best medical and surgical care available to maximise the chance of a successful outcome of pregnancy for both mother and child.

Ehlers–Danlos syndrome

Ehlers–Danlos syndrome includes at least ten separate entities.[17] Classic type I is inherited as an autosomal dominant trait characterised by hyperextensible skin, joint hypermobility, fragile tissues, and a bleeding diathesis. During pregnancy, women may show increased bruisability, hernias, varicosities, or rupture of large blood vessels.[18] Delivery may cause separation of the symphysis pubis, and postpartum haemorrhage may be severe. Episiotomy and laparotomy incisions heal slowly, and perineal haematoma may occur despite episiotomy. It is suggested that retention sutures be used and that the sutures not be removed for at least 14 days, to avoid wound dehiscence.

Prematurity and precipitous deliveries are common complications, partly because of lax cervical connective tissues.[19] If the fetus is affected, the membranes are involved; premature rupture of the membranes often occurs at 32 to 36 weeks. Affected infants tend to be hyperextensible and may have congenitally dislocated hips. Neonates may even be misdiagnosed as having neurological problems because of floppiness and bleeding disorders.

Gynaecological problems also are more common in women with Ehlers–Danlos syndrome type I. Menorrhagia may be secondary to the bleeding diathesis. Uterine and bladder prolapse or abdominal hernias occur because of abnormal connective tissue. There is insufficient experience with the effects of other forms of the syndrome on reproduction to draw conclusions. Ehlers–Danlos type IV, which is characterised by greater bleeding tendencies and vascular rupture, is inherited as a dominant trait. Menorrhagia has been reported, and vessel rupture during pregnancy is of particular concern in these women.

Osteogenesis imperfecta

Osteogenesis imperfecta is a rare disease with an incidence in the region of one in 40 000 births. There are at least four different types of osteogenesis imperfecta, all of which result in osteoporosis and fracture of long bones with minimal trauma. Type I is an autosomal dominant form with blue sclerae; type II is a lethal autosomal dominant (new mutations) or rarely autosomal recessive form; type III is an autosomal dominant (uncommonly autosomal recessive) form with white sclerae and progressive deformities; and type IV is an autosomal dominant variety with mild to moderate bone deformity with white sclerae and variable severity of fractures. The expressivity of the autosomal dominant forms may vary greatly among family members.

Women with osteogenesis imperfecta tarda may have blue sclerae, multiple fractures after trivial injuries, short stature with scoliosis and bowing of the femur and tibia, and gradual onset of otosclerosis and deafness. Complications during pregnancy include increasing respiratory compromise, especially in women with short stature and kyphoscoliosis, cephalopelvic disproportion as a result of previous pelvic fractures, uterine rupture, and separation of the symphysis pubis.[20] General anaesthesia is associated with an increased risk of malignant hyperthermia,[21] and spinal or epidural anaesthesia may lead to fracture of osteoporotic vertebrae. A fetogram in the late third trimester is advisable to diagnose an affected fetus with healing fractures, in which case caesarean section to avoid fetal trauma is indicated. Forceps must be avoided, as wormian bones fracture and cause intracranial bleeding. Delivery by caesarean section is probably the method of choice because of the increased risk of cephalopelvic disproportion, pelvic fractures, uterine rupture, and intrapartum or postpartum haemorrhage associated with this condition.[22]

Endotracheal intubation may be difficult because of limited cervical spine movement, brittle teeth, and receding mandible. If technically possible, epidural anaesthesia may be preferable. An arterial line can be inserted for blood pressure monitoring if arterial blood-gas analysis is also required. Otherwise, digital blood pressure monitoring is adequate. Temperature should be monitored continuously, and a cooling blanket and cold intravenous fluids be available.

Pseudoxanthoma elasticum

Pseudoxanthoma elasticum is a rare disorder of elastic fibres with a prevalence of six per million population. Two types are inherited as autosomal dominant traits, and two as autosomal recessive traits.[23] It affects mainly the skin, cardiovascular system, and eye. Progressive yellow maculopapular areas resembling "plucked chicken skin" affect the lax skin of flexural areas such as the side of the neck, elbow crease, and arm pit. Early arteriosclerotic changes in medium-sized arteries lead to hypertension, congestive cardiac failure, and stroke. The retina demonstrates angioid streaks, retinal haemorrhage, and macular degeneration, and the patient eventually becomes blind.

Despite the potential maternal and fetal hazards, most pregnancies in women with this disease have a normal course and outcome. Progression of cardiovascular and ophthalmic features during pregnancy has not been reported. In 1983 Berde et al reported a total of 24 pregnancies in seven women.[24] Gastrointestinal haemorrhage was a prominent feature in eight of 20 pregnancies in five women.

Viljoen et al described 54 pregnancies in 20 women, all of whom inherited the trait in autosomal recessive manner, the diagnosis being established by skin biopsy.[25] Twelve pregnancies miscarried between six and 14 weeks' gestation. Two of these losses occurred in the same woman and were attributed to cervical incompetence. Hypertension complicated seven pregnancies. One baby died at 4 days of age from a complex congenital cardiac anomaly. Abdominal wall striae developed in all patients. No abnormal maternal vaginal or gastrointestinal bleeding was recorded.

Achondroplasia

This rare (four/million population) dominantly inherited condition is the most common form of short-limbed dwarfism, inherited as an autosomal dominant trait. As many as 75% to 80% of cases are the result of new mutations. Gynaecological problems, including premature menarche, leiomyomata uteri, enlarged breasts, and premature menopause, are common. Pregnancy causes glucosuria, great reduction in mobility because of awkwardness, and cardiorespiratory compromise (due to the small chest cavity). All women with achondroplasia should be delivered by caesarean section because of a contracted pelvis, and general anaesthesia should be used because spinal stenosis, osteophytes, short pedicles or a small epidural space make conduction anaesthesia difficult. This increases the risk of dural puncture, and may limit the spread of local anaesthetic. If epidural anaesthetic is necessary, attempting puncture above the lordotic lumbar spine may permit easier location and catheterisation of the epidural space. A low dose of epidural anaesthetic is usually sufficient. Cervical spine instability can lead to increased difficulty with tracheal intubation, necessitating the use of a small tracheal tube.[26-29]

Other short-stature syndromes

A number of other chondrodystrophies are compatible with pregnancy. Asphyxiating thoracic dystrophy may be complicated by cystic renal tubular dysplasia or glomerulosclerosis, and careful monitoring of renal status during pregnancy is required. A few women with diastrophic dysplasia have had children without complications. Chondroectodermal dysplasia (Ellis–van Creveld syndrome) is often associated with cardiac defects, and appropriate monitoring and prophylactic antibiotics are required. Women with Kniest dysplasia have delivered without complications. Morquio syndrome (spondyloepiphyseal dysplasia congenita) may be associated with retinal detachments, and this should be considered during pregnancy. Odontoid hypoplasia may make neck manipulation during general anaesthesia dangerous. Many women with chondrodysplasia punctata (Conradi–Hunermann syndrome) have borne children without incident. Cartilage-hair hypoplasia syndrome may cause such a short trunk that there is severe cardiac and respiratory compromise; periodic pulmonary function tests during pregnancy may be of value.

A few general statements may be made about pregnancy in women with chondrodystrophies.[30] Caesarean section is usually required for cephalopelvic disproportion, and a trial of labour is often not advisable. General anaesthesia must be undertaken with special care because of odontoid hypoplasia with secondary instability of C1 and C2, and risk of spinal cord damage. Subluxation of C1 on C2 can occur during general anaesthesia. Unfortunately, conduction anaesthesia also may be problematic because of altered vertebral configurations.[4] Cardiorespiratory compromise may occur as a result of a small chest cavity. Despite these potential problems, most women with chondrodystrophies do remarkably well during pregnancy.

References

1 Royce PM, Steinmann B, eds. *Connective tissue and its heritable disorders*. New York: Wiley-Liss, 1993.

161

2 Beighton P, de Paepe A, Danks D, *et al*. International nosology of heritable disorders of connective tissue. *Am J Med Genet* 1988; **29**: 581–94.

3 White MB, Carvalho M, Derse D, O'Brien SJ, Dean M. Detecting single base substitutions as heteroduplex polymorphisms. *Genomics* 1992; **12**: 301–6.

4 Godfrey M, Vandermark N, Want M, *et al*. Prenatal diagnosis and a donor splice site mutation in fibrillin in a family with Marfan syndrome. *Am J Hum Genet* 1993; **53**: 472–80.

5 Pyeritz RE. Maternal and fetal complications of pregnancy in the Marfan syndrome. *Am J Med* 1981; **71** 784–90.

6 Child AH, Poloniecki J, Camm AJ. Reproductive decisions and the potential demand for prenatal diagnosis. *Am J Med Genet* 1993; **47**: 145.

7 Pinosky ML, Hopkins RA, Pinckert TL, Suyderhoud J. Anaesthesia for simultaneous cesarean section and acute aortic dissection repair in a patient with Marfan's syndrome. *J Cardiothorac Vasc Anesth* 1994; **8**: 451–4.

8 Gordon CF, Johnson MD. Anaesthetic management of the pregnant patient with Marfan syndrome. *J Clin Anesth* 1993; **5**: 248–51.

9 Greaves M. Anticoagulants in pregnancy. *Pharmacol Ther* 1993; **59**: 311–27.

10 Ginsberg JS, Hirsh J, Turner DC, Levine MN, Burrows R. Risks to the fetus of anticoagulant therapy during pregnancy. *Thromb Haemost* 1989; **61**: 197–203.

11 Irons DW, Pollard K. Postpartum haemorrhage secondary to Marfan's disease of the uterine vasculature. *Br J Obstet Gynaecol* 1993; **100**: 279–81.

12 Gott VL, Pyeritz RE, Magovern GJ Jr, Cameron OE, McKusick VA. Surgical treatment of aneurysms of the ascending aorta in the Marfan syndrome: results of composite-graft repair in 50 patients. *N Engl J Med* 1986; **314**: 1070–4.

13 Svensson LG, Crawford ES, Coselli JS, Safi HJ, Hess KR. Impact of cardiovascular operation on survival in the Marfan patient. *Circulation* 1989; **80(suppl)**: 233–42.

14 Crawford EJ, Crawford JL, Stowe CL, Safi HJ. Total aortic replacement for chronic aortic dissection occurring in patients with and without Marfan's syndrome. *Ann Surg* 1984; **199**: 358–62.

15 Pyeritz RE, Fishman EK, Bernhardt BA, Siegelman SS. Dural ectasia is a common feature of the Marfan syndrome. *Am J Hum Genet* 1988; **43**: 726–32.

16 Sloper JC, Storey G. Aneurysms of the ascending aorta due to medial degeneration associated with arachnodactyly (Marfan's disease). *J Clin Pathol* 1953; **6**: 299–303.

17 Steinmann B, Royce PM, Superti-Furga A. The Ehlers–Danlos syndrome. In: Royce PM, Steinmann B, eds. *Connective tissue and its heritable disorders*. New York: Wiley-Liss, 1993.

18 Beighton P. *The Ehlers–Danlos syndrome*. London: William Heinemann Medical, 1970.

19 Barabas AP. Ehlers–Danlos syndrome: associated with prematurity and premature rupture of the foetal membranes; possible increase in incidence. *BMJ* 1966; **2**: 682.

20 Young BK, Gorstein F. Maternal osteogenesis imperfecta. *Obstet Gynecol* 1968; **31**: 461.

21 Solomons CC, Myers DN. Hyperthermia of osteogenesis imperfecta and its relationship to malignant hyperthermia. In: Gordon RA, Gritt BA, Kalow W, eds. *International symposium on malignant hyperthermia*. 1971: 319.

22 Cunningham AJ, Donnelly M, Comerford J. Osteogenesis imperfecta: Anesthetic management of a patient for cesarean section: A case report. *Anesthesiology* 1984; **61**: 91–3.

23 Neldner KH. Pseudoxanthoma elasticum. In: Royce PM, Steinmann B, eds. *Connective tissue and its heritable disorders*. New York: Wiley-Liss, 1993.

24 Berde C, Willis DC, Sandberg EC. Pregnancy in women with pseudoxanthoma elasticum. *Obstet Gynecol Surv* 1983; **38**: 339–44.

25 Viljoen DL, Beighton P, Mabin T, Woods K, Saxe N, Bonafede P. Pseudoxanthoma elasticum in South Africa—genetic and clinical implications. *S Afr Med J* 1984; **66**: 813–16.

26 Kalla GN, Fening E, Obiaya MO. Anaesthetic management of achondroplasia. *Br J Anaesth* 1986; **58**: 117–19.

27 Wardall GJ, Frame WT. Extradural anaesthesia for caesarean section in achondroplasia. *Br J Anaesth* 1990; **64**: 367–70.

28 Brimacombe JR, Caunt JA. Anaesthesia in a gravid achondroplastic dwarf. *Anaesthesia* 1990; **45**: 132–4.

29 Carstoniu J, Yee I, Halpern S. Epidural anaesthesia for caesarean section in an achondroplastic dwarf. *Can J Anaesth* 1992; **33**: 708–11.

30 Allanson JE, Hall JG. Obstetric and gynecologic problems in women with chondrodystrophies. *Obstet Gynecol* 1986; **67**: 74–8.

13: Autoimmune diseases

CELIA OAKLEY

The collagen vascular diseases are characterised by multiorgan dysfunction, predominantly affecting the joints, skin, and connective tissues but often also the heart and lungs. In most of them specific autoantibodies have been identified and so they are often known as systemic autoimmune diseases. All of these disorders have in common vasculitis, exudation, fibrosis, and immunological phenomena. Many of them affect young women who become pregnant or seek advice about pregnancy.

The heart can be involved in any of these conditions and the cardiologist must be alert to recognise underlying collagen vascular disease in any patient with a pericardial syndrome, myocardial disorder, conduction system failure, aortitis, valve disease, systemic or pulmonary hypertension, or even myocardial infarction. Any of these manifestations can develop first during pregnancy but more usually the immune depression which protects the fetus from rejection provides the mother with a welcome remission of her disease. Although remission of activity is common, pre-existing compromise of cardiovascular reserve may first cause difficulties during pregnancy. Since the use of echocardiography became widespread in clinical practice, it has become apparent that the prevalence of cardiovascular involvement in patients with collagen vascular disease is much higher than had previously been appreciated. Fitness for pregnancy depends on disease activity, cardiovascular reserve, involvement of other organ systems, and prognosis. It is individually highly variable and both the literature and personal experience of pregnancy in patients with cardiac involvement in some of the syndromes is sparse.

Rheumatic fever

Rheumatic fever is still common in developing countries, particularly India,[1] and South America but in the Arabian Peninsula,[2] Hong Kong, and Singapore[3] the prevalence of rheumatic fever and its sequelae is now comparable to that in the West. A resurgence of acute rheumatic fever was reported in 1992 from eight locations in the United States when largely middle-class children were affected.[4] Because spread of the responsible streptococcus is facilitated by poverty and overcrowding, as well as by lack of prompt penicillin treatment of pharyngitis, this was a surprise but perhaps caused by changes in streptococcal antigenicity. Rheumatic fever is a serious

163

complication of pregnancy which is now rarely seen in developed countries but which should be remembered in new immigrants. It usually represents reactivation and there may be pre-existing valve disease. Long term penicillin prophylaxis following rheumatic fever in childhood should prevent recurrence of rheumatic activity during early adulthood and be continued up to the age of 25 or for at least five years following the last evidence of activity.

In the past chorea was regarded as a peculiarly common manifestation of rheumatic activity during pregnancy and for this reason was termed "chorea gravidarum".[5] Rheumatic activity during pregnancy has been associated with spontaneous abortion and fetal death[6] and if rheumatic activation or reactivation leads to congestive heart failure during pregnancy the risk of maternal death is high.[5,6,7]

The treatment of active rheumatic fever during pregnancy is by rest, penicillin, paracetamol analgesia if needed, and selective use of steroids.[6,7,8] Aspirin, usually the mainstay of treatment outside pregnancy, should, like other non-steroidals, be avoided in analgesic dosage because it may cause premature closure of the ductus arteriosus.[9]

Women with rheumatic activity during pregnancy usually already have mitral stenosis or other valve lesions causing risk of pulmonary oedema. The mitral stenosis may previously have been asymptomatic and undiagnosed (Chapter 8).

Rheumatoid arthritis

Pericarditis is much the commonest cardiological manifestation of rheumatoid arthritis. The histological features are non-specific usually in the form of a fibrous adhesive pericarditis seen in more than one third of necropsy cases.[10,11] The pericarditis may be patchy but may obliterate the pericardial cavity and cause constriction of the heart.

Strangely, pericarditis in rheumatoid arthritis is often painless and not recognised clinically.[10,12] Chest pain is unusual despite a friction rub being heard. Clinical pericarditis is most often seen in patients with active seropositive disease but can occur at any time during the course of rheumatoid arthritis and occasionally may even precede the development of joint manifestations.[13]

Echocardiography is a sensitive technique for the detection of pericardial involvement, particularly pericardial effusion.[14] Tamponade is rare. The outcome of pericardial effusion in rheumatoid pericarditis is usually clinical resolution but a minority have persistent or recurrent effusions or go on to constrictive pericarditis.

Rare patients are troubled by recurrent pericardial effusions which may be loculated. The size of pericardial effusion that can be tolerated without producing a rise in intra-pericardial pressure (tamponade) is usually small because of the indistensibility of a thickened fibrous pericardium and tolerance is lessened in pregnancy. This "effusive constrictive" picture is also seen in tuberculous pericarditis (Chapter 17). Such chronic tamponade, like constrictive pericarditis without effusion is best treated by pericardiectomy. Surgery can be carried out safely during pregnancy.

Chronic pericardial involvement with limitation of cardiac filling either with or without residual effusion may first cause symptoms during pregnancy. As blood volume and stroke input rise, so does the venous pressure rise, ultimately with the development of hepatomegaly and peripheral oedema but pulmonary congestion is absent unless there are other cardiac problems such as mitral regurgitation.

Electrocardiographic changes are non-specific. Echocardiography may show a small and sometimes loculated pericardial effusion and pericardial thickening may be recognised. The important echocardiographic signs of pericardial constriction are diagnostic but may be quite subtle. There is typically a trembling appearance of the septum which lacks its normal curvature towards the right ventricle because of the equal diastolic pressures in the two ventricles but with an early diastolic jerk towards the left ventricle. An abrupt halt to ventricular filling is seen both on imaging of the posterior wall and septum and on continuous wave Doppler inflow studies. The latter show reciprocal changes with respiration and there may be dramatic inspiratory swings of the septum towards the left ventricle explaining the pulsus paradoxus usually but not invariably found.

The pathognomonic rheumatoid granuloma is not seen in the pericardium but occurs in the myocardium where it does not usually cause impairment of myocardial function.[11] Apart from granulomas, the myocardium may show interstitial collections of lymphocytes, plasma cells, and histiocytes.[15]

Granulomas may involve the cardiac valves but it is rare for the functional integrity of the valves to be compromised. Rarely, severe aortic regurgitation may develop associated with an aortitis or even rupture of a sinus of valsalva, and acute mitral regurgitation may be caused by chordal rupture in severe seropositive disease.[16–18]

Coronary arteritis may develop as part of a generalised vasculitis in a few rheumatoid patients and this may also involve the pulmonary vascular bed giving rise to primary type pulmonary hypertension.[12,19]

Rheumatoid granulomas may rarely involve the conduction system causing sinoatrial or atrioventricular conduction abnormality.[13]

Adult Still's disease

Rheumatoid arthritis associated with marked systemic symptoms is usually given the eponym "adult Still's disease". This may present with acute pericarditis similar to acute idiopathic pericarditis, but constitutional features with prolonged fever, continued raised acute phase reactants, and hypoalbuminaemia with developing diffuse arthritis make the true diagnosis clear. Progression to constriction is much more common in Still's disease than it is in rheumatoid arthritis. This may be subclinical until pregnancy brings it to light.

It is important for young women with rheumatoid arthritis or a history of Still's disease to have a full cardiovascular examination including echocardiography if they are contemplating pregnancy. An effusive constrictive or constrictive syndrome not previously symptomatic may be discovered. Although this is unlikely to be dangerous during pregnancy, it may cause considerable discomfort and prepregnancy pericardiectomy is usually advisable. This is a low risk procedure with gratifying results and avoids the development of tachycardia, high venous pressure, and oedema associated with progressive fatigue and breathlessness. This development during pregnancy can also cause considerable concern if the pericardial cause is not recognised and the picture falsely ascribed to a restrictive cardiomyopathy.

Primary type pulmonary hypertension is a rare but recognised complication of rheumatoid arthritis which can be progressive and endanger the mother's life during pregnancy (Chapter 7).[19] In general the presence of pulmonary hypertension is a contraindication to pregnancy. It is a difficult diagnosis to make clinically and an important reason for including a comprehensive echocardiographic examination in the prepregnancy cardiovascular evaluation of patients with autoimmune diseases.

Systemic lupus erythematosus (SLE) and the anticardiolipin antibody syndrome

Systemic lupus erythematosus (SLE) is characterised by multiorgan involvement with damage to skin, kidneys, lungs, and heart caused by a microvasculitis. The disorder is recognised serologically by the presence of antinuclear or antiphospholipid antibodies or both. These form antigen antibody complexes and are responsible for the widespread vasculitis that occurs.

The heart is a major target in SLE with clinical features in more than half the cases and autopsy involvement in almost all.[20] The endocarditis described by Libman and Sacks in 1924 was one of the first well defined autopsy findings in SLE and was then regarded as pathognomonic.[21] The pericardium, myocardium, endocardium, cardiac valves, and coronary or pulmonary vessels may be involved and systemic hypertension secondary to renal vascular involvement may be a further serious complication.[22–25]

Pericarditis is the most common and may be the first clinical manifestation of cardiac involvement and occurs in about one half of patients with SLE but is found echocardiographically or at autopsy in many more.[20,23] This is usually painful in contrast to pericarditis in rheumatoid arthritis and it varies from an acute serofibrinous pericarditis to a continuing process with obliteration of the pericardial space, though constriction is rare. The effusion in SLE is exudative with low complement levels.

166

Evidence of endocarditis may be found only on echocardiography or there may be clinical mitral regurgitation sometimes slowly evolving to mitral stenosis or mixed mitral disease resembling that in rheumatic disease and eventually needing valve replacement.[25–27] Valvular abnormalities are found on echocardiography in up to one third of patients ranging from localised leaflet thickening to distinct vegetations (Figure 13.1).[28,29,32] These are of variable size, usually ovoid, either isolated or occurring as mulberry like clusters at the tips of the leaflets. Rarely they can be large enough to affect leaflet mobility. They consist of lymphocytes, plasma cells, and fibrous tissue with platelets. Severe involvement of the tricuspid valve has also been described.[30]

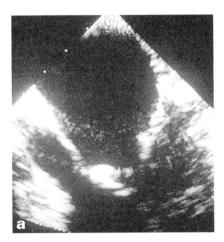 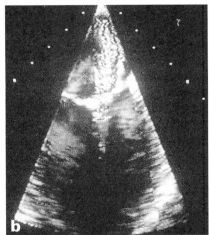

FIGURE 13.1—*Transoesophageal echocardiographic images of Libman-Sacks vegetation on the anterior leaflet of the mitral valve of a 23 year old woman with systemic lupus erythematosus. The valve was moderately regurgitant and gradually also became stenotic. She eventually died of staphylococcal endocarditis. (a) The mitral valve in diastole. The valve is domed and the large vegetation is clearly seen. (b) The mitral regurgitant jet is shown with Doppler in systole. (Both figures: left atrium above and left ventricle below)*

Myocardial involvement is uncommon particularly if the disease has been diagnosed early and immunosuppressive agents have been given.[31,32] The most common cause of myocardial dysfunction in SLE is occlusive coronary artery disease caused either by arteritis or by atheroma.[33] The atheroma may itself be secondary to a previous arteritis, possibly accelerated by the use of steroids in treatment. Thrombosis of a major epicardial coronary artery may be responsible for acute myocardial infarction in SLE. A high prevalence of coronary atherosclerosis has been found in young women dying with SLE, though of course these are patients with the most severe disease who often have pericardial and valvular involvement. Intensive immunosuppressive treatment appropriate for suppression of extra cardiac vasculitis may paradoxically aggravate coronary lesions.[35] Complete coronary occlusion by thrombosis may be followed by lysis with

167

an angiographically normal appearance although this may go on later to stricture formation, angiographically identical to the appearance in ordinary atheroma. The intravascular ultrasound appearances may differ.

Pulmonary hypertension is a rare but important complication of SLE which may appear suddenly during the course of the disease.[34-37] Death often occurs within two or three years but regression has also been observed. Progressive right heart failure is the usual cause of death, which may also be sudden. The true prevalence of pulmonary hypertension in SLE is difficult to ascertain but recent studies using Doppler techniques have shown pulmonary hypertension in as many as 14% of patients with SLE.[35] The pulmonary hypertension may progress to a plexiform arteriopathy without evidence of thromboembolism or veno-occlusive disease. A few patients, however, have large vessel pulmonary arterial thrombosis and occlusion, perhaps related to the lupus anticoagulant and a hypercoagulable state or vasculitis which was fatal in a patient in the postpartum period.[38] Medial hypertrophy and intimal fibrosis are seen in all.

Young women with SLE contemplating pregnancy need to be screened specifically for anticardiolipin antibodies and particularly for the presence of pulmonary hypertension and other cardiovascular complications of their disease including lupus nephritis and systemic hypertension. Pulmonary hypertension may lead to rapid deterioration in pregnancy with progressive dyspnoea, fatigue, and right heart failure. As lupus patients often complain of fatigue, particularly in pregnancy, the presence of pulmonary hypertension may be missed if it is not remembered, and may lead to a fatal outcome. If it is first recognised during pregnancy the pregnancy should be terminated if it is early but if it is more advanced or the mother refuses termination her admission for in-hospital rest, observation, oxygen, subcutaneous heparin, and readiness for early delivery are important. Fetal growth may slow or stop, usually in association with compromise of maternal output and oxygenation. Delivery is best accomplished by caesarean section under general anaesthesia (Chapter 7).

The prevalence of antibodies to phospholipids in SLE has been recognised for many years and lupus "anticoagulant" is responsible for the well known false positive test for syphilis. In the anticardiolipin syndrome (the Hughes syndrome), described in 1986, antibodies to cardiolipin are associated with venous and arterial thrombosis, labile and malignant hypertension, pulmonary hypertension, cerebral vasculitis, migraine, and recurrent abortion.[39] Raised anticardiolipin antibodies can cause placental vessel thrombosis and should be remembered particularly as a cause for recurrent mid-trimester miscarriage.[39,40] Patients with anticardiolipin antibody syndrome typically have livedo reticularis and thrombocytopenia but not necessarily other features of lupus. Endothelial injury by anticardiolipin antibodies leads to platelet adhesion and thrombus formation. An association has been described between raised anticardiolipin antibodies and cardiac involvement in SLE[39-41] but valvular involvement is not always found to be related to antiphospholipid autoimmunisation. In a study of

168

20 women with primary antiphospholipid syndrome all had increased levels of serum IgG anticardiolipin antibodies and recurrent miscarriages with or without thromboses and thrombocytopenia but none had cardiac valvular involvement on echocardiographic study. Conversely in 39 consecutive patients with SLE high levels of anticardiolipin antibodies were found in 73% of the patients with valvular lesions and in 67% of the patients whose valves appeared to be normal.[42]

Pregnancy in patients with antiphospholipid antibodies may be complicated by thrombocytopaenia, thromboembolic episodes, pre-eclampsia, intra-uterine growth retardation, and fetal death. Recent reports have also described postpartum cardiac, pulmonary, and renal failure. ·

Patients with antiphospholipid antibodies are at risk of thromboembolic events and sometimes show striking livedo reticularis, strokes, or vascular dementia (Sneddon's syndrome).[43] Pregnancy is often interrupted by repeated early and mid-trimester abortions. One such patient who had severe aortic regurgitation from aortitis with widening of the aortic root, underwent aortic valve replacement with a mechanical valve.[44] Subsequently, after treatment with aspirin, she brought a pregnancy to full term for the first time. She was converted from warfarin to heparin at 38 weeks (as was then the usual practice) but there was an unavoidable break in anticoagulant control following delivery between cessation of full doses of heparin and resumption of warfarin with achievement of an adequate international normalised ratio. During this time she had a stroke which has left her with considerable residual impairment. It was especially important for anticoagulant control to be uninterrupted in this vulnerable patient and she should have had elective caesarean section after temporary reversal of warfarin with fresh frozen plasma followed by rapid resumption thereafter. This syndrome may be an indication for a bioprosthesis because of the increased thromboembolic risk. A similar patient with an aortic bioprosthesis has had a successful pregnancy without complications.

The mechanism by which anticardiolipin antibodies promote thrombosis is still unclear and it is uncertain also whether immunosuppressive treatment reduces this risk. Anticoagulants need to be given long term to patients who have had thrombotic events, especially if imaging shows cerebral infarction, but individual judgement is needed after a single thrombosis and in patients with thrombocytopenia. Doubt has been expressed about the efficacy of aspirin unless combined with high intensity warfarin in these patients.[45]

Infants born to mothers with active SLE may have congenital atrioventricular block, pericarditis, and a lupus like syndrome which is attributable to transplacental transfer of maternal antibodies.[46,47] This neonatal lupus syndrome comprises congenital heart block or neonatal skin rash and is specifically associated with maternal anti Ro/SS-A autoantibodies.[47,48] Sera from all 14 mothers of children with isolated heart block were positive for Ro/SS-A auto antibodies but these antibodies may also present in mothers with SLE whose children are healthy. However, acquired heart block has been seen in mothers with SLE whose serum is negative for the Ro/SS-A antibodies.[46,49] The heart block may appear as early as the middle trimester of pregnancy or may not be recognised until the peripartum period. It may give rise to heart failure and hydrops fetalis. Fetal heart pacing has been used successfully to treat it. The heart block remains throughout life. Fetal bradycardia from this cause should not be mistaken for fetal distress.

Progressive systemic sclerosis (scleroderma)

Progressive systemic sclerosis (PSS) is a chronic fibrosing disorder of insidious onset and with a prolonged course.[50] It usually does not develop until childbearing is over but occasionally Raynaud's phenomenon and evidence of visceral involvement affecting gastrointestinal tract, lungs, heart, and kidneys may develop earlier. Involvement of small renal arteries may cause severe systemic hypertension as well as renal failure.

A variety of PSS with a milder and more slowly evolving course has been given the acronym CREST syndrome. This stands for calcinosis, Raynaud's phenomenon, oesophageal dysfunction, sclerodactily, and telangiectasia. Patients with CREST syndrome have a high incidence of primary type pulmonary hypertension which may be associated with pulmonary interstitial fibrosis and a restrictive lung syndrome. The anti-centromere antibody is found in more than half the patients with CREST syndrome.[53]

The pathophysiology is one of diffuse vascular and microvascular destruction, leading to a state of under-perfusion and chronic ischaemia of involved organs with low grade inflammation. Pulmonary[51] and renal hypertension contribute to mortality and morbidity but cardiac involvement can lead to heart failure even in the absence of pulmonary or systemic arterial hypertension.[52] When pericarditis occurs it is usually asymptomatic. Conduction system abnormalities are common.

Pregnancy is rare in PSS or CREST syndrome because the patients are usually older. Pregnant women should have full assessment, particularly of myocardial integrity, remembering pulmonary hypertension, renal function, and systemic hypertension.

Mixed connective tissue disease (MCTD)

This is an overlap syndrome with elements of rheumatoid arthritis, SLE, systemic sclerosis and polymyositis.[53] The disorder is characterised by high titres of anti-ribonuclear protein (RNP) antibodies.[54] Although the presence of the RNP antibody is not in itself diagnostic, the absence of antibodies to native DNA differentiates MCTD from SLE. Cardiovascular abnormalities are common, including acute pericarditis, myocarditis, and pulmonary hypertension.[55] The incidence of pericarditis is up to 38% usually with a small asymptomatic effusion, though large effusions and tamponade can occur. The fluid is often sero-sanguineous with fibrin deposition and infiltration with polymorphonuclear leucocytes.

Valvular involvement, myocardial inflammation with patchy fibrosis, coronary artery involvement, and systemic hypertension may individually or together contribute to left ventricular failure.[56] Both the epicardial and intramyocardial coronary arteries may develop intimal hyperplasia distinct from the abnormality described in SLE or polymyositis. Unlike patients with systemic sclerosis, no contraction band necrosis or widespread fibrosis is found in the myocardium.

Pulmonary hypertension is a common complication, which determines fitness for pregnancy and prognosis.[55,57] The pathology is similar to that in primary pulmonary hypertension. Interstitial pulmonary fibrosis is less prominent than in systemic sclerosis. Valvular and endocardial abnormalities are non-specific without the vegetations seen in SLE.

Polyarteritis nodosa

This belongs to a group of diseases characterised by systemic necrotising vasculitis whose clinical features depend on the size and site of the involved arteries, associated granuloma formation, and variable eosinophilia. These variations distinguish the clinical presentation as polyarteritis nodosa (PAN), the Churg–Strauss variant, Wegener's granulomatosis, allergic granulomatosis, giant cell arteritis, or hypsersensitivity vasculitis. The distinctive features often overlap and defy precise classification.

Veins and venules are involved as well as muscular arteries in a focal necrotising inflammation, leading to aneurysm formation and sometimes rupture. Thrombosed vessels with and without recanalisation, and healed lesions with fibrous replacement are seen. The angiographic demonstration of multiple aneurysms of small arteries in the liver or kidneys is important for diagnosis.

Aneurysmal dilatation may also occur in the coronary arteries with occlusion. Renal involvement can lead to systemic hypertension. Haemorrhage into any organ from rupture of aneurysms can lead to many clinical syndromes. Hepatitis B surface antigen is present in up to half the patients with PAN. PAN is most common in young and middle aged men but the Churg–Strauss variant is more common in women.

Churg–Strauss syndrome

The Churg–Strauss syndrome is associated with considerable eosinophilia. These patients usually have an atopic history of asthma, allergic rhinitis, and nasal polyps.[58] The hypereosinophilia can occasionally mimic Loeffler's syndrome or a primary eosinophilic syndrome but rarely reaches as high concentrations and is associated with a life-threatening vasculitic illness with high concentrations of IgE and immune complexes containing IgE.[59] Pericarditis may occur and progress to constriction, and endomyocardial fibrosis has been described leading to overlap with hypereosinophilic syndrome.[60–61] Myocardial failure may develop from microvascular involvement with patchy myocardial necrosis. The Churg–Strauss variant does not usually relapse after remission.

Pregnancy during the acute phase is rare but can occur if there has been spontaneous remission. Fitness for pregnancy in a patient with a history of Churg–Strauss syndrome depends on the residual integrity of vital organs.

Patients who have recovered from the Churg–Strauss syndrome continue to have asthma and nasal polyps but otherwise may remain as well as they were before the illness. One such patient who developed jaundice from hepatic vascular involvement at age 22 was then found to have pulmonary eosinophilia with a long atopic history of asthma and nasal polyps. She was referred to us because she had developed peripheral oedema with persistent hepatomegaly. She was found to have a raised venous pressure from constrictive pericarditis. This was successfully resected. She subsequently had three children and more than 20 years later remains well.

Wegener's granulomatosis

Wegener's granulomatosis usually causes a necrotising granulomatous vasculitis of the upper respiratory tract including the para nasal sinuses, middle ear, nasal pharynx, and bronchial tree with renal involvement.[62] Raised titres of antineutrophil cytoplasmic antibodies (ANCA) are a specific marker for Wegener's granulomatosis. ANCA titres can also be helpful in following disease activity during treatment. Cardiac complications are rare, though coronary arteritis and pericarditis are found in half the cases at autopsy. Myocardial infarction and heart block are rare complications.[63]

Wegener's is rarely seen during pregnancy as it is most common at an older age. It responds particularly well to cyclophosphamide, so women are likely to have been rendered infertile unless ova have been stored.

Kawasaki disease (mucocutaneous lymph node syndrome)

This acute febrile illness of infancy and early childhood was first described in Japan in 1967 but before that it was probably known in the West as the rare "infantile polyarteritis nodosa". It is known that although still more prevalent in the Orient, Kawasaki disease can affect any ethnic group.

The clinical features in childhood are distinctive. They include fever, conjunctival injection, strawberry tongue, erythema and swelling of the hands and feet, an erythematous rash, and lymphadenopathy. This is followed by desquamation of the skin of the hands and feet, arthritis, defervescence, and thrombocytosis. A widespread systemic vasculitis affects arterioles, capillaries, and venules with a propensity for involvement of the proximal epicardial coronary arteries.[64,65] A widespread panarteritis of medium sized muscular arteries tends to develop in the second and third weeks of illness. The major coronary arteries may undergo aneurysmal dilatation, thrombotic occlusion, or rupture. The small vessel vasculitis resolves with scarring and considerable intimal fibrosis. Survivors may be left with chronic ischaemic heart disease and a risk of sudden death. They may subsequently develop angina or late infarction and need coronary artery bypass surgery.[66,67,68] Kawasaki disease is an important though rare cause of ischaemic heart disease in young women who have no other risk factors.[69] There is not always a history of the distinctive febrile illness in childhood.

The coronary artery aneurysms are usually readily seen on echocardiography during the active phase of the illness in childhood but may regress after treatment with immunoglobulin. Later coronary angiography usually shows abnormalities that are confined to the proximal two or three cm of the main left and right coronary arteries with sparing of the more distal parts. This is distinct from the appearance of coronary ectasia which is a manifestation of advanced coronary atherosclerosis and therefore usually seen in older people with conventional risk factors. Old Kawasaki disease is one of the rare causes of myocardial infarction during pregnancy or the puerperium (Chapter 18).

Takayasu's arteritis

First described by a Japanese ophthalmologist this large vessel arteritis is not confined to the Orient, but it is seen far less frequently in the West. In contrast to temporal arteritis which is a disorder of the elderly, Takayasu's arteritis affects children or young adults of either sex.[70] Large to medium sized arteries are the seat of the arteritis, from the aortic root (where it may lead to aortic regurgitation) to the more distal aorta. At any site it causes acquired coarctations or linear narrowing. The brachiocephalic, coronary, mesenteric, and renal arteries may become occluded at their origins. The major pulmonary artery branches may be affected in a similar manner (Figures 13.2 and 13.3). If the aorta and its branches are spared the patient may present with pulmonary hypertension as a result of large vessel stenoses or occlusions (Chapter 7).

The duration of active inflammatory arteritis may be quite short and is often obscured in apparently non-specific constitutional illness, the patient presenting later with the effects of regional arterial occlusion such as stroke, subclavian steal syndrome, and systemic or pulmonary hypertension.

Widespread involvement of the aorta and major conducting arteries can lead to systolic hypertension with a greatly widened pulse pressure even in the absence of aortic regurgitation. The systolic hypertension tends to increase on exercise and pharmacological control is difficult, particularly if the rigidity of the aorta is complicated by acquired thoracic or abdominal coarctation. Localised disease can sometimes be remedied surgically and renal artery stenosis by angioplasty, but the results are often poor. The arteries become thick walled and eventually widespread calcification may result.

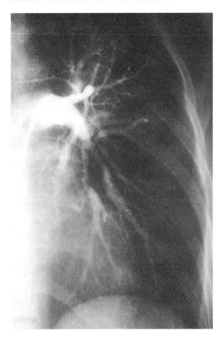

FIGURE 13.2—*Left pulmonary arteriogram from a young English woman with moderately severe pulmonary hypertension from burnt out Takayasu arteritis involving also the origins of carotid, subclavian, and renal arteries. Multiple linear stenoses are present. Despite this she has had two successful pregnancies.*

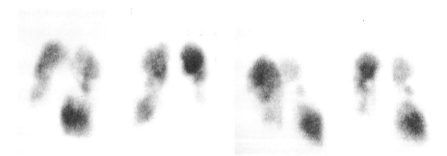

FIGURE 13.3—*Perfusion lung scans from a Chinese woman who developed haemoptysis during a pregnancy and was found to have severe pulmonary hypertension with murmurs over the lungs caused by branch stenoses. She also had systemic hypertension from renal artery stenosis. Now, 30 years later, she is well at age 65 and still has pulmonary hypertension at systemic level, marked pulmonary regurgitation and systemic hypertension controlled on nifedipine. The perfusion lung scan has not changed over the years and shows multiple defects.*

Pregnancy in women with Takayasu's arteritis has led to fatalities, cerebral haemorrhage, and heart failure.[71-74] Problems usually stem from poor blood pressure control particularly during labour when systolic blood pressure may rise considerably during contractions.[71] Low birth weights have been reported in patients with hypertension. Management in pregnancy should be focused on blood pressure control to avoid these maternal complications but excessive reduction in blood pressure may compromise placental perfusion in patients with acquired aortic coarctations.

A good response to steroids can be anticipated only if patients are seen during the acute phase as indicated by fever and raised acute phase reactants, and steroid treatment should be given only to patients who become pregnant during the active phase of the disease.[72]

Advice about future pregnancy depends on the sequelae of the burnt out disease. Digital subtraction angiography may show previously silent occlusions of major arteries. One symptom-free patient was found to have only a single vertebral arterial supply to the brain after silent occlusion of both carotids and one vertebral artery. She subsequently had a successful pregnancy with no complications. Another patient with a history of acute disease at the age of 9 was left with a blood pressure of 200/20 without aortic regurgitation but associated with evidence of previous widespread aortitis and distal aortic occlusion. She became pregnant against advice and survived. Another patient underwent Dacron tube bypass grafting of a thoraco-abdominal stenosis with relief of hypertension and no complications in a subsequent successful pregnancy.

Delivery by caesarean section should be considered for patients with severe hypertension or heart failure, and epidural anaesthesia should be avoided in patients with considerable aortic narrowing because the vasodilatation may greatly reduce blood pressure in the distal segment and compromise placental blood flow. An accelerated second stage of labour may be suitable for less severely affected patients.

Relapsing polychondritis

This is a rare syndrome in which no specific autoantibodies have been identified. It is characterised by chronic inflammatory changes in cartilage, particularly of the nose and ears, often associated with scleritis and episcleritis and sometimes with aortitis leading to aortic regurgitation. Mitral regurgitation caused by chordal rupture has also been described in this condition which may overlap with other collagen vascular disorders or with Takayasu's arteritis.[75]

Judgement about the safety of pregnancy must take into account the severity of aortic regurgitation and the systemic hypertension if aortitis is widespread. Aortic regurgitation is well tolerated during pregnancy in patients with good left ventricular function, and activity of the disease is likely to remit during pregnancy.

The sero-negative spondyloarthropathies

These disorders are distinguished by association with HLA B27 haplotype and by the absence of rheumatoid factor. They include ankylosing spondylitis, Reiter's syndrome, and psoriatic arthritis. Cardiovascular involvement when it occurs is similar in all three syndromes.

The B27 antigen is present in 4–8% of the normal population but in over 90% of patients with ankylosing spondylitis or Reiter's syndrome and in half the patients with a spondyloarthropathy associated with psoriasis. More than 80% of patients with inflammatory bowel disease complicated by spondyloarthropathy are B27 positive.

Men develop ankylosing spondylitis and Reiter's syndrome more commonly than women but as many women as men get psoriatic arthritis. Cardiac involvement when it occurs is usually associated with a long history of disease. Aortitis is similar to that in syphilis, affecting the aortic root and valve[76] but, unlike syphilis, may extend down into the proximal ventricular septum so involving the conducting system and rarely also the anterior leaflet of the mitral valve.[77] Aortic regurgitation results from scarring, thickening and shortening of the aortic cusps and from dilatation of the aortic root.[76,77] Mitral regurgitation is rare. Heart block may develop. Cardiac involvement is uncommon in women of childbearing age.

Behçet's disease

Behçet's disease is a multi-system vasculitic disorder which mainly affects young adults. Men are involved more often than women, usually in the third or fourth decade and more often in Mediterranean or Oriental people than in the West. Cardiovascular and pulmonary involvement is common. It was originally identified by the triad of oral and genital ulceration with relapsing uveitis.[79,80] Oral ulceration and erythema nodosum remain major diagnostic pointers. The disease has been divided into mucocutaneous, arthritic, and ocular types and skin pathergy has come to be regarded as pathognomonic but is not present in all patients. Pathergy is the development of sterile abscesses following even mild skin trauma such as venepuncture.

Reports of pregnancy are rare.[81–83] Among 27 pregnant women with Behçet's disease reported from a single centre in Korea the activity of the disease was exacerbated in 18 women and reduced in nine. Deterioration usually occurred during the first trimester in those who did poorly but no predictive features emerged. The newborn were healthy.[84]

Vascular Behçet's disease is characterised by venous and arterial thromboses and large vessel aneurysms involving any major arteries including the pulmonary arteries. Death may follow massive haemoptysis. Polymorphonuclear infiltration of the arterial wall with degeneration of elastica and medial muscle are seen.

There is no known autoantibody and the diagnosis is based on the typical constellation of abnormalities with polymorphonuclear leucocytosis, circulating immune complexes, and skin pathergy.

References

1 Vijaykumar M, Narula J, Srinath Reddy K, Kaplan EL. Incidence of rheumatic fever and prevalence of rheumatic heart disease in India. *Int J Cardiol* 1994; **43**: 221–8.

2 Agarwal AK. Rheumatic fever and rheumatic heart disease in Arabia. *Int J Cardiol* 1994; **43**: 229–30.

3 Sanderson JE, Woo KS. Rheumatic fever and rheumatic heart disease—declining but not gone. *Int J Cardiol* 1994; **43**: 231–2.

4 Ayoub EM. Resurgence of rheumatic fever in the United States: the clinical picture of a preventable disease. *Postgrad Med J* 1992; **92**: 133–6.

5 Lewis BV, Parson M. Chorea gravidarum. *Lancet* 1966; **i**: 284–6.

6 Ueland K, Metcalfe J. Acute rheumatic fever in pregnancy. *Am J Obstet Gynecol* 1966; **95**: 586–7.

7 Ueland K. Rheumatic heart disease in pregnancy. In: Elkayam U, Gleicher N, eds. *Cardiac problems in pregnancy*. New York: Alan R Liss, 1990.

8 Sullivan JM, Ramanathan KB. Management of medical problems in pregnancy. *N Engl J Med* 1985; **313**: 304.

9 Rudolph AM. Effects of aspirin and acetaminophen in pregnancy and in the newborn. *Arch Intern Med* 1981; **141**: 358–63.

10 Lebowitz WB. The heart in rheumatoid arthritis (rheumatoid disease). A clinical and pathological study of sixty-two cases. *Ann Intern Med* 1963; **58**: 102–23.

11 Bonfiglio T, Atwater EC. Heart disease in patients with seropositive rheumatoid arthritis. A controlled autopsy study and review. *Arch Intern Med* 1969; **124**: 714–9.

12 Gordon DA, Stein JL, Broder I. The extra-articular features of rheumatoid arthritis. A systemic analysis of 127 cases. *Am J Med* 1973; **54**: 445–52.

13 Cathcart ES, Spodick DH. Rheumatoid heart disease. A study of the incidence and nature of cardiac lesions in rheumatoid arthritis. *N Engl J Med* 1962; **266**: 959.

14 Bacon PA, Gibson DG. Cardiac involvement in rheumatoid arthritis. An echocardiographic study. *Ann Rheum Dis* 1974; **33**: 20–4.

15 Weintraub AM, Zvaifler NJ. The occurrence of valvular and myocardial disease in patients with chronic joint deformity. A spectrum. *Am J Med* 1963; **35**: 145–62.

16 Zvaifler NJ, Weintraub AM. Aortitis and aortic insufficiency in the chronic rheumatic disorders—a reappraisal. *Arthritis Rheum* 1963; **6**: 241–56.

17 Roberts WC, Kehoe JA, Carpenter DF, Golden A. Cardiac valvular lesions in rheumatoid arthritis. *Arch Intern Med* 1968; **122**: 141–6.

18 Howell A, Say J, Hedworth-Whitty R. Rupture of the sinus of valsalva due to severe rheumatoid heart disease. *Br Heart J* 1972; **34**: 537–40.

19 Asherson RA, Morgan SH, Hackett D, *et al*. Rheumatoid arthritis and pulmonary hypertension. *J Rheumatol* 1984; **12**: 154–9.

20 Ansari A, Lardon PH, Bates HD. Cardiovascular manifestations of systemic lupus erythematosus. Current perspective. *Prog Cardiovasc Dis* 1985; **27**: 421.

21 Libman E, Sacks B. A hitherto undescribed form of valvular and mural endocarditis. *Arch Intern Med* 1924; **33**: 701–37.

22 Bergen S. Pericardial effusion as manifestation of systemic lupus erythematosus. *Circulation* 1960; **22**: 144–50.

23 Heijtmancik M, Wright JC, Quint R, Jennings FL. The cardiovascular manifestations of systemic lupus erythematosus. *Am Heart J* 1964; **68**: 118–30.

24 Borenstein DG, Fye B, Arnett FC, Stevens MB. Myocarditis in systemic lupus erythematosus. Association with myositis. *Ann Intern Med* 1978; **89**: 619–24.

25 Galve E, Candell-Riera J, Pigrau C, Permanyer-Miralda G, Garcia-del-Castillo H, Soler-Soler J. Prevalence, morphologic types and evolution of cardiac valvular disease in systemic lupus erythematosus. *N Engl J Med* 1988; **319**: 817–23.

26 Dajee H, Hurley EJ, Szarnicky RJ. Cardiac valve replacement in systemic lupus erythematosus. *J Thorac Cardiovasc Surg* 1983; **85**: 718–26.

27 Ford PM, Ford SE, Lillicrap DP. Association of lupus anticoagulant with severe valvular heart disease in systemic lupus erythematosus. *J Rheumatol* 1988; **15**: 597–600.

28 Crozier G, Li E, Milne MJ, Nicholls MG. Cardiac involvement in systemic lupus erythematosus detected by echocardiography. *Am J Cardiol* 1990; **65**: 1145–8.

29 Enomoto K, Kaji Y, Mayumi T, *et al*. Frequency of valvular regurgitation by colour Doppler echocardiography in systemic lupus erythematosus. *Am J Cardiol* 1991; **15**: 209–11.

30 Laufer J, Frand M, Milo S. Valve replacement for severe tricuspid regurgitation caused by Libman-Sacks endocarditis. *Br Heart J* 1982; **48**: 294–7.

31 Bulkley BH, Roberts WC. The heart in systemic lupus erythematosus and the changes induced in it by corticosteroid therapy: a study of 36 necropsy patients. *Am J Med* 1975; **58**: 243–64.

32 Been M, Thomson BJ, Smith MA, *et al*. Myocardial involvement in systemic lupus erythematosus detected by magnetic resonance imaging. *Eur Heart J* 1988; **9**: 1250–6.

33 Homcy CJ, Liberthson RR, Fallon JT, *et al*. Ischemic heart disease in systemic lupus erythematosus in the young patient: report of six cases. *Am J Cardiol* 1982; **49**: 478–84.

34 Asherson RA, Oakley CM. Pulmonary hypertension and systemic lupus erythematosus. *J Rheumatol* 1986; **13**: 1–5.

35 Simonson JS, Schiller NB, Petri M, Hellmann DB. Pulmonary hypertension in systemic lupus erythematosus. *J Rheumatol* 1989; **16**: 918–25.

36 Morelli S, Giordano M, De Marzio P, Priori R, Sgreccia A, Valesini G. Pulmonary arterial hypertension responsive to immunosuppressive therapy in systemic lupus erythematosus. *Lupus* 1993; **2**: 367–9.

37 Perez HD, Kramer N. Pulmonary hypertension in systemic lupus erythematosus: report of four cases and review of the literature. *Semin Arthr Rheum* 1981; **11**: 177–81.

38 Hubscher O, Eimon A, Elsner B, *et al*. Fatal postpartum vasculitis in systemic lupus erythematosus. *J Rheumatol* 1989; **16**: 918–25.

39 Hughes GRV, Gharavi AE. The anticardiolipin syndrome. *J Rheumatol* 1986; **13**: 486–9.

40 Hughes GRV. The antiphospholipid syndrome: ten years on. *Lancet* 1993; **342**: 341–4.

41 Nihoyannopoulos P, Gomez PM, Joshi J, Loizou S, Walport MJ, Oakley CM. Cardiac abnormalities in systemic lupus erythematosus. Association with raised anticardiolipin antibodies. *Circulation* 1990; **82**: 369–75.

42 Gabrielli F, Alcini E, Di Prima MA, Mazzacurati G, Masala C. Cardiac valve involvement in systemic lupus erythematosus and primary antiphospholipid syndrome: lack of correlation with antiphospholipid antibodies. *Int J Cardiol* 1995; **51**: 117–26.

43 Antoine JC, Michel D, Garnier P, Genin C. Rheumatic heart disease and Sneddon's syndrome. *Stroke* 1994; **25**: 689–91.

44 Chartash EK, Lans DM, Paget SA, *et al*. Aortic insufficiency and mitral regurgitation in patients with systemic lupus erythematosus and the antiphospholipid syndrome. *Am J Med* 1989; **86**: 407.

45 Ducceschi V, Sarubbi B, Iacono A. Primary antiphospholipid syndrome and cardiovascular disease. *Eur Heart J* 1995; **16**: 441–5.

46 Meilof JF, Frohn-Mulder IM, Stewart PA, *et al*. Maternal autoantibodies and congenital heart block: no evidence for the existence of a unique heart block associated anti-Ro/SS-A autoantibody profile. *Lupus* 1993; **2**: 239–46.

47 Reed BR, Lee LA, Harmon C. Autoantibodies to SS-A/Ro in infants with congenital heart block. *J Pediatr* 1983; **103**: 889–91.

48 Buyon JP, Ben-Chetrit E, Karp S, *et al*. Acquired congenital heart block: pattern of maternal antibody response to biochemically defined antigens of the SSA/Ro-SSB La system in neonatal lupus. *J Clin Invest* 1989; **84**: 627–34.

49 Bilazarian SD, Taylor AJ, Brezinski D, *et al*. High-grade atrioventricular heart block in an adult with systemic lupus erythematosus: the association of nuclear RNP (U1 RNP) antibodies, a case report, a review of the literature. *Arthritis Rheum* 1989; **32**: 1170–4.

50 Sackner AM, Akgun N, Kimbel P, *et al*. The pathophysiology of scleroderma involving the heart and respiratory system. *Ann Intern Med* 1964; **60**: 611–30.

51 Salerni R, Rodnan GP, Leon DF, Shaver JA. Pulmonary hypertension in the CREST syndrome: variant of progressive systemic sclerosis (scleroderma). *Ann Intern Med* 1977; **86**: 394–9.

52 Follansbee WP, Curtiss EI, Medsger TA, *et al*. Myocardial function and perfusion in the CREST variant of progressive systemic sclerosis. *Am J Med* 1984; 77: 489–96.

53 Miller MH, Littlejohn GO, Davidson A, *et al*. The clinical significance of the anticentromere antibody. *Br J Rheumatol* 1987; **26**: 17–21.

54 Sharp GS, Irvin WS, Tan EM, Gould RG, Holman HR. Mixed connective tissue disease. An apparently distinct rheumatic disease syndrome with a specific antibody to extractable nuclear antigen. *Am J Med* 1972; **52**: 148–59.

55 Oetgen WJ, Mutter ML, Davia JE, Lawless OJ. Cardiac abnormalities in mixed connective tissue disease. *Chest* 1983; **83**: 185–8.

56 Alpert MA, Goldberg SH, Singsen BH, *et al*. Cardiovascular manifestations of mixed connective tissue disease in adults. *Circulation* 1983; **68**: 1182–93.

57 Jones MG, Osterholm RK, Wilson RB, *et al*. Fatal pulmonary hypertension and resolving immune-complex glomerulonephritis in mixed connective tissue disease: a case report and review of the literature. *Am J Med* 1978; **65**: 855–63.

58 Lonham JG, Elkon KB, Pusey CD, Hughes GRV. Systemic vasculitis with asthma and eosinophilia: a clinical approach to the Churg–Strauss syndrome. *Medicine* 1984; **63**: 65–81.

59 Manger BJ, Krape FE, Gramatzki M, *et al*. IgE containing circulating immune complexes in Churg–Strauss vasculitis. *Scand J Immunol* 1985; **21**: 369–73.

60 Lanham JG, Cooke S, Davies J, Hughes GRV. Endomyocardial complications of the Churg–Strauss syndrome. *Postgrad Med J* 1985; **61**: 341–4.

61 Spry CJF, Davies J, Tai PC, Olsen EGJ, Oakley CM, Goodwin JF. Clinical features of fifteen patients with hypereosinophilic syndrome. *Q J Med* 1983; **52**: 1–22.

62 Fauci AS, Wolf SM. Wegener's granulomatosis: studies in eighteen patients and review of the literature. *Medicine* 1973; **52**: 535–61.

63 Allen DC, Doherty PA, Neufeld GK, Harmon CE, Forstot SL. Cardiac complications of Wegener's granulomatosis. *Br Heart J* 1984; **52**: 674–8.

64 Lupi-Herrera E, Sanchez-Torres G, Marcushamer J, *et al*. Takayasu's arteritis: clinical study of 107 cases. *Am Heart J* 1977; **93**: 94–103.

65 Hiraishi S, Yashiro K, Oguchi K, Makazawa K. Clinical course of cardiovascular involvement in the mucocutaneous lymph node syndrome. *Am J Cardiol* 1981; **47**: 323–30.

66 Onouchi, Shimazu S, Takamatsu T, Hamaoka K. Aneurysms of the coronary arteries in Kawasaki disease: an angiographic study of 30 cases. *Circulation* 1982; **66**: 6–13.

67 Kato H, Ichinose E, Matsunaga S, *et al*. Fate of coronary aneurysms in Kawasaki disease: serial coronary angiography and long-term follow-up study. *Am J Cardiol* 1982; **49**: 1758–66.

68 Suma K, Takeuchi Y, Shiroma K, *et al*. Early and late postoperative studies in coronary arterial lesions in Kawasaki disease in children. *J Thorac Cardiovasc Surg* 1982; **84**: 224–9.

69 Suzuki A, Kamiya T, Yasuo O, Kuroe K. Extended long-term follow-up study of coronary arterial lesions in Kawasaki disease. *J Am Coll Cardiol* 1991; **17**: 33A.

70 Schelhamer JH, Volkman DJ, Parillo JE, *et al*. Takayasu's arteritis and its therapy. *Ann Intern Med* 1985; **103**: 121–6.

71 Ishikawa K, Matsuura S. Occlusive thromboaortopathy (Takayasu's disease) and pregnancy: clinical course and management of 33 pregnancies and deliveries. *Am J Cardiol* 1982; **50**: 1293–300.

72 Wong VCW, Wang RYE, Tse TF. Pregnancy and Takayasu's arteritis. *Am J Med* 1983; **75**: 597–601.

73 Sise MJ, Couniham CM, Shackford ST, *et al*. The clinical spectrum of Takayasu's arteritis. *Surgery* 1988; **104**: 905–10.

74 Winn HN, Setaro JF, Mazor M, *et al*. Severe Takayasu's arteritis in pregnancy: the role of central hemodynamic monitoring. *Am J Obstet Gynecol* 1988; **159**: 1135–6.

75. Balsa-Criado A, Garcia-Fernandez F, Roldan I. Cardiac involvement in relapsing polychondritis. *Int J Cardiol* 1987; **14**: 381–3.

76 Bulkley BH, Roberts WC. Ankylosing spondylitis and aortic regurgitation: description of characteristic cardiovascular lesion from study of eight necropsy patients. *Circulation* 1973; **48**: 1014–27.

77 Roberts WC, Hollingsworth JF, Bulkley BH, *et al*. Combined mitral and aortic regurgitation in ankylosing spondylitis: angiographic and anatomic features. *Am J Med* 1974; **56**: 237–43.

78 Paulus HE, Pearson CM, Pitts W. Aortic insufficiency in 5 patients with Reiter's syndrome. *Am J Med* 1972; **53**: 464–72.

79 Matsumoto T, Uekusa T, Fukuda Y. Vasculo-Behçet's disease: a pathologic study of eight cases. *Hum Pathol* 1991; **22**: 45–51.

80 International Study Group for Behçet's disease. Criteria for diagnosis of Behçet's disease. *Lancet* 1990; **335**: 1078–80.

81 Hurt WG, Cooke CL, Jordan WP, Bullock JP, Rodriguez GE. Behçet's syndrome associated with pregnancy. *Obstet Gynecol* 1979; **53** (**suppl**): 31S–3S.

82 Hamza M, Elleuch M, Zribi A. Behçet's disease and pregnancy. *Ann Rheum Dis* 1988; **47**: 350.

83 Madkour M, Kudwah A. Behçet's disease. *BMJ* 1978; **ii**: 1786.

84 Bang D, Haam IB, Lee ES, Lee S. The influence of pregnancy on Behçet's disease. In: Godeau P, Wechsler B, eds. *Behçet's disease*. Amsterdam: Excerpta Medica, 1993: 403–6.

14: Pulmonary disease and cor pulmonale

J M B HUGHES, CLAIRE SHOVLIN,
ANITA K SIMONDS

In this chapter, we will focus on diffuse lung diseases which are associated with secondary pulmonary hypertension (PHT), as a consequence of destructive bronchial or alveolar pathology and/or alveolar hypoxia, rather than primary pathology of the heart or pulmonary vessels. We discuss pulmonary arteriovenous malformations in which there is severe arterial hypoxaemia but no secondary PHT and pulmonary compromise from extrapulmonary disease. The effects of asthma, tuberculosis, and bacterial and viral pneumonias on pregnancy are covered elsewhere.[1,2]

Effects of pregnancy on the normal lung

The effects of pregnancy on lung mechanics, pulmonary gas exchange, and control of ventilation have been extensively studied and reviewed.[3,4,5]

Lung mechanics

Lung volume is not affected until the second half of pregnancy when the uterus enlarges, raising intra-abdominal pressure and altering the configuration of the diaphragm and chest wall. There is a 20% reduction in the relaxed end-expiratory volume (functional residual capacity, FRC) so that breathing at rest takes place closer to residual volume than normal—changes similar to those seen in ascites and obesity.[6] This may lead to an increase in the closing capacity, which is the absolute lung volume at which small bronchi in the dependent lung zones collapse.[7] The increase in closing capacity and decrease in FRC means that dependent zone bronchi may collapse during tidal breathing and mild hypoxaemia may ensue, particularly in the supine position.[8]

The vital capacity, VC, (erect and supine) and total lung capacity (and therefore residual volume) are unchanged in pregnancy. Lung compliance is normal but airway resistance at resting lung volume is reduced by 50%;[9] this is surprising as the low FRC should be associated with airway narrowing and higher resistance. Thus, mean (SD) specific airway conductance (the reciprocal of resistance, corrected for lung volume) is increased (0·44 (0·28) sec cmH$_2$O^{-1} compared with 0·3 (0·1) in the non-pregnant state). It is thought that the hormonal changes in pregnancy cause smooth muscle relaxation of the bronchi. The oxygen cost of breathing is increased in pregnancy by about 25% probably as a result of extra work required to displace the chest wall and abdominal contents.[10] No measurements of the actual work of breathing have been reported; the static pressure–volume curve of the thorax (in one subject) was right-shifted (to higher pressures), consistent with mass loading of the rib cage.[11]

Resting minute ventilation (V̇E) increases in pregnancy by 10% at 3 months, 30% at 6 months and 45% near term as a result of an increase in tidal volume, not respiratory frequency.[3,4,5] Oxygen consumption (VO$_2$) also increases in a linear fashion throughout pregnancy ($+20\%$ near term) but to a lesser extent so that the ventilatory equivalent (V̇E/V̇O$_2$) increases.[3] The V̇E/V̇CO$_2$ ratio also increases, so that arterial PCO$_2$ falls progressively to 27–32 mm Hg (3·6–4·3 kPa).[3,4,5] This hyperventilation of pregnancy raises alveolar and arterial PO$_2$ especially in the erect posture.[12] While this has little effect normally on arterial oxygen saturation (SaO$_2$) at sea level, it plays an important part in raising SaO$_2$ at altitude (see below) or in the presence of lung disease at sea level. The increase in V̇O$_2$ in the first two trimesters reflects the extra renal and cardiac work in pregnancy, although there must be additional causes of increases in oxygen consumption. In the last trimester, the uterus, placenta and fetus account for 50% of the additional V̇O$_2$.[3]

The early literature on the changes in pulmonary diffusing capacity (DLCO) was rather confusing; the most definitive study involving 21 pregnant women was published in 1977.[13] It is important to correct the DLCO for the fall in haemoglobin concentration [Hb] which occurs during pregnancy. There was no difference in DLCO in the second and third trimesters of pregnancy compared with 3–5 months postpartum, but there was a significant increase (10%) in the first trimester. The explanation for these changes is probably complex with positive and negative effects cancelling. Resting cardiac output rises early in pregnancy (by 1·5–2·0 l/min) and reaches a steady level.[14] Total blood volume increases by 40% in pregnancy (plasma expansion exceeding red cell volume increase, so that haemoglobin concentration falls slightly) but there are no reliable measurements of pulmonary blood volume. Pulmonary capillary volume (Vc) (obtained by partitioning DLCO into its membrane diffusing capacity (DM) and microvascular volume components) reputedly does not change during pregnancy, but would have increased by about 10% had changes in [Hb] been taken into account.[15] Thus, expansion of the pulmonary capillary bed, secondary to the increase in cardiac output, explains the increase in DLCO in the first trimester. This is offset in the second and third trimesters by a fall in lung volume[13] and alveolar surface area or DM, because of the enlarging uterus.[15]

181

Control of breathing

The increase in minute ventilation which begins early in pregnancy is greater than the increased metabolic demands require. Increased progesterone levels are the main factor driving ventilation; $PaCO_2$ is linearly and inversely related to the log of serum progesterone concentration both during the menstrual cycle and during pregnancy,[16] and there is a reduction in resting ventilation in postmenopausal and amenorrhoeic women.[17] Oestrogen and its receptors act synergistically with progesterone at central (hypothalamus) and peripheral (carotid body) sites to stimulate ventilation. Both hypoxic and hypercapnic ventilatory responsiveness increase during pregnancy.[17]

Pregnancy and the pulmonary circulation

The rise in cardiac output in pregnancy is associated with a fall in pulmonary vascular resistance $-0·51$ mm Hg l^{-1} min in 11 healthy women at 16 weeks of pregnancy compared with $0·76$ mm Hg l^{-1} min in 15 non-pregnant controls.[18] There was no change in pulmonary blood volume (somewhat surprising, and unexplained)[19] but a fall in mean pulmonary artery pressure from 13 to 10 mm Hg. Moore in an extensive review pointed out that in animals there is a reduced vascular reactivity in pregnancy to alveolar hypoxia, prostaglandin $F_2\alpha$, noradrenaline and angiotensin II.[20] Chronic infusion of oestradiol-17β in sheep reproduces many of the cardiovascular responses associated with pregnancy, such as systemic vasodilatation and a blunted pressure response to angiotensin II.[21] Potential mechanisms have been reviewed recently.[22]

In summary (Table 14.1) the most important physiological changes in the respiratory system during pregnancy are an increase in minute ventilation (mostly hormonally induced) leading to hypocapnia, and a low end-expiratory lung volume (related to the enlarging uterus). Apart from causing dyspnoea, these pregnancy-induced changes do not significantly compromise the normal respiratory system.

Effect of high altitude

The increase in arterial PO_2 during a normal pregnancy at sea level ($+8$ to $+13$ mm Hg [$+1·07$ to $+1·73$ kPa])[12] is unimportant in terms of increasing arterial oxygen content because of the flatness of the oxygen disassociation curve.[12] In Leadville, Colorado, altitude 3100 m, arterial oxygen saturation (SaO_2) was only 92% in the non-pregnant state (normal 97% to 98%) in 33 subjects but SaO_2 increased to 94% during pregnancy as a result of the accompanying hyperventilation.[23] In a further study in the Andes at 4300 m SaO_2 was 83% in the non-pregnant state and 87% in the 36th week of pregnancy.[24] In spite of an average 9 g/l fall in [Hb] in pregnancy, arterial oxygen *content* remained the same as before pregnancy. There was a 25% increase in resting ventilation and a fourfold increase in

TABLE 14.1—*Cardiorespiratory changes in pregnancy.*

Minute ventilation	$+10$ to $+40\%$
Functional residual capacity	-20%
Oxygen consumption	$+5$ to $+20\%$
PaO_2	$+8$ to $+13\,\text{mm Hg}$ ($1 \cdot 07$ to $1 \cdot 73\,\text{kPa}$)
$PaCO_2$	-7 to $-12\,\text{mm Hg}$ ($0 \cdot 93$ to $1 \cdot 6\,\text{kPa}$)
Cardiac output	$+20$ to $+40\%$
Pulmonary artery pressure	$-3\,\text{mm Hg}$ (-23%)
Pulmonary vascular resistance	-33%
No change in vital capacity or diffusing capacity	

hypoxic ventilatory responsiveness [HVR] (because of chronic altitude exposure, a blunted response was present in the non-pregnant state). Compared with sea level the pregnancy-induced increase in cardiac output was reduced ($+13\%$), possibly as a result of pulmonary hypertension (pulmonary pressures were not measured). There was a fair correlation ($r = 0 \cdot 44$, p<$0 \cdot 05$) between HVR and infant birth weight. These studies show that the hyperventilation of pregnancy can compensate to some extent for the hypoxaemia of altitude and, by extrapolation, lung disease at sea level. It is also possible that the higher PaO_2 and low $PaCO_2$ in the pregnant state increases oxygen and carbon dioxide tension gradients across the placenta to the benefit of the fetus. The fetus also benefits at altitude from a persistence of fetal haemoglobin and a leftward shift in the oxygen dissociation curve.

Pregnancy and lung resection

In a review by Gaensler *et al*, 17 women after pneumonectomy underwent 34 pregnancies without any increase in complications.[25] Women with extensive resections, provided they are not breathless at rest, tolerate pregnancy without difficulty. Extensive bronchiectasis (rarely associated with pregnancy nowadays) can be tolerated satisfactorily. Three patients with vital capacities ranging from 60% to 80% of predicted and FEV_1 from 43% to 70% of predicted delivered normal infants without special assistance.[26] In a different context, emphysema from α_1-antitrypsin deficiency was associated with a successful outcome in a single case report.[27]

Pregnancy and cystic fibrosis

Increased medical supervision and improvements in the management of recurrent chest infections and pancreatic insufficiency have meant that more women with cystic fibrosis are sufficiently healthy in adult life to become pregnant. Unlike men who have atresia of the vas and epididymis, women with cystic fibrosis are not infertile. In contrast to the earlier literature, recent reports of pregnancy in cystic fibrosis are more encouraging. Canny *et al* reported 38 pregnancies in 25 patients, half of whom were pancreatic-sufficient.[28] Pregnancy was well tolerated without excess fetal prematurity or neonatal mortality. Two patients had had lobectomies. Before pregnancy, FEV_1 ranged from 24% to 124% (mean 66%) of predicted and vital capacity from 46% to 124% (mean 80%) of predicted. There was a 4% to 8% drop in function after pregnancy. There was moderately severe hypoxaemia in some (range 67 to 94 mm Hg, mean 75 mm Hg), but no significant hypercapnia ($PaCO_2$ 37 mm Hg, range 32–42 mm Hg). There were two terminations, one at 14 weeks in a patient with an acute exacerbation of her chest disease, increasing hypoxaemia and a fall in vital capacity from 53% to 39% of predicted. This patient died two years later. In the second case, pregnancy was terminated at ten weeks because of poor nutritional status (weight for height ratio 71% of predicted) and poor respiratory status (VC 57% of predicted). Nevertheless, this patient had a successful pregnancy 4 years later at the same weight for height ratio and at a *lower* VC (46% of predicted).

The good results in Canny's series were probably influenced by a satisfactory overall nutritional status (weight for height 95%, SD 12% of predicted).[28] This seems to be as important as respiratory status in determining the outcome of pregnancy.

Two short reports briefly review current experience with 79 pregnancies in 44[29] and 27 women,[30] respectively. There was one maternal death in the seventh month,[29] three miscarriages[29] and a total of 14 terminations.[29,30] Thus, 77% of pregnancies were completed successfully. These series are somewhat biased towards milder cases. In another report of 22 pregnancies in 20 patients, 82% were successfully completed (one spontaneous and three therapeutic abortions).[31] Those six pregnancies in which the mother's FEV_1 was <50% of predicted had a considerably more complicated outcome. Four of the women died (0·5 to 3·2 years postpartum), and four were delivered by caesarean section. There was also one therapeutic abortion (FEV_1 32% of predicted), one rib fracture, and one pneumothorax. The most incapacitated patient (FEV_1 1·01 [28% of predicted]) was alive 0·9 years after delivery; the baby required assisted ventilation, but did well. Only 2/18 infants were light in weight for their dates.

Because of the 33% rise in resting cardiac output in pregnancy, pulmonary hypertension is likely to put a considerable strain on the right ventricle. In many respiratory diseases, hypoxaemia and abnormal pulmonary function reflects the extent of lung destruction and, by implication, the severity of the pulmonary hypertension stemming from it. It would seem reasonable to screen women with cystic fibrosis in early pregnancy (or before pregnancy) with measurements of pulmonary function (FEV_1), vital capacity, transfer factor (T_LCO), SaO_2, PaO_2, and $PaCO_2$; values less than 50% of predicted for pulmonary function, <90% for SaO_2, <60 mm Hg (8 kPa) for PaO_2 and more than 45 mm Hg (6 kPa) for $PaCO_2$ call for an indirect measurement of pulmonary artery pressure with an echocardiogram. If substantial pulmonary hypertension is suspected a flow-directed Swan–Ganz catheter should be inserted to measure the pressures directly.[1] The higher the systolic pressure, above a threshold of 40 mm Hg, the greater the risk of right ventricular failure during pregnancy.

Geddes has given a concise review.[32] A mother with cystic fibrosis will only pass the disease to her child if the father is a cystic fibrosis carrier (1 in 25 chance), when the risk of the child being affected is 1 in 2. The issue of lung transplantation in cystic fibrosis and a subsequent pregnancy is addressed in a recent editorial, the consensus being that pregnancy should not be attempted.[33]

Pulmonary arteriovenous malformations (PAVMs) and pregnancy

PAVMs are abnormal connections between pulmonary arteries and pulmonary veins in which the interposed capillary network has been replaced by a sac. They are a developmental abnormality, 80% being associated with hereditary haemorrhagic telangiectasia (HHT) (Rendu–Osler–Weber syndrome). HHT is caused by mutations in at least three genes, endoglin or chromosome 9[34], ALK-1 on chromosome 12[35], and there is at least one other locus for PAVMs associated with HHT (C L Shovlin, personal communication). Endoglin and ALK-1 are part of the transforming growth factor (TGF)-β receptor system on endothelial cells. The remaining 20% of PAVMs are idiopathic developmental abnormalities confined to the lung. There are fewer arteriovenous communications than in the PAVMs associated with HHT, and their response to the hormonal stimuli of pregnancy may be different.

Pulmonary arteriovenous malformations act as intrapulmonary anatomic shunts. The size of the PAVM sacs varies from 1–30 mm, and the number of PAVMs ranges from one to over 100 in some cases of HHT. They are accompanied by hypoxaemia, which may be severe and is associated with cyanosis, polycythaemia, clubbing, and pulmonary bruits. Despite profound hypoxaemia in some instances, patients with PAVMs are well adapted and retain a remarkably good exercise tolerance compared with patients with other respiratory conditions who are less cyanosed.[36] We attribute their well-preserved exercise ability to the absence of pulmonary hypertension (they have a lower than normal pulmonary vascular resistance) which enables them to increase their cardiac output on exercise to supernormal levels to compensate for the right to left shunt.[37]

Another consequence of the right to left shunting in PAVMs, more serious in practice than the cyanosis, is the liability to paradoxical embolisation through the shunts, bypassing the normal filtering function of the pulmonary microvasculature. The brain is particularly at risk. The incidence of transient ischaemic attacks (TIAs) or strokes in patients with

185

PAVMs (pregnant or non-pregnant) is about 40% and of cerebral abscess 9% to 20%.[38,39] A third complication of PAVMs is life-threatening pulmonary haemorrhage which has an incidence (in combination with HHT) of 8%.[40]

Fifteen to twenty percent of patients with hereditary haemorrhagic telangiectasia have lung involvement with PAVMs, but in some HHT families the incidence of PAVMs is much higher.[41] Patients with PAVMs are particularly prone to develop complications during or after pregnancy. The clinical data relating to this originates from patients who also have HHT (PAVMs without HHT being relatively uncommon). Shovlin *et al* reviewed 161 pregnancies in 47 women.[42] In 138 pregnancies in 35 women where PAVMs had not been shown, there was only one significant complication (a cerebrovascular event). In contrast, in 23 pregnancies in 12 women (from 8 different families) with known PAVMs, there were 10 complications (Table 14.2) including increases in shunt, cardiovascular incidents, and fatal pulmonary haemorrhages. In the report by Ference *et al* on pulmonary haemorrhage from PAVMs, three of the seven women were pregnant at the time.[40]

The case history presented in Table 14.2 shows that a normal pregnancy and delivery of a normal baby can occur in the presence of severe arterial hypoxaemia. In spite of extremely low SaO_2 concentrations the patient was able to lead an active life, nearly keeping up with her peers, passed national examinations, and attended a college of technology. Only some of her numerous PAVMs had feeding vessels large enough to be embolised, so that the improvement in her oxygenation and right to left shunt after treatment (aged 14–16 years) was quite modest. She became pregnant aged 19 years and decided to proceed with the pregnancy, after being counselled of the hazards to her health. She attended an antenatal clinic every week from 22 weeks gestation, and arterial oxygen saturations were measured on each occasion. Her SaO_2 in the sitting or erect posture actually increased somewhat during her pregnancy (from 67% to 73% to 80% to 82%), but fell to low levels in the postpartum period (71% to 65% to 53% subsequently 58%) with an increase in R-L shunt from 38% to 50%. There was some recovery at nine months postpartum. The baby was perfectly healthy and had a normal weight for his gestational age.

We know from previous studies that this patient has a good cardiovascular response to exercise, the cardiac output at 30 watts being $12·8–16·5 \, l \, min^{-1}$ (140% to 180% of predicted) at a SaO_2 of 61% to 67%.[37] Thus, she could respond to the cardiovascular stress of pregnancy in the same manner and maintain a normal oxygen delivery to her tissues, including the placenta.

A similar case was reported by Swinburne *et al*, the right to left shunt being 38% (supine) at 31 weeks gestation (SaO_2 sitting was 84%).[43] The patient, 21 years old, was delivered by caesarean section at 35 weeks of a healthy infant. Two weeks postpartum, she had become more breathless with a deterioration in her shunt (sitting) to 57% and in SaO_2 (68% [sitting] and 50% [standing]). The improvement in SaO_2 during pregnancy might be related to a reduction in shunt flow caused by the low functional

TABLE 14.2—*Case history of pregnancy with pulmonary arteriovenous malformations.*

Diagnosis: **Hereditary haemorrhage telangiectasia**

Age 13—	Cyanosis, dyspnoea and epistaxes
	FH: mother and grandmother had epistaxes
	Pulmonary angiography: extensive pulmonary arteriovenous malformations (PAVM)
	SaO_2 65% (erect) 78% (supine) 53% (on exercise)
	Right to left shunt 48%
Age 14–16 —20	PAVMs occluded with steel coils in 5 sessions
	SaO_2 73% (erect), 84% (supine): **R–L shunt 38%**. Hb 151 g/l
Age 18—	Quite active life in spite of SaO_2 67% (erect) 82% (supine)
Age 19—	18 weeks pregnant $\quad\quad$ SaO_2 74% (sitting)
	25 weeks pregnant $\quad\quad$ SaO_2 80% (erect)
	32 weeks pregnant $\quad\quad$ SaO_2 82% (sitting)
	Fetal well being confirmed on ultrasound scans, Hb 130 g/l
	33 weeks (premature labour) $\quad$ SaO_2 83% (recumbent)
	during labour $\quad\quad\quad\quad\quad\quad$ SaO_2 77–78% (sitting)
	$\quad\quad\quad\quad\quad\quad\quad\quad\quad\quad$ *HR 120/min;*
	$\quad\quad\quad\quad\quad\quad\quad\quad\quad\quad$ *Fetal HR 130–110/min*
	Vaginal elective forceps delivery under epidural anaesthesia of healthy 1900 g male baby
	12 hours postpartum $\quad\quad$ SaO_2 71% (sitting)
	48 hours postpartum $\quad\quad$ SaO_2 65% (sitting)
Age 20—	13 weeks postpartum $\quad\quad$ SaO_2 53% (erect) 71% (supine)
	$\quad\quad\quad\quad\quad\quad\quad\quad\quad\quad$ **R–L shunt 50%**
	19 months postpartum $\quad\quad$ SaO_2 58% (erect) 70% (supine)

residual capacity in pregnancy (right to left shunting in PAVMs is volume dependent)[44] or direct compression of the lower lobes where PAVMs are most commonly situated,[38] by the gravid uterus. Alternatively, the improvement in SaO_2 during pregnancy may reflect the increase in arterial or mixed venous PO_2, resulting from pregacy-induced changes in minute ventilation and cardiac output, which can exceed metabolic demands. This would account for part of the postpartum deterioration in SaO_2. The continued fall below the pre-pregnancy values may reflect persistent remodelling of the abnormal vascular bed,[45] as seen in other vessels such as the aorta following normal pregnancy.[46]

The practical points are as follows: all families in whom hereditary haemorrhagic telangiectasia has been detected should be screened for the presence of HHT in other family members. Recurrent epistaxis is an early and common finding in affected members.[47] Affected family members should be screened for PAVMs with chest radiographs and measurements of arterial oxygen saturation (SaO_2) in the erect and supine positions.[38] A fall of 2% or more in SaO_2 on standing suggests the presence of PAVMs.

What advice should be given to women with HHT and PAVMs who are pregnant or wish to become pregnant? First, the mother can be reassured that her condition, even if it is associated with severe arterial hypoxaemia, will not harm the baby in utero. Her cardiac output can increase sufficiently to keep the growing fetus well supplied with oxygen. Although infant birth weights are low in the presence of maternal cyanotic congenital heart disease and in severe respiratory disease with associated pulmonary hypertension, the birth weights of three babies born to mothers with severe hypoxaemia from PAVMs (Table 14.2,[43] J M B Hughes, personal communication) were not low for their dates.

Secondly, she should be warned that the main risk of a pregnancy is to her own health. Serious deterioration in oxygenation occurs in those with substantial shunts before pregnancy. Our impression is that all PAVMs increase in size when exposed to the altered haemodynamics and hormone concentrations in pregnancy. It appears that in spite of the reduced pulmonary vascular resistance, the fragile nature of PAVM walls render them more prone to haemorrhage.[40,42] If the PAVMs and right to left shunt are small, then one or two pregnancies could be undertaken at relatively little risk. Where the right to left shunt (measured with 100% oxygen or ^{99m}Tc-albumin macroaggregates) exceeds 20%, pregnancy is potentially hazardous for the mother.[48]

As regards the anaesthetic management of labour in PAVMs, there are strong grounds for considering epidural anaesthesia in a primigravida.[49] General anaesthesia with positive pressure ventilation may increase shunt flow; intravenous injections and caesarean delivery increase the hazard of paradoxical air embolism. Lastly, the incidence of spinal cord AVMs is only about 0·4% in HHT.[50] Nevertheless, an experienced obstetric anaesthetic team should be involved. Multigravidae can be managed with N_2O/air mixtures for analgesia (W A R Davies, personal communication). Forceps-assisted delivery is the rule.

Extrapulmonary disease

Table 14.3 lists the extrapulmonary disorders that may be associated with ventilatory insufficiency and cor pulmonale in pregnancy. Chest wall disorders including scoliosis and kyphosis, neuromuscular diseases affecting the respiratory muscles, and central drive disorders can progress to ventilatory failure and ultimately cor pulmonale if the load placed on the respiratory system exceeds the capacity to accommodate this, or if the ventilatory drive is inadequate. In chest wall disease and respiratory muscle weakness a restrictive ventilatory defect characterised by reduced forced vital capacity, FEV_1, and total lung capacity, with normal FEV_1/FVC ratio is seen. Many neuromuscular disorders are complicated by scoliosis.

Scoliosis

Scoliosis is the commonest of chest wall disorders, and lateral curves of more than 70 degrees affect 0·01% of the population. Eighty percent

188

TABLE 14.3—*Extrapulmonary conditions that may be associated with ventilatory insufficiency during pregnancy.*

A Chest wall disorders

Scoliosis: Idiopathic (majority), neuromuscular, osteogenic, associated with inherited
    disorders eg neurofibromatosis, Marfan's syndrome
Kyphosis: Spinal tuberculosis, idiopathic

B Neuromuscular disorders

- Muscular dystrophies: Limb girdle muscular dystrophy
                             Congenital muscular dystrophy
                             Facioscapulohumeral muscular dystrophy

- Myopathies
  Congenital: Nemaline
               Acid maltase deficiency (Pompe's disease)
               Mitochondrial
               Central core
  Acquired: Polymyositis
             Myasthenia gravis

- Spinal muscular atrophy: Anterior horn cell disease

- Combined muscle weakness and ventilatory drive disorder: Myotonic dystrophy

C Ventilatory drive disorders

    Primary alveolar hypoventilation
    Central sleep apnoea

D Obstructive sleep apnoea

---

of thoracic scolioses are idiopathic, the remainder being the result of neuromuscular disease, osteogenic causes, or thoracic surgery, or associated with congenital disease. Adolescent onset curves occur more commonly in women, whereas early onset curves show no sex preference. The presence of a scoliosis has important implications in pregnancy, as a substantial thoracic curvature can cause ventilatory insufficiency and cor pulmonale, and lumbar curves can cause obstetric complications. Menarche tends to be delayed in girls with scoliosis.[51]

The frequency of pregnancy in patients with chest wall disorders has been variously reported. In a series from Johannesburg, 50 women with chest wall disease (predominantly Pott's kyphosis) were identified in a total of 119 678 deliveries.[52] This high figure (1:2394) reflects the prevalence of tuberculosis in South Africa. Other studies have recorded an incidence of kyphoscoliosis in pregnancy varying from 1:1471 to 1:12 000, an average figure being 1:5253.[52] From a different perspective, Siegler and Zorab reported pregnancies in 64 patients with thoracic scoliosis in 205 women with scoliosis who were attending a respiratory clinic.[53] The outcome of pregnancy differs between groups with previously identified respiratory problems and those presenting de novo in pregnancy.

Early work suggested a relatively good outcome of pregnancy in chest wall disorders.[54] This is probably because most affected women have a modest (less than 50 degree) thoracic scoliosis, which is unlikely to cause cardiopulmonary or obstetric problems. Some patients are, however, at high risk of cardiorespiratory decompensation during pregnancy, labour, and the postpartum period.[55,56]

While women with a thoracic spinal curvature of less than 50 degrees experience minimal effects on chest wall mechanics, a reduction in chest wall compliance is seen in those with more pronounced curves.[57] Ventilatory insufficiency is exacerbated during sleep. This is because in rapid eye movement (REM) sleep, intercostal inhibition occurs leading to a reliance on the diaphragm to generate tidal volume. Ventilatory drive is also reduced in both non-REM and REM sleep.[58] As a consequence, marked hypoventilation can occur during sleep if diaphragm function is limited. This causes hypoxaemia with potential adverse effects on maternal and fetal health. Monitoring of respiration during sleep is therefore important when ventilatory insufficiency is suspected. If untreated, severe nocturnal hypoventilation progresses to daytime hypoxaemia and hypercapnia, pulmonary hypertension, and right heart failure.

In scoliotic patients with a vital capacity of less than a litre, pulmonary artery pressure may rise on exercise in the absence of hypoxaemia.[59] This rise is the result of the increased cardiac output passing through a low capacity pulmonary vascular bed. It is not known if the increased cardiac output in pregnant women with scoliosis can provoke pulmonary hypertension by a similar mechanism, or whether oestrogenic effects on the pulmonary vasculature in pregnancy can offset this process.

Longitudinal studies have shown that patients with idiopathic scoliosis who are at risk of cardiopulmonary decompensation have a vital capacity of less than 50% of predicted.[60] This risk is enhanced if VC is less than about 1 litre. Early onset scoliosis (age of onset less than 5 years) is associated with an increased incidence of cardiorespiratory failure and high mortality.[60] This is thought to be because the onset of chest wall deformity inhibits alveolar duplication and growth of the pulmonary vasculature.

The converse of these observations is that women with adolescent onset scoliosis and vital capacity of more than 50% of predicted can be reassured that they are unlikely to experience respiratory difficulties.

Outcome of pregnancy in scoliosis

Phelan *et al* estimated that maternal mortality was 2·6% and perinatal mortality 3·8% in scoliotic patients.[55] However, these statistics depend on patient selection and the underlying disease.

In a series of 50 pregnant kyphoscoliotic women presenting to Baragwanath Hospital in South Africa over a nine year period, 42 had spinal tuberculosis, three had previously had poliomyelitis, one a spinal tumour, and the cause of the deformity was unknown in four.[52] There were two maternal deaths from cardiorespiratory failure, three patients survived cardiac or respiratory failure, and two developed bronchitis postpartum.

There were five perinatal deaths, but malpresentation was uncommon. Lung function data were unavailable, but the most important prognostic factors were the severity of the deformity and a thoracic site.

By contrast, in European and American series scoliosis is usually idiopathic. Manning *et al* reviewed the outcome of 35 pregnancies in 14 patients.[54] In all the thoracic curvature was severe with a Cobb angle of greater than 90 degrees. Pulmonary function tests were done in nine subjects. Mean vital capacity was 1365 mls (range 33% to 61% of predicted). No maternal complications or fetal loss occurred.

Data on 118 pregnancies in 64 patients with thoracic scoliosis (mainly idiopathic) were reported from the Royal Brompton Hospital.[53] 42 patients had curves which exceeded 60 degrees and 12 patients had vital capacities of less than one litre. Disproportionate breathlessness occurred during pregnancy in 17% of patients, but none developed cardiorespiratory decompensation. Vaginal delivery was successful in 83%. A deficiency of this retrospective postal questionnaire survey addressed to the patients is that maternal deaths are missed. However, the authors thought that continued follow up excluded this possibility in non-responders.

Several workers have confirmed that stable mild to moderate thoracolumbar curves are unlikely to progress during or after pregnancy.[61,62] Neurogenic or myopathic scolioses, particularly if unstable, may be adversely affected.

The factors which contribute to respiratory insufficiency in pregnancy have been examined by Sawicka *et al* in a study of six patients with chest wall diseases.[56] Four had idiopathic scoliosis and two previous poliomyelitis. All had developed scoliosis before the age of eight years. Mean vital capacity was 920 mls (33% of predicted). One woman also had asthma. Five developed progressive dyspnoea in the second or third trimester. Four progressed to respiratory failure and cor pulmonale before term; two were managed with negative pressure ventilation, one with non-invasive positive pressure support, and the fourth with controlled oxygen therapy. Early elective caesarean section was carried out in four patients. Three experienced acute cardiopulmonary distress postpartum, requiring mechanical ventilation. All patients survived and there was no neonatal loss, but five mothers have subsequently required non-invasive respiratory support at night.

While negative pressure ventilation using the iron lung was successful in the above study, the newer non-invasive technique of nasal intermittent positive pressure ventilation (NIPPV) is more widely available and easier to apply. NIPPV has been used effectively in this unit (Table 14.4 and Figure 14.1) and elsewhere[63] to maintain arterial blood gases in pregnant scoliotic women.

Outcome of pregnancy in neuromuscular disease

Although neuromuscular disorders are relatively uncommon it is estimated that at least 200 0000 individuals in Europe have inherited or acquired neuromuscular disease.

TABLE 14.4—*Case history of pregnancy with congenital scoliosis and cor pulmonale.*

Born with thoracic idiopathic scoliosis which progressed through childhood. No cardiac disease.

Age 12—Harrington rod spinal fusion

Age 25—First pregnancy. Vital capacity 1000 ml (35% of predicted value)

    35 weeks pregnant. Developed cor pulmonale
    Rapid deterioration despite treatment with diuretics and O_2

    37 weeks *Emergency caesarean section* Infant survived

    Postpartum: Continued deterioration in cardiorespiratory state
    10 days after caesarean section: cardiac arrest necessitating IPPV
    Resuscitation complicated by gastric aspiration causing ARDS

    1 month postpartum weaned from IPPV using negative pressure ventilation (iron lung)

Age 26—Continued to use nocturnal negative pressure ventilation with a cuirass at home for 1 year after delivery

Age 29—Second pregnancy (against medical advice)

    13 weeks pregnant. Vital capacity 930 ml; PaO_2 8·9 kPa; $PaCO_2$ 8·1 kPa

    Overnight monitoring: Minimum SaO_2 40%
    Maximum transcutaneous $PaCO_2$ 11 kPa

    Started on nocturnal nasal ventilation (NIPPV) using Lifecare PLV 100 ventilator (tidal volume 810 ml)
    14 weeks pregnant PaO_2 10·7 kPa $PaCO_2$ 7·2 kPa

    Overnight monitoring on NIPPV
    Mean SaO_2>90%. Few dips to 77%

    20 weeks pregnant. More dyspnoeic. No evidence cardiac failure.
    Used NIPPV for rest periods during day as well as at night
    Tidal volume on NIPPV increased to improve $PaCO_2$ control

    35 weeks pregnant. Spontaneous labour

    Caesarean section with elective sterilisation
    No obstetric or medical complications
    Extubated after delivery on to NIPPV
    Infant healthy, no growth retardation
    Two weeks postpartum. Discharged home using nocturnal NIPPV

Age 36—Continues to use nocturnal NIPPV. Works part-time
    Vital capacity 890 ml PaO_2 10·2 kPa $PaCO_2$ 6·4 kPa
    No progression in scoliosis during either pregnancy

Alterations in chest wall properties may also occur in patients with respiratory muscle weakness in the absence of spinal or rib cage deformity. Estenne *et al* showed that chest wall compliance was reduced in 75% of patients without scoliosis and with a vital capacity between 50% and 60% of predicted.[64] Pulmonary compliance may also be reduced as a result of a low tidal volume pattern of respiration and shift in the pulmonary pressure volume curve.[65] In chest wall disorders the respiratory muscles work at a mechanical disadvantage, thereby increasing the work of breathing. While there is no evidence that respiratory muscle function is impaired during pregnancy, weak inspiratory muscles may be unable to sustain the additional

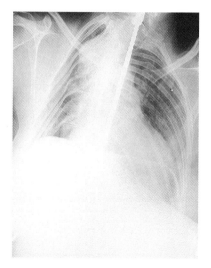

FIGURE 14.1—*Chest radiograph of the patient with congenital thoracic scoliosis and Harrington rod instrumentation (see Table 14.4).*

workload of increased thoracic impedance which occurs in pregnancy.[66] Patients with respiratory muscle weakness, particularly if the diaphragm is involved, are liable to develop hypercapnia if respiratory muscle strength is less than 30% of predicted.

Microatelectasis and more generalised atelectasis with a tendency to recurrent chest infections occurs in individuals with low inspiratory muscle strength, and poor ability to cough results from expiratory muscle weakness. Basal atelectasis may be exacerbated by a low functional residual capacity which becomes lower as the uterus enlarges. Bulbar insufficiency increases the risk of chest infections from aspiration.

There are a number of reports of successful maternal and fetal outcome in spinal muscular atrophy,[67] limb girdle muscular dystrophy,[68] and an undefined muscular dystrophy,[69] despite a marked restrictive ventilatory defect in each case. In all, careful monitoring of maternal and fetal oxygenation was carried out with early elective delivery. Respiratory support was not required in these cases.

Primary alveolar hypoventilation and pregnancy

This condition (also known as Ondine's curse) is characterised by absent or reduced ventilatory responses to hypercapnia or hypoxia or both. Lung volumes are normal. Without intervention, gross hypoventilation occurs during sleep, as the voluntary control of breathing is removed. Affected people progress to decompensated hypercapnic failure and cor pulmonale. The condition may be present at birth or acquired (for unknown reasons) in later life. Pieters *et al* reported a female who developed primary alveolar hypoventilation in her 20s, presenting with hypercapnic respiratory failure, polycythaemia and pulmonary hypertension (pulmonary arterial pressure 100 mm Hg).[70] Respiratory failure was controlled with NIPPV and cardiac findings reverted to normal after several months of nocturnal ventilatory support. The patient subsequently became pregnant and continued to use nocturnal NIPPV throughout the pregnancy. No change in ventilatory settings was required. Fetal growth was normal. Labour was induced at 39 weeks and uncomplicated delivery was achieved by vacuum extraction. At 27 month follow up both infant and mother were in good health.

Obstructive sleep apnoea and pregnancy

Obstructive sleep apnoea (OSA) has recently been recognised as a major cause of respiratory insufficiency during sleep. Initially thought to be uncommon in premenopausal women, OSA complicating pregnancy has been reported, and is probably under-recognised.[71,72]

Overnight monitoring shows multiple dips in arterial oxygen saturation as a result of recurrent periods of upper airway obstruction during sleep. The fall in functional residual capacity which accompanies late pregnancy is likely to result in a greater degree of desaturation during apnoeas or periods of hypoventilation when compared with the non-pregnant state, as alveolar oxygen stores are more rapidly depleted.[73] Each apnoea is terminated by arousal which results in sleep fragmentation and somnolence during the day. Arousals are associated with increased sympathetic outflow which causes swings in systemic blood pressure.[74,75]

High levels of progesterone in pregnancy do not prevent sleep disordered breathing in women with moderate or severe obstructive sleep apnoea. The incidence of OSA in pregnancy is not known, although many women report snoring and poor sleep quality.[76] Monitoring of respiration during sleep is essential to diagnose OSA,[77] which can be successfully managed, as described below.

A 32 year old woman presented with severe OSA (apnoea/hypopnoea index 159/hour) in the last trimester.[71] The patient was obese (weight 155 kg, body mass index 55) and gained 12 kg during pregnancy. There was a past history of heavy snoring, with daytime somnolence getting worse in the first two trimesters. A sleep study at 36 weeks showed that apnoeas provoked marked maternal desaturation to a minimum level of 40%, and bradycardia during REM sleep. Cardiotocography showed normal fetal heart rate during the apnoeas. The patient was treated with continuous positive airway pressure (CPAP) at 15 cmH$_2$O during sleep, and delivered electively at 39 weeks. The infant survived but showed signs of growth retardation, suggesting that earlier intervention with CPAP might have been helpful. A repeat maternal sleep study two months postpartum (weight loss 10 kg) showed persistent apnoeas with a slightly reduced apnoea/ hypopnoea index (122/hour). In this case OSA clearly preceded pregnancy, but was probably exacerbated by weight gain, and increased thoracic and upper airway impedance. Weight gain may precipitate OSA and it is possible that mild to moderate OSA may present de novo in pregnancy, triggered at least in part by these mechanisms.

Assessment and management of extrapulmonary ventilatory insufficiency in pregnancy

Pre-pregnancy genetic counselling and discussion of potential medical and obstetric risks is of great importance in patients with restrictive disorders. Prenatal diagnosis is available in an increasing number of inherited neuromuscular conditions. Clinical examination of a woman with chest wall disease should establish the extent of the deformity, degree of respiratory muscle involvement, and pulmonary function. Global respiratory muscle strength can be measured with a simple mouth pressure meter. A significant fall in vital capacity on assuming the supine position is seen in patients with diaphragmatic weakness.

A vital capacity of a litre or less indicates a high risk of respiratory insufficiency during pregnancy. Arterial blood gases should be checked, together with monitoring of overnight SaO_2 and PCO_2, and breathing pattern. A sleep study should also be carried out in women with snoring, disturbed sleep, witnessed apnoeas, or daytime somnolence. The risk of OSA is likely to be increased in obese people.

Severe pulmonary hypertension from whatever cause is a major contraindication to pregnancy.[78] The loudness of the pulmonary component of the second heart sound (P2) may be unreliable in scoliosis because of rotation of the heart, but if P2 is louder than the aortic component pulmonary hypertension is likely.[79] Any suspicion of pulmonary hypertension should be confirmed by ECG and echocardiogram. It should be remembered that congenital heart disease is more common in patients with congenital scoliosis than in the rest of the population.[80,81]

Labour or caesarean section may be managed best by spinal epidural as this reduces the risks of atelectasis.[78] Surprisingly, spinal epidural does not appear to be less effective or associated with more complications in patients who have had previous spinal surgery.[82] The successful use of a spinal microcatheter to provide anaesthesia for caesarean section in a patient with cervical deformity and scoliosis due to Klippel–Feil syndrome has been described.[83] Lumbar and lumbar-sacral scoliosis were associated with a comparatively low rate of obstetric complications in one series.[54] However, in a review of 77 cases with spinal deformity, 71% of deliveries required caesarean section or forceps assistance.[55] As expected, caudal deformities were associated with a higher rate of pelvic disproportion.

The case history in Table 14.4 outlines the clinical course throughout two pregnancies in a woman with severe early onset scoliosis. With medical management, particularly NIPPV to relieve hypoxaemia and hypercapnia, the second pregnancy was well-tolerated in contrast to the first pregnancy in which non-invasive ventilation was not used before delivery.

195

Extrapulmonary disorders: summary

Patients with adolescent onset scoliosis are generally at low risk of cardiorespiratory problems in pregnancy. For those with early onset scoliosis and stable mild respiratory muscle weakness a successful outcome may be achieved if vital capacity is in excess of 1–1·25 litres and there is no evidence of pulmonary hypertension.[56] If hypercapnic respiratory failure or cor pulmonale develop in pregnancy or the postpartum period, the woman may be saved by non-invasive nasal intermittent positive pressure ventilation or negative pressure ventilation. Continuous airway pressure therapy is effective in obstructive sleep apnoea. In high risk cases it is essential to use a multidisciplinary approach with the early involvement of a respiratory team familiar with non-invasive ventilatory support, together with close monitoring of nocturnal and diurnal oxygenation.

General conclusions

- A normal pregnancy stresses the respiratory system less than the cardiovascular system.[1] Resting ventilation rises in pregnancy to about $10 \, \text{l.min}^{-1}$ (probably only $8 \, \text{l.min}^{-1}$ if the equipment dead space is taken away), which is perhaps 25% of a chronically sustainable level. Cardiac output, on the other hand, rises to $6 \, \text{l.min}^{-1}$, up to 50% of the tolerable limit. A threefold increase of pulmonary artery pressure before pregnancy leads to 2·6-fold increase in pulmonary vascular resistance in pregnancy (assuming no change in left atrial pressure). But even with a threefold reduction in ventilatory capacity (forced expired volume in one second of say 0·8 l), a patient can sustain a minute ventilation of $8 \, \text{l.min}^{-1}$ easily.
- The pulmonary hypertension of respiratory disease is more of a hazard to the pregnant woman than a reduction in ventilatory capacity. The severity of arterial hypoxaemia is a guide to the severity of pulmonary hypertension. The risk of cor pulmonale in pregnancy is probably linked to the level of pulmonary arterial pressure, with a watershed at 40 mm Hg. Fortunately, the pulmonary hypertension associated with residence at altitude, cystic fibrosis, and neuromuscular and chest wall disorders is generally of moderate severity, and pulmonary artery systolic pressures of 40 mm Hg are rarely exceeded.
- The development of cor pulmonale in pregnancy is a possibility in any mother whose pulmonary function is <50% predicted, or whose respiratory muscle power or gas exchange is severely compromised. Pulmonary function and arterial oxygen saturation (measured by pulse oximeter) and arterial blood gases (where necessary) should be monitored closely throughout pregnancy. The standard medical treatment for cor pulmonale comprises: (*a*) control of respiratory infection with antibiotics and physiotherapy; (*b*) avoidance of fluid retention; (*c*) relief of deteriorating hypoxaemia with additional inspired oxygen; (*d*) support of ventilatory failure with nasal positive pressure ventilation; and (*e*)

relief of airflow obstruction with nebulised bronchodilators. There is no indication for additional vasodilator drugs because the PHT of primary respiratory disease is not particularly severe, and because beta-agonist bronchodilator preparations are also pulmonary vasodilators. Patients with cystic fibrosis should be managed jointly with a cystic fibrosis clinic.

- Pulmonary arteriovenous malformations with right to left shunting, usually associated with hereditary haemorrhagic telangiectasia, are a special case, because pulmonary artery pressures are normal or low, even though arterial hypoxaemia may be severe. Cardiac output increases to supernormal levels to compensate for the arterial hypoxaemia, and the fetus develops normally. But the mother runs the risk of paradoxical embolism, pulmonary haemorrhage and a permanent increase in the right to left shunt.

Acknowledgements

We thank W A R Davies and S Krishnamurthy (obstetrics), R P Wroth (anaesthesia), and D M Geddes and M E Hodson (cystic fibrosis) for helpful suggestions, and M de Swiet for his advice and review of the text.

References

1 de Swiet, M. Diseases of the respiratory system. In: de Swiet M, ed. *Medical disorders in obstetric practice.* 3rd ed. Oxford: Blackwell, 1995: 1–32.
2 Cunningham FG, MacDonald PC, Leveno KJ, Gant NF, Gilstrap LC. *Pulmonary disorders.* 19th ed. New York: Prentice-Hall, 1993: 1105–26.
3 de Swiet, M. The respiratory system. In: Hytten F, Chamberlain G, eds. *Clinical physiology in obstetrics.* Oxford: Blackwell, 1991: 83–100.
4 Weinberger SE, Weiss ST, Cohen WR, Weiss JW, Johnson TS. Pregnancy and the lung. *Am Rev Respir Dis* 1980; **121**: 559–81.
5 Gaensler EA. Lung displacement: abdominal enlargement, pleural space disorders, deformities of the thoracic cage. In: Fenn WO, Rahn H, eds. *Handbook of physiology, section 3. Respiration. Vol 2.* Washington DC: American Physiological Society, 1965: 1624–8.
6 Cugell DW, Frank NR, Gaensler EA, Badger TL. Pulmonary function in pregnancy I. Serial observations in normal women. *American Review of Tuberculosis and Pulmonary Diseases* 1953; **67**: 568–97.
7 Bevan DR, Holdcroft A, Loh L, MacGregor WG, O'Sullivan JC, Sykes MR. Closing volume and pregnancy. *BMJ* 1974; **i**: 13–15.
8 Awe RJ, Nicotra MB, Newson TD, Viles R. Arterial oxygenation and alveolar–arterial gradients in term pregnancy. *Obstet Gynecol* 1979; **53**: 182–6.
9 Gee JBL, Packer BS, Millen JE, Robin ED. Pulmonary mechanics during pregnancy. *J Clin Invest* 1967; **46**: 945–52.
10 Bader RA, Bader ME, Rose DI. The oxygen cost of breathing in dyspnoeic subjects as studied in normal pregnant women. *Clin Sci* 1959; **18**: 223–35.
11 Sharp JT. The chest wall and respiratory muscles in obesity, pregnancy and ascites. In: Roussos C, Macklem PT, eds. *The Thorax.* New York: Marcel Dekker, 1985: 1014. (Lung biology in health and disease series 29B)
12 Templeton A, Kelman GR. Maternal blood gases (PaO_2-PaO_2), physiological shunt and VD/VT in pregnancy. *Br J Anaesth* 1976; **48**: 1001–4.
13 Milne JA, Mills RJ, Coutts JRT, MacNaughton MC, Moran F, Pack AI. The effect of human pregnancy on the pulmonary transfer factor for carbon monoxide as measured by the single breath method. *Clin Sci Mol Med* 1977; **53**: 271–6.

14 Lees MM, Taylor SH, Scott DB, Kerr MG. A study of cardiac output at rest during pregnancy. *Journal of Obstetrics and Gynaecology of the British Commonwealth* 1967; **74**: 319–28.

15 Gazioglu K, Kaltreider NL, Rosen M, Yu PN. Pulmonary function during pregnancy in normal women and in patients with cardiopulmonary disease. *Thorax* 1970; **25**: 445–50.

16 Machida H. Influence of progesterone on arterial blood and CSF acid-base balance in women. *J Appl Physiol* 1981; **51**: 1433–6.

17 Tatsumi K, Hannhart B, Moore LG. Influences of sex steroids on ventilation and ventilatory control. In: Dempsey JA, Pack AI, eds. *Regulation of Breathing*. New York: Marcel Dekker, 1994: 829–64. (Lung Biology in Health and Disease Series 79)

18 Werko L. Pregnancy and heart disease. *Acta Obstet Gynaecol Scand* 1954; **33**: 162–210.

19 Lagerlöf H, Werko L, Bucht H, Holmgren A. Separate determination of the blood volume of the right and left heart and the lungs in man with the aid of the dye injection method. *Scand J Clin Lab Invest* 1949; **i**: 114–25.

20 Moore LG. Circulation in the pregnant and non pregnant state. In: Weir EK, Reeves JT, eds. *Pulmonary vascular physiology and pathophysiology*. New York: Marcel Dekker, 1989: 135–72. (Lung Biology in Health and Disease Series 38)

21 Magness RR, Parker CR, Rosenfeld CR. Systemic and uterine responses to chronic infusion of estradiol-17 β. *Am J Physiol* 1993; **265**: E690–8.

22 Gerhard M, Ganz P. How do we explain the clinical benefits of estrogen? *Circulation* 1995; **92**: 5–8.

23 Moore LG, Jahniggen D, Rounds SS, Reeves JT, Grover RF. Maternal hyperventilation helps preserve arterial oxygenation during high-altitude pregnancy. *J Appl Physiol* 1982; **52**: 690–4.

24 Moore LG, Brodeur P, Clunbe O, D'Bvot J, Hofmeister S, Monge C. Maternal hypoxic ventilatory response, ventilation, and infant birth weight at 4300 m. *J Appl Physiol* 1986; **60**: 1401–6.

25 Gaensler EA, Patton WE, Verstraeten JM, Badger TL. Pulmonary function in pregnancy. III. Serial observations in patients with pulmonary insufficiency. *American Review of Tuberculosis and Pulmonary Diseases* 1953; **67**: 779–97.

26 Howie AO, Milne JA. Pregnancy in patients with bronchiectasis. *Br J Obstet Gynaecol* 1978; **85**: 197–200.

27 Giesler CF, Buehler JH, Depp R. Alpha₁-antitrypsin deficiency. Severe obstructive disease and pregnancy. *Obstet Gynecol* 1977; **49**: 31–4.

28 Canny GJ, Corey M, Livingstone RA, Carpenter S, Green L, Levison H. Pregnancy and cystic fibrosis. *Obstet Gynecol* 1991; **77**: 850–3.

29 Halpin DMG, Hodson ME, Geddes DM. Sex of children born to women with cystic fibrosis. *Lancet* 1992; **339**: 990.

30 Metz O. Sex of children born to women with cystic fibrosis. *Lancet* 1992; **339**: 739–40.

31 Edenborough FP, Stableforth DE, Webb AK, Mackenzie WE, Smith DL. Outcome of pregnancy in women with cystic fibrosis. *Thorax* 1995; **50**: 170–4.

32 Geddes DM. Cystic fibrosis and pregnancy. *J R Soc Med* 1992; **85(suppl 19)**: 36–7.

33 Edenborough FP, Stableforth DE, Mackenzie WE. Pregnancy in women with cystic fibrosis. *BMJ* 1995; **311**: 822–3.

34 McAllister KA, Grogg KM, Johnson DW, *et al.* Endoglin, a TGF-β binding protein of endothelial cells, is the gene for hereditary haemorrhagic telangiectasia type I. *Nature Genet* 1994; **8**: 345–51.

35 Johnson DW, Berg JN, Baldwin MA, *et al.* Mutations in the activin receptor-like kinase 1 gene in hereditary haemorrhagic telangiectasia type 2. *Nature Genet* 1996; **13**: 189–95.

36 Chilvers ER, Whyte MKB, Jackson JE, Allison DJ, Hughes JMB. Effect of percutaneous transcatheter embolisation on pulmonary function, right to left shunt and arterial oxygenation in patients with pulmonary arteriovenous malformations. *Am Rev Respir Dis* 1990; **142**: 420–5.

37 Whyte MKB, Hughes JMB, Jackson JE, *et al.* Cardiopulmonary response to exercise in patients with intrapulmonary vascular shunts. *J Appl Physiol* 1993; **75**: 321–8.

38 Dutton JAE, Jackson JE, Hughes JMB, *et al.* Pulmonary arteriovenous malformations: results of treatment with coil embolisation in 53 patients. *AJR* 1995; **165**: 1119–25.

39 White RI, Lynch-Nyhan A, Terry P, *et al.* Pulmonary arteriovenous malformations: techniques and long term outcome of embolotherapy. *Radiology* 1988; **169**: 663–9.

40 Ference BA, Shannon TM, White RI, Zawin M, Burdge CM. Life-threatening pulmonary haemorrhage with pulmonary arteriovenous malformations and hereditary hemorrhagic telangiectasia. *Chest* 1994; **106**: 1387–90.

41 Hughes JMB. Intrapulmonary shunts: coils to transplantation. *J R Coll Phys Lond* 1994; **28**: 247–53.

42 Shovlin CL, Winstock AR, Peters AM, Jackson JE, Hughes JMB. Medical complications of pregnancy in hereditary haemorrhagic telangiectasia. *Q J Med* 1995; **88**: 879–87.

43 Swinburne AJ, Fedulla AJ, Gangemi R, Mijangos JA. Hereditary telangiectasia and multiple pulmonary arteriovenous fistulas. Clinical deterioration during pregnancy. *Chest* 1986; **89**: 459–60.

44 Ueki J, Hughes JMB, Peters AM, *et al.* Oxygen and ^{99m}Tc-MAA shunt estimations in patients with pulmonary arteriovenous malformations: effects of postural and lung volume change. *Thorax* 1994; **49**: 327–31.

45 Shovlin CL, Scott J. Inherited diseases of the vasculature. *Annual Review of Physiology* 1996; **58**: 483–507.

46 Hart MV, Morton MJ, Hosenpud JD, Metcalf J. Aortic function during normal human pregnancy. *Am J Obstet Gynecol* 1986; **154**: 887–91.

47 Plauchu H, de Chadarevian JP, Bideau A, Robert CM. Age-related clinical profile of hereditary hemorrhagic telangiectasia in an epidemiologically recruited population. *Am J Med Genet* 1989; **32**: 291–7.

48 Whyte MKB, Peters AM, Hughes JMB, *et al.* Quantification of right-to-left shunt at rest and during exercise in patients with pulmonary arteriovenous malformations. *Thorax* 1992; **47**: 790–6.

49 Wroth RP, Alderson JD. The anaesthetic management of a labouring woman with pulmonary arteriovenous malformations. *Int J Obstet Anesth* 1996.

50 Roman G, Fisher M, Perl DP, Poser CM. Neurological manifestations of hereditary haemorrhagic telangiectasia (Rendu–Osler–Weber disease): report of two cases and review of the literature. *Ann Neurol* 1978; **4**: 130–44.

51 King TE. Restrictive lung disease in pregnancy. *Clin Chest Med* 1992; **13**: 607–22.

52 Kopenhager T. A review of 50 pregnant patients with kyphoscoliosis. *Br J Obst Gynaecol* 1977; **84**: 585–7.

53 Siegler D, Zorab PA. Pregnancy in thoracic scoliosis. *Br J Dis Chest* 1981; **75**: 367–70.

54 Manning CW, Prime FJ, Zorab PA. Pregnancy and scoliosis. *Lancet* 1967; **ii**: 792–5.

55 Phelan JP, Dainer MJ, Cowherd DW. Pregnancy complicated by thoracolumbar scoliosis. *Southern Med J* 1978; **71**: 76–8.

56 Sawicka EH, Spencer GT, Branthwaite MA. Management of respiratory failure complicating pregnancy in severe kyphoscoliosis: a new use for an old technique? *Br J Dis Chest* 1986; **80**: 191–6.

57 Bergofsky EH. Respiratory failure in disorders of the thoracic cage. *Am Rev Respir Dis* 1979; **119**: 643–69.

58 Orem J. The wakefulness stimulus for breathing. In: Saunders NA, Sullivan CE, eds. *Sleep and breathing.* New York: Marcel Dekker, 1994: 113–55.

59 Shneerson JM. Pulmonary artery pressure in thoracic scoliosis during and after exercise while breathing air and pure oxygen. *Thorax* 1978; **33**: 747–54.

60 Branthwaite MA. Cardiorespiratory consequences of unfused idiopathic scoliosis. *Br J Dis Chest* 1986; **80**: 360–9.

61 Blount WP, Mellencamp DD. The effect of pregnancy on idiopathic scoliosis. *J Bone Joint Surg* (A) 1980; **62**: 1083–7.

62 Betz RR, Bunnell WP, Lambrecht-Mulier E, MacEwen GD. Scoliosis and pregnancy. *J Bone Joint Surg* (A) 1987; **69**: 90–5.

63 Gaucher P, Gerard M, Prud'hon MC, Gelas M, Robert D. Insuffisance respiratoire chronique severe et grossesse: nouvel essai therapeutique. *J Gynecol Obstet Biol Reprod* 1990; **19**: 197–201.

64 Estenne M, Heilporn A, Delhez L, Yernault J-C, De Troyer A. Chest wall stiffness in patients with chronic respiratory muscle weakness. *Am Rev Respir Dis* 1983; **128**: 1002–7.

65 Gibson GJ, Pride NB, Newsom-Davis JN, Loh LC. Pulmonary mechanics in patients with respiratory muscle weakness. *Am Rev Respir Dis* 1977; **115**: 389–95.

66 Contreras G, Gutierrez M, Beroiza T, *et al.* Ventilatory drive and respiratory muscle function in pregnancy. *Am Rev Respir Dis* 1995; **144**: 837–41.

67 Dahl B, Norregard FO, Juhl B. Pregnancy and delivery in a woman with neuromuscular disease. (Spinal muscular atrophy and severely reduced pulmonary function). *Ugeskr Laeger* 1995; **157**: 750–1.

68 Ville Y, Barbet JP, Pompidou A, Tournaire M. Limb girdle dystrophy and pregnancy: a case report. *J Gynecol Obstet Biol Reprod* 1991; **20**: 973–7.

69 Ekblad U, Kanto J. Pregnancy outcome in an extremely small woman with muscular dystrophy and respiratory insufficiency. *Acta Anaesth Scand* 1993; **37**: 228–30.

70 Pieters Th, Amy JJ, Burrini D, Aubert G, Rodenstein DO, Collard Ph. Normal pregnancy in primary alveolar hypoventilation treated with nocturnal nasal intermittent positive pressure ventilation. *Eur Respir J* 1995; **8**: 1424–7.

71 Charbonneau M, Falcone T, Cosio MG, Levy RD. Obstructive sleep apnea during pregnancy. Therapy and implications for fetal health. *Am Rev Respir Dis* 1991; **144**: 461–3.

72 Sherer DM, Caverly CB, Abramowicz JS. Severe obstructive sleep apnea and associated snoring documented during external tocography. *Am J Obstet Gynecol* 1991; **165**: 1300–1.

73 Cheun JK, Choi KT. Arterial oxygen desaturation rate following obstructive apnea in parturients. *J Korean Med Sci* 1992; 7: 6–10.

74 Noda A, Okada T, Hayashi H, Yasuma F, Yokota M. 24 hour ambulatory blood pressure variability in obstructive sleep apnea syndrome. *Chest* 1993; **103**: 1343–7.

75 Davies RJO, Vardi-Visy K, Clarke M, Stradling JR. Identification of sleep disruption and sleep disordered breathing profile from systolic blood pressure profile. *Thorax* 1993; **48**: 1242–7.

76 Feinsilver SH, Hertz G. Respiration during sleep in pregnancy. *Clin Chest Med* 1992; **13**: 637–44.

77 Simonds AK. Sleep studies of respiratory function and home respiratory support. *BMJ* 1994;**309**:35–40.

78 de Swiet M. Chest diseases in pregnancy. In: Weatherall DJ, Ledingham JGG, Warrell DA, eds. *Oxford textbook of medicine.* Oxford: Oxford University Press, 1987: 27–9.

79 Shneerson JM. Deformities of the thoracic cage. II. Acquired deformities. In: Emerson P, ed. *Thoracic medicine.* London: Butterworth, 1981: 363–4.

80 Reckles LN, Peterson HA, Bianco AJ, Weidman WH. The association of scoliosis and congenital heart disease. *J Bone Joint Surg* (A) 1975; **57**: 449–55.

81 Simonds AK, Carroll N, Branthwaite MA. Kyphoscoliosis as a cause of cardiorespiratory failure: pitfalls of diagnosis. *Respir Med* 1989; **83**: 149–50.

82 Daley MD, Rolbin SH, Hew EM, Morningstar BA, Stewart JA. Epidural anesthesia for obstetrics after spinal surgery. *Reg Anesth* 1990; **15**: 280–4.

83 Dresner MR, Maclean AR. Anaesthesia for caesarean section in a patient with Klippel–Feil syndrome. *Anaesthesia* 1995; **50**: 807–9.

15: Hypertrophic cardiomyopathy

CELIA OAKLEY

Hypertrophic cardiomyopathy (HCM) is an autosomal dominant disease characterised by hypertrophy of the undilated left and sometimes also the right ventricle in the absence of an abnormal haemodynamic load and with underlying myocytic and myofibrillar disarray.[1,2] It has fascinated cardiologists ever since the disorder was rediscovered as a clinical entity after Donald Teare described an autopsy series of eight patients who had died suddenly.[3] These included a young brother and sister, so suggesting the genetic nature of the condition. Symptoms include exertional chest pain, dyspnoea, fatigue, palpitations, and syncope, but sudden death may be the first manifestation. Early attention was on the labile left ventricular flow tract obstruction (even though the surviving two sisters and a brother of the dead siblings did not have this) but since then it has been realised that outflow tract obstruction is present in only a minority of patients, may persist for only part of the natural history, and is a predictor neither of disability nor of death.[4–10]

Family studies, now sometimes aided by genetic identification of mutant gene, have indicated the broad spectrum of morphological and phenotypic abnormality that exists not only between individuals at different ages but within families.[11] The development of echocardiography and its general availability has aided diagnosis, indeed has sometimes led to over-diagnosis, but has made it clear that a previously rare disorder with a grave prognosis may be a more common disorder with a better prognosis especially in older patients.[4,12,13] Series from specialist centres are highly skewed towards bad risk patients because patients have been referred on account of disabling symptoms or a family history of sudden death. In the early years before echocardiography only gross examples of the disease were identified but even without this limitation 40 years is too short a time in which to learn the natural history of a disorder which can be seen at almost any age.

Myocardial hypertrophy as shown by thickening of the ventricular wall may accelerate rapidly during the adolescent growth spurt,[14] then remain stable for years[15] or even gradually diminish as a result of myocyte fallout and replacement fibrosis. This may lead to wall thinning and systolic failure but with only relative cavity dilatation.[16]

Sudden death is a risk that has been widely publicised because it is a tragedy that occurs most commonly in young people either previously undiagnosed or members of known hypertrophic cardiomyopathy families (Figure 15.1).[17] This risk was thought to be higher in patients who showed bursts of ventricular tachycardia on ECG ambulatory monitoring[18,19] and led to the prescription of amiodarone for these patients. More recent work, however, has found no such prognostic significance and no difference in survival between patients with and without arrhythmias.[20] Children and young people at greatest risk are notably free from arrhythmias on monitoring.[21] The risk of sudden death is estimated as up to 6% per annum in the affected children of "malignant" families,[22] but is only a fraction of 1% in patients attending non-selective cardiac centres[11,12] and less than the risk of sudden death in patients with coronary artery disease.

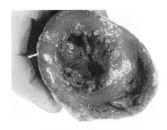

FIGURE 15.1—*The risk of sudden death is highest in young people. This heart is from a young woman who had not previously been known to have heart disease. It shows an undilated slightly thick walled left ventricle with the ventricular septum nearly twice as thick as the free wall, exaggerated trabeculation and a normal right ventricle. No macroscopic fibrosis is visible.*

Diagnosis in pregnancy

Most young patients with hypertrophic cardiomyopathy are symptom-free and are found through family screening or after a routine medical examination, which showed a murmur which led to ECG and echocardiography. The diagnosis may be made in this way during routine examination at the antenatal clinic.

Hypertrophic cardiomyopathy is sometimes first recognised during pregnancy when many physiological systolic murmurs lead to cardiological referral. Conversely the diagnosis may be missed if patients are murmur-free or the murmur may be mistaken for an innocent one or indeed may be a physiological murmur in a usually murmur-free patient. If suspicion is aroused the increase in the length and loudness of a late systolic ejection murmur on standing and its transient disappearance on squatting should lead to further investigation.

The ECG takes various forms but is almost always abnormal in patients beyond the first decade (Figure 15.2).[23,24] It often shows such bizarre features that no other diagnosis would fit. In other patients the changes may be mild and non-specific but in the context of family screening such changes are a more sensitive marker than echocardiography and if the patient is young they have high specificity also (Table 15.1). The abnormal ECG leads to echocardiography which will usually show symmetrical or asymmetrical left ventricular wall thickening (Figure 15.3). If hypertrophic cardiomyopathy is confirmed, ventricular arrhythmias should be sought by Holter ambulant ECG monitoring and an exercise test should be done to assess tolerance and with special attention to blood pressure. Failure of blood pressure to rise on exercise may indicate inability to raise stroke volume and risk of syncope.[25]

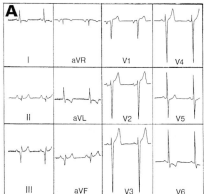

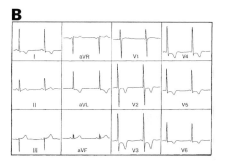

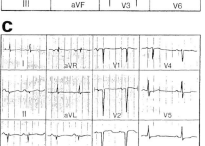

FIGURE 15.2—*Three electrocardiograms all showing different abnormalities but all incompatible with any diagnosis other than hypertrophic cardiomyopathy. In (A) are seen left atrial P waves, deep Q waves in leads III and AVF but upright T waves, high voltage in the chest leads with deep S waves in V₁ to V₄, tall R waves in V₆, absent Q waves with T wave inversion in the left ventricular leads I, AVL and V₆ but preserved R waves in V₁ to V₃. In (B) is again seen pronounced evidence of left ventricular hypertrophy with absent Q and T wave inversion in the left ventricular leads but also tall R waves in the right chest leads with T wave inversion starting in V₂. In (C) the voltage is not increased. There are left atrial P waves and QS waves in V₁ to V₃ suggestive of anteroseptal infarction.*

Risks in pregnancy

Symptom-free young women with HCM usually go through pregnancy without difficulty[29] and even those who complain of some shortness of breath or angina may do well. The increased blood volume and stroke volume of pregnancy may be beneficial if the left ventricle dilates to accommodate an increased stroke in a normal way. Sudden death has rarely

TABLE 15.1—*Results of electrocardiogram and echocardiogram analysis in 159 patients with confirmed hypertrophic cardiomyopathy and calculated sensitivities. Figures are number (%) of patients*

	Abnormal electrocardiogram	Normal electrocardiogram	Total
Abnormal echocardiogram	145 (91)	1	146 (92)
Normal echocardiogram	9 (6)	4 (3)	13 (8)
Total	154 (97)	5	159

Sensitivity of electrocardiogram alone 97%; sensitivity of echocardiogram alone 92%; and sensitivity of electrocardiogram and echocardiogram 97%.

The electrocardiogram can be a more sensitive marker of hypertrophic cardiomyopathy than the echocardiogram. It is also cheap, easy, and available unlike echocardiography which requires a skilled technician. (Reprinted with permission from American Journal of Cardiology.)[24]

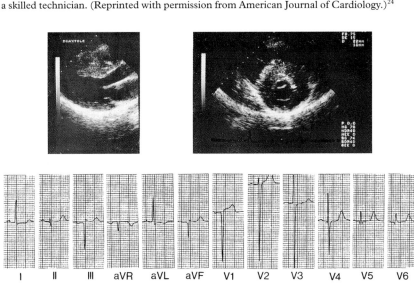

FIGURE 15.3—*Echocardiogram from a young woman with hypertrophic cardiomyopathy showing asymmetrical left ventricular wall thickening most pronounced in the septum (long axis view on the left and short axis on the right). Her electrocardiogram (below) shows abnormal Q waves in leads II, III and V, with deep S waves in V_1 to V_4 with abnormal T waves.*

been reported during pregnancy[30,31] but the information is too sparse to assess disease severity, any effect of drug treatment, and whether the death was haemodynamic or as a result of a primary arrhythmia. The strong impression is that the risk is not increased by pregnancy.

A family history of sudden death at a young age is the most potent indicator of risk,[22] particularly if a patient from such a family is having syncopal or near syncopal attacks. Apart from this the amount and disposition of hypertrophy, the presence or absence of outflow tract obstruction, and even the severity of symptoms of dyspnoea or angina are not predictive.[7-10] Syncopal attacks are usually ominous even in the absence of a bad family history although a few patients with syncopal attacks continue to have them for many years. Ventricular ectopy (other than bursts of ventricular tachycardia) on Holter monitoring may be predictive (as it is in coronary heart disease, dilated cardiomyopathy, and corrected tetralogy of Fallot) but the predictive accuracy is low. There is thus no proven relationship between prognosis, symptoms, and cardiac phenotype and no investigations including aggressive invasive electrophysiological tests have added prognostic information.

The main haemodynamic abnormality is a low stroke volume, a high ejection fraction, and diastolic stiffness. Relaxation is slow in early cases and progresses to a restrictive picture of early curtailment of filling in later cases. Hypertrophic cardiomyopathy is said to be the commonest cause of sudden death in athletes under the age of 30[32] but successful athletes need to have a supernormal maximal stroke volume and rapid diastolic filling. Not all patients with hypertrophic cardiomyopathy have a diastolic fault or indeed any haemodynamic impairment, at least while they are young.

Management of pregnancy

Even though the outcome is usually favourable, many women develop symptoms for the first time during pregnancy, or pre-existing symptoms get worse. These symptoms are often hard to interpret especially if the heart disorder is newly diagnosed, but dyspnoea, palpitation, or chest pain are usually an indication for starting beta-blocking drugs. Propranolol or metoprolol are good choices. The bradycardia induced augments coronary blood flow and aids left atrial emptying. If dizziness and syncope become troublesome or congestive features develop admission to hospital is required. The mechanism of syncope or pre-syncope should be investigated to find out whether the basis is haemodynamic or due to primary arrhythmia. A decision may need to be made about anti-arrhythmic drug treatment.

The data concerning the efficacy of anti-arrhythmic drugs including amiodarone in prevention of sudden death are very soft, based on amiodarone's undoubted ability to remove "short burst" ventricular tachycardia from the Holter tape, and clinical impression. Because of the heterogeneity of the disease no randomised controlled trial has been carried out and studies of efficacy have necessarily been based on historical controls. Sudden deaths still occur in amiodarone treated patients.[33] Amiodarone has been used safely in pregnancy. Fetal hypothyroidism may be induced but no congenital abnormality has been attributed to its use in pregnancy (Chapter 19). Verapamil is safe for use in pregnancy but a drug which augments systemic vasodilatation is probably unwise in case it precipitates a fall in blood pressure or syncope.

If supraventricular tachycardia or atrial fibrillation develop haemodynamic deterioration may be abrupt and threaten the fetus. The former can be corrected by intravenous adenosine and prevented by verapamil if this is tolerated.

If atrial flutter or fibrillation develop and persist DC cardioversion should be advised because of the deterioration in cardiovascular efficiency which tachycardia causes. To avoid the need to start warfarin an alternative is to carry out a transoesophageal echocardiographic study and if no intra-cavitary thrombus is seen in the left atrium or its appendage to follow this immediately by cardioversion. This is preferable to the conventional four weeks of anticoagulant treatment before cardioversion but heparin prophylaxis should be given for some days afterwards or until atrial contraction has been seen to have returned. Digoxin may be used to control the ventricular rate in atrial fibrillation if the arrhythmia returns or becomes permanent. Although through its inotropic effect it can increase the outflow tract gradient, such a gradient is unusual when atrial fibrillation develops. It usually occurs in more advanced disease associated with deterioration in left ventricular systolic function, increased diastolic abnormality, and loss of left atrial contractile force. The main reason for the fall in cardiovascular efficiency with onset of atrial fibrillation is the loss of regularity in these patients who need an optimal diastolic interval for maximum cardiac output.

Surgical septal myotomy is less popular now than it used to be when outflow tract gradients were considered more important, and there is renewed interest in DDD pacing which can reduce outflow tract gradients by pre-excitation of the ventricular septum.[34,35] This causes paradoxical posterior movement of the septum which widens the outflow tract. Some advocate an ultrashort atrioventricular delay to ensure capture of the ventricle and maximum pre-excitation of the septum. Increased doses of beta-blocking drugs or even atrioventricular nodal ablation may be needed to programme a longer atrioventricular delay and thereby harness a maximal atrial contribution to improve ventricular filling. Pacing can reduce outflow tract gradients but objective evidence of functional improvement is sparse and patients may be unable to tell whether the pacemaker is switched on or off. Others complain of the increased drug dosage and this is obviously undesirable in pregnancy.

Mitral valve replacement with a low profile valve relieves outflow tract obstruction and used to be used for this purpose but is now largely reserved for patients with substantial mitral regurgitation usually caused by structural changes in the valve, particularly after infective endocarditis. Alcohol injection into a septal branch of the anterior descending coronary artery has been suggested as a non-surgical means of ablating the ventricular septum[36] but creation of an infarct of necessarily uncontrolled size to reduce an outflow gradient of uncertain significance is unappealing and no long term results are available.[37]

Management of delivery

Delivery should take place in hospital with continuous ECG and blood pressure monitoring. Normal vaginal delivery is safe. The use of prostaglandins for induction of labour is inadvisable because of their vasodilator effect but oxytocic agents are well tolerated. For the same reason epidural anaesthesia should be avoided and blood loss replaced promptly. The patient should be sat up after completion of the third stage to avoid pulmonary congestion. If there is concern about this, 20 mg or 40 mg frusemide should be given intravenously at the start of labour. In some patients with severe disease there is only a narrow margin between enough left ventricular filling pressure to maintain output and pulmonary oedema. Conversely loss of venous return can lead to cardiogenic shock.

Antibiotic prophylaxis is needed for dental procedures during pregnancy or to cover surgical delivery.

The infants

It is unusual to find hypertrophy in the infants of mothers with hypertrophic cardiomyopathy. Hypertrophy recognised echocardiographically in neonates is usually part of the macrosomia shown by the infants of diabetic mothers or caused by glycogen storage disease, particularly type II (Pompe's disease). The echocardiographic appearances are indistinguishable from those of hypertrophic cardiomyopathy but regress spontaneously in the infants of diabetic mothers. No fetal problems can be attributed to the use of beta-adrenergic blocking drugs during pregnancy. Despite a large experience we have not encountered growth retardation, low Apgar scores or neonatal hypoglycaemia[26,27]. Breast feeding is not contraindicated but atenolol, acebutalol, nadolol and sotalol are secreted in breast milk in greater amounts than other beta-blockers which should therefore be preferred.

Advice to patients contemplating pregnancy

With the broad spectrum of clinical abnormality made more complex by the wide genetic heterogeneity of the disorder, how do we advise a young woman with the disorder who wishes to become pregnant? It is necessary to assess her cardiovascular reserve by taking into account symptoms, examination, and testing of her exercise tolerance. She should be fully informed about the risks to the child.

The genetic risk is not straightforward. The disorder is inherited as an autosomal dominant but with variable penetrance. In any affected family there is a 50% risk of any child inheriting the mutation but because of the great variation in its expression the condition may never be recognised clinically and the prognosis is normal. Conversely, the phenomenon of anticipation may be seen, the disease being manifest earlier and in more severe form in successive generations. A detailed family history may show no other known affected relatives, or several sudden deaths in young people. The pedigree may be incomplete because the family is far flung, or there has been a family rift, or the family may be small. Family screening should be initiated if this has not already been done. ECG alone is sufficient in the first instance. Those with abnormal or equivocal ECGs should be studied by echocardiography. A genetic diagnosis can now be made in nearly half of hypertrophic cardiomyopathy families and in people from families in whom a mutation has been identified.[38] Linkage to the beta-myosin heavy chain gene on chromosome 14 is expected in about 30% of pedigrees, linkage to the cardiac troponin T gene on chromosome 1 in approximately 15%, and linkage to the α-tropomysin gene on chromosome 15 in less than 3%. Linkage has also been found to chromosome 11.[39] The influence of yet other genes or environmental factors controlling expression of the hypertrophic cardiomyopathy phenotype will no doubt become known in the next few years.

References

1 Maron BJ, Gottdiener JS, Epstein SE. Patterns and significance of left ventricular hypertrophy in hypertrophic cardiomyopathy. A wide angle, two-dimensional echocardiographic study of 125 patients. *Am J Cardiol* 1981; **48**: 418–28.

2 Davies MJ. The current status of myocardial disarray in hypertrophic cardiomyopathy. *Br Heart J* 1984; **51**: 361–3.

3 Teare RD. Asymmetrical hypertrophy of the heart in young adults. *Br Heart J* 1958; **20**: 1–8.

4 Kofflard MJ, Waldstein DJ, Voz J, Ten Cate FJ. Prognosis in hypertrophic cardiomyopathy observed in a large clinic population. *Am J Cardiol* 1993; **72**: 939–43.

5 Braunwald E, Labrew CT, Rockoff SD, Ross J, Morrow AG. Idiopathic hypertrophic subaortic stenosis. I. Description of the disease based upon an analysis of 64 patients. *Circulation* 1964; **29** (**suppl 4**): 3–119.

6 Cohen J, Effat H, Goodwin JF, Oakley CM, Steiner RE. Hypertrophic obstructive cardiomyopathy. *Br Heart J* 1964; **26**: 16–32.

7 Romeo F, Pelliccia F, Cristofani R, Martuscelli E, Reale A. Hypertrophic obstructive cardiomyopathy: is a left ventricular outflow tract gradient a major prognostic determinant? *Eur Heart J* 1990; **11**: 233–40.

8 Maron BJ, Roberts WC, Epstein SE. Sudden death in hypertrophic cardiomyopathy. A profile of 78 patients. *Circulation* 1982; **65**: 1388–94.

9 Spirito P, Maron BJ. Relation between extent of left ventricular hypertrophy and occurrence of sudden cardiac death in hypertrophic cardiomyopathy. *J Am Coll Cardiol* 1990; **15**: 1521–6.

10 Fananapazir L, Chang AC, Epstein SE, McAreavey D. Prognostic determinants in hypertrophic cardiomyopathy. *Circulation* 1992; **86**: 730–40.

11 Shapiro LM, Zezulka A. Hypertrophic cardiomyopathy a common disease with a good prognosis. Five year experience of a district general hospital. *Br Heart J* 1983; **50**: 530–3.

12 Spirito P, Chiarella F, Carrantino L, *et al*. Clinical course and prognosis of hypertrophic cardiomyopathy in an outpatient population. *N Engl J Med* 1989; **320**: 749–55.

13 Maron BJ, Spirito P. Impact of patient selection biases on the perception of hypertrophic cardiomyopathy and its natural history. *Am J Cardiol* 1993; **72**: 970.

14 Maron BJ, Spirito P, Wesley Y, Arce J. Development and progression of left ventricular hypertrophy in children with hypertrophic cardiomyopathy: identification by two-dimensional echocardiography. *N Engl J Med* 1986; **315**: 610–14.

15 Spirito P, Maron BJ. Absence of progression of left ventricular hypertrophy in adult patients with hypertrophic cardiomyopathy. *Am J Cardiol* 1987; **9**: 1013–17.

16 Spirito P, Maron BJ, Bonow RO, Epstein SE. Occurrence and significance of progressive left ventricular wall thinning and relative cavity dilatation in patients with hypertrophic cardiomyopathy. *Am J Cardiol* 1987; **60**: 123–9.

17 Maron BJ, Roberts WC, Epstein SE. Sudden death in hypertrophic cardiomyopathy: a profile of 78 patients. *Circulation* 1982; **65**: 1388.

18 Maron BJ, Savage DD, Wolfson JK, *et al.* Prognostic significance of 24 hour ambulatory electrocardiographic monitoring in patients with hypertrophic cardiomyopathy: a prospective study. *Am J Cardiol* 1981; **48**: 252.

19 McKenna WJ, England D, Doi YL *et al.* Arrhythmia in hypertrophic cardiomyopathy. I. Influence on prognosis. *Br Heart J* 1981; **46**: 168.

20 Spirito P, Rapezzi C, Autore C, *et al.* Prognosis of asymptomatic patients with hypertrophic cardiomyopathy and non-sustained ventricular tachycardia. *Circulation* 1994; **90**: 2743.

21 McKenna WJ, Franklin RCG, Nihoyannopoulos P, Robinson KC, Deanfield JE. Arrhythmia and prognosis in infants, children and adolescents with hypertrophic cardiomyopathy. *J Am Coll Cardiol* 1988; **11**: 147–53.

22 Maron BJ, Lipson LC, Roberts WC, Savage DD, Epstein SE. "Malignant" hypertrophic cardiomyopathy: identification of a subgroup of families with unusually frequent premature deaths. *Am J Cardiol* 1978; **41**: 1133.

23 Al Mahdawi S, Chamberlain S, Chojnowska L, *et al.* The electrogram is a more sensitive indicator than echocardiography of hypertrophic cardiomyopathy in families with a mutation in the MYH7 gene. *Br Heart J* 1994; **72**: 105–11.

24 Ryan MP, Cleland JGF, French JA, *et al.* The standard electrocardiogram as a screening test for hypertrophic cardiomyopathy. *Am J Cardiol* 1995; **76**: 689–94.

25 Frenneaux P, Counihan PJ, Calforio ALP, *et al.* Abnormal blood pressure response during exercise in hypertrophic cardiomyopathy. *Circulation* 1991; **82**: 1995–2002.

26 Turner GM, Oakley CM, Dixon HG. Management of pregnancy complicated by hypertrophic cardiomyopathy. *BMJ* 1968; **ii**: 281.

27 Oakley GDG, McGarry K, Limb DG, Oakley CM. Management of pregnancy in patients with hypertrophic cardiomyopathy. *BMJ* 1979; **37**: 305–12.

28 Evans-Jones JC. Hypertrophic cardiomyopathy in pregnancy. *J R Soc Med* 1983; **76**: 524.

29 Kumar A, Elkayam U. Hypertrophic cardiomyopathy in pregnancy. In: Elkayam U, Gleicher N eds. *Cardiac problems in pregnancy: diagnosis and management of maternal and fetal disease.* 2nd ed. New York: Alan R Liss, 1990: 129.

30 Shah DM, Sunderji SG. Hypertrophic cardiomyopathy and pregnancy: report of a maternal mortality and review of the literature. *Obstet Gynecol Surv* 1985; **40**: 444.

31 Pelliccia F, Gainfrocca C, Gandio C, Reale A. Sudden death during pregnancy in hypertrophic cardiomyopathy. *Eur Heart J* 1992; **13**: 421–3.

32 Maron BJ, Epstein SE, Roberts WC. Causes of sudden death in competitive athletes. *J Am Coll Cardiol* 1986; **7**: 204.

33 Fananapazir L, Leon MB, Bonow RD, Tracy CM, Cannon RO, Epstein SE. Sudden death during empiric amiodarone therapy in symptomatic hypertrophic cardiomyopathy. *Am J Cardiol* 1991; **67**: 169–75.

34 Kappenberger L. Pacing for obstructive hypertrophic cardiomyopathy. *Br Heart J* 1995; **73**: 107–8.

35 Slade AKB, Sadoul N, Shapiro L, *et al.* DDD pacing in hypertrophic cardiomyopathy: a multicentre clinical experience. *Heart* 1996; **75**: 44–9.

36 Sigwart U. Non surgical myocardial reduction for hypertrophic obstructive cardiomyopathy. *Lancet* 1995; **346**: 211–13.

37 Oakley CM. Non-surgical ablation of the ventricular septum for the treatment of hypertrophic cardiomyopathy. *Br Heart J* 1995; **74**: 479–80.

38 Ryan MP, French J, Al-Mahdawi S, Nihoyannopoulos P, Cleland JGF, Oakley CM. Genetic testing for familial hypertrophic cardiomyopathy in newborn infants. *BMJ* 1995; **310**: 856–7.

39 Schwartz K, Carrier L, Guicheney P, Komajda M. Molecular basis of familial cardiomyopathies. *Circulation* 1995; **91**: 532–40.

16: Peripartum cardiomyopathy and other heart muscle disorders

CELIA OAKLEY

Peripartum cardiomyopathy describes unexplained heart failure that develops in temporal relation to pregnancy and is usually defined as heart failure occurring within a month before or six months after childbirth in women who were not previously known to have heart disease.[1,2] The worst cases develop explosively in the puerperium most often within a few days of parturition and patients may die. Milder cases may first be seen a few weeks after delivery. Much less commonly symptoms are first noticed during the last weeks of pregnancy. The condition is rare and the true incidence is unknown. It has been variously reported as from 1 in 1300 to 1 in 15 000 deliveries in the United States but minor cases go unrecognised.[3-5] It is alleged to cause 5% of the cardiac deaths that occur in relation to pregnancy but less than 1% of the cardiovascular problems encountered in pregnancy.[6]

Clinical features

Peripartum cardiomyopathy presents with all degrees of severity from catastrophic to mild left ventricular dysfunction that is discovered only fortuitously by echocardiography when attribution is difficult and further investigation inappropriate. In the worst cases fulminating pulmonary oedema and congestive failure develop in the first days after delivery with severe dyspnoea, orthopnea, tachycardia, hypotension, fluid overload, a third heart sound gallop, and sometimes a mitral regurgitant murmur. Embolism from mural thrombus in the left ventricle, or ventricular tachycardia, may precede the onset of clinical heart failure. The new mother and her family are catapulted from delight to desperate illness.

Investigations

The electrocardiogram shows sinus tachycardia. Supraventricular and ventricular ectopic beats or sustained atrial or ventricular arrhythmias are

210

common. The QRS complexes may be normal, low voltage, or show an intraventricular conduction defect or fascicular block. The changes may appear focal and suggest myocardial infarction (Figure 16.1). The chest radiograph shows an enlarged heart with pulmonary congestion or oedema and often bilateral pleural effusions (Figure 16.2). Echocardiography shows dilatation which usually involves all four chambers but is dominated by left ventricular hypokinesia which may be global or most pronounced in a particular territory, again suggesting possible infarction. A small pericardial effusion may be seen. Doppler ultrasound shows mitral, tricuspid, and pulmonary regurgitation through structurally normal valves, all minor and secondary to generalised dilatation (but this on its own is not diagnostic because such regurgitation is not uncommon in normally functioning volume-loaded hearts in pregnancy). Laboratory blood studies are largely unhelpful but there may be release of cardiac enzymes and high levels are reached in severe cases, again raising the possibility of myocardial infarction. Since the myometrium contains the MB isoenzyme of creatinine phosphokinase increased plasma concentrations of this enzyme are a normal postpartum finding after normal delivery[7] so other cardiac enzymes should be measured.

The diagnosis is by exclusion. Cardiac catheterisation should be instituted rapidly to establish the integrity of the coronary arteries and to take right ventricular endomyocardial biopsies. The cardiac output is sometimes surprisingly well maintained with a normal mixed venous saturation despite overwhelming heart failure and pronounced fluid overload, but in most cases the cardiac output is low. Although the left atrial pressure (usually

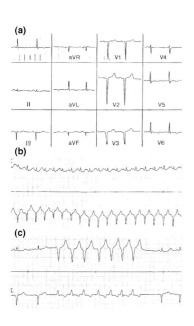

FIGURE 16.1—(a) Electrocardiogram from a patient with peripartum cardiomyopathy showing low voltage and QS waves in leads V1 to V3 with poor T wave development suggesting possible anteroapical infarction. (b) & (c) are rhythm strips from the same patient showing supraventricular tachycardia (b) and a burst of ventricular tachycardia (c).

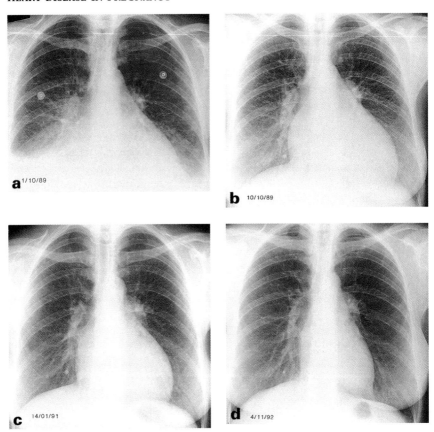

FIGURE 16.2—(a) Chest radiograph from a patient who developed fulminant heart failure two days after delivery of twins. Nine days later (b) shows a globally enlarged heart. (c) The heart was still considerably dilated after 15 months but three years after the onset the heart size is normal and remains so (d) although echocardiography still shows depressed contractile indices.

measured indirectly) is high there is little pulmonary hypertension. This implies a recent onset of the condition.

When the myocardium is biopsied within a month of the onset examination of the specimen nearly always shows an acute myocarditis with myocytolysis and infiltration by T lymphocytes (Figure 16.3).[8-10]

When heart failure occurs shortly after delivery, initial diagnosis and treatment are necessarily within the same hospital, which may well not have full cardiac facilities. Because of this many patients do not undergo cardiac biopsy until much later if at all, especially as the frequency of underlying myocarditis has been appreciated only relatively recently. Although death may occur during the acute phase subsequent recovery of myocardial function may be considerable as is the experience when acute myocarditis occurs outside pregnancy.[10,11]

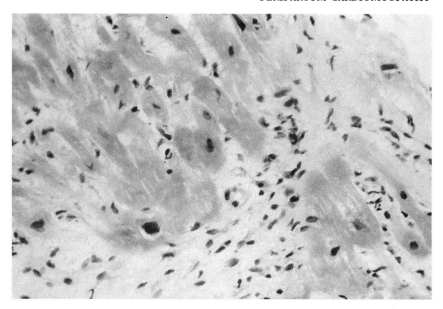

FIGURE 16.3—*Endomyocardial biopsy specimen showing acute myocarditis. There is pronounced myocytolysis with sheets of pale staining, dead myocytes and infiltration with T lymphocytes and some macrophages (identified by immunohistochemical staining)*

Incidence and causation

Peripartum cardiomyopathy is particularly common in women with multiple pregnancies and this may be because of the greater haemodynamic burden—higher blood volume and stroke output—than in single pregnancies. Diminished cardiovascular reserve may account for cases of peripartum cardiomyopathy complicating organic heart disease, which perhaps caused the development of clinical symptoms that might not have developed if the heart had previously been normal.[12,13] This could also explain an association with pre-eclamptic toxaemia.[14] There is no convincing evidence that the disorder is more common in socially deprived, multiparous, older, or black mothers.

Physiological pregnancy-related changes conducive to fluid overload and heart failure are maximal in the peripartal period. Blood volume and cardiac output are at a peak, serum aldosterone increases in the last trimester causing sodium and water retention, and when the low resistance arteriovenous fistula created by the placenta closes after delivery there is an abrupt rise in systemic vascular resistance which could result in heart failure. But this does not explain the myocarditis. Return of blood from the placenta to the circulation "placental auto-transfusion" may add further to the cardiovascular load and it may be that normal women suffer some temporary deterioration in left ventricular function postpartum.[1]

The aetiology seems to be immunological. Evidence of an infective origin is rarely found. Occasionally a family history of dilated cardiomyopathy is

213

obtained and, as this is also immunologically based, it may be that pregnancy was a trigger for the development of myocarditis and heart failure in a genetically predisposed woman at a haemodynamically vulnerable time. Cell mediated immunity is reduced in pregnancy. This prevents rejection of the fetus but increases maternal susceptibility to virus infection. Three cases of peripartum cardiomyopathy with biopsy-proven myocarditis were reported.[15] Two had a history of influenza and one had elevated antibody titres to Coxsackie B2. As evidence of viral or other infection is usually absent in peripartum cardiomyopathy, which usually develops postpartum, the antigen is more likely to be fetal than viral.

Postpartum heart failure in Nigeria

The development of postpartum heart failure which is common among the Hausa women of northern Nigeria seems to be of different origin, related to traditional practices with overheating and fluid loading. This is caused by an excessive salt intake from eating "kanwa" (traditional salt) while reclining on a heated mud bed, resulting in high output failure which usually resolves after withdrawal of the causative factors.[16,17]

Differential diagnosis

The clinical differential diagnosis includes pre-existing dilated cardiomyopathy, pulmonary thromboembolism, amniotic fluid embolism, myocardial infarction, and beta-2-agonist-associated pulmonary oedema in patients who have been given an agent such as ritodrine to postpone premature delivery (Table 16.1). Echocardiography firmly places the fault within the left ventricle and is an essential early investigation.

TABLE 16.1—*Differential diagnosis of peripartum cardiomyopathy*

- Pre-existing dilated cardiomyopathy
- Peripartum myocardial infarction
- Pulmonary embolism: thrombus or amniotic fluid
- Overtransfusion
- Ritodrine associated pulmonary oedema (premature delivery)

It may be difficult or impossible to distinguish peripartum cardiomyopathy from dilated cardiomyopathy exacerbated by pregnancy.[5] Such patients are perhaps more likely to develop heart failure before delivery as the cardiovascular load becomes maximal rather than after it; they are less likely to release cardiac enzymes or show acute myocarditis in biopsy specimens (though acute myocarditis may have been superimposed on pre-existing dilated cardiomyopathy), and are more likely to have pulmonary hypertension as well as symptoms of dyspnoea and fatigue early in the pregnancy.

Myocardial infarction, though rare, is the major complication of the peripartum period which needs to be distinguished.[15,16] A history of preceding angina is uncommon because peripartal infarction is not usually caused by underlying atherosclerotic disease except in diabetic smokers or patients with other risk factors for premenopausal coronary disease, including familial hypercholesterolaemia. The commonest cause is spontaneous coronary artery dissection (Chapter 18).

Pulmonary embolism may complicate peripartum cardiomyopathy but by itself causes only right ventricular dilatation. The origin of the postpartum patient's sudden dyspnoea is quickly confirmed by echocardiography (Chapter 20).

Pulmonary oedema may be caused by ritodrine given to postpone premature labour while steroids are given to mature the fetal lungs. The cause seems to be the infusion of the drug in saline instead of dextrose and so leading to fluid overload. Echocardiography shows normal left ventricular function. Recovery is usually prompt but in one case ritodrine-induced pulmonary oedema unmasked an underlying peripartum cardiomyopathy.[18]

Management

Patients with peripartum heart failure should be given oxygen, diuretics, angiotensin converting enzyme (ACE) inhibitors (if postpartum), digoxin, and warfarin. Cautious addition of a beta-adrenergic blocking drug may be beneficial particularly when cardiac output is well preserved. The most gravely ill patients need intubation, ventilation, Swan-Ganz catheterisation for monitoring, intravenous dobutamine, renal doses of dopamine, and sometimes temporary support by an intra-aortic balloon pump. Arrhythmias may precipitate cardiogenic shock and should be treated promptly by DC reversion or if recurrent, by overdrive pacing. Appropriate anti-arrhythmic drug treatment will be needed. Amiodarone is usually the safest and most effective of these because it is a mild vasodilator, has no myocardial depressant effect when given orally, and has the least pro-arrhythmic effect of the major anti-arrhythmic drugs (Chapter 22). Cardiac transplantation sometimes offers the only hope and has been reported in such patients but only rarely does a suitable organ become available.[19] If the patient survives and improves everyone is relieved that no transplant was made during the emergency.

In severe cases and particularly when florid myocarditis is found on biopsy,[20] immunosuppressive treatment should be started early using prednisolone in a dose of 1·5 mg/kg/day plus azathioprine as a steroid sparer in a dose of 1 mg/kg/day.[8] This should be continued until there is clear evidence of improvement. The duration of treatment must be discretionary in the individual case as there are no data. Serial cardiac biopsy is carried out by some to provide guidance. Loss of cellular infiltration together with clinical and haemodynamic improvement is encouraging but because the severity of myocarditis may vary considerably within small areas the results are not necessarily helpful. Recruitment into the American trial of immunosuppressive treatment in acute myocarditis was exceedingly slow and the results unconvincing.[21] No randomised prospective trial of treatment of peripartum cardiomyopathy is ever likely to be conducted because the condition is so rare.

Patients should remain on an ACE inhibitor for as long as left ventricular function remains abnormal as judged by serial echocardiography rather than clinically.[22] The benefit may be enhanced by low doses of a diuretic. Digoxin and warfarin may be stopped once the left ventricle has improved but in patients who had intracavitary thrombus or had had an embolic complication it is tempting to continue warfarin until there is a reason to stop it. ACE inhibitors should be stopped if a patient becomes pregnant again because of the risk of causing fetal renal failure and oligohydramnios.

Breast feeding is often proscribed for nutritional reasons but there is little logic to this. It is often easier for the mother than preparing bottles and the amount of maternal drugs secreted in the milk is not sufficient to have any adverse effect on the baby.

Prognosis

Although early improvement must be rapid for the most sick patients to survive, further gains can be anticipated during the subsequent weeks or months. Patients may recover even from profound failure to apparently normal or near normal function and this improvement may continue for one or two years after delivery (Figure 16.2). Sometimes the condition may appear depressingly static with persistently impaired left ventricular function for many months, only to start recovering a year or more after the acute episode (Figure 16.4). Not all patients do well. Some show progressive left ventricular dysfunction and gradually deteriorate and die or have a cardiac transplant.

Progress should be followed by serial echocardiography. Left ventricular function often remains subnormal even in patients who have made a complete clinical recovery.[18]

Because cardiac biopsy specimens obtained in the acute phase show myocytolysis it is clear that even patients with apparently complete recovery must have lost some cardiovascular reserve and it may be prudent for them to avoid subsequent pregnancy. The propensity to deteriorate in a future pregnancy is much greater in patients with severe initial illness or with persisting abnormality of left ventricular function than in patients whose left ventricular function has apparently returned to normal. Patients whose first pregnancy was complicated by peripartum cardiomyopathy may want a second child but they should be advised to wait several years before embarking on further pregnancy. The condition does not necessarily recur

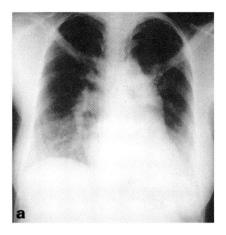
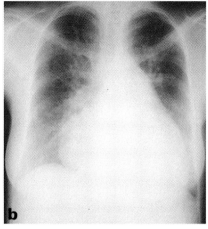
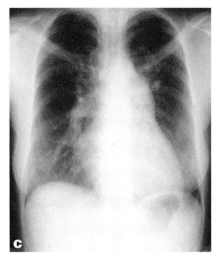

FIGURE 16.4—*Chest radiographs from a patient with a non-restrictive ventricular septal defect and severe pulmonary vascular disease (a) when she was first seen at 24 weeks' gestation, (b) when she developed severe postpartum heart failure and cyanosis due to shunt reversal and four years later (c) she was again well, acyanotic and with good left and right ventricular function. (The echocardiograms of this patient are shown in Chapter 4)*

in patients who have made a complete echocardiographic recovery but such patients clearly need careful serial echocardiographic monitoring during subsequent pregnancy and should be delivered in hospital.[18] Further pregnancy should be discouraged in any patient with persistent left ventricular dysfunction, and in patients who have apparently fully recovered the possibility of relapse in a subsequent pregnancy should be discussed.

Psychosocial

Patients who have survived peripartum cardiomyopathy often become depressed. After the elation of a successful birth or delivery of twins they experience the trauma of a life threatening illness which makes them unable for some time to look after or enjoy the new baby or their other children.

Husbands and grandparents have to deal with domestic chores and the children in the family feel deprived. It is a difficult time for everyone.

Women who have previously been employed outside the home may well find it easier to return to a job which is not physically demanding than to take up increased domestic chores together with the extra work caused by the new baby. Crêches and child minders are usually not available until the baby is more than three months old and the mother will need home helps and other social services together with considerable moral support from her partner, doctors, and friends.

Dilated cardiomyopathy

Dilated cardiomyopathy is characterised by reduced contraction of the left or right or both ventricles with consequent dilatation. Usually the left ventricle is involved, right ventricular failure being a later development, but occasionally it is the other way around with a dilated right ventricle and preserved function of the left ventricle. Mild disease may not change for years or even improve but patients who have severe left or right or biventricular failure when they are first seen tend to do badly.[23] There has been an improvement in survival attributable to use of ACE inhibitors and beta-blockers and recognition of milder cases in women who do not necessarily deteriorate.[24,25] Right ventricular failure may be delayed for many years after the first development of left ventricular failure and is then often a consequence of the development of pulmonary hypertension secondary to the left ventricular failure. A poor prognosis is indicated by severe effort intolerance (NYHA class III or IV), the onset of right ventricular failure, the development of mitral regurgitation, atrial fibrillation, or systemic hypotension, and by hyponatraemia and raised plasma noradrenaline and adrenaline concentrations.[23] Pregnancy is unlikely in such patients and carries high risk.

Dilated cardiomyopathy may be seen at any age and in either sex. Mild cases are usually asymptomatic unless complicated by arrhythmia or thromboembolism. They are identified by routine health screening or family studies but still escape detection in the absence of echocardiographic examination because the ECG may be normal and a chest radiograph does not show mild left ventricular dilatation or reduced contraction. They may be detected after referral to a physician or a cardiologist if the patient is worried because of a relative or friend with heart trouble, or if the patient has symptoms which even after recognition of left ventricular dysfunction may seem to have been coincidental rather than caused by the cardiomyopathy.

Dilated cardiomyopathy is familial in about 20% of cases as shown by family studies. The autosomal dominant inheritance may be obscured because of subclinical cases. The prognosis in such mildly affected cases is unknown but in women the cardiac disorder may first become manifest as a peripartum cardiomyopathy.

About 10% of patients with dilated cardiomyopathy complain of chest pain, either typical angina or atypical chest pain, which may lead to investigation. Among them are some younger women. Echocardiography shows mild or moderate left ventricular hypokinesia. This is usually global but may be regionally more marked with preservation of normal or near normal contraction of part of the left ventricle.

Dilated cardiomyopathy may be associated with ventricular arrhythmia as its only clinical feature and ambulatory ECG monitoring should be carried out in all patients[26]. Ventricular tachycardia may first develop in pregnancy (Chapter 19).

Most patients with dilated cardiomyopathy are first diagnosed because of the unexpected development of left ventricular failure with symptoms which are at first attributed to a chest infection and treated accordingly. Only when the condition fails to respond and it is realised that breathlessness without fever is not the hallmark of a chest infection is the patient given a diuretic. This provides immediate relief of dyspnoea and it is then that the patient is usually referred to a specialist. Such patients usually already have considerably dilated left ventricles measuring 6 cm or more, with depressed contractile indices. They are usually advised firmly against pregnancy and there is little experience of pregnancy in patients with previously diagnosed dilated cardiomyopathy. A few patients have a stable dilated cardiomyopathy over many years during which they are relatively or absolutely without symptoms, usually on a small dose of diuretic and an ACE inhibitor with or without digoxin.

Such patients need individual decisions but some will tolerate pregnancy. ACE inhibitors should be withdrawn and substituted by an alternative vasodilator such as hydralazine, together with a long-acting nitrate. A diuretic may be unavoidable or the dose may need to be increased. Tachycardia at rest reflects failure to increase stroke volume and indicates cautious introduction of a beta-blocker such as metoprolol in an initially low dose such as 12·5 mg twice daily. Such a patient would be at risk of peripartum heart failure caused by the haemodynamic changes or on account of real deterioration due to a superadded peripartum cardiomyopathy. There is little experience to draw upon because most physicians and cardiologists err on the side of caution and tend to advise against pregnancy.

Phaeochromocytoma

Phaeochromocytoma may be associated with frequent ventricular ectopic beats or ventricular tachycardia and needs to be excluded. Rarely it can cause failure or pulmonary oedema without hypertension and with catecholamine-induced myocardial necrosis in pregnancy.[27] The tumour should be removed in pregnancy after preliminary treatment with phenoxybenzamine followed by labetolol. Considerable improvement in myocardial function can be anticipated.

Other causes of depressed left ventricular function

Young women with mild or moderate depression of left ventricular function can go through pregnancy without difficulty and there is more experience of dealing with residual impairment of left ventricular function following previous surgery than because of dilated cardiomyopathy. Examples are patients who have had operations for the relief of discrete subaortic stenosis, sometimes more than once, and are left with globally impaired contraction often with some mitral regurgitation. Occasional patients are seen who have had surgery for coarctation associated with endocardial fibroelastosis.

Left ventricular dysfunction may follow previous irradiation or chemotherapy in childhood for Hodgkin's lymphoma or other malignancy. Radiation to the thorax can damage the pericardium, coronary arteries or myocardium in the exposed field and although cardiac protection is much better now with highly focused radiation, this was not the case 20 years ago. Previous treatment with doxorubicin (Adriamycin) may cause cardiac damage which is important in long term survivors. Restrictive features predominate and may not be apparent for some years afterwards. These patients are rare and each needs to be considered on her merits. Most who have mild or no symptoms (NYHA class II) negotiate pregnancy successfully but they should be closely monitored, admitted to hospital before delivery for rest, avoid excessive weight gain with a calorie controlled low salt diet, avoid fluid overload, and be given ACE inhibitors after delivery.

Restrictive cardiomyopathy

Restrictive cardiomyopathy is characterised by diastolic indistensibility with preserved left ventricular systolic function and no increase in wall thickness. The cavity is therefore not dilated but the diastolic pressure is raised with an excessive increment in pressure for each increment in filling. It is rare but sometimes familial and is seen in children and young adults. Some families show an associated progressive conduction system fault with sinoatrial and atrioventricular conduction failure developing either before or at the same time as the cardiomyopathy.[28] Marked dilatation of both atria sometimes develops and is associated with atrial standstill with or without a disorder of atrioventricular conduction. A skeletal myopathy may be associated in some families with Noonan syndrome in which both restrictive[29] and hypertrophic cardiomyopathies have been described.[30] Noonan syndrome is dominantly inherited and has a normal chromosome pattern and normal fertility.

The underlying pathology may be of a fine interstitial myocardial fibrosis and sometimes myocyte hypertrophy without disarray.[30,31] Endocardial fibroelastosis may also be familial and exist in mild form. Infiltrations and storage disease may also cause a restrictive clinical picture.[31]

In some of these patients the signs mimic those of constrictive pericarditis though differentiating features include a higher diastolic pressure in the left than in the right ventricle resulting in dissimilar left and right atrial pressures, pulmonary hypertension, and tricuspid regurgitation. Pulsus paradoxus does not occur and continuous wave Doppler echocardiography does not show reciprocal changes in mitral and tricuspid inflow velocities with respiration. In constrictive pericarditis increased tricuspid inflow with inspiration is associated with reduced mitral inflow (and therefore a paradoxical pulse) and the ventricular septum moves posteriorly towards the left ventricle with inspiration. In constrictive pericarditis the ventricular septum is straight in diastole because of equal pressures each side of it and shows a typical shuddering movement with early posterior kick (Chapter 17). This marked ventricular interdependence in constrictive pericarditis is not seen in restrictive cardiomyopathy in which the ventricular septum is convex towards the right ventricle through all phases of the cardiac cycle but, as in constrictive pericarditis, ventricular filling is rapid and curtailed early. A normal pericardial space and absence of thickening of the fibrous pericardium may be seen in good echocardiograms.

Patients with restrictive cardiomyopathy may go through pregnancy successfully but with increasing tachycardia and fluid retention. Tachycardia is well tolerated because ventricular filling is rapid but it reflects limited stroke volume. The heart fails to dilate to accommodate increased volume and the left atrial pressure rises causing pulmonary congestion or oedema. Loss of sinus rhythm with the onset of a supraventricular arrhythmia may cause abrupt deterioration.

Patients with severely compromised cardiovascular function from restrictive cardiomyopathy are best served by early admission to hospital and delivery by elective caesarean section. After delivery there is usually brisk improvement back to their pre-pregnancy state and no permanent deterioration is observed though the condition is a progressive one and eventually fatal.

Family studies should be arranged. The phenomenon of anticipation with earlier onset in succeeding generations seen in some families will terminate the disease line in that family.

Arrhythmogenic right ventricular dysplasia

This disorder in which parts of the myocardium of the free wall of the right ventricle are replaced by fibro-adipose tissue is associated with ventricular tachycardia of right ventricular origin, and sudden death. It seems to be much more common in Northern Italy and parts of France than in the UK but should be suspected in any patient with ventricular ectopic beats or recurrent tachycardia with a left bundle branch block pattern. Many familial cases have been described with a predominance of young men affected.[32]

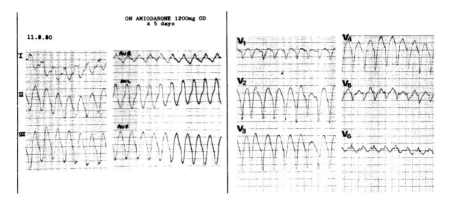

FIGURE 16.5—*Ventricular tachycardia in a young woman with right ventricular dysplasia. The wide complexes show a left bundle branch block configuration.*

X-linked cardiomyopathies

A number of x-linked disorders are associated with cardiomyopathy and in most of these the female carriers may be affected to a milder extent. The best known and most extensively studied is Duchenne's progressive muscular dystrophy. The gene was identified in 1987 and the disease is caused by deficiency of the corresponding protein dystrophin (Figure 16.5). Although dilated cardiomyopathy is often seen and may be severe[33-35] symptomatic cardiac involvement is less probably because of the patients' greatly restricted activity and eventual immobility.[33-35] Previously scoliosis made examination difficult but nowadays this is prevented by a spinal brace. Cardiac involvement is common also in the later onset and more slowly progressive Becker's muscular dystrophy. Distinctive electrocardiographic findings include tall right precordial R waves with increased RS ratio and deep Q waves in leads I AVL and the left precordial leads. These features have been associated with lesions in the posterolateral wall of the left ventricle. Abnormal left ventricular function is shown on echocardiography with diminished posterior wall thickening and activity. When investigated by positron emission tomography metabolic abnormalities have been found to be most prevalent in the same region. The left ventricular dysfunction is progressive with dilatation and generally diminished contractile indices.

The female carriers of Duchenne and Becker's muscular dystrophy show dystrophin defects in 50% of myocardial cells and can be identified by endomyocardial biopsy.[36,37] They show ECG abnormalities similar to those found in male subjects, though the abnormalities are usually less severe.

Echocardiography confirms occult myocardial involvement in many female carriers despite a lack of clinical manifestations. They may have raised serum concentrations of creatinine phosphokinase and a small number may show a mild form of pseudohypertrophic skeletal myopathy. These abnormalities in the female carriers of Duchenne's muscular dystrophy allow them to be identified.

The dystrophin gene is genetically lethal to male possessors so that cases of Duchenne's dystrophy must arise either as a result of a new mutation or from transmission of the gene through the female. Rarely a female carrier of Duchenne's dystrophy may be seen in whom there is no family history of affected males and recognition of the female carrier is then of great importance. In vitro fertilisation can now ensure that such women give birth only to unaffected children.

Emery-Dreifuss muscular dystrophy is a rare x-linked dystrophy associated with severe cardiac involvement characterised by myocardial fibrosis and atrophy, bradycardias, conduction abnormalities, atrial arrhythmias, and atrial standstill. Symptom-free female carriers may also show cardiac abnormalities and need an implanted pacemaker. Genetic counselling is obviously important.[38]

X-linked storage diseases

Fabry's disease must also be considered in women with evidence of a cardiomyopathy.[39] Fabry's disease is an x-linked disorder in which a glycosphingolipid accumulates in all tissues. The disease is caused by deficiency of alpha-galactosidase A. The major clinical manifestations include progressive cardiac and renal failure, with corneal dystrophy and angiokeratoma. Female carriers show a mild form of the disease with later onset and particularly with cardiac involvement. Thickening of the left and right ventricular walls is associated with mild or moderate depression of contractile function. Cerebrovascular disease and renal failure develop later.

Hunter's syndrome results from deficiency of a lysosomal enzyme iduronate sulfatase. The clinical features are similar to those in the autosomal recessive Hurler's syndrome (dwarfism, coarse facies, hepato-splenomegaly, and mental and skeletal deterioration) except that they are milder in Hunter's syndrome and allow survival into early or mid adulthood. Heart failure is progressive and caused by mucopolysaccharide infiltration of the myocardium, valves, and the walls of the coronary arteries. No abnormalities have been reported in female carriers.[38]

Until the genes are identified, female carriers of these severe storage diseases may wish to have male fetuses aborted.

References

1 Julian DG, Szekely P. Peripartum cardiomyopathy. *Prog Cardiovasc Dis* 1985; **27**: 223–40.
2 Homans DC. Peripartum cardiomyopathy. *N Engl J Med* 1985; **312**: 1432–7.

3 Woolford RM. Postpartum myocardosis. *Ohio State Med J* 1952; **48**: 924–30.

4 Meadows WR. Idiopathic myocardial failure in the last trimester of pregnancy and the puerperium. *Circulation* 1957; **15**: 903–24.

5 Cunningham FG, Pritchard JA, Hankin GDV, *et al.* Peripartum heart failure: idiopathic cardiomyopathy or compounding cardiovascular events? *Obstet Gynecol* 1986; **67**: 157–68.

6 Veille JC. Peripartum cardiomyopathies: a review. *Am J Obstet Gynecol* 1984; **148**: 805–18.

7 Leiserowitz GS, Evans AT, Samuels SJ, Omand K, Kost GJ. Creatinine kinase and its MB isoenzyme in the third trimester and the peripartum period. *J Reprod Med* 1992; **37**: 910–16.

8 Midei MG, DeMent SH, Feldman AM, Hutchins GM, Baughman KL. Peripartum myocarditis and cardiomyopathy. *Circulation* 1990; **81**: 922–8.

9 Sanderson JE, Olsen EGJ, Gatei D. Peripartum heart disease: an endomyocardial biopsy study. *Br Heart J* 1986; **56**: 285–91.

10 O'Connell JC, Costanzo-Nordin MR, Subramanian R, *et al.* Peripartum cardiomyopathy: clinical, haemodynamic, histologic and prognostic characteristics. *J Am Coll Cardiol* 1986; **8**: 52–6.

11 Demakis JG, Rahimtoola SH, Sutton GC, *et al.* Natural course of peripartum cardiomyopathy. *Circulation* 1971; **44**: 1053–61

12 Oakley CM, Nihoyannopoulos P. Peripartum cardiomyopathy with recovery in a patient with coincidental Eisenmenger ventricular septal defect. *Br Heart J* 1992; **67**: 190–2.

13 Purcell IF, Williams DO. Peripartum cardiomyopathy complicating severe aortic stenosis. *Int J Cardiol* 1995; **52**: 163–6.

14 Brockington IF. Postpartum hypertensive heart failure. *Am J Cardiol* 1971; **27**: 650–8.

15 Melvin KR, Richardson PJ, Olsen EGJ, Daly K, Jackson G. Peripartum cardiomyopathy due to myocarditis. *N Engl J Med* 1982; **307**: 731–4.

16 Davidson NM, Parry EHO. Peripartum cardiac failure. *Q J Med* 1978; **47**: 431–61.

17 Sanderson JE, Adesanya CO, Anjorin FI, Parry EHO. Postpartum cardiac failure – heart failure due to volume overload? *Am Heart J* 1979; **97**: 613–21.

18 Blickstein I, Zaleb Y, Katz Z, Lancet M. Ritodrine induced pulmonary oedema unmasking peripartum cardiomyopathy. *Am J Obstet Gynecol* 1988; **159**: 332–3.

19 Aravot JJ, Banner NR, Dhalla N. Heart transplantation for peripartum cardiomyopathy. *Lancet* 1987; **ii**: 1024.

20 Aretz HT, Billingham ME, Edwards WD, *et al.* Myocarditis: a histopathologic definition and classification. *Am J Cardiovasc Pathol* 1986; **1**: 3–14.

21 Mason JW, O'Connell JB, Herskowitz A, *et al.* A clinical trial of immunosuppressive therapy for myocarditis. *N Engl J Med* 1995; **333**: 269–75.

22 Cole P, Cook F, Plappert T, Saltzman, Sutton M St. J. Longitudinal changes in left ventricular architecture and function in peripartum cardiomyopathy. *Am J Cardiol* 1987; **60**: 871–6.

23 Komajda M, Iais JP, Reeves F, *et al.* Factors predicting mortality in idiopathic dilated cardiomyopathy. *Eur Heart J* 1990; **11**: 824–31.

24 Diaz RA, Obasohan A, Oakley CM. Prediction of outcome in dilated cardiomyopathy. *Br Heart J* 1987; **58**: 393–9.

25 Di Lenarda A, Secoli G, Perkan A, *et al.* Changing mortality in dilated cardiomyopathy. *Br Heart J* 1994; **72** (**suppl**): S46–51.

26 Mestroni L, Krajinovic M, Severini GM, *et al.* Familial dilated cardiomyopathy. *Br Heart J* 1994; **72** (**suppl**): S35–41.

27 Sardesai SH, Mourant AJ, Sivathandon Y, Farrow R, Gibbons DO. Phaeochromocytoma and catecholamine induced cardiomyopathy presenting as heart failure. *Br Heart J* 1990; **63**: 234–7.

28 Fitzpatrick AP, Shapiro LM, Rickards AF, Poole-Wilson PA. Familial restrictive cardiomyopathy with atrioventricular block and skeletal myopathy. *Br Heart J* 1990; **63**: 114–18.

29 Cooke RA, Chambers JB, Curry PVL. Noonan's cardiomyopathy: a non-hypertrophic variant. *Br Heart J* 1994; **71**: 561–5.

30 Wilmshurst PT, Katritsis D. Restrictive and hypertrophic cardiomyopathy in Noonan syndrome: the overlap syndromes. *Heart* 1996; **75**: 94–7.

31 Katritsis D, Wilmshurst PT, Wendon JA, Davies MJ, Webb-Peploe MM. Primary restrictive cardiomyopathy: clinical and pathologic characteristics. *J Am Coll Cardiol* 1991; **18**: 1230–5.

32 Buiq GF, Nava A, Martini B, Canciani B, Thiene G. Right ventricular dysplasia: a familial cardiomyopathy? *Eur Heart J* 1989; **10 (suppl D)**: 13–15.

33 Oldfors A, Eriksson BO, Kyllerman M, Martinsson T, Wahlstrom J. Dilated cardiomyopathy and the dystrophin gene: an illustrated review. *Br Heart J* 1994; **72**: 344–8.

34 Bies RD. X-linked dilated cardiomyopathy. *N Engl J Med* 1994; **330**: 368–9.

35 Towbin JA, Ortizlopez R. X linked dilated cardiomyopathy. *N Engl J Med* 1994; **330**: 369–70.

36 Schmidt-Achert M, Fischer P, Mullerteiber W, Mudra H, Pongratz D. Heterozygotic gene expression in endomyocardial biopsies – a new diagnostic tool confirms the Duchenne carrier status. *Clin Invest* 1994; **71**: 247–53.

37 Michels VV, Pastores GM, Moll PP, *et al.* Dystrophin analysis in idiopathic dilated cardiomyopathy. *J Med Genet* 1993; **30**: 955–7.

38 Ziter FA, Tyler FH. Neuromuscular disorders In: Pierpont ME, Moller JH, eds. *Genetics of cardiovascular disease.* Boston: Martinus Nijhoff, 1986: 241.

39 Broadbent JC, Edwards WD, Gordon H, *et al.* Fabry cardiomyopathy in the female confirmed by endomyocardial biopsy. *Mayo Clin Proc* 1981; **56**: 623–8.

17: Pericardial disease

CELIA OAKLEY

Pericardial disease has been known since the time of Galen. It forms a major part of the cardiology of the other medical and surgical specialties because the pericardium can become involved in all kinds of medical and surgical diseases. Pericardial syndromes are not rare but tend to be underdiagnosed. The physical signs of acute pericarditis, "adherent pericardium", pericardial tamponade, and constrictive pericarditis were worked out in the 19th century. Acute pericarditis has a wide differential diagnosis in pregnancy, particularly in older women who are now seen more frequently as pregnancy is increasingly postponed into the 30s and early 40s.

From its inception echocardiography provided a reliable means of recognising pericardial effusion and has since shown an even higher incidence of pericardial involvement in rheumatology, renal, and oncology patients than was ever previously realised. With Doppler ultrasound it has clarified the pathophysiology of tamponade and constriction.

Tuberculosis is rare in the indigenous population but relatively common in immigrants from Asia and there has been a major resurgence of tuberculosis and tuberculous pericarditis as a complication of HIV infection.

Pericarditis syndromes

As septic pericarditis became rarer, acute "idiopathic" pericarditis of presumed viral origin became the commonest type of acute pericarditis. It may progress rapidly to constriction of which it is now the commonest cause. Pericarditis of any cause from foreign bodies (it was first described in soldiers with retained shrapnel) to myocardial infarction, cardiac surgery and other trauma, as well as after acute idiopathic pericarditis may be followed by a relapsing syndrome of presumed immunological origin. The autoimmune diseases have a high incidence of pericarditis and any pericarditis may heal with shrinkage, scarring, and constriction (Table 17.1).[1]

TABLE 17.1—*Pericardial syndromes.*

- Acute pericarditis
- Relapsing pericarditis
- Subacute effusive constrictive pericarditis
- Tamponade
- Chronic lax pericardial effusion
- Constrictive pericarditis

Pregnancy and pericardial disease

The fibrous pericardium is indistensible and pericardial constraint is important in limiting cardiac dilatation in acute cardiac failure such as after massive pulmonary embolism. The increase in blood volume of up to 50% and associated greater cardiac volume and stroke output increases the pregnant woman's vulnerability to the haemodynamic consequences of pericardial disease but these involve systemic rather than pulmonary congestion, so they are uncomfortable rather than dangerous. However, the pregnant woman may suffer tamponade from a relatively small accumulation of pericardial fluid.

Acute pericarditis

Precordial pain, a pericardial friction rub and concordant ST-segment elevation on the electrocardiogram are the well known features of acute pericarditis. The causes are numerous (Table 17.2) but acute idiopathic pericarditis is the most common. This usually transient acute illness may occur in pregnancy[2] when the pericardial friction rub has to be distinguished from physiological systolic murmurs and continuous venous or mammary souffles.[3] It is important to exclude a tuberculous cause in any patient presenting with acute pericarditis. The fibrous pericardium has an important role in protecting the heart from spread of infection or malignancy from adjacent structures.[4] Pericarditis caused by pyogenic bacteria has become rare but should not be forgotten particularly in patients with rheumatoid arthritis or who are on steroid treatment.[5]

The chest pain is usually associated with fever. The pain may be similar to the pain of myocardial infarction and the ECG changes are also similar to those of early acute anterior myocardial infarction. The pain differs from that of myocardial ischaemia in having a pleuritic component and it often radiates to the tips of the shoulders because the pericardium is supplied by the phrenic nerves. The pain can be predominantly epigastric and simulate an acute abdomen. It is characteristically increased by coughing, swallowing or movement, particularly twisting of the thorax and is eased by sitting up and leaning forward. Other constitutional symptoms such as

TABLE 17.2—*Important causes of pericarditis.*

   I **Idiopathic** (previously called acute benign)

  II **Infective**
        Viral: Coxsackie group B
             Echovirus type 8
             Mumps
             Epstein Barr
             Varicella
             Rubella

        Bacterial: Pneumococcal
                Meningococcal
                Haemophilus
                Gonococcal
                Tuberculous

        Fungobacterial: Actinomyces
                    Nocardia asteroides

        Fungal: *Candida*
              Histoplasma

        Parasitic: *Entamoeba histolytica*
                Echinococcus
                Toxoplasma

 III **Immunological**
        Relapsing pericarditis

        Postinfarction (Dressler's syndrome)

        Postcardiotomy syndrome

        Associated with autoimmune disorders:
             Rheumatic fever
             SLE
             Rheumatoid arthritis
             Scleroderma
             Mixed connective tissue disease
             Polyarteritis and the Churg–Strauss variant
             Wegener's granulomatosis

 IV **Neoplastic**

  V **Post irradiation**

 VI **Traumatic**

VII **Uraemic**

sweating, anorexia, and fatigue are usual but may point to an underlying autoimmune disorder if prolonged (Chapter 13).

The pericardial friction rub results from grating of the roughened visceral and parietal pericardial surfaces with cardiac movement and is superficial and out of phase with the heart sounds. It is usually both systolic and diastolic but occasionally only systolic and it may be quite transient, disappearing as an effusion develops, then reappearing as it resolves. Tamponade is rare in idiopathic pericarditis but vigilance is especially necessary in a pregnant patient. Pulsus paradoxus is a late sign and indicates severe compression of the heart.

The electrocardiogram usually shows characteristic changes with ST-segment elevation. This is a current of injury coming from the superficial layers of the myocardium. Because acute pericarditis is usually diffuse, the changes are generalised and concordant. The QRS is normal unless accumulation of fluid results in lowered voltage. With healing the ST-segment becomes isoelectric, often with T wave inversion which is usually transient but sometimes permanent even in the absence of constriction. Rhythm disturbances are common, particularly paroxysmal flutter or fibrillation.

Echocardiography permits detection, quantification, and serial evaluation of the effusion, of left and right ventricular function, and of the development of constriction. Occasionally acute pericarditis develops in association with myocarditis and depression of left or right ventricular function, or both, may be a surprise finding. An echo-free space is seen both anterior and posterior to the heart whose width varies with the heart beat and, when the effusion is large, also cyclically as a result of the heart swinging within the fluid sac. This movement may cause electrical alternans. The space should be visible both anteriorly and posteriorly to avoid error caused by excessive epicardial fat, an enlarged thymus anteriorly, or a pleural effusion posteriorly.

Admission to hospital for rest and investigation is usually needed. Arrhythmias can be treated as in the non-pregnant state with digoxin, with or without DC cardioversion for atrial fibrillation or flutter.[6] Although these arrhythmias are usually transient and self reverting, they may cause haemodynamic embarrassment if the heart rate is fast and thus disturb the pregnancy, so DC reversion should be resorted to without delay if this occurs. Adenosine can be given to revert paroxysmal supraventricular tachycardia.

Analgesia may be provided by aspirin or other non-steroidal anti-inflammatory drugs if the patient is not close to term. The pain responds to steroids but these are usually not necessary. Occasionally when fever, malaise, and tachycardia persist the acute pericarditis may turn out to be the first sign of adult Still's disease, systemic lupus erythematosus (SLE), or mixed connective tissue disease and steroid treatment will be needed to achieve resolution.

Pericardiocentesis can be carried out by the sub-xiphoid route for diagnostic purposes if there is an effusion of at least moderate size. Echocardiographic guidance is helpful and is now considered an essential adjunct for safety, and the ECG should be recorded continuously. Attachment of a chest electrode to the needle allows a current of injury to be recognised if the needle touches the epicardium but availability of echocardiography makes this redundant.

Pericardiocentesis is not necessary in typical cases with rapid improvement but should always be done when there is a possibility of a

229

tuberculous or malignant cause or of course if there is haemodynamic compromise. If tuberculous pericarditis is suspected, all available fluid should be drained and centrifuged to concentrate the mycobacteria. Even so, failure to culture the organism is all too common and does not in any way refute the diagnosis.

Although involvement of the superficial myocardial layers is the cause of the ECG changes in acute pericarditis, evidence of an associated generalised myocarditis with myocardial depression is unusual. Collapse with cardiogenic shock has happened uncommonly after aspiration of a pericardial effusion for relief of tamponade when associated myocarditis was unsuspected. Some involvement of the myocardium in acute pericarditis is however quite usual as shown by release of the creatinine phosphokinase MB isoenzyme although the concentrations are not as high as after myocardial infarction.[7]

If the pericardial fluid shows bacteria on Gram stain or if it is opaque or frankly purulent, antibiotics should be given to cover staphylococcal and Gram negative organisms. If there is a strong suspicion of a tuberculous cause triple therapy should be started without waiting for confirmation of the diagnosis. Purulent pericarditis may develop silently in patients with rheumatoid arthritis or in diabetic patients. In any patient with a purulent pericarditis constriction may develop quickly and a strong case can be made for early pericardiectomy, which hastens resolution. Sometimes pericardiectomy can be avoided by continued antiseptic lavage of the pericardium combined with appropriate antibiotic treatment (Chapter 22).

Acute idiopathic pericarditis usually improves rapidly though a few patients relapse and a few constrict.[8,9] Constriction may develop within days or weeks of the acute illness. Pericardiectomy is technically easy and curative at low risk. It can be carried out safely in pregnancy.[10,11]

Relapsing pericarditis

Relapsing pericarditis can cause great distress and can continue for years. Steroids should be avoided because although acute flares are quickly suppressed they do not prevent relapses and there is a tendency to need a gradually climbing maintenance dose. It is better to use non-steroidal anti-inflammatory drugs.

Colchicine is effective both for the treatment of acute relapses and to prevent recurrence[9] but is said to be contraindicated in pregnancy which is a pity because unlike the non-steroidals, it does not cause fluid retention.

Few cases of acute pericarditis have been reported during pregnancy but most are probably not written up. The course is likely to be benign with rapid response to aspirin but occasionally steroids are required or surgical intervention for tamponade or constriction. Physicians should be alert to the occasional associated myocarditis which is then the more important aspect of the illness and may lead to heart failure, spontaneous abortion, or the need for termination if the pregnancy is at an early stage.

Cardiac tamponade

If a patient with an illness carrying the risk of pericardial tamponade is in hospital, the effusion is usually sought and recognised by echocardiogram which gives early warning of tamponade. If not suspected and chest pain is absent, it is commonly missed and can be fatal. Clinically tamponade is recognised by tachycardia, pulsus paradoxus, and faint heart sounds. The venous pressure is raised and there is a brisk systolic x descent but blunting or loss of the diastolic y descent, giving a diagnostic flow velocity pattern in the superior vena cava. This is because the right atrium can fill during ventricular ejection but right ventricular filling after the tricuspid valve opens quickly ceases as the intrapericardial pressure rises and the walls of the right atrium and ventricle buckle inwards.[12-15]

Tamponade may complicate pericarditis of any cause but is relatively uncommon in idiopathic or post-infarction pericarditis. It is usual in pyogenic, tuberculous, and malignant pericarditis. Acute haemopericardium may cause tamponade following trauma or rupture of an aortic root dissection into the pericardium. It is a common early complication of cardiac surgery. Rare pericardial tumours such as primary mesothelioma may present with tamponade, as may lymphoma or metastatic carcinoma. Chronic tamponade may occur in tuberculosis, uraemia, and after irradiation (subacute effusive constrictive pericarditis) (Table 17.3).[16]

TABLE 17.3—*Important causes of cardiac tamponade.*

I **Purulent**
    Acute: Bacterial

        Tuberculous

II **Haemorrhagic**
    Dissection of the aorta

    Post-infarction: Rupture
                  Anticoagulant-induced haemopericardium

    Traumatic: Stab wounds
            Iatrogenic—cardiac catheter
                       central venous line
            Post-cardiac surgery

    Uraemic

    Neoplastic: Primary mesothelioma
              Lymphoma
              Secondary carcinoma
III **Serous**
    Idiopathic acute pericarditis (rare)

    Tuberculous

    SLE or drug-induced lupus syndrome (rare)

    Rheumatoid and other connective tissue disorders (rare)

Patients usually complain of shortness of breath and heaviness in the chest. Pulsus paradoxus is an exaggeration of the normal respiratory variation in arterial pressure. Inspiratory increase in blood flow into the right ventricle is accommodated at the expense of left ventricular volume because the total diastolic volume of the heart cannot increase. The ventricular septum moves sharply towards the left ventricle on inspiration and this is readily seen on echocardiography. The electrocardiogram may show electrical "alternans" caused by the heart swinging about. The alteration in voltage may therefore be variable. In typical cases the diagnosis is obvious and urgent pericardiocentesis is needed. Diastolic collapse of the free walls of the right atrium and right ventricle provide early warning of impending haemodynamic compromise and is caused by a rise in intrapericardial pressure during diastolic filling.[17]

Chronic pericardial effusions are sometimes seen without compressive features or any indication of a cause.[18] Hypothyroidism should be excluded (Table 17.4).

TABLE 17.4—*Chronic pericardial effusion.*

- Idiopathic
- Post pericarditic
- Post infarction
- Post irradiation
- Myxoedema
- Chylous effusion

Subacute effusive constrictive pericarditis

Cardiac compression results from thickening of the visceral pericardium or indistensibility of the fibrous pericardium associated with effusion.[16] The compression may not improve after pericardiocentesis if the visceral pericardium is involved. This condition occurs in tuberculous pericarditis and also in rheumatoid patients. It may also be seen after mediastinal irradiation and as a result of neoplastic pericardial involvement.

Constrictive pericarditis

Constriction develops when thickening and scarring of the parietal or visceral pericardium results in restriction of cardiac filling as a result of compression of the heart. Usually the entire pericardium is involved but occasionally constriction is localised to a calcified constricting band at one or other atrioventricular groove or around the superior or inferior vena cava. Most cases of constrictive pericarditis are not calcified and probably follow idiopathic pericarditis but other causes include previous mediastinal irradiation,[11] rheumatoid arthritis and other collagen vascular diseases, chronic uraemia, and cardiac surgery (Table 17.5).[19] Patients with severe constriction are chronically ill and unlikely to be pregnant. Pregnancy may cause occult constriction to become manifest for the first time because the increase in blood volume in pregnancy with fixed cardiac volume leads to a rise in venous pressure.[20] Early in pregnancy such a patient may develop dependent oedema with a high venous pressure, hepatomegaly, and a persistent tachycardia often with pulsus paradoxus. The venous pressure tracing is M-shaped as a result of exaggerated x and y descents. The cardiac impulse is usually impalpable but there is an early third heart sound (often erroneously called a pericardial knock). Ascites may develop.

TABLE 17.5—*Causes of constrictive pericarditis*

- Postacute or idiopathic pericarditis
- Tuberculous
- Post pyogenic
- Rheumatoid (or rarely other connective tissue disorders)
- Post irradiation
- Post cardiac surgery
- Neoplastic
- Uraemic (rare)

Pulmonary oedema is not a risk and compensation is provided by tachycardia, but the congestive features may be distressing. Surgical pericardiectomy carried out without cardiopulmonary bypass is safe and effective except in a few cases of tuberculous constriction in which adequate dissection cannot safely be obtained without bypass.

The diagnosis of pericardial constriction is often missed because it is relatively rare.[21] Cardiomyopathy is more common and is usually the preferred diagnosis. In other cases the cardiac abnormality is missed and the symptoms and oedema are attributed to the pregnancy, anaemia, or lack of rest.

The ECG usually shows sinus tachycardia with non-specific inferior axis, low voltage, and repolarisation changes. The heart is not enlarged on the chest radiograph but there may be pleural effusions.

Pericardial constriction used to be thought of as an echocardiographic weak spot but the features of constriction are in fact highly characteristic. Left and right ventricular systolic functions are normal. The small pericardial echo free space that is usually seen is absent and there may be a high signal from the pericardium or actual evidence of thickening. On inspiration the ventricular septum may move towards the left ventricle, compromising its size. On short axis views the ventricular septum is straight in diastole, resuming its normal convexity towards the right ventricle in systole. Apical four chamber views show a "shivering septum" typical of this condition, and continuous wave Doppler images show an increase in tricuspid inflow velocity on inspiration, with a reciprocal decrease in left ventricular inflow velocity. This is caused by the fixed total volume of the

233

heart in diastole and the interdependence of the two ventricular chambers.

Cardiac catheterisation is unnecessary for the diagnosis of typical cases of constrictive pericarditis and should be avoided in pregnancy. A Swan-Ganz floatation catheter can be used in cases of clinical doubt to show that the wedged pulmonary artery and right atrial pressures are similar, and to show the absence of significant pulmonary hypertension. This is not as accurate as right and left heart catheterisation with simultaneous measurement of right atrial and left ventricular diastolic pressures, which should be similar at all times. The cardiac output is reduced with a low mixed venous saturation which reflects the severity of the constriction.

Constrictive pericarditis has to be differentiated from restrictive cardiomyopathies either primary or from endomyocardial fibrosis or amyloid heart disease.[21] Immunological (AL) amyloid is usually a disorder of older people but amyloid heart disease may rarely be encountered in younger patients with AA amyloid in Crohn's disease or familial Mediterranean fever or genetic amyloid. Endomyocardial fibrosis is rare. It is seen in the tropics years after parasitic infection in childhood or associated with the hypereosinophilic syndrome in western countries. The thickened ventricular walls, valves, and atrial septum seen in amyloid heart disease and the apical obliteration and atrioventricular valve involvement of endomyocardial fibrosis are readily recognised on echocardiography. Primary restrictive cardiomyopathy may be more difficult to distinguish from constrictive pericarditis, but it tends to involve the left heart more than the right with higher diastolic filling pressures on the left than on the right. Doppler inflow velocities show no respiratory reciprocity between the left and right ventricles.[22]

Tuberculous pericarditis

Tuberculous pericarditis has re-emerged as a problem in association with the AIDS epidemic but is also seen in young Asians. The pericardium is usually infected by direct spread from paratracheal lymph nodes or in the young by haematogenous spread from primary infection.[23,24]

Acid fast bacilli are numerous within the pericardial fluid only during the acute phase and later on are hard to find. The effusion may be bloodstained but is usually serous and contains polymorphonuclear leucocytes early on but lymphocytes later. Tamponade may occur and constriction is common. The illness may be acute and severe with constitutional symptoms, fever, malaise, weight loss, and sweating. Pulmonary tuberculosis is not usually associated.

Tuberculous pericarditis should be suspected particularly in a patient with pyrexia of unknown origin and unexplained ECG abnormality or cardiomegaly, but the clinical presentation is highly variable and a tuberculous origin should always be sought even in patients with a relapsing syndrome or in the absence of fever.

The tuberculin skin test is sometimes negative during the acute illness but becomes positive later on. If fluid is obtained a raised adenosine deaminase concentration has high specificity for the diagnosis. Anti-tuberculous drugs should be prescribed when there is doubt and in patients who are more ill than expected in acute idiopathic pericarditis while the results of cultures are awaited.

The use of prednisolone in addition to anti-tuberculous drugs has been controversial for the prevention of constriction which is recognised by the combination of a rise in venous pressure with a reduction in heart size.[25]

Constrictive pericarditis should be managed medically in pregnancy provided the symptoms and the haemodynamic compromise are not severe. If necessary pericardiectomy can be undertaken with low risk to mother and fetus, in anticipation of an excellent result and no problem in subsequent pregnancies.[10,11]

References

1 Permanyer-Miralda G, Sagrista-Sauleda J, Soler-Soler J. Primary acute pericardial disease: a prospective series of 231 consecutive patients. *Am J Cardiol* 1985; **56**: 623–30.
2 Krausz Y, Naparstek E, Eliakim ML. Idiopathic pericarditis and pregnancy. *Aust NZ J Obstet Gynaecol* 1978; **18**: 86–9.
3 Cutforth R, MacDonald CB. Heart sounds and murmurs in pregnancy. *Am Heart J* 1966; **71**: 741–7.
4 Crobok H, Ogorzal L, Zajiczek J. Suppurative pericarditis during pregnancy as a complication of pleural emphysema. *Przegl Lek* 1996; **22**: 417–19.
5 Probst R, Mier T. Acute pericarditis complicating pregnancy. *Obstet Gynecol* 1963; **22**: 393–5.
6 Schroeder JS, Harrison DC. Repeated cardioversion during pregnancy. *Am J Cardiol* 1971; **27**: 445–6.
7 Tiefe N, Brunn AJ, Roberts R. Elevation of plasma MB creatinine kinase and the development of new Q-waves in association with pericarditis. *Chest* 1980; **77**: 438–40.
8 Fowler NO, Harbin AD. Recurrent acute pericarditis: follow-up study of 31 patients. *J Am Coll Cardiol* 1986; **7**: 300–5.
9 Guindo J, Rodrigues de la Serna A, Rarnio J. Recurrent pericarditis. Relief with colchicine. *Circulation* 1990; **82**: 1117–20.
10 Richardson PM, LeRoux BT, Rogers MA, Gotsman MS. Pericardiectomy in pregnancy. *Thorax* 1970; **25**: 627–30.
11 Watson P, Havelda C, Sorosky J, Kochenour NK, Sohi GS, Gray L. Irradiation-induced constrictive pericarditis requiring pericardiectomy during pregnancy. *J Reprod Med* 1980; **24**: 127–30.
12 Fowler NO, Gabel M. The haemodynamic effects of cardiac tamponade: mainly the result of atrial, not ventricular, compression. *Circulation* 1985; **71**: 154–7.
13 Fast J, Wielenga RP, Jansen E, Schuurmans Stekhoven JH. Abnormal wall movements of the right ventricle and both atria in patients with pericardial effusion as indicators of cardiac tamponade. *Eur Heart J* 1986; **7**: 431–6.
14 Appleton CP, Hatle LK, Popp RL. Superior vena cava flow velocity patterns can diagnose cardiac tamponade in patients with pericardial effusions. *J Am Coll Cardiol* 1987; **9**: 118A.
15 Reddy PS, Curtiss EI, Uretsky BF. Spectrum of haemodynamic changes in cardiac tamponade. *Am J Cardiol* 1990; **66**: 1487–91.
16 Hancock EW. Subacute effusive constrictive pericarditis. *Circulation* 1971; **43**: 183–92.
17 Klopfenstein HS, Schuchard GH, Wann LS, *et al.* The relative merits of pulsus paradoxus and right ventricular diastolic collapse in the early detection of cardiac tamponade: an experimental echocardiographic study. *Circulation* 1985; **71**: 829–33.
18 Haiat R, Halphan C, Clement F, Michelson B. Silent pericardial effusion in late pregnancy. *Chest* 1981; **79**: 717 (letter).

19 Cameron J, Oesterle SN, Baldwin JC, Hancock EW. The etiologic spectrum of constrictive pericarditis. *Am Heart J* 1987; **113**: 354–60.
20 Buch CA, Stang TM, Wooley CG, Kilman J. Occult constrictive pericardial disease. Diagnosis by rapid volume expansion and correction by pericardiectomy. *Circulation* 1977; **56**: 924–30.
21 Oakley CM. Pericardial disease. In: Julian DG, Camm AJ, Fox, Hall RJC, Poole-Wilson PAL, eds. *Diseases of the heart.* London: Bailliere Tindall, 1989: 974–1000.
22 Vaitkus PT, Kussmaul WG. Constrictive pericarditis versus restrictive cardiomyopathy: a reappraisal and update of diagnostic criteria. *Am Heart J* 1991; **122**: 1431–41.
23 Sagrista-Sauleda J, Permanyet-Miralda G, Soler-Soler J. Tuberculosis pericarditis: 10 year experience with a prospective protocol for diagnosis and treatment. *J Am Coll Cardiol* 1988; **11**: 724–8.
24 Fowler NO. Tuberculous pericarditis. *JAMA* 1991; **266**: 99–103.
25 Strang JIG, Kakaza HHS, Gibson DG, *et al.* Controlled clinical trial of complete open surgical drainage and of prednisolone in treatment of tuberculous pericardial effusion in Transkei. *Lancet* 1988; **ii**: 759–64.

18: Coronary artery disease

CELIA OAKLEY

Atheromatous coronary artery disease is still uncommon in women of childbearing age but is becoming more common. This has been attributed to changes in women's lifestyle, the use of oral contraceptives, smoking, sometimes abuse of other drugs, going out to work, and postponing pregnancy. Oral contraceptives containing hyperphysiological doses of synthetic hormones may cause adverse changes in lipids and predispose to thrombosis.[1] This is in contrast to the beneficial changes in the lipids of postmenopausal women on hormone replacement therapy using physiological doses of largely natural hormones.

Although the rest of the population is smoking less, young women, particularly young professional women, are smoking more. Premenopausal smokers have three times the risk of heart attack of non-smokers and women who smoke more than 40 cigarettes a day increase their risk 20 fold. Diabetic women who smoke have a particularly high risk.[2] Most young women nowadays work outside the home and many do sedentary jobs in contrast to the more active lives of housewives even in this age of washing machines and fast food.

Women, thinking that they are immune from heart disease, tend to eat imprudently. Clustering of risk factors including abdominal obesity, insulin resistance or overt non-insulin dependent diabetes, and hypertension (Reaven's syndrome X) predispose to early onset of coronary disease in some relatively young women.[3,4] Women with familial hypercholesterolaemia also develop early coronary atheroma with angina or myocardial infarction but women with angina-like chest pain and angiographically normal coronary arteries, (Kemp's syndrome X), are usually middle-aged and are rarely seen during the childbearing years.[5] Rare causes of coronary disease or of myocardial ischaemia which may be seen during pregnancy include congenital coronary anomalies and inflammatory disease.

Myocardial infarction

Myocardial infarction is rare during pregnancy or the puerperium. Its true incidence is unknown but has been estimated to be less than 1 in

237

10 000 pregnancies.[6] Only about 100 cases have been reported but most are probably not published.

Myocardial infarction usually develops out of the blue in pregnancy without preceding angina or other evidence of ischaemic heart disease. This is because atheromatous coronary disease is usually not the underlying cause. The most common mechanism is dissection but numerous other pathogenic factors may contribute.[7] These may be peculiar to or aggravated by pregnancy or coincidental (Tables 18.1 and 18.2). Dissection of the aorta is well recognised during pregnancy. Spontaneous dissection may also develop in a coronary artery and cause myocardial infarction (Figure 18.1), severe chest pain, unstable angina or sudden death.[8-11] The site is usually the left anterior descending artery but multiple dissections affecting all three main coronary artery branches have been described.[11-13]

TABLE 18.1—*Causes of myocardial infarction during pregnancy predisposed to by pregnancy or peculiar to it.*

- Spontaneous coronary artery dissection

- Oxytocic drugs
  Ergot derivatives
  Bromocriptine

- Embolism from the placenta
  Hydatidiform mole
  Metastases from chorion carcinoma

- Hypercoagulable states
  Coronary embolism
  —from prosthetic aortic or mitral valves
  —in mitral stenosis
  —paradoxical   in atrial septal defect, or patent foramen ovale
                 or in cyanotic congenital heart disease

- Maternal pre-eclampsia

- Coronary artery spasm

Two thirds of myocardial infarcts reported occurred during the third trimester and most developed peripartum or postpartum.[6] Nearly all involved the anterior wall of the left ventricle. Myocardial infarction has been reported in association with multiple pregnancy and has been followed by the development of pre-eclampsia.[14,15] The anterior descending artery seems to be most at risk both from coronary dissection and possibly also from coronary embolism, the two most frequently reported causes of infarction associated with pregnancy.

Reviews of necropsy diagnosed coronary artery dissections have shown a predominance of women who were commonly postpartum. Among 134 reported cases of spontaneous coronary artery dissections over two thirds had occurred in women, half of whom were either pregnant or puerperal between one day and four months following delivery.[7,11] Haemodynamic stress, changes in collagen, and hyper-coagulability are probably all maximal late in pregnancy. Hormonal influences on vessel wall collagen synthesis

TABLE 18.2—*Coincidental causes of myocardial infarction during pregnancy.*

- Coronary atheroma

- Coronary arteritis:
    Systemic lupus erythematosus
    Antiphospholipid syndrome
    Polyarteritis nodosa
    Still's disease
    Takayasu arteritis
    Old Kawasaki disease

- Coronary embolism:
    In infective endocarditis
    Left atrial myxoma

- Cocaine misuse

- Phaeochromocytoma-induced

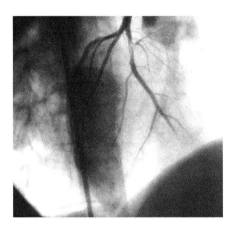

FIGURE 18.1—*A left coronary angiogram (right anterior oblique view) of a 37 year old woman with a spontaneous dissection in the proximal anterior descending coronary artery which caused acute anterior myocardial infarction (reproduced with permission from the British Journal of Cardiology).*[24]

may lead to weakening of the integument and predispose to dissection at times of haemodynamic stresses related especially to pregnancy, labour, and delivery particularly in women with the Marfan syndrome or other hereditary connective tissue defect. Reduced collagen synthesis was shown in vitro in cultured skin fibroblasts of one patient.[16] Eosinophilic infiltration in the adventitia was described in eight fatal cases[17] but was not found in two cases treated by heart transplantation.[18,19] Cystic medial necrosis at the dissection site has been suggested[20] but not consistently found.[21] The dissection typically arises within 2 cm of the coronary ostium.[22] As the diagnosis has hitherto usually been made at autopsy the preponderance of anterior descending artery dissections may reflect the higher mortality of anterior infarction rather than a true difference in vulnerability between the coronary arteries.

Spontaneous coronary artery dissections are now being recognised at angiography sometimes at the site of coronary spasm, sometimes in patients with coronary atheroma but with a prediction for young healthy women and most commonly in the puerperium.[8,11,22–24] Hypertension did not seem to be a risk factor in an Italian series in which 74 out of 97 cases were women and 24 were in the puerperium.[25]

The association with coronary artery spasm probably explains infarction precipitated by ergot derivatives used for prevention of postpartum haemorrhage or for termination of pregnancy. These may cause acute chest pain sometimes followed by myocardial infarction[26,27] as happened in one of our patients, previously apparently perfectly healthy, who developed a fatal infarct after routine ergotamine. Bromocriptine is another ergot derivative which has been reported to cause spasm and infarction when used to suppress lactation.[28,29] These are vasoconstrictor agents. They can cause constriction of coronary arteries resulting in endothelial breaches leading to haemorrhagic dissection of the media but also attracting platelets and subsequent thrombus formation.

Although patients with myocardial infarction complicating pregnancy are now fully investigated by coronary angiography, most reported cases have not been so studied and suggestions about causation have been speculative when the infarct was associated with maternal pre-eclamptic toxaemia and hypertension. Coronary artery spasm with thrombosis had previously been suggested, vasospasm being triggered by renin release from the chorion, but dissection now seems to be the more likely mechanism.

Myocardial infarction has also been reported from coronary embolism during curettage for hydatidiform mole[30] and from metastases from chorion carcinoma.[31]

Myocardial infarction is a well recognised complication of collagen vascular disease in polyarteritis nodosa, systemic lupus, and the antiphospholipid syndrome, as well as in old Kawasaki disease.[32–34] Angiographically proved coronary thrombosis has also been described in a patient with adult Still's disease who had a myocardial infarction 12 weeks following delivery.[35]

Misuse of cocaine should be considered in any young person with a sudden coronary event and is increasingly prevalent particularly in some inner cities. Myocardial infarction in a pregnant woman who had used "crack" cocaine has been reported.[36]

Coronary embolism from prosthetic valves, from infective endocarditis, or from mitral stenosis, may cause myocardial infarction during pregnancy.[37,38] The hypercoagulable state associated with pregnancy may be responsible for left atrial thrombosis in patients with mitral stenosis even with persistent sinus rhythm and possibly predisposes to embolism from prosthetic valves or in infective endocarditis. Myocardial infarction was the presenting event in a 19 year old immigrant Asian with previously undiagnosed mitral stenosis when she was only 8 weeks pregnant. The coronary arteries were normal angiographically and the left atrium was free from thrombus. The mitral stenosis was successfully relieved and she continued the pregnancy without further events while on treatment with warfarin. Seven years later she is still in sinus rhythm and has had two further uneventful pregnancies.

Premature atherosclerotic coronary disease has probably been under-reported in journals because it is less exotic. It accounted for only nine out of 70 cases reviewed by Hankins et al[6] but is seen in women with familial hypercholesterolaemia and in association with multiple risk factors. Women with familial hypercholesterolaemia develop symptoms on average 10 years later than men with similar cholesterol concentrations. Pregnancy may be complicated by angina or infarction but may be undertaken successfully after coronary bypass surgery, as in a patient who had coronary surgery at the age of 32 after multiple lipid lowering drugs and partial ileal bypass before the "statin" era. She then had a successful pregnancy and now has four sons, three of whom are affected. She took only cholestyramine during the last pregnancy but is now well controlled on 40 mg simvastatin daily. Phaeochromocytoma has also been reported in association with myocardial infarction in pregnancy and if found should be removed during the pregnancy after appropriate treatment with phenoxybenzamine followed by labetalol.[39]

Reports of coronary angiograms following myocardial infarction in pregnancy have usually described normal appearances but this is probably because only a minority of such angiograms were done sufficiently early after the event. Healed coronary dissections may not always have been recognised but the dissection sites were still visible in a patient with three dissections who had repeat angiography after six months.[11] Occlusive thrombi may lyse. Normal coronary arteries following myocardial infarction were found at angiography in 74 patients of whom 32 were women and 11 either peripartum or taking oral contraceptives.[40] The reported mortality of myocardial infarction associated with pregnancy has been extremely high, 25% to 50%,[6] but these were not recent patients treated in a modern way. Mortality has been highest when the infarct occurred late, particularly if it occurred during delivery or in the early postpartum period.

Management of myocardial infarction in pregnancy

The diagnosis should be confirmed from ECG changes and cardiac enzyme release. Both total creatinine kinase and creatinine kinase MB isoenzyme concentrations rise postpartum because they are released from the myometrium[41] so other cardiac enzymes should be measured if the infarct occurred peripartum or postpartum as the majority do.

The cause of the infarct should, whenever possible, be clarified by immediate coronary angiography. Thrombolytic agents are only relatively contraindicated during pregnancy and should be used without hesitation for life threatening conditions such as large anterior infarcts. We have used streptokinase without interruption of the pregnancy. Delivery of a lytic agent locally into an occluded thrombosed coronary artery allows the dose to be minimised and efficiency maximised. Primary angioplasty would be the choice in the case of pre-existing disease but is probably not necessary as most coronary thromboses occur in previously normal arteries. Coronary dissection is not helped by thrombolytic therapy, but intracoronary streptokinase may be useful when thrombus in the false lumen compresses the true lumen and causes obstruction. Thrombolytic treatment had been given to three patients before coronary angiography revealed dissection. All survived with normal ejection fractions.[23] It may be possible to seal off a dissection by stenting but they may heal naturally with preservation of the lumen.[8,12] For major dissections threatening the entire territory of the anterior descending artery, urgent coronary bypass is indicated despite the risk to the fetus which should be delivered first if it is viable. Individual decisions have to be made dependent on the patient's clinical condition and the appearance of the coronary artery at angiography. Both percutaneous angioplasty and coronary bypass grafting have been performed safely during pregnancy.[42–44]

Beta-blockers should be started as soon as possible after the infarct to reduce the risk of arrhythmias, limit infarct size, and reduce the risk of rupture. ACE inhibitors should also be given. They are relatively contraindicated during pregnancy but should be considered if there has been major infarction. Two patients with postpartum myocardial infarction needed transplantation.[18,19] Management of arrhythmias is largely the same as in non-pregnant patients and DC cardioversion can be carried out safely without risk to the fetus. In patients with good cardiac function invasive central monitoring is unnecessary and the mode of delivery should be based on obstetric indications.[9,14]

If ventricular fibrillation occurs resuscitation should be carried out with the uterus displaced laterally to avoid aorto-caval compression. If resuscitation fails and the infant is viable emergency caesarean section needs to be carried out within 15 minutes.

Every effort should be made to maintain the pregnancy until the infarct has healed and to deliver at term. Beta-blockers should be continued to reduce myocardial oxygen demand and caesarean section is preferred to expedite delivery and reduce maternal physical stress especially if the left ventricle is compromised. The anaesthetist should avoid anaesthetic agents that cause myocardial depression. General anaesthesia can maintain haemodynamic stability and minimise haemodynamic stress. Prophylactic heparin should be given after delivery. Epidural anaesthesia is an acceptable alternative to general anaesthesia in these patients.

Following delivery venous return to the heart increases because of blood returned to the circulation by the contracting uterus. Vasoconstricting oxytocic agents also contribute to an increase in venous return and venous filling pressure and are contraindicated because of the possibility of inducing coronary artery constriction.

Angina

Angina caused by myocardial ischaemia is extremely uncommon in pregnancy but may be caused by premature coronary atherosclerosis particularly in older women with major risk factors. It is obviously desirable for the diagnosis to be made before pregnancy and the patient should have full investigation including coronary angiography so that she can receive the best possible advice and treatment. Angina caused by coronary artery obstructive disease gets worse in pregnancy and the patient runs the risk of coronary thrombosis and infarction. Full anti-anginal treatment with beta-blockade or a calcium antagonist or both, nitrates, aspirin, and rest are needed.

Exercise testing is notoriously unreliable in women and Bayes Theorem may be applied. Thus: "in patients from a population with a low prevalence of disease and with atypical symptoms (of angina) a negative exercise test is unlikely to be a false negative". Positive tests are less useful. False positives are common and exercise tests in young women with chest pain and no risk factors tend to confound rather than clarify.

Congenital coronary anomalies

Congenital coronary anomalies are occasionally encountered in pregnancy (Figure 18.2).[45] A continuous murmur caused by a coronary cameral fistula may be detected during antenatal examination. Anomalous origin of a coronary artery (usually the left) from the pulmonary artery with poor left ventricular function due to previous (neonatal) infarction or acquired ischaemia (caused by fistulous flow from right to left coronary artery) has been reported with successful pregnancy after surgical correction. The patient illustrated (Figure 18.3) had undergone two uneventful pregnancies before she was referred with angina, mitral regurgitation and failure. She did well after ligation of the left coronary at its ostium and left internal mammary artery bypass into the anterior descending artery, together with mitral valve replacement.

Coronary arteritis either old in Kawasaki disease (with aneurysm formation and thrombosis which may be new) or ongoing in systemic lupus erythematosus are occasionally seen during pregnancy or in patients requiring advice about conception. All depends upon left ventricular function, severity of ischaemia, and activity of disease.

The occurrence of myocardial infarction during pregnancy is deeply traumatic and likely to be followed by considerable depression and insecurity even if the woman makes a good recovery. Little is known about pregnancies undertaken after previous myocardial infarction. Both patients and their doctors may be fearful of risking a further pregnancy. Patients with impaired left ventricular function may develop heart failure and increased angina occurred in five of 24 reported cases but there were no fatalities.[46]

Summary

Coronary artery disease is a rare complication of pregnancy but is becoming more common as a result of the increased use of oral

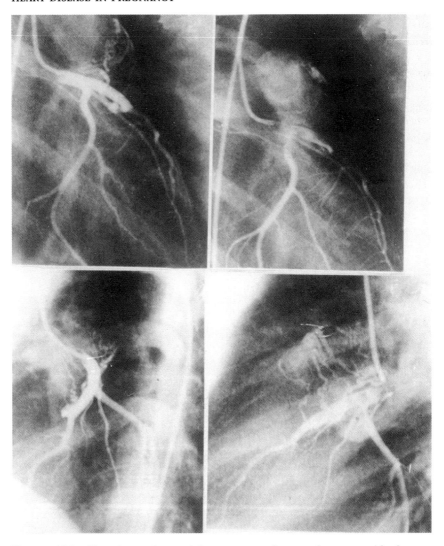

FIGURE 18.2—*Four frames from a left coronary angiogram of a young girl who was found to have a murmur at a routine examination. This was continuous and placed maximally at the third left interspace too low for a patent ductus. Echocardiography showed flow into the main pulmonary artery just distal to the valve. Coronary angiography showed a coronary artery fistula with abnormal branches from the anterior descending coronary artery draining into the main pulmonary artery which is opacified from the left coronary injection. This rare abnormality carries no adverse prognostic significance.*

contraceptives, the increase in smoking among women, and the trend towards postponement of pregnancy. Precise diagnosis with early coronary angiography contributes to individual and optimal management. Myocardial infarction is usually caused by primary dissection rather than pre-existing disease and usually occurs postpartum or peripartum. Fully

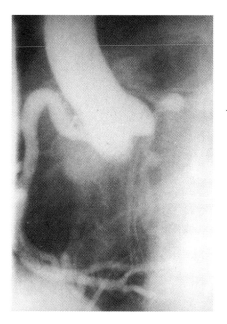

FIGURE 18.3—*Aortogram showing the dilated right coronary artery in a patient with anomalous origin of the left coronary artery from the pulmonary artery (described in the text). The left coronary artery is faintly opacified by fistulous flow from the right coronary artery but has no connection with the aorta.*

recovered patients after a small infarct can anticipate normal delivery at low risk but women with large infarcts should be delivered by caesarean section. Large infarcts, particularly those occurring peripartum, carry highest risk.

References

1 Mann JI, Vessey MP, Thorogood M, *et al*. Myocardial infarction in young women with special reference to oral contraceptive practice. *BMJ* 1975; **ii**: 241–5.
2 Jackson G. Coronary artery disease and women. *BMJ* 1994; **309**: 555–6.
3 Reaven GM. Role of insulin resistance in human disease. *Diabetes* 1988; **37**: 1595–1607.
4 Hauner H, Bognar E, Blum A. Body fat distribution and its association with metabolic and hormonal risk factors in women with angiographically assessed coronary artery disease: evidence for the presence of a metabolic syndrome. *Atherosclerosis* 1994; **105**: 209–16.
5 Kemp HG, Kronmal RA, Vlietstra RE. Seven year survival of patients with normal or near normal coronary angiograms. A CASS Registry Study. *J Am Coll Cardiol* 1986; **7**: 479–83.
6 Hankins GDV, Wendel GD, Leveno KL, Stoneham J. Myocardial infarction during pregnancy: a review. *Obstet Gynecol* 1985; **65**: 139–46.
7 Kearney P, Singh H, Hutter J, Khan S, Lee G, Lucey J. Spontaneous coronary artery dissection: a report of three cases and review of the literature. *Postgrad Med J* 1993; **69**: 940–5.
8 DeMaio SJ, Kinsella SH, Silverman ME. Clinical course and long-term prognosis of spontaneous coronary artery dissection. *Am J Cardiol* 1989; **64**: 471–4.
9 Hands ME, Johnson MD, Saltzman DH, Rutherford JD. The cardiac, obstetric and anaesthetic management of pregnancy complicated by acute myocardial infarction. *J Clin Anesth* 1990; **2**: 258–68.
10 Samra D, Samra Y, Hertz M, Maier M. Acute myocardial infarction in pregnancy and puerperium. *Cardiology* 1986; **76**: 455–60.

11 Bac DJ, Lotgering FK, Verkaaik APK, Deckers JE. Spontaneous coronary artery dissection during pregnancy and postpartum. *Eur Heart J* 1995; **16**: 136–8.

12 Antoniucci D, Magidiligenti I. Spontaneous dissection of the three major coronary arteries. *Eur Heart J* 1990; **11**: 1130–4.

13 Black MD, Catzavelos C, Boyd D, Walley VM. Simultaneous spontaneous dissections in three coronary arteries. *Can J Cardiol* 1991; 7: 34–6.

14 Sheikh AU, Harper MA. Myocardial infarction during pregnancy: management and outcome of two pregnancies. *Am J Obstet Gynecol* 1993; **163**: 279–83.

15 Badui, E, Rangel A, Enciso R, *et al*. Acute myocardial infarction during pregnancy and puerperium in athletic women. Two case reports. *Angiology* 1994; **45**: 897–902.

16 Bonnet J, Aumailley M, Thomnas D, Grosgogeat Y, Broustet JP, Bricaud H. Spontaneous coronary artery dissection: case report and evidence for a defect in collagen metabolism. *Eur Heart J* 1986; 7: 904–9.

17 Robinowitz M, Virmani R, McAllister H. Spontaneous coronary dissection and eosinophilic inflammation: a cause and effect relationship? *Am J Med* 1982; **72**: 923–8.

18 Curiel P, Spinelli G, Petrella A, *et al*. Postpartum coronary artery dissection followed by heart transplantation. *Am J Obstet Gynecol* 1990; **163**: 538–9.

19 Movsesian MA, Wray RB. Postpartum myocardial infarction. *Br Heart J* 1989; **62**: 154–6.

20 Dowling GP, Buja LM. Spontaneous coronary artery dissection occurs with and without peri-adventitial inflammation. *Arch Pathol Lab Med* 1987; **111**: 470–2.

21 Chanler Smith J. Dissecting aneurysms of coronary arteries. *Archives of Pathology* 1975; **99**: 1127–31.

22 Thayer JO, Healy RW, Maggs PR. Spontaneous coronary artery dissection. *Ann Thorac Surg* 1987; **44**: 97–102.

23 Zampieri P, Aggio S, Roncon L, *et al*. Follow up after spontaneous coronary artery dissection: a report of five cases. *Heart* 1996; **75**: 206–9.

24 Goodfellow J, Hutter JA, Walker PR. Spontaneous dissection of the left anterior descending artery in a young woman. Case report. *Br J Cardiol* 1995; 2: 260–1.

25 Coco P, Thiene G, Corrado D, Lodovichetti G, Pennelli N. Ematoma (aneurisma) dissecante spontaneo delle coronarie e morte imporovvisa. *G Ital Cardiol* 1990; **20**: 795–800.

26 Fujiwara Y, Yamanaka O, Nakamura T, Yokoi H, Yamaguchi H. Acute myocardial infarction induced by ergonovine administration for artificially induced abortion. *Jpn Heart J* 1993; **34**: 803–8.

27 Liao JK, Cockrill BA, Yurchak PM. Acute myocardial infarction after ergonovine administration for uterine bleeding. *Am J Cardiol* 1991; **68**: 823–4.

28 Ruch A, Duhring JL. Postpartum myocardial infarction in a patient receiving bromocriptine. *Obstet Gynecol* 1989; **74**: 448–9.

29 Iffy L, TenHove W, Frisoli G. Acute myocardial infarction in the puerperium in patients receiving bromocriptine. *Am J Obstet Gynecol* 1986; **155**: 371–2.

30 Asada M, Nakayama K, Yamaguchi O, Kudoh I. A case of myocardial infarction associated with pulmonary edema during curettage for hydatidiform mole. *Japanese Journal of Anesthesiology* 1991; **40**: 113–18.

31 Akaike A, Ito T, Sada T, *et al*. Myocardial infarction due to metastasis of choriocarcinoma in a 29 year old woman. *Jpn Circ J* 1977; **41**: 1257–63.

32 Malillos-Perez M, Ortega-Carnicer O, Gutierrez-Millet V, Pazmino-Narvaez L. Postpartum acute myocardial infarction associated with polyarteritis nodosa. *Med Clin* 1982; **78**: 32–4.

33 Nolan TE, Savage RW. Peripartum myocardial infarction from presumed Kawasaki's disease. *Southern Med J* 1990; **83**: 1360–1.

34 Rallings P, Exner T, Abraham R. Coronary artery vasculitis and myocardial infarction associated with antiphospholipid antibodies in a pregnant woman. *Aust NZ J Med* 1989; **19**: 347–50.

35 Parry G, Goudevenos J, Williams DO. Coronary thrombosis postpartum in a young woman with Still's disease. *Clin Cardiol* 1992; **15**: 305–7.

36 Liu SS, Forrester RM, Murphy GS, Chen K, Glassenberg R. Anaesthetic management of a parturient with myocardial infarction related to cocaine use. *Can J Anaesth* 1992; **39**: 858–61.

37 Ottman EH, Gall SA. Myocardial infarction in the third trimester of pregnancy secondary to an aortic valve thrombus. *Obstet Gynecol* 1993; **81**: 804–5.

246

38 Janion M, Kurzawski J, Konstantynowicz H, Wozakowska Kaplon B, Tracz W. Myocardial infarction in pregnancy. *Kardiologia Polska* 1993; **38**: 351–3.
39 Jessurun CR, Adams K, Moise KJ Jr, Wilansky S. Pheochromocytoma-induced myocardial infarction in pregnancy. A case report and literature review. *Texas Heart Inst J* 1993; **20**: 120–2.
40 Raymond R, Lynch J, Underwood D, Leatherman J, Razavi M. Myocardial infarction and normal coronary arteriography: a 10 year clinical and risk analysis of 74 patients. *J Am Coll Cardiol* 1988; **11**: 471–7.
41 Leiserowitz GS, Evans AT, Samuels SJ, Omand K, Kost GJ. Creatinine kinase and its MB isoenzyme in the third trimester and the peripartum period. *J Reprod Med* 1992; **37**: 910–16.
42 Razavi M. Unusual forms of coronary artery disease. *Cardiovascular Clinics* 1975; 7: 25–46.
43 Saxena R, Nolan TE, von Dohlen T, Houghton JL. Postpartum myocardial infarction treated by balloon angioplasty. *Obstet Gynecol* 1992; **79**: 810–12.
44 Gonzalez JI, Hill JA, Conti CR. Spontaneous coronary artery dissection treated with percutaneous transluminal angioplasty. *Am J Cardiol* 1989; **63**: 885–6.
45 Ruszkiewicz A, Opeskin K. Sudden death in pregnancy from congenital malformation of the coronary arteries. *Pathology* 1993; **25**: 236–9.
46 Frenkel Y, Barkai G, Reisin L, Rath S, Mashiach S, Battle A. Pregnancy after myocardial infarction: are we playing safe? *Obstet Gynecol* 1991; 77: 822–5.

19: Rhythm disorders

MARK H ANDERSON

The cardiovascular system undergoes dramatic changes during pregnancy. There is a 50% increase in cardiac output, a 30% rise in stroke volume, and a 25% increase in heart rate.[1] Despite these changes, the incidence of significant arrhythmias during pregnancy is low because there is a low prevalence of serious cardiac disease in young women. None the less, existing arrhythmias can become worse and new arrhythmias can arise during pregnancy. All pharmacological agents used for the control of arrhythmias have potentially adverse effects on the mother and fetus and interventional antiarrhythmic treatment generally requires the use of radiographic screening which is contraindicated, so the management of cardiac arrhythmias during pregnancy presents a difficult challenge to the physician.

In this chapter I will review the impact of pregnancy on existing arrhythmias, the incidence of new arrhythmias, the means of diagnosis, and choice of management with the aim of aiding the physician faced with the management of the pregnant patient with an arrhythmia. I will also review the investigation and treatment of arrhythmias involving the fetus.

The scale of the problem

There are few data on the prevalence of arrhythmias in young women of reproductive age. Nevertheless, some form of cardiac arrhythmia (including atrial or ventricular ectopic beats) can be identified on Holter recordings in up to 60% of patients under 40 years of age, even in the absence of cardiac disease.[2] The incidence of myocardial infarction in women aged 20–40 is only 0·03/1000 so ventricular arrhythmias due to ischaemic heart disease are rare.[3] Wolff–Parkinson–White syndrome has a prevalence of 1·2/1000 in women aged 20–40 and declines with age. About 60% of these patients have episodes of tachycardia. The prevalence of supraventricular arrhythmias secondary to atrioventricular nodal re-entry is similar.[4] The prevalence of atrial fibrillation and flutter reflect the local incidence of rheumatic heart disease which is low in the developed world. Overall the prevalence of sustained tachyarrhythmias in women of reproductive age is around 2–3/1000.

Sustained symptomatic bradyarrhythmias are rare in women of childbearing age. They are mostly patients with congenital complete heart block, the prevalence being about 1/20 000.[5] Over 70% of these patients present before reaching child-bearing age so the incidence of newly discovered congenital heart block during pregnancy is low.[6]

Over the 12 year period from 1979 to 1990 there were no maternal deaths from primary tachyarrhythmias in the United Kingdom although some deaths involved tachyarrhythmias in association with structural heart disease.[7] One death 26 days after a termination at 13 weeks in a patient with congenital heart block was probably unrelated to the pregnancy.

Diagnosis and investigation of arrhythmias

Correct diagnosis of arrhythmias is of vital importance because of the potentially adverse effects of antiarrhythmic strategies in pregnancy. There is no place for empirical treatment in pregnant patients.

Paroxysmal arrhythmias

Diagnostically, these present a challenge as, being generally short-lived, they are rarely present when the patient seeks medical attention. Paroxysmal tachyarrhythmias may present with episodic palpitations, breathlessness, chest pain, and rarely syncope. A full history of the frequency, duration, and type of attack should be taken. Patients often find it easier to "tap out" their heart beat and this may help to decide whether they have a regular or irregular rhythm and give a rough idea of heart rate. A 12 lead ECG is usually normal but may show evidence of frequent atrial or ventricular extrasystoles, pre-excitation (Wolff–Parkinson–White syndrome), bundle branch block, or conduction abnormalities.

Further investigation of arrhythmias is guided by the history. Episodes that occur daily are best investigated by 24 or 48 hour recording of the ECG using a Holter monitor. However, episodes which occur much less frequently often evade detection and for these the use of a patient triggered ECG event-recorder is more appropriate. Such devices may take the form of a continuous recording Holter monitor (sloop), a solid state recorder with metal "feet" which can be placed on the chest during an attack ("Cardiomemo"), or even a wristwatch incorporating recording electrodes (Heart Watch). All share the facility to transmit a short period (about 30 seconds) of ECG by telephone to a central recording station, thus enabling the patient's arrhythmia to be documented without a visit to hospital, and allowing the recording of multiple events. Because the patients have to use these devices when they have symptoms the quality of the recording may be poor. A "low technology" strategy can be surprisingly successful in patients whose paroxysmal arrhythmias last for more than a few minutes and who live near a hospital accident department. The patient carries a letter from her physician requesting that an ECG be done immediately she arrives at the hospital. This strategy should be chosen only for patients in whom the conscious level is unaffected by the arrhythmia and if a friend or relative can take them to the hospital.

Sustained arrhythmias

Where a sustained arrhythmia can be documented by ECG the diagnostic problem is reduced to one of correct ECG interpretation. Diagnostic features of the ECG which help to classify narrow complex arrhythmias are summarised in Figure 19.1 and broad complex arrhythmias in Table 19.1.

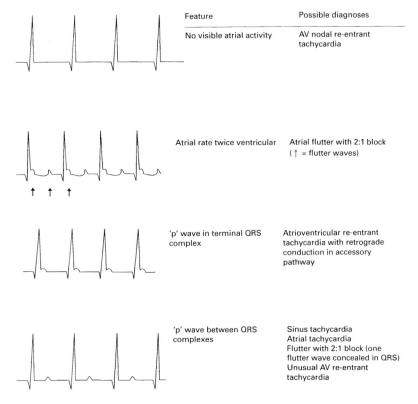

Feature	Possible diagnoses
No visible atrial activity	AV nodal re-entrant tachycardia
Atrial rate twice ventricular	Atrial flutter with 2:1 block (↑ = flutter waves)
'p' wave in terminal QRS complex	Atrioventricular re-entrant tachycardia with retrograde conduction in accessory pathway
'p' wave between QRS complexes	Sinus tachycardia Atrial tachycardia Flutter with 2:1 block (one flutter wave concealed in QRS) Unusual AV re-entrant tachycardia

FIGURE 19.1—*Diagnostic features of narrow complex arrhythmias.*

Previously documented arrhythmias

A proportion of arrhythmias in pregnancy occur in patients already known to have a sustained or paroxysmal arrhythmia. The frequency of supraventricular tachycardias in patients with the Wolff–Parkinson–White syndrome is thought to increase during pregnancy and a similar increase in other arrhythmias may occur.[8] It is important not to assume that

TABLE 19.1—*Diagnostic features of broad complex arrhythmias*

Fusion beats

Capture beats

Atrioventricular dissociation (independent P wave activity)

Left axis deviation

QRS duration >140 ms

QRS morphology:
   Concordance (all complexes upright or inverted) V1–V6
   Right bundle branch block pattern:
      R wave in V1>R'
      Deep S wave in V6
   Left bundle branch block pattern:
      R wave >30 ms duration
      Any Q wave in V6
      >60 ms from onset of the QRS to nadir of the S wave in V1 or V2
      Notching of the downstroke of the S wave in V1 or V2

---

symptoms occurring in pregnancy are necessarily a recurrence of a previously documented arrhythmia. Whilst they may be, it is important to investigate and document the arrhythmia associated with symptoms.

Role of electrophysiological studies in pregnancy

Diagnostic electrophysiology has established a major role in the diagnosis of supraventricular and ventricular arrhythmias and a more controversial role in the risk stratification of ventricular arrhythmias and selection of appropriate antiarrhythmic drug therapy.[9–11] It is useful, not only in obtaining a definitive diagnosis in those cases where an arrhythmia has already been shown, but also in establishing the presence of a substrate and an inducible arrhythmia in patients with palpitations in whom the arrhythmia itself has remained elusive. With the development of radiofrequency ablation invasive electrophysiology has acquired a therapeutic role.

During pregnancy the role of invasive electrophysiology is limited. Physicians have been understandably cautious because of the significant exposure to x rays involved in diagnostic and therapeutic electrophysiological studies.[12,13] The vast majority of patients with an ECG diagnosed tachyarrhythmia can be managed with antiarrhythmic drugs alone, even if a precise diagnosis cannot be reached. In patients with palpitations in whom no arrhythmia can be shown the likelihood of a life threatening arrhythmia being present is low and diagnostic electrophysiological evaluation is not indicated.

It is possible to do electrophysiological studies using echocardiographic guidance of electrode catheters during pregnancy[14] and this may allow avoidance or reduction of x ray exposure when invasive electrophysiological studies are essential.[15,16]

Management of tachyarrhythmias: emergencies and acute-onset sustained tachycardias

Cardiac arrest

Cardiac arrest in pregnant women is fortunately rare and a number of special considerations apply to its management.[7] There is a considerable body of evidence that in late pregnancy resuscitation in the supine position may be unsuccessful because of aortocaval obstruction that reduces venous return.[17] There are a number of reports of immediate caesarean section being accompanied by successful resuscitation, presumably as a result of relief of aortocaval obstruction.[18-20] Resuscitation may be possible without immediate caesarean section by using a wedge[21] or the knees of an assistant to tilt the patient from the supine position.[22] Otherwise, resuscitation should proceed in accordance with the established guidelines of the European Resuscitation Council.[23] A successful maternal and fetal outcome may follow even prolonged attempts at resuscitation.[24] Cardioversion and defibrillation may be needed. There are many reports of successful cardioversion during pregnancy without adverse effect on the fetus at energies of up to 300 J.[25-27] It is important to obtain good central venous access to ensure prompt delivery of drugs,[28] or failing this to give drugs by the intra-tracheal route.

Ventricular tachycardia

Sustained ventricular tachycardia is an unusual arrhythmia in pregnancy. If the tachycardia is associated with hypotension or circulatory insufficiency immediate cardioversion is the most appropriate treatment. For haemo-dynamically stable ventricular tachycardia intravenous antiarrhythmic drugs may be used. Lignocaine is the drug for which there is the most experience in pregnancy because of its use as a local anaesthetic. It is known to cross the placenta and result in fetal concentrations 50%–60% of maternal concentrations. Disopyramide has been reported to stimulate uterine contractions and is probably best avoided.[29] Sotalol has been used in pregnancy for control of hypertension and arrhythmias without reports of problems[30,31] but there are no reports of its use to terminate ventricular tachycardia. Therefore lignocaine is the drug of choice. As the efficacy of intravenously administered antiarrhythmic drugs is 50% or less[32] it may still be necessary to proceed to cardioversion. A final option is to use a flotation pacing wire which may be positioned without the use of radiographic screening.[33] Antitachycardia pacing has an efficacy of at least 55%[34] and it may be the safest way to treat repeated episodes of tachycardia.

Atrioventricular re-entrant and AV nodal re-entrant tachycardias

In a population with a low incidence of rheumatic heart disease these are the most common sustained arrhythmias seen in pregnancy. Presenting with a narrow complex tachycardia and heart rates in the 140–220 range they may be asymptomatic, may cause palpitations alone, or at more rapid rates may give rise to haemodynamic symptoms such as dizziness, syncope, and chest pain. These arrhythmias should be managed in accordance with the recommendations of the Advanced Life Support Group (Table 19.2).[35] Intravenous adenosine has an efficacy approaching 100% for terminating supraventricular tachycardias.[36] It works best when delivered as a rapid bolus injection and is most effective when delivered through a central line.[37] It appears to be effective during pregnancy without impact on the fetal heart rate as a result of its rapid metabolism in the maternal circulation, resulting in a half-life of just a few seconds.[38–41] With the increasing use of adenosine, verapamil has been relegated to being a second-line drug for acute treatment of supraventricular tachycardias. It is effective given in a bolus of up to 10 mg without effect on fetal heart rate.[42,43]

TABLE 19.2—*Management of supraventricular tachycardia.*

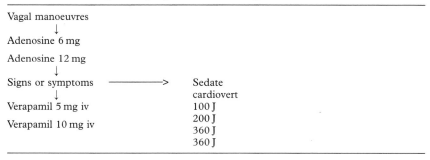

Vagal manoeuvres may prove useful in terminating supraventricular arrhythmias with reported success rates ranging from 17% to 92%.[44,45] Some studies have reported carotid sinus massage to be most effective whilst others favour the valsalva manoeuvre.[45,46] Atrioventricular nodal arrhythmias are more likely to terminate than those which use an accessory pathway. Since vagal manoeuvres offer the opportunity to avoid the use of antiarrhythmic drugs they should be attempted first for narrow complex arrhythmias. An electrocardiogram should be recorded during the vagal manoeuvres or while giving adenosine or verapamil, as useful diagnostic information may be obtained even when the arrhythmia fails to terminate.

Atrial fibrillation and atrial flutter

These rhythms occur relatively rarely in women of childbearing age, in the absence of underlying rheumatic heart disease. In the absence of underlying cardiac disease the most appropriate strategy for acute onset atrial fibrillation is early cardioversion, avoiding the need for chronic anticoagulation. There is no published experience of using antiarrhythmic drugs such as flecainide or amiodarone to achieve pharmacological cardioversion of atrial fibrillation in pregnancy. The issue of heart rate control in established atrial fibrillation is considered below.

Management of tachyarrhythmias: chronic sustained and paroxysmal arrhythmias

Recurring arrhythmias are perhaps the most difficult management problem because of the desire to avoid long term antiarrhythmic drug treatment during pregnancy. The issues of antiarrhythmic drugs, fetal toxicity, and teratogenicity are considered in more detail in chapter 22. In young women of childbearing age who suffer from recurrent arrhythmias of whatever type it is important to consider the implications of pregnancy before conception. Radiofrequency catheter ablation may be used to cure atrial tachycardias (>85%),[47] atrioventricular nodal tachycardias (>95%),[48] atrioventricular re-entrant tachycardias (>95%),[49] atrial flutter (>70%)[50] and some types of ventricular tachycardia (>70%). The need for chronic antiarrhythmic drug treatment is removed, thus making pregnancy safer and reducing anxiety levels for the patient and the physician. All women with arrhythmias of these types contemplating pregnancy should be referred to a cardiologist with an interest in arrhythmias so that all the issues may be considered. If continued antiarrhythmic drugs are required, a drug of which there is more experience in pregnancy should be given. Patients whose arrhythmias are infrequent and not life-threatening may be managed best by withdrawal of drugs for the duration of pregnancy. If the arrhythmias become more frequent treatment can always be reinstated.

Ventricular extrasystoles

Ventricular extrasystoles are common and at rates less than 30/hour are found in more than a third of Holter recordings in adults. In patients with previous myocardial infarction the presence of ventricular premature contractions and particularly of complex multimorphic forms is associated with an increased risk of sudden cardiac death.[51,52] But they are generally benign. When frequent they may cause palpitations. These can usually be alleviated by removal of precipitants such as caffeine and alcohol, and by reassurance. Pharmacological treatment of isolated ventricular premature contractions is not justified during pregnancy.

Ventricular tachycardia

Recurrent ventricular tachycardia may result from a number of causes (Table 19.3) and a knowledge of the mechanism in the individual patient is helpful in determining the choice of treatment.

TABLE 19.3—*Causes of recurrent ventricular tachycardia during pregnancy*

Idiopathic/normal heart

Hypertrophic cardiomyopathy

Right ventricular dysplasia

Preexisting dilated cardiomyopathy

Peripartum cardiomyopathy

Coronary artery disease

Idiopathic ventricular tachycardia

This diagnosis implies the absence of any evidence of ischaemic heart disease on the electrocardiogram or any evidence of myocardial disease on the echocardiogram. There are a number of reports in the literature of patients developing ventricular tachycardia of this type for the first time during pregnancy.[53-55] It is not clear whether pregnancy is the cause or whether they are purely coincidental. Four different patterns of idiopathic ventricular tachycardia have been described based on the bundle–branch block pattern and frontal QRS axis.[56] These are summarised in Table 19.4. The right bundle branch block right axis group appear to have a different mechanism from the other groups, involving bundle branch re-entry. This type of tachycardia is responsive to verapamil but rarely occurs during exercise.[57] The remaining patterns of normal heart ventricular tachycardia are often induced by exercise (40%–75%), suggesting a role for catecholamines. Autonomic nervous system abnormalities have been found in some "normal heart" ventricular tachycardia patients.[58] No randomised prospective study of patients with normal heart ventricular tachycardia has been published. Lemery et al studied 47 such patients and found no mortality from sudden cardiac death or arrhythmias after a mean follow-up of 96 months.[59] There are, however, isolated reports of sudden death.[60] Recurrence of arrhythmia is common despite medical treatment[56] (Figure 19.2) but radiofrequency ablation has been reported to be successful in most of these patients.[61]

TABLE 19.4—*Different ECG patterns in 47 patients with "normal heart" ventricular tachycardia.*[56]

Bundle branch block pattern	Frontal QRS axis	No (%)	Group
Right	Left or superior	9 (19)	RBBBLA
Right	Normal or right axis	9 (19)	RBBBRA
Left	Left or superior	5 (11)	LBBBLA
Left	Normal or right	24 (51)	LBBBRA

RBBB: Right bundle branch block; LBBB: Left bundle branch block; RA: Right axis; LA: Left axis.

Gill et al compared flecainide (200 mg or 300 mg/day), sotalol (240 or 320 mg/day), and verapamil (360 mg/day) for normal heart ventricular

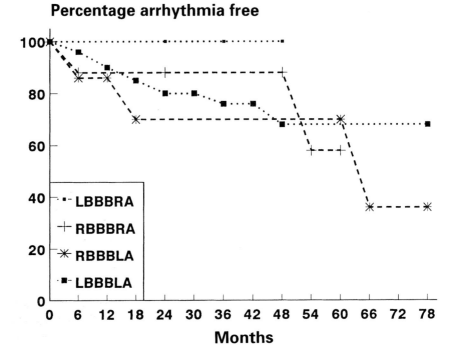

Percentage arrhythmia free

FIGURE 19.2—*Recurrence rate of ventricular tachycardia for different patterns of "normal heart" ventricular tachycardia*[56] *(RBBBRA—right bundle branch block right axis, RBBBLA—right bundle branch block left axis, LBBBRA—left bundle branch block right axis, LBBBLA—left bundle branch block left axis).*

tachycardia.[62] Although all three drugs were active sotalol was the most effective (89% of patients). There may also be a role for conventional beta-blockers in these patients and this should be first-line treatment in view of the relative safety of beta-blockers in pregnancy.[63,64] Brodsky *et al* reported favourable outcomes in six patients with new-onset ventricular tachycardia during pregnancy treated with beta-blockers.[65] The outcome of patients with ventricular tachycardia with a normal heart in 16 recent publications are summarised in Table 19.5.

Ventricular tachycardia in hypertrophic cardiomyopathy

Spontaneous sustained monomorphic ventricular tachycardia occurs in less than 1% of patients with hypertrophic obstructive cardiomyopathy.[66,67] By contrast non-sustained ventricular tachycardia is relatively common in patients with hypertrophic cardiomyopathy and is found in about 25% of adult patients.[68,69] Data from two studies suggest that non-sustained ventricular tachycardia is the single best indicator of risk of sudden death in patients with hypertrophic obstructive cardiomyopathy.[68,70] Amiodarone has been reported to reduce mortality by some[71] but not all[72] workers. There are 43 case reports in the literature of amiodarone in pregnancy, in

TABLE 19.5—*Case reports of "normal heart" ventricular tachycardia during pregnancy.*

First author	Case No. (No. of pregnancies)	Treatment	Maternal outcome	Fetal outcome
McMillan[235]	1	Dig, quin	OK	Unknown
Peters[236]	1	None	OK	Unknown
Hair[237]	1	Quin	OK	OK
Adams[238]	1 (2)	Quin	OK	Unknown
	2 (4)	Quin	OK	Unknown
	3 (1)	Quin	OK	Unknown
Rally[239]	1	Proc	+	+
Pine[240]	1	Quin, proc, phen	OK	OK
Gettes[241]	1	Quin, prop	Unknown	Unknown
Russell[242]	1 (1)	Quin, proc, dig	OK	OK
	1 (2)	Quin, ligno, phen	OK	OK
Reed[243]	1	Ligno, proc, phen, prop	OK	IUGR
Timmis[244]	1	Mex, prop	OK	Brady
Alpert[245]	1	None	Unknown	Unknown
Menon[246]	1	Ligno	OK	OK
Brodsky[247]	1	Meto	OK	OK
	2	Meto	OK	OK
Vlay[248]	1	Prop	OK	OK
Connaughton[249]	1	Flec	OK	OK
Chandra[250]	1	None	OK	OK
	2	None	OK	OK

dig: digoxin. quin: quinidine. proc: procainamide. phen: phenytoin. prop: propranolol. ligno: lignocaine. mex: mexiletine. meto: metoprolol. flec: flecainide. IUGR: intrauterine growth retardation. brady: bradycardia. +: died.

17 cases the drug being used throughout pregnancy. Substantial abnormalities of fetal thyroid function occurred in seven of the 43 cases and in one case were associated with delayed motor development (see Table 24.4). There are isolated reports of sudden death during pregnancy in patients with hypertrophic cardiomyopathy[73,74] but other large series have reported few problems with pregnancy in patients with hypertrophic cardiomyopathy.[75] The sudden deaths probably represent the yearly 2% to 3% sudden death rate of adults with hypertrophic cardiomyopathy,[76] and there is no evidence that pregnant women are at increased risk. In the absence of conclusive data about the most appropriate way to manage hypertrophic cardiomyopathy during pregnancy the risks and benefits should be discussed with each patient before making a decision whether or not to continue amiodarone.

Ventricular tachycardia in right ventricular dysplasia

Arrhythmogenic right ventricular dysplasia is a disorder of the muscle of the right ventricular free wall which is progressively replaced by fibro adipose tissue and may be responsible for up to 50% of ventricular tachycardias of right ventricular origin.[77] The prognosis is not clear because so few patients have been reported. The incidence of cardiac arrest ranges between 0% and 13% at 8 years.[78,79] Recurrent episodes of ventricular tachycardia, particularly on exercise, are common, occurring in at least 70% of patients often before overt signs or symptoms of cardiac dysfunction. In others the development of progressive right ventricular failure may be the most important factor affecting eventual outcome.[80] Right ventricular dysplasia differs from a right ventricular cardiomyopathy resembling dilated cardiomyopathy but confined to the right ventricle and in which ventricular tachycardias are not usually a feature. These may result from a congenital partial absence of muscle (Uhl's Anomaly) in which a favourable outcome of pregnancy has been reported.[81]

Ventricular tachycardia in pre-existing dilated cardiomyopathy

Between 40% and 80% of patients with congestive heart failure and dilated cardiomyopathy have non-sustained ventricular tachycardia on Holter monitoring.[82] Whether or not these patients should receive antiarrhythmic drugs and how that treatment should be evaluated remains controversial. Nearly half of all deaths in patients with congestive heart failure are thought to be the result of arrhythmias[82,83] although an unknown number of these may be the result of bradyarrhythmias.[84,85] In patients without a history of ventricular arrhythmias left ventricular function is a better predictor of outcome than conventional Holter monitoring or electrophysiological study.[86,87] Three year survival falls from 92% in patients with an ejection fraction greater than 40% to 71% in patients with an ejection fraction of 30% or less.[86] The signal-averaged electrocardiogram has poor sensitivity for identifying patients with ventricular arrhythmias and the role of heart rate variability remains to be established.[88]

Two non-randomised trials of electrophysiology-guided drug treatment in patients with dilated cardiomyopathy presenting with ventricular arrhythmias suggest it may be effective at preventing recurrences[89,90] but less so in patients without a history of sustained ventricular arrhythmias.[91]

On balance pregnant women who have not had a sustained symptomatic ventricular arrhythmia should not be given antiarrhythmic medication. Patients who are taking antiarrhythmic drugs for sustained ventricular arrhythmias should be counselled about the risk of drug withdrawal compared with the risks of drug treatment before considering pregnancy. Patients with overt heart failure should be advised against pregnancy anyway, and these patients are at highest risk of serious arrhythmias. Patients who develop heart failure during pregnancy should have this well controlled by drugs throughout.

Ventricular tachycardia in peripartum cardiomyopathy

This should be treated in the same way as that associated with pre-existing dilated cardiomyopathy.

Ventricular tachycardia in coronary artery disease

The rarity of myocardial infarction in women of child-bearing age makes this an uncommon cause of ventricular tachycardia during pregnancy. Ventricular tachycardia is an important marker of increased risk of future life-threatening arrhythmias after myocardial infarction.[92] In patients in whom antiarrhythmic drugs have been effective before conception they should be continued. If a change of drugs is required to minimise fetal risk this should be considered carefully before conception and the new drug assessed formally by invasive electrophysiological studies or Holter monitoring.

The long QT syndrome

The idiopathic long QT syndrome is characterised by a prolonged QT interval on the surface ECG, syncopal episodes, and sudden cardiac death from ventricular arrhythmias. Inheritance may be autosomal dominant or recessive.[93,94] Beta-blockers and left stellate ganglionectomy may be effective in reducing the risk of sudden death.[95] Patients have also been treated with pacemakers and the implantable defribrillator.[96,97] There are a few reports of successful pregnancy in patients with the long QT syndrome.[98–101] Beta-blockade should be continued in these patients throughout pregnancy to prevent recurrence of life-threatening arrhythmias.

Special considerations: the implantable defibrillator in pregnancy

At least one patient with an implantable defibrillator has completed an uneventful pregnancy[102] and it has also been used to treat ventricular tachycardia in peripartum cardiomyopathy.[103] Given the proven safety of cardioversion during pregnancy the problems are similar to those of having a pacemaker, complicated by the additional bulk of these devices, potentially increasing the risk of erosion and infection.

Supraventricular arrhythmias

Sinus tachycardia

During normal pregnancy the heart rate increases by about 10 beats a minute with further increases during labour.[104–105] Sinus rhythm with a rate above 100 beats a minute (sinus tachycardia) has no particular obstetric implications. It may be from exercise, anxiety, anaemia, fever, hypotension, hypoxia, heart failure, or thyrotoxicosis. Correction of the cause will restore a normal sinus rate. Sinus node re-entry can cause a persistent tachycardia with normal P wave morphology but is extremely unusual during pregnancy.

Atrial premature beats

Atrial premature beats are common, being present on over a third of adult Holter recordings.[2] Although they may produce troublesome symptoms they are rarely of any haemodynamic consequence and pharmacological therapy for this benign arrhythmia should be avoided during pregnancy. Removal of possible causes including smoking, caffeine, alcohol, anxiety, or fatigue may be effective.

Atrioventricular re-entrant and AV nodal re-entrant tachycardias

Both of these arrhythmias can cause recurrent attacks of palpitations. Patients with occasional attacks may be managed without drugs and the frequency of attacks can be reduced by avoiding precipitants such as caffeine and alcohol. However, arrhythmias of this type may become more common or may present for the first time in pregnancy.[106]

If the arrhythmia is well tolerated and occurs relatively infrequently it may be best not to prescribe any drugs and to terminate the attacks when they occur with vagal manoeuvres (which the patient can perform herself), or adenosine or even repeated cardioversion.[26] Because these arrhythmias rely on conduction through the atrioventricular node they may be controlled by drugs which affect AV nodal conduction.[107] If preventive antiarrhythmic drugs are required, low doses of beta-blockers, verapamil or digoxin can be used, increased as necessary. In patients with evident pre-excitation, digoxin and verapamil should be avoided. There is extensive experience with these drugs in pregnancy (Chapter 22) and although they are not completely without adverse effects they do not appear to be teratogenic. Drugs such as flecainide with which experience is limited, or amiodarone, with its well documented potential for fetal thyroid dysfunction, should be reserved for cases where the arrhythmia remains uncontrolled despite use of established agents alone or in combination. In patients with evident pre-excitation digoxin and verapamil should be avoided because of the risk of rapid conduction through the accessory pathway should atrial fibrillation occur.

Atrial flutter and atrial fibrillation

Chronic atrial flutter is unusual in pregnancy. Rate control with digoxin or verapamil is usually effective and conversion to sinus rhythm should be considered. It is not associated with an increased risk of embolism and anticoagulation is not indicated.

Chronic atrial fibrillation in women of child-bearing age is almost always the result of rheumatic mitral valve disease.[108] In patients with established atrial fibrillation the primary aim of treatment is to achieve adequate control of heart rate to optimise cardiac output. The precise heart rate that is required to do this remains the subject of controversy and certainly varies among patients.[109] In practice the resting heart rate should be 90 beats a minute or less and 140 beats a minute or less on exercise. There is no necessity to use any rate control medication if these figures are met and the patient has no symptoms. Digoxin has traditionally been used to control the heart rate in patients with atrial fibrillation, but because it is primarily a vagotonic drug[110] its effect may be overridden by increased sympathetic tone, leading to poor heart rate control on exercise.[111] Rate control on exercise and at rest may be improved by the use of a beta-blocker, either alone[112,113] or in combination with digoxin.[114-116] Neither regimen has been shown to increase exercise tolerance or oxygen uptake. The calcium antagonists verapamil and diltiazem are better than digoxin for the control of rate on exercise and their effect is additive to digoxin.[113,117,118] When acute control of rapid atrial fibrillation is required intravenous verapamil achieves quicker control of the ventricular rate than intravenous digoxin.

Patients with chronic atrial fibrillation and mitral valve disease have a 17-fold increased risk of cardiac thrombus and cerebral embolisation making continued anticoagulation during pregnancy mandatory.[119]

Atrial fibrillation in the absence of organic heart disease is uncommon in pregnancy. It may be the result of excessive alcohol intake, thyroid disease, infection, or sick sinus syndrome but usually no cause can be found. In the absence of risk factors (previous stroke, hypertension, or heart failure) the incidence of embolic stroke in patients under 65 is less than 1·0% a year and the risk of anticoagulation during pregnancy outweighs any potential benefits.[120,121] The presence of any one risk factor increases the risk to 7·2% a year and with two or three risk factors it rises to 17%. In these higher risk patients anticoagulation is justified throughout pregnancy. The use of aspirin in place of warfarin would be attractive in these patients as aspirin is well tolerated during pregnancy.[122] However, there is conflicting data on whether aspirin alone reduces the risk of stroke.[123,124] The use of subcutaneous heparin in the early stage of pregnancy is justified in these patients to avoid the teratogenic effects of warfarin.

An isolated episode of atrial fibrillation is best treated by cardioversion. Anticoagulation is required for all patients undergoing cardioversion to minimise the risk of thromboembolism which is otherwise about 5%.[125] The absence of atrial thrombus or "smoke" on transoesophageal echocardiography may identify a group of patients in whom prolonged precardioversion anticoagulation is unnecessary.[126] Thromboembolism may occur in the weeks after cardioversion due to the gradual return of atrial mechanical function and therefore anticoagulation should be maintained for at least three weeks after cardioversion.[127] The precardioversion transoesophageal echocardiogram does not help to identify people who are not at risk during this period.[128] The one exception to this requirement for postcardioversion anticoagulation is in patients with normal hearts and short lived atrial fibrillation (<48 hours). Therefore cardioversion of recent onset atrial fibrillation should be done as soon as possible. Because of the requirement for anticoagulation after cardioversion of atrial fibrillation that has been present for more than 48 hours it may be preferable to defer cardioversion during the early weeks of pregnancy or near term.

Recurrent episodes of paroxysmal atrial fibrillation may be treated with a variety of drugs. The best data are for the type Ic antiarrhythmic drugs such as flecainide.[129] Although there are no controlled trials in pregnancy it is most appropriate to start treatment with a simple beta-blocker or quinidine if this fails. Quinidine has a long history of obstetric use without teratogenic effects.[130] There are also data to suggest that sotalol may be as effective as propafenone.[131] Digoxin is commonly prescribed for paroxysmal atrial fibrillation but only marginally reduces the frequency of attacks and the heart rate during them.[132] However, in patients who are well controlled on this drug it is reasonable to continue it during pregnancy.

Bradyarrhythmias and pregnancy

The heart rate increases by 10 or more beats a minute during pregnancy[105,106] and profound bradycardia (<50 beats/minute) is uncommon. Potential causes of intermittent and permanent bradycardia are summarised in Table 19.6.

TABLE 19.6—*Causes of bradycardia during pregnancy.*

Arrhythmia	Causes
Sinus bradycardia:	Vasovagal syncope
Intermittent	Sick sinus syndrome
Permanent	Idiopathic
	Familial
	Drugs (beta-blockade)
	Physical training
Heart block:	
Congenital	With or without congenital heart disease
Acquired	Valve disease, infection, sarcoidosis

Sinus bradycardia, sick sinus syndrome and the malignant vasovagal syndrome

Persistent sinus bradycardia (heart rate <50/minute) is generally benign and does not require specific therapy.[133] Sick sinus syndrome is a degenerative disorder comprising intermittent profound bradycardia and episodic atrial tachyarrhythmia (the tachy-brady syndrome). It is rare in women of child-bearing age. It requires treatment with AAI or DDD pacing and drugs for the tachyarrhythmia. Neurally mediated syncope, also known as the malignant vasovagal syndrome appears to be the result of a combination of abnormalities of vasoregulation on standing, together with a cardiodepressant vagal reflex.[134-136] It may be responsible for over 20% of unexplained syncope.[137] The relative contribution of cardiodepression and abnormal vasoregulation varies in different patients and may explain the variable response to pacing and drugs. Given its frequency it is perhaps surprising that there is no reference to its occurrence during pregnancy. It may be that the alterations in cardiovascular regulation during pregnancy protect these patients from syncope.

262

Complete heart block

Complete heart block in pregnant women differs from that in the general population, in whom acquired complete heart block, most commonly the result of aging or coronary artery disease, is the commonest form. Because of their youth and the absence of coronary disease congenital heart block is relatively more common as a cause of bradycardia in pregnant women. In a review Mendelson quoted 53 cases of which 28 were acquired and 25 congenital.[138] Congenital complete heart block is a condition of unknown aetiology although it is known to be associated with maternal connective tissue disease.[139] Most cases present in childhood but about 30% remain undiscovered until adulthood so it may present for the first time during pregnancy.[140]

Management of unpaced pre-existing complete heart block

There are no reliable criteria for the prediction of sudden death or syncope in patients with complete heart block.[141] Patients with a slower escape rhythm are more likely to have syncope.[142] A patient with congenital complete heart block may be managed conservatively, but then the increasing cardiac output requirements of pregnancy will have to be met by an increase in stroke volume. Before the availability of pacing reports suggested a substantial mortality—four maternal deaths in 42 pregnancies.[108,143] Other reports of uneventful pregnancy and labour abound.[132,144] The presence of underlying structural heart disease such as corrected congenital transposition in addition to complete heart block is certainly an adverse risk factor during pregnancy. However, such patients are likely to have been discovered before pregnancy and to have had pacemakers inserted. In patients who have previously been symptom-free the first Stokes–Adams attacks commonly occur during pregnancy.[145,146] This includes patients with previously undetected corrected transposition (Chapter 6).

On balance it seems sensible to suggest that patients with asymptomatic isolated complete heart block in whom a decision has been made not to pace, or who present for the first time during pregnancy, should be managed conservatively. If they develop Stokes–Adams attacks they should be paced permanently, except in the last week of pregnancy when temporary pacing may be more appropriate.[147] Patients with symptomatic heart block who are considering pregnancy should have pacemakers inserted before conception.

Pacemaker insertion in pregnancy

Because of the potential risks of fetal irradiation all possible steps should be taken to avoid the need for radiographic screening during pregnancy. Permanent atrial and ventricular pacing leads can be inserted using echocardiography and ECG guidance alone.[148-150]

The pregnant patient with a pacemaker

Patients with pacemakers tolerate pregnancy well.[151-155] Serious complications are rare, the most common being irritation or ulceration at the implantation site, particularly with the more bulky pacemaker generators used in previous decades.[156,157] For this reason submammary implantation has been advised for pacemaker implantation in women of childbearing age.

With the exception of patients with chronic atrial arrhythmias all patients with conduction disorders should have a physiological (DDD) pacemaker[158] and assuming normal sinus node function they will show a normal heart rate response to pregnancy. Young patients with chronic atrial arrhythmias and conduction disease should have a rate responsive pacemaker (VVI-R). However these patients do not show the normal heart rate response to pregnancy. Even pacemakers with metabolic sensors have algorithms that maintain a constant heart rate in response to the gradual increase of metabolic rate during pregnancy. As there are many reports of successful pregnancy with fixed rate ventricular pacing this is not a problem but it is always possible to increase the basic pacing rate should the patient develop symptoms.

Fetal arrhythmias

The quoted incidence of fetal arrhythmias varies from 1:25 000 to 1:50, the first figure reflecting substantial underdiagnosis from times when diagnostic tools were less well developed and the latter reflecting the inclusion of even minor variations in rhythm.[159-161]

Diagnosis

The presence of a fetal arrhythmia should be considered when the heart rate is outside the range 110–180 bpm, when the heart beat is repeatedly

TABLE 19.7—*Differential diagnosis of fetal arrhythmias.*

Tachycardia (>80 bpm)
  Sinus tachycardia
  Atrial tachycardia
  AV re-entrant tachycardia
  Atrial flutter with 2:1 block

Irregular rhythms
  Atrial extrasystoles
  Ventricular extrasystoles
  Atrial flutter/fibrillation

Bradycardia (<110 bpm)
  Sinus bradycardia
  Heart block (2nd and 3rd degree)
  Non-conducted atrial extrasystoles

irregular, or in the presence of unexplained hydrops fetalis. Originally the fetal electrocardiogram was used for the diagnosis of arrhythmias but the P wave is usually not recorded and even the QRS amplitude may be too low for interpretation.[162] The development of ultrasound and fetal echocardiography has revolutionised the diagnosis of fetal arrhythmias by allowing independent visualisation of atrial and ventricular contraction and the flow of blood through the atrioventricular valves and great vessels.[163,164] The differential diagnoses of fetal arrhythmias are shown in Table 19.7. It is important to remember that, as in adults, fetal arrhythmias may be paroxysmal and may not be present at the time of the first examination.[165]

Aetiology

Pooled data from three published series (Table 19.8) show that a structural cardiac defect is present in 50% of fetuses with bradycardia but in less than 5% of those with supraventricular arrhythmias or extrasystoles of atrial or ventricular origin.[160,166,167] Many conditions can occasionally be associated with tachyarrhythmias, including cardiac tumours,[168] cardio-myopathies, and a persistent connective tissue membrane in the right atrium (Chiari's network).[169] Atrial fibrillation or flutter may be idiopathic or in association with an overt accessory pathway (Wolff–Parkinson–White syndrome).[170] There is evidence from echocardiographic studies of atrioventricular timing that most other supraventricular tachycardias are atrioventricular re-entrant, employing a retrogradely conducting concealed accessory pathway.[171] Fetal heart block is associated in a third of cases with structural congenital heart disease and in most of the others with transplacental transfer of antibodies from the mother.

TABLE 19.8—*Incidence of structural cardiac defects associated with cardiac arrhythmias.*

	Bradycardia	Tachycardia	APC/VPC
Allan[167]	3/9	0/7	0/15
Stewart[166]	4/8	0/5	2/17
Rajadurai[160]	0/1	0/4	0/2

Management

There has been no controlled trial of conservative management of fetal arrhythmia but some consensus emerged in the late 1970s that arrhythmias associated with heart rates above 250 beats per minute or with heart failure require treatment.[172,173] The primary aim of management is to allow the development of the fetus to a stage of maturity when survival is assured, minimising the impact of arrhythmia on fetal growth.

Fetal supraventricular tachycardias

Pharmacotherapy

Digoxin

The first attempt at intrauterine treatment of fetal tachyarrhythmia using digoxin was reported in 1978.[172] A series of case reports of the use of digoxin for this purpose followed.[170,174-181] Of the 19 patients who received digoxin alone termination of the arrhythmia occurred in 12 (63%). There was a non-significant trend towards a higher success rate (9/11) in the fetuses without hydrops than in those with hydrops (3/8). This may be related to reduced placental transfer of the drug in fetuses with hydrops. The dosages of digoxin used in these cases varied greatly between 0·125 mg and 0·75 mg daily. These studies were uncontrolled, so spontaneous reversion of the arrhythmia might have occurred in some cases. Although digoxin appears to be safe to use during pregnancy important alterations in its pharmacokinetics occur, which must be considered. Increased renal excretion of digoxin mean that higher than usual doses are required to achieve therapeutic levels in the mother. Additionally production of endogenous digoxin-like substances by the placenta or fetus may lead to an underestimation of digoxin requirements.[182,183] In patients taking digoxin mean gestation was reduced from 39·9 weeks in a control group to 38·5 weeks, and the mean duration of labour was reduced from 8 to 4 hours, possibly as a result of a stimulant effect on the drug on the myometrium.[184]

Because about a third of fetuses fail to respond to digoxin monotherapy a number of combinations of digoxin with other agents have been evaluated.

Verapamil

The first report of successful intrauterine control of a supraventricular tachycardia using verapamil dates back to 1980[185] and was followed by a series of case reports.[186-190] In Maxwell's series of 23 fetuses with tachycardia 15 women received verapamil (in increasing doses up to 480 mg/day) in addition to digoxin.[165] Full control of the arrhythmia was achieved in nine, partial control in three and failure occurred in three. In another series of 14 cases successful control of fetal arrhythmia was achieved in 6 out of 6 patients in whom digoxin alone had failed.[181] However, verapamil had to be discontinued in one case because of maternal second-degree heart block. Verapamil increases plasma concentrations of digoxin and this may explain its efficacy in some cases. However, in these two series the plasma concentrations of digoxin were closely controlled and the dose adjusted as necessary, so the benefit obtained is likely to have been directly attributable to the verapamil.

Verapamil has been widely used in pregnant women for control of arrhythmias,[191,192] for hypertension[193] and to limit the adverse effect of sympathomimetic drugs used for tocolysis[194] without reported adverse effect. A single case of fetal death has been reported four weeks after successful termination of a supraventricular arrhythmia with a combination of digoxin and verapamil (360 mg/day).[189] No anatomical cause for the fetal death could be found, so a drug related effect could not be ruled out.

Propranolol

Despite the observation that fetal concentrations of propranolol are well below those achieved in the mother[195-199] this drug has been used as a first and second line agent for treatment of fetal tachyarrhythmias both alone and in combination with digoxin.[181,197,200-203] The success rate of propranolol seems to be below 50% although many of the case reports have not specified the dosage used.

Procainamide

There are six case reports of the use of procainamide, always after the failure of conventional treatment with digoxin and sometimes other agents. The first report was in 1992 by Dumesnic et al in a patient who had failed to respond after six days of digoxin and propranolol.[201] Fetal cardioversion occurred after a slow maternal intravenous infusion of 340 mg procainamide and was maintained by an infusion of 4 mg a minute reducing to 2 mg a minute. At 31 weeks the patient was discharged taking 0·5 mg digoxin daily and oral procainamide 4 g/day. Fetal tachycardia recurred at 33 weeks and was impossible to control despite further doses of procainamide. A caesarean section was performed and the arrhythmia was controlled in the newborn with digoxin and propranolol. Sometimes the use of procainamide has been associated with only transient control of the arrhythmia[190,204] or an increase in the time spent in sinus rhythm.[205] In other cases procainamide has failed to achieve control of the arrhythmia despite adequate dosage and the achievement of therapeutic levels in the fetus.[159,181]

Amiodarone

There are a few case reports of the use of amiodarone in the maternal treatment of fetal arrhythmias.[187,203,206] In one woman in whom control of the fetal tachycardia had not been achieved by digoxin, propranolol, lignocaine, and procainamide amiodarone was infused intravenously (900 mg) for 24 hours.[187] The following day two 5 mg intravenous boluses of verapamil achieved control of the heart rate, which was subsequently maintained by the combination of oral verapamil 240 mg/day and oral amiodarone (1200 mg/day). Reduction of the oral amiodarone to 200 mg/day after 20 days resulted in a steady rise in fetal heart rate which was controlled by increasing the dose back to 400 mg/day.

The fetus was successfully delivered at 33 weeks gestation and cardioverted from atrial flutter to sinus rhythm. Another report of the use of amiodarone described five cases in which amiodarone was given in doses of 800–1200 mg/day because fetal heart rate had not been controlled after 12–48 hours of digoxin treatment.[203] Two of the five fetuses converted to sinus rhythm after 5 days but the arrhythmia continued in the others. The precise duration of treatment and the impact of amiodarone on the concentrations of digoxin was not stated. Arnoux et al reported successful use of the combination of digoxin (0·25 mg/day) with amiodarone (1600 mg/day for 4 days, 1200 mg/day for 3 days and 800 mg/day for 6 weeks).[206] Fetal heart rate was controlled after 14 days. Digoxin alone and in combination with verapamil and sotalol had previously failed in this case. Wladimiroff et al reported the death two days after birth of a baby in whom amiodarone had successfully controlled the heart rate but hydrops had continued to worsen and elective caesarean section was done at 31 weeks.[159] Further details of amiodarone dosage were not given but digoxin, verapamil, procainamide, and propranolol had already failed in this case.

The major restriction on the use of amiodarone therapy in pregnancy is the development of fetal hypothyroidism from the large iodine load (see Chapter 22). This is sometimes associated with permanent retardation of psychomotor development even though thyroid replacement therapy is begun immediately.[207]

Flecainide

Use of flecainide to terminate a fetal tachycardia which presented at 28 weeks' gestation and was resistant to digoxin (which achieved therapeutic maternal levels) was first reported in 1988.[208] The tachycardia stopped abruptly after flecainide 110 mg had been infused over five minutes (Figure 19.3). Oral flecainide 300 mg daily was continued throughout the remainder of an uneventful pregnancy without recurrence of the arrhythmia. Other reports of successful second-line treatment with flecainide used oral doses of between 100 mg and 300 mg daily.[209–211] Smoleniec et al reported successful use of flecainide given as an infusion of 2 mg/kg over 30 minutes followed by 300 mg daily orally.[212] Fetal tachycardia ceased within 12 hours and the subsequent course of the pregnancy was uneventful. Ten cases of oral flecainide for supraventricular tachycardia were reported by van Engelen et al.[213] Daily dosage was 200–300 mg and arrhythmia was terminated in 5/5 (100%) of non-hydropic fetuses and 2/5 (40%) when hydrops was present. A single fetal death was reported after 3 days of flecainide treatment but cordocentesis had been performed within the previous 24 hours and may have been responsible.[214] Flecainide can cause hepatic damage in adults and a single case of conjugated hyperbilirubinaemia in a newborn after seven weeks of intrauterine flecainide treatment has been reported.[211]

Sotalol

There are isolated reports of sotalol use for fetal arrhythmias but despite its apparent safety in pregnancy it has yet to be formally evaluated.[215]

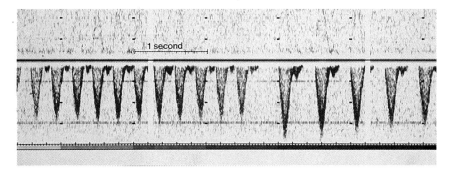

FIGURE 19.3—*Aortic flow pattern showing termination of fetal tachycardia after maternal administration of flecainide.*[208] *Reproduced with permission.*

Direct fetal drug administration

Most antiarrhythmic drugs achieve fetal:maternal concentration ratios of less than unity. Transplacental drug transfer may further be inhibited by the oedema associated with fetal hydrops. For this reason it may be impossible to achieve control of fetal arrhythmia by giving antiarrhythmic drugs to the mother. In these cases there may be a role for direct intramuscular or intraumbilical vein injections. Weiner *et al* reported the intramuscular administration of digoxin using ultrasound imaging to locate the injection site.[190] Fetal venous sampling enabled a digoxin half-life of 15·9 hours to be calculated and administration of 200 μg per day in divided doses led to control of arrhythmia. Because of the potential risks of frequent fetal dosing the injections were abandoned and spontaneous labour ensued at 39 weeks' gestation and a normal infant was born. The short half-life of digoxin also proved limiting in the other case report of direct treatment.[205]

The long tissue half-life of amiodarone might make it more suitable for direct treatment of the fetus and it has been given by cordocentesis in divided doses to a total of 21 mg over 3 weeks, achieving partial control of a resistant supraventricular arrhythmia.[216] The potential for disturbances in thyroid function means that it should be reserved for resistant life-threatening arrhythmias.

Adenosine is effective for the termination of maternal supraventricular arrhythmias but has no effect on the fetal heart rate because of its rapid metabolism within the maternal circulation.[38-41] Kohl *et al* reported the effectiveness of 0·2 mg/kg of adenosine given into the umbilical vein in terminating a supraventricular tachycardia in a fetus with hydrops.[217] Adenosine may allow short term control of the arrhythmia and improve transplacental passage of maternally administered long-acting anti-arrhythmic drugs.

Non-pharmacological manoeuvres

There are reports of successful termination of supraventricular arrhythmias by transabdominal compression of the fetal cephalic pole[218] or by compression of the umbilical cord under ultrasound guidance.[219] Such manoeuvres may allow short term control of arrhythmias.

Summary of management of fetal supraventricular tachyarrhythmias

In the absence of controlled trials of treatment of fetal supraventricular tachycardia no single strategy can be advocated as superior. When fetal tachycardia is identified accurate diagnosis by the use of ultrasound is imperative. Once a tachycardia has been identified it should be observed for one or two days to see if it is sustained or paroxysmal. Paroxysmal tachycardias can reasonably be monitored without treatment. If fetal hydrops develops the tachycardia should be treated. Sustained tachycardias should be treated unless the fetus is close to term when elective induction of labour or caesarean section may be considered. No single antiarrhythmic drug has emerged as pre-eminent in the treatment of supraventricular arrhythmias. Although the supraventricular arrhythmias can be subdivided into atrioventricular re-entrant arrhythmias, atrial flutter, and atrial fibrillation no clear guidelines can be given as to which antiarrhythmic drug may most appropriately be used for which arrhythmia. The volume of experience with digoxin means that it is still a reasonable choice as a first line agent but dosage must be monitored carefully to ensure maternal concentrations at the upper end of the therapeutic range. The effectiveness of digoxin appears to be considerably reduced in the presence of fetal hydrops and it may be appropriate to use flecainide or verapamil instead. In future sotalol may emerge as a safe and useful agent. If the first drug tried fails it is appropriate to change to a second agent and to use combinations of agents. Combinations with potential adverse effects on fetal ventricular function, such as beta-blockers and verapamil, should be avoided. Direct fetal administration of drugs should be reserved for those cases associated with hydrops in which tachycardia persists. In these circumstances, once the tachycardia is controlled delivery is appropriate when the fetus is sufficiently mature.

Fetal ventricular arrhythmias

Ventricular tachycardia in utero is unusual although there are sporadic reports of treatment with quinidine[220] or flecainide.[213] Ventricular tachycardia in neonates is often associated with other medical problems.[221] By contrast, ventricular extrasystoles causing irregularity of the pulse are more common, and less likely to be associated with other disease.[222]

Fetal bradycardias

Persistent fetal bradycardia is 10–20 times less common than supraventricular tachyarrhythmias. In a series of 113 cases of fetal arrhythmia detected over a five year period in six hospitals in southern Sweden only five had bradycardia.[223] Two of these had second-degree heart block and converted to sinus rhythm in utero, the remaining three had complete heart block. In a study of 12 fetuses presenting with bradycardia <100 bpm, 10 were found to have complete heart block and two had close coupled atrial extrasystoles.[224] Structural heart disease is more common in fetuses with heart block, and four of the 10 patients in this series had atrioventricular septal defects. In fetuses with structurally normal hearts there is a high incidence of maternal anti-SSA/Ro and anti-SSB/La antibodies, which may occur in association with Sjögren's syndrome (40%), systemic lupus erythematosus (25%) and rheumatoid arthritis (5%).[225,226] Over half of these patients have no clinical evidence of connective tissue disease although they may later develop it.

Steroids and plasmapheresis for the mother have been used in uncontrolled trials to prevent or treat fetal heart block with mixed success.[227–230] The feasibility of short term direct ventricular pacing in the fetus using a pacing wire placed through the maternal abdomen has been shown but it seems unlikely to be a practical method of managing fetal bradycardia for several weeks.[231,232] The major determinant of survival of neonates with heart block is the presence of structural cardiac disease; the mortality in this group is over 30%.[145] Factors which decide whether permanent pacing is required in the neonate are beyond the scope of this chapter but heart rate and other ECG features are important predictors of later mortality.[145,233] Despite the autoimmune nature of many of these cases of fetal heart block the incidence of recurrence in subsequent pregnancies is less than 10%.[234]

Summary

Rhythm disorders in pregnancy are a major challenge to the physician because of the need to balance the risks of the arrhythmia against the possible risks of treatment for the mother and the fetus. The relative rarity of serious arrhythmias during pregnancy means that there are few data to help rational decision making. Sensible management depends on accurate diagnosis of the arrhythmia, followed by consideration of all therapeutic options. Where possible strategies should be considered before rather than during pregnancy. All pregnant patients with significant arrhythmias should be referred to a cardiologist.

Fetal arrhythmias in the absence of congenital structural heart disease generally have a good prognosis but may require drugs to control the heart rate if hydrops develops. Interventional treatment for fetal arrhythmias is in its infancy and maternal antiarrhythmic drug treatment remains the mainstay of treatment. Careful selection of single or multiple antiarrhythmic drugs usually allows successful control of the arrhythmia.

References

1 Hunter S, Robson SC. Adaptation of the maternal heart in pregnancy. *Br Heart J* 1992; **68**: 540–3.
2 Turner AS, Watson OF, Adey HS, Cottle LP, Spence R. The prevalence of disturbance of cardiac rhythm in randomly selected New Zealand adults. *NZ Med J* 1981; **93**: 253–5.
3 Mant D, Villard-Mackintosh L, Vessey MP, Yeates D. Myocardial infarction and angina pectoris in young women. *J Epidemiol Community Health* 1987; **41**: 215–9.
4 Rodriguez L, de Chillou C, Schläpfer J, *et al.* Age at onset and gender of patients with different types of supraventricular tachycardias. *Am J Cardiol* 1992; **70**: 1213–15.
5 Michaëlsson M, Engle MA. Congenital complete heart block: an international study of the natural history. *Cardiovasc Clin* 1972; **4**: 86–101.
6 Reid JM, Coleman EN, Doig W. Complete congenital heart block. Report of 35 cases. *Br Heart J* 1982; **42**: 236–9.
7 *Reports on confidential enquiries into maternal deaths in England and Wales.* London: HMSO, 1979–1981, 1982–1984, 1985–1987, 1988–1990.
8 Widerhorn J, Widerhorn AL, Rahimtoola SH, Elkayam U. WPW syndrome during pregnancy: increased incidence of supraventricular arrhythmias. *Am Heart J* 1992; **123**: 796–8.
9 Mason JW, Winkle RA. Accuracy of the ventricular tachycardia-induction study for predicting long-term efficacy and inefficacy of antiarrhythmic drugs. *N Engl J Med* 1980; **303**: 1073–7.
10 Fogoros RN, Elson JJ, Bonnet CA, Fielder SB, Chenarides JG. Reproducibility of successful drug trials in patients with inducible sustained ventricular tachycardia. *PACE* 1992; **15**: 295–303.
11 Mason JW for the Electrophysiologic Study versus Electrocardiographic Monitoring Investigations. A comparison of electrophysiologic testing with Holter monitoring to predict antiarrhythmic-drug efficacy for ventricular tachyarrhythmias. *N Engl J Med* 1993; **329**: 445–51.
12 Calkins H, Nikalson L, Sousa J, El-Atassi R, Langberg J, Morady F. Radiation exposure during radiofrequency catheter ablation of accessory atrioventricular connections. *Circulation* 1991; **84**: 2376–82.
13 Lindsay BD, Eichling JO, Ambos D, Cain M. Radiation exposure to patients and medical personnel during radiofrequency catheter ablation for supraventricular tachycardia. *Am J Cardiol* 1992; **70**: 218–23.
14 Lee MS, Evans SJ, Blumberg S, Bodenheimer MM, Roth SL. Echocardiography guided electrophysiologic testing in pregnancy. *J Am Soc Echocardiogr* 1994; 7: 182–6.
15 Drinkovic N. Subcostal echocardiography to determine right ventricular pacing catheter position and control advancement of electrode catheters in intracardiac electrophysiologic studies. *Am J Cardiol* 1981; **47**: 1260–5.
16 Goldman AP, Irwin JM, Glover MU, Mick W. Transoesophageal echocardiography to improve positioning of radiofrequency ablation catheters in left-sided Wolff–Parkinson–White syndrome. *PACE* 1991; **14**: 1245–50.
17 Kerr MG, Scott DB, Samuel E. Studies of the inferior vena cava in late pregnancy. *BMJ* 1964; **1**: 532–3.
18 Marx GF. Cardiopulmonary resuscitation of late-pregnant women [letter]. *Anesthesiology* 1982; **56**: 156.
19 Depace NL, Betesh JS, Kotler MN. "Postmortem" cesarian section with recovery of both mother and offspring. *JAMA* 1982; **248**: 971–3.
20 Lindsay SL, Hanson GC. Cardiac arrest in near-term pregnancy. *Anaesthesia* 1987; **42**: 1074–7.
21 Rees GAD, Willis BA. Resuscitation in late pregnancy. *Anaesthesia* 1988; **43**: 347–9.
22 Goodwin APL, Pearce AJ. The human wedge. A manoeuvre to relieve aortocaval compression during resuscitation in late pregnancy. *Anaesthesia* 1992; **47**: 433–4.

23 European Resuscitation Council Working Party. Adult advanced cardiac life support: the European Resuscitation Council guidelines 1992 (abridged). *BMJ* 1993; **306**: 1589–93.

24 Selden BS, Burke TJ. Complete maternal and fetal recovery after prolonged cardiac arrest. *Ann Emerg Med* 1988; **17**: 346–9.

25 Finlay AY, Edmunds V. DC cardioversion in pregnancy. *Br J Clin Pract* 1979; **33**: 88–94.

26 Schroeder JS, Harrison DC. Repeated cardioversion during pregnancy. Treatment of refractory paroxysmal atrial tachycardia during 3 successive pregnancies. *Am J Cardiol* 1971; **27**: 445–6.

27 Grand A, Bernard J. Cardioversion and pregnancy. Fetal consequences. *La Nouvelle Presse Medicale* 1973; **2**: 2327–9.

28 Kuhn GJ, White BC, Swetnam RE, *et al*. Peripheral vs central circulation times during CPR: a pilot study. *Ann Emerg Med* 1981; **10**: 417–19.

29 Leonard RF, Braun TE, Levy AM. Initiation of uterine contractions by disopyramide during pregnancy. *N Engl J Med* 1978; **299**: 84–5

30 Wagner X, Jouglard J, Moulin M, Miller AM, Petitjean J, Pisapia A. Coadministration of flecainide acetate and sotalol during pregnancy: lack of teratogenic effects, passage across the placenta, and excretion in human breast milk. *Am Heart J* 1990; **119**: 700–2.

31 O'Hare MF, Murnaghan GA, Russell CJ, Leahey WJ, Varma MP, McDevitt DG. Sotalol as a hypotensive agent in pregnancy. *Br J Obstet Gynaecol* 1980; **87**: 814–20.

32 Griffith MJ, Linker NJ, Garratt CJ, Ward DE, Camm AJ. Relative efficacy and safety of intravenous drugs for termination of sustained ventricular tachycardia. *Lancet* 1990; **336**: 670–3.

33 Harvey JR, Wyman RM, McKay RG, Baim DS. Use of balloon flotation pacing catheters for prophylactic temporary pacing during diagnostic and therapeutic catheterization procedures. *Am J Cardiol* 1988; **62**: 941–4.

34 Oldroyd K, Rankin A, Rae A, Cobbe S. Pacing termination of spontaneous ventricular tachycardia in the coronary care unit. *Int J Cardiol* 1992; **36**: 223–6.

35 Advanced Life Support Group. *Advanced cardiac life support—the practical approach*. London: Chapman and Hall, 1993.

36 Garratt C, Linker N, Griffith M, Ward D, Camm AJ. Comparison of adenosine and verapamil for termination of paroxysmal junctional tachycardia. *Am J Cardiol* 1989; **64**: 1310–16.

37 McIntosh-Yellin N, Drew BJ, Scheinman MM. Safety and efficacy of central intravenous bolus administration of adenosine for termination of supraventricular tachycardia. *J Am Coll Cardiol* 1993; **22**: 741–5.

38 Harrison JK, Greenfield RA, Wharton JM. Acute termination of supraventricular tachycardia by adenosine during pregnancy. *Am Heart J* 1992; **123**: 1386–8.

39 Leffler S, Johnson DR. Adenosine use in pregnancy: lack of effect on fetal heart rate. *Am J Emerg Med* 1992; **10**: 548–9.

40 Afridi I, Moise KJ Jr, Rokey R. Termination of supraventricular tachycardia with intravenous adenosine in a pregnant woman with Wolff–Parkinson–White syndrome. *Obstet Gynecol* 1992; **80**: 481–3.

41 Podolsky SM, Varon J. Adenosine use during pregnancy. *Ann Emerg Med* 1991; **20**: 1027–8.

42 Klein V, Repke JT. Supraventricular tachycardia in pregnancy: cardioversion with verapamil. *Obstet Gynecol* 1984; **63**: 16S–18S.

43 Byerly WG, Hartmann A, Foster DE, Tannenbaum AK. Verapamil in the treatment of maternal paroxysmal supraventricular tachycardia. *Ann Emerg Med* 1991; **20**: 552–4.

44 Ornato JP, Hallagan LF, Reese WA, *et al*. Treatment of paroxysmal supraventricular tachycardia in the emergency department by clinical decision analysis. *Am J Emerg Med* 1988; **6**: 555–60.

45 Waxman MB, Wald RW, Sharma AD, Huerta F, Cameron DA. Vagal techniques for termination of paroxysmal supraventricular tachycardia. *Am J Cardiol* 1980; **46**: 655–64.

46 Mehta D, Wafa S, Ward DE, Camm AJ. Relative efficacy of various physical manoeuvres in the termination of junctional tachycardia. *Lancet* 1988; **i**: 1181–5.

47 Lesh MD, Van Hare GF, Epstein LM, *et al*. Radiofrequency catheter ablation of atrial arrhythmias. *Circulation* 1994; **89**: 1074–89.

48 Kadish A, Goldberger J. Ablative therapy for atrioventricular nodal reentry arrhythmias. [Review] *Prog Cardiovasc Dis* 1995; **37**: 273–93.

49 Manolis AS, Wang PJ, Estes NA 3rd. Radiofrequency ablation of left-sided accessory pathways: transaortic versus transseptal approach. *Am Heart J* 1994; **128**: 896–902.

50 Fischer B, Haissaguerre M, Garrigues S, *et al.* Radiofrequency catheter ablation of common atrial flutter in 80 patients. *J Am Coll Cardiol* 1995; **25**: 1365–72.
51 Bigger JT, Fleiss JL, Kleiger R, Miller JP, Rolnitzky LM. The relationships among ventricular arrhythmias, left ventricular dysfunction and mortality in the 2 years after myocardial infarction. *Circulation* 1984; **69**: 250–8.
52 Ruberman W, Weinblatt E, Goldberg JD, Frank CW, Chaudhary BS, Shapiro S. Ventricular premature complexes and sudden death after myocardial infarction. *Circulation* 1981; **64**: 297–305.
53 Russell RO Jr. Paroxysmal ventricula tachycardia associated with pregnancy. *Alabama Journal of Medical Sciences* 1969; **6**: 111–20.
54 Brodsky M, Doria R, Allen B, Sato D, Thomas G, Sada M. New-onset ventricular tachycardia during pregnancy. *Am Heart J* 1992; **123**: 933–41.
55 Braverman AC, Bromley BS, Rutherford JD. New onset ventricular tachycardia during pregnancy. *Int J Cardiol* 1991; **33**: 409–12.
56 Mont L, Seixas T, Brugada P, *et al.* The electrocardiographic, clinical, and electrophysiological spectrum of idiopathic monomorphic ventricular tachycardia. *Am Heart J* 1992; **124**: 746–53.
57 Okumura K, Matsuyama K, Miyagi H, Tsuchiya T, Yasue H. Entrainment of idiopathic ventricular tachycardia of left ventricular origin with evidence for reentry with an area of slow conduction and effect of verapamil. *Am J Cardiol* 1988; **62**: 727–32.
58 Gill JS, Hunter GJ, Gane J, Ward DE, Camm AJ. Asymmetry of cardiac [123] meta-iodobenzyl-guanidine scans in patients with ventricular tachycardia and "clinically normal" heart. *Br Heart J* 1993; **69**: 6–13.
59 Lemery R, Brugada P, Bella PD, Dugernier T, van den Dool A, Wellens HJJ. Nonischemic ventricular tachycardia; clinical course and long-term follow-up in patients without clinically overt heart disease. *Circulation* 1989; **79**: 990–9.
60 Yamamoto K, Bando S, Nishikado A, Ikefuji H, Shinohara A, Ito S. Two sudden death cases of idiopathic ventricular tachycardia. *Tokushima J Exp Med* 1992; **39**: 127–34.
61 Coggins DL, Lee RJ, Sweeney J, *et al.* Radiofrequency catheter ablation as a cure for idiopathic tachycardia of both left and right ventricular origin. *J Am Coll Cardiol* 1994; **23**: 1333–41.
62 Gill JS, Mehta D, Ward DE, Camm AJ. Efficacy of flecainide, sotalol and verapamil in the treatment of right ventricular tachycardia in patients without overt cardiac abnormality. *Br Heart J* 1992; **68**: 392–7.
63 Buxton AS, Marchlinski FE, Goherty JU, *et al.* Repetitive monomorphic ventricular tachycardia: clinical and electrophysiologic characteristics in patients with and patients without organic heart disease. *Am J Cardiol* 1984; **54**: 997–1002.
64 Brodsky MA, Allen BJ, Luckett CR, Capparelli EV, Wolff LJ, Henry WL. Antiarrhythmic effect of solitary beta-adrenergic blockade for patients with sustained ventricular tachyarrhythmias. *Am Heart J* 1989; **118**: 997–1002.
65 Brodsky M, Doria R, Allen B, Sato D, Thomas G, Sada M. New-onset ventricular tachycardia during pregnancy. *Am Heart J* 1992; **123**: 933–41.
66 Geibel A, Brugada P, Zehender M, Stevenson W, Waldecker B, Wellens HJ. Value of programmed electrical stimulation using a standardized ventricular stimulation protocol in hypertrophic cardiomyopathy. *Am J Cardiol* 1987; **60**: 738–9.
67 Alfonso F, Frenneaux M, McKenna WJ. Clinical sustained monomorphic ventricular tachycardia in hypertrophic cardiomyopathy. *Am J Cardiol* 1987; **60**: 738–9.
68 McKenna WJ, England D, Doi YL, Deanfield JE, Oakley CE, Goodwin JF. Arrhythmia in hypertrophic cardiomyopathy. 1. Influence on prognosis. *Br Heart J* 1981; **46**: 168–72.
69 Savage DD, Seides SF, Maron BJ, Myers DJ, Epstein SE. Prevalence of arrhythmia during 24-hour electrocardiographic monitoring and exercise testing in patients with obstructive and non obstructive hypertrophic cardiomyopathy. *Circulation* 1979; **59**: 866–75.
70 Maron BJ, Savage DD, Wolfson JK, Epstein SE. Prognostic significance of 24-hour ambulatory electrocardiography monitoring in patients with hypertrophic cardiomyopathy. A prospective study. *Am J Cardiol* 1981; **48**: 252–7.
71 McKenna WJ, Oakley CM, Krikler DM, Goodwin JF. Improved survival with amiodarone in patients with hypertrophic cardiomyopathy and ventricular tachycardia. *Br Heart J* 1985; **53**: 412–6.
72 Fananapazir L, Leon MB, Bonow RO, Tracy CM, Cannon RO, Epstein SE. Sudden death during empiric amiodarone therapy in symptomatic hypertrophic cardiomyopathy. *Am J Cardiol* 1991; **67**: 169–75.

274

73 Pelliccia F, Cianfrocca C, Gaudio C, Reale A. Sudden death during pregnancy in hypertrophic cardiomyopathy. *Eur Heart J* 1992; **13**: 421–3.

74 Shah DM, Sunderji SG. Hypertrophic cardiomyopathy and pregnancy: report of a maternal mortality and review of literature. *Obstet Gynecol Surv* 1985; **40**: 444–8.

75 Oakley GD, McGarry K, Limb DG, Oakley CM. Management of pregnancy in patients with hypertrophic cardiomyopathy. *BMJ* 1979; **1**: 1749–50.

76 McKennna W, Deanfield J, Faruqui A, England D, Oakley C, Goodwin J. Prognosis in hypertrophic cardiomyopathy: role of age and clinical electrocardiographic and hemodynamic features. *Am J Cardiol* 1981; **47**: 532–8.

77 Iesaka Y, Hiroe M, Aonuma K, *et al*. Usefulness of electrophysiologic study and endomyocardial biopsy in differentiating arrhythmogenic right ventricular dysplasia from idiopathic right ventricular tachycardia. *Heart Vessels* 1990; **5** (**suppl**): 65–9.

78 Blomstrom-Lundqvist C, Sabel KG, Olsson SB. A long term follow up of 15 patients with arrhythmogenic right ventricular dysplasia. *Br Heart J* 1987; **58**: 477–88.

79 Lemery R, Brugada P, Janssen J, Cheriex E, Dugernier T, Wellens HJ. Nonischemic sustained ventricular tachycardia: clinical outcome in 12 patients with arrhythmogenic right ventricular dysplasia. *J Am Coll Cardiol* 1989; **14**: 96–105.

80 Leclercq JF, Coumel P. Characteristics, prognosis and treatment of the ventricular arrhythmias of right ventricular dysplasia. *Eur Heart J* 1989; **10**: 61–7.

81 Koenig C, Katz M, Gertsch M, Schaer HM, Schneider H. Pregnancy and delivery in a patient with Uhl anomaly. *Obstet Gynecol* 1991; **78**: 932–4.

82 Francis GS. Should asymptomatic ventricular arrhythmias in patients with congestive heart failure be treated with antiarrhythmic drugs. *J Am Coll Cardiol* 1988; **12**: 274–83.

83 Packer M. Sudden unexpected death in patients with congestive heart failure: a second frontier. *Circulation* 1985; **72**: 681–5.

84 Ando S, Koyanagi S, Muramatsu K, Itaya R, Takeshita A, Nakamura M. Clinical characteristics of patients with dilated cardiomyopathy and bradyarrhythmias. *J Cardiol* 1991; **21**: 53–91.

85 Radhakrishnan S, Kaul U, Bahl VK, Talwar KK, Bhatia ML. Sudden bradyarrhythmic death in dilated cardiomyopathy: a case report. *PACE* 1988; **11**: 1369–72.

86 Olshausen KV, Stienen U, Schwarz F, Kubler W, Meyer JSO. Long-term prognostic significance of ventricular arrhythmias in idiopathic dilated cardiomyopathy. *Am J Cardiol* 1988; **61**: 146–51.

87 Kron J, Hart M, Schual-Berke S, Niles NR, Hosenpud JD, McAnulty JH. Idiopathic dilated cardiomyopathy. Role of programmed electrical stimulation and Holter monitoring in predicting those at risk of sudden death. *Chest* 1988; **93**: 85–90.

88 Keeling PJ, Kulakowski P, Yi G, Slade AKB, Bent SE, McKenna WJ. Usefulness of signal-averaged electrocardiogram in idiopathic dilated cardiomyopathy for identifying patients with ventricular arrhythmias. *Am J Cardiol* 1993; **72**: 78–84.

89 Liem LB, Swerdlow CD. Value of electropharmacologic testing in idiopathic dilated cardiomyopathy and sustained ventricular tachyarrhythmias. *Am J Cardiol* 1988; **62**: 611–6.

90 Rae AP, Spielman SR, Kutalek SP, Kay HR, Horowitz LN. Electrophysiologic assessment of antiarrhythmic drug efficacy for ventricular tachyarrhythmias associated with dilated cardiomyopathy. *Am J Cardiol* 1987; **59**: 291–5.

91 Kron J, Hart M, Schual-Berke S, Nile NR, Hosenpud JD, McAnulty JH. Idiopathic dilated cardiomyopathy. Role of programmed electrical stimulation and Holter monitoring in predicting those at risk of sudden cardiac death. *Chest* 1988; **93**: 85–90.

92 Willems AR, Tijssen JGP, van Cappelle FJL, *et al*. Determinants of prognosis in symptomatic ventricular tachycardia or ventricular fibrillation late after myocardial infarction. *J Am Coll Cardiol* 1990; **16**: 521–30.

93 Jervell A, Lange-Nielse F. Congenital deaf-mutism, functional heart disease with prolongation of the QT interval and sudden death. *Am Heart J* 1957; **54**: 59–68.

94 Garza LA, Vick RL, Nora JJ, McNamara DG. Heritable Q-T prolongation without deafness. *Circulation* 1970; **41**: 39–48.

95 The idiopathic long QT syndrome: pathogenetic mechanisms and therapy. *Eur Heart J* 1985; **6**: D103–D114.

96 Breithardt G, Witcher T, Haverkamp W, Borgrefe M, Block M, Hammel D. Implantable cardioverter defibrillator therapy in patients with arrhythmogenic right ventricular cardiomyopathy, long QT syndrome, or no structural heart disease. *Am Heart J* 1994; **127**: 1151–8.

97 Moss AJ, Liu JE, Gottlieb S, Locati EH, Schwartz PJ, Robinson JL. Efficacy of permanent pacing in the management of high-risk patients with the long QT syndrome. *Circulation* 1991; **84**: 1524–9.

98 O'Callaghan AC, Normandale JP, Morgan M. The prolonged QT syndrome: a review with anaesthetic implications and a report of two cases. *Anaesth Intensive Care* 1982; **10**: 50–5.

99 Ryan H. Anaesthesia for caesarean section in a patient with Jervell, Lange-Nielsen syndrome. *Can J Anaesth* 1988; **35**: 422–4.

100 Bruner JP, Barry MJ, Elliott JP. Pregnancy in a patient with idiopathic long QT syndrome. *Am J Obstet Gynecol* 1984; **149**: 690–1.

101 McCurdy CM Jr, Rutherford SE, Coddington CC. Syncope and sudden arrhythmic death complicating pregnancy. *J Reprod Med* 1993; **38**: 233–4.

102 Isaacs JD, Mulholland DH, Hess LW, Allbert JR, Martin RW. Pregnancy in a woman with an automatic implantable cardioverter-defibrillator. *J Reprod Med* 1993; **38**: 487–8.

103 Bwer M, Freeman LJ, Rickards AF, Rowland E. The automatic implantable cardioverter/defibrillator for a life threatening arrhythmia in a case of post-partum cardiomyopathy. *Postgrad Med J* 1989; **65**: 932–5.

104 Mendelson CL, Pardee HEB. The pulse and respiratory rate during labor as a guide to the onset of cardiac failure in women with rheumatic heart disease. *Am J Obstet Gynecol* 1942; **44**: 370–83.

105 Pradee HEB, Mendelson CL. The pulse and respiratory variations in normal women during labor. *Am J Obstet Gynecol* 1941; **41**: 36–44.

106 Tawam M, Levine J, Mendelson M, Goldberger J, Dyer A. Effect of pregnancy of paroxysmal supraventricular tachycardia. *Am J Cardiol* 1993; **72**: 838–40.

107 Manz M, Luderitz B. Supraventricular tachycardia and pre-excitation syndromes: pharmacological therapy. *Eur Heart J* 1993; **14**: 91–8.

108 Mendelson CL. Disorders of the heart beat during pregnancy. *Am J Obstet Gynecol* 1956; **72**: 1268–1301.

109 Rawles JM. What is meant by a "controlled" ventricular rate in atrial fibrillation? *Br Heart J* 1990; **63**: 157–61.

110 Smith TW. Digitalis. Mechanisms of action and clinical use. *N Engl J Med* 1988; **318**: 358–65.

111 Falk RH, Knowlton AA, Bernard SA, Gotlieb NE, Batinelli NJ. Digoxin for converting recent-onset atrial fibrillation to sinus rhythm. A randomized double-blind trial. *N Engl J Med* 1991; **325**: 1621–9.

112 Matsuda M, Matsuda Y, Tamagishi T, *et al.* Effects of digoxin, propranolol, and verapamil on exercise in patients with chronic isolated atrial fibrillation. *Cardiovasc Res* 1991; **25**: 453–7.

113 Ahuja RC, Sinha N, Saran RK, Jain AK, Hasan M. Digoxin or verapamil or metoprolol for heart rate control in patients with mitral stenosis—a randomised cross-over study. *Int J Cardiol* 1989; **25**: 325–31.

114 Khalsa A, Edvardsson N, Olsson SB. Effects of metoprolol on heart rate in patients with digitalis treated chronic atrial fibrillation. *Clin Cardiol* 1978; **1**: 91–5.

115 DiBianco R, Morganroth J, Freitag JA, Ronan JA Jr, Lindgren KM. Effects of nadolol on the spontaneous and exercise-provoked heart rate of patients with chronic atrial fibrillation receiving stable dosages of digoxin. *Am Heart J* 1984; **108**: 1121–7.

116 Lewis RV, McMurray J, McDevitt DG. Effects of atenolol, verapamil, and xamoterol on heart rate and exercise tolerance in digitalised patients with chronic atrial fibrillation. *J Cardiol Pharmacol* 1989; **13**: 1–6.

117 Lewis RV, Lakhani M, Moreland TA, McDevitt DG. A comparison of verapamil and digoxin in the treatment of atrial fibrillation. *Eur Heart J* 1987; **8**: 148–53.

118 Roth A, Harrison E, Mitani G, Cohen JD, Rahimtoola SH, Elkayam U. Efficacy and safety of medium- and high-dose diltiazem alone and in combination with digoxin for control of heart rate at rest and during exercise in patients with chronic atrial fibrillation. *Circulation* 1986; **73**: 316–24.

119 Wolf PA, Dawber TR, Thomas HE, Kannel WB. Epidemiological assessment of chronic atrial fibrillation and risk of stroke: the Framingham study. *Neurology* 1978; **28**: 973–7.

120 The Stroke Prevention in Atrial Fibrillation Investigators. Predictors of thromboembolism in atrial fibrillation. I. Clinical features of patients at risk. *Ann Intern Med* 1992; **116**: 1–5.

121 The Stroke Prevention in Atrial Fibrillation Investigators. Predictors of thromboembolism in atrial fibrillation. II. Echocardiographic features of patients at risk. *Ann Intern Med* 1992; **116**: 6–12.

122 Low-dose aspirin in prevention and treatment of intrauterine growth retardation and pregnancy-induced hypertension. *Lancet* 1993; **341**: 396–400.

123 Petersen P, Boysen G, Godtfredsen J, Andersen ED, Andersen B. Placebo-controlled randomised trial of warfarin and aspirin for prevention of thromboembolic complications in chronic atrial fibrillation. The Copenhagen AFASAK study. *Lancet* 1989; **1**: 175–9.

124 Anonymous. Stroke prevention in Atrial Fibrillation Study: final results. *Circulation* 1991; **84**: 527–39.

125 Bjerkelund CJ, Orning OM. The efficacy of anticoagulant therapy in preventing embolism related to DC electrical conversion of atrial fibrillation. *Am J Cardiol* 1969; **23**: 208–16.

126 Manning WJ, Silverman DI, Gordon SPF, Krumholz HM, Douglas PS. Cardioversion from atrial fibrillation without prolonged anticoagulation with use of transesophageal echocardiography to exclude the presence of atrial thrombi. *N Engl J Med* 1993; **328**: 750–5.

127 Manning WJ, Leeman DE, Gotch PJ, Come PC. Pulsed doppler evaluation of atrial mechanical function after electrical cardioversion of atrial fibrillation. *J Am Coll Cardiol* 1989; **13**: 617–23.

128 Black IW, Fatkin D, Sagar KB, Khandheria BK, Leung DY, Galloway JM. Exclusion of atrial thrombus by transesophageal echocardiography does not preclude embolism after cardioversion of atrial fibrillation. *Circulation* 1994; **89**: 2509–13.

129 Anderson JL, Gilert EM, Alpert BL, Henthorn RW, Waldo AL, Bhaudari AK. Prevention of symptomatic recurrences of paroxysmal atrial fibrillation in patients initially tolerating antiarrhythmic drug therapy. A multicenter, double-blind, crossover study of flecainide and placebo. *Circulation* 1989; **80**: 1557–70.

130 Rotmensch HH, Elkayam E. Antiarrhythmic drug therapy during pregnancy. *Ann Intern Med* 1983; **98**: 487–97.

131 Reimold SC, Cantillon CO, Friedman PL, Antman EM. Propafenone versus sotalol for suppression of recurrent symptomatic atrial fibrillation. *Am J Cardiol* 1993; **71**: 558–63.

132 Murgatroyd FD, O'Nunain S, Gibson SM, Poloniecki JD, Ward DE, Camm AJ. The results of CRAFT-I: a multi-center, double-blind, placebo-controlled crossover study of digoxin in symptomatic paroxysmal atrial fibrillation. *J Am Coll Cardiol* 1993; **21**: 478A.

133 Abramovici H, Faktor JH, Gonen Y, Brandes JM, Amikam S. Maternal permanent bradycardia: pregnancy and delivery. *Obstet Gynecol* 1984; **63**: 381–3.

134 Sneddon JF, Counihan PJ, Bashir Y, Haywood GA, Ward DE, Camm AJ. Impaired immediate vasoconstrictor responses in patients with recurrent neurally mediated syncope. *Am J Cardiol* 1993; **71**: 72–6.

135 Maloney JD, Jaeger FJ, Rizo-Patron C, Zhu DW. The role of pacing for the management of neurally mediated syncope: carotid sinus syndrome and vasovagal syncope. *Am Heart J* 1994; **127**: 1030–7.

136 Sneddon JF, Counihan PJ, Bashir Y, Haywood GA, Ward DE, Camm AJ. Assessment of autonomic function in patients with neurally mediated syncope: augmented cardiopulmonary baroreceptor responses to graded orthostatic stress. *J Am Coll Cardiol* 1993; **21**: 1193–8.

137 Fitzpatrick A, Theodorakis G, Vardas P, *et al.* The incidence of malignant vasovagal syndrome in patients with recurrent syncope. *Eur Heart J* 1991; **12**: 389–94.

138 Mendelson CL. *Cardiac disease in pregnancy.* Philadelphia: Davis, 1960.

139 McCue CM, Mantakas ME, Tingelstad JB, Ruddy S. Congenital heart block in newborns of mothers with connective tissue disease. *Circulation* 1977; **56**: 82–90.

140 Michaelson M, Engle MA. Congenital complete heart block: an international study of the natural history. *Cardiovasc Clin* 1972; **4**: 85–101.

141 Odemuyiwa O, Camm J. Prophylactic pacing for prevention of sudden death in congenital complete heart block? *PACE* 1992; **15**: 1526–30.

142 Karpawich PP, Gillette PC, Garson A Jr, Hesslein PS, Porter C, McNamara DG. Congenital complex atrioventricular block: clinical and electrophysiological predictions of need for pacemaker insertion. *Am J Cardiol* 1981; **48**: 1098–1102.

143 Epstein JR, Altman HE. Heart block in pregnancy. *Medical Annals of the District of Columbia* 1951; **20**: 6660–3.

144 Kenmure ACF, Cameron AJV. Congenital complete heart block in pregnancy. *Br Heart J* 1967; **29**: 910–12.

145 Esscher E. Congenital complete heart block. *Acta Paediatr Scand* 1981; **70**: 131–6.
146 Dalvi BV, Chaudhuri A, Kulkarni HL, Kale PA. Therapeutic guidelines for congenital complete heart block presenting in pregnancy. *Obstet Gynecol* 1992; **79**: 802–4.
147 Ramsewak S, Persad P, Perkins S, Narayansingh G. Twin pregnancy in a patient with complete heart block. *Clin Exp Obstet Gynecol* 1992; **19**: 166–7.
148 Gudal M, Kervancioglu C, Oral D, Gurel T, Erol C, Sonel A. Permanent pacemaker implantation in a pregnant woman with the guidance of ECG and two-dimensional echocardiography. *PACE* 1987; **10**: 543–5.
149 Jordaens LJ, Vancenbogaerde JF, Van de Bruaene P, De Buyzere M. Transesophageal echocardiography for insertion of a physiological pacemaker in early pregnancy. *PACE* 1990; **13**: 955–7.
150 Lau CP, Lee CP, Wong CK, Cheng CH, Leung WH. Rate responsive pacing with a minute ventilation sensing pacemaker during pregnancy and delivery. *PACE* 1990; **13**: 158–63.
151 Eddy WA, Frankenfeld RH. Congenital complete heart block in pregnancy. *Am J Obstet Gynecol* 1977; **128**: 223–5.
152 Amikam S, Abramovici H, Brandes JM, Peleg H, Riss E. Pregnancy in the presence of an implanted pacemaker. *Int Surg* 1981; **66**: 369–71.
153 Laurens P, Haiat R, Gavelle P, Maurice P, Chiche P. Isotope cardiac pacemaker during pregnancy. *Nouvelle Presse Medicale* 1976; **5**: 2997–3000.
154 Matorras R, Diez J, Saez M, Montoya F, Aranguren G, Rodriguez-Escudero FJ. Repeat pregnancy associated with cardiac pacemaker. *Int J Gynaecol Obstet* 1991; **36**: 323–7.
155 Jaffe R, Gruber A, Fejgin M, Altaras M, Ben-Aderet N. Pregnancy with an artificial pacemaker. *Obstet Gynecol Surv* 1987; **42**: 137–9.
156 Berestka SA, Spellacy WN. Complete heart block associated with pregnancy and treated with an internal pacemaker. *Lancet* 1967; **87**: 461–3.
157 Ginns HM, Hollinrake K. Complete heart block in pregnancy treated with an internal cardiac pacemaker. *Journal of Obstetrics & Gynaecology of the British Commonwealth* 1970; **77**: 710–12.
158 British Pacing and Electrophysiology Group. Recommendations for pacemaker prescription for symptomatic bradycardia. *Br Heart J* 1991; **66**: 185–91.
159 Wladimiroff JW, Stewart PA. Treatment of fetal cardiac arrhythmias. *Br J Hosp Med* 1985; **34**: 134–40.
160 Rajadurai VS, Menahem S. Fetal arrhythmias: a 3-year experience. *Aust NZ J Obstet Gynaecol* 1992; **32**: 28–31.
161 Elkayam U, Gleicher N. *Cardiac problems in pregnancy. Diagnosis and management of maternal and fetal disease.* New York: Alan R Liss, 1982: 535–64.
162 Shenker L. Fetal electrocardiography. *Obstet Gynecol Surv* 1966; **21**: 367–88.
163 Fyfe DA, Meyer KB, Case CL. Sonographic assessment of fetal cardiac arrhythmias. *Semin Ultrasound CT MRI* 1993; **14**: 286–97.
164 Chan FY, Woo SK, Ghosh A, Tang M, Lam C. Prenatal diagnosis of congenital fetal arrhythmias by simultaneous pulsed doppler velocimetry of the fetal abdominal aorta and inferior vena cava. *Obstet Gynecol* 1990; **76**: 200–5.
165 Maxwell DJ, Crawford DC, Curry PV, Tynan MJ, Allan LD. Obstetric importance, diagnosis, and management of fetal tachycardias. *BMJ* 1988; **297**: 107–10.
166 Stewart PA, Tonge HM, Wladimiroff JW. Arrhythmia and structural abnormalities of the fetal heart. *Br Heart J* 1983; **50**: 550–4.
167 Allan LD, Crawford DC, Anderson RH, Tynan M. Evaluation and treatment of fetal arrhythmias. *Clin Cardiol* 1984; **7**: 467–73.
168 Wedemeyer AL, Breitfeld V. Cardiac neoplasm, tachyarrhythmia, and anasarca in an infant. *American Journal of Diseases of Children* 1975; **129**: 738–41.
169 Clements J, Sobotka-Plojhar M, Exalto N, van Geijn HP. A connective tissue membrane in the right atrium (Chiari's network) as a cause of fetal cardiac arrhythmia. *Am J Obstet Gynecol* 1982; **142**: 709–12.
170 Belhassen B, Pauzner D, Blieden L, Sherez J, Zinger A, David M. Intrauterine and postnatal atrial fibrillation in the Wolff–Parkinson–White syndrome. *Circulation* 1982; **66**: 1124–8.
171 Clinical and electrophysiologic features of fetal and neonatal paroxysmal atrial tachycardia resulting in congestive heart failure. *Am J Cardiol* 1988; **62**: 225–8.
172 Valerius NH, Jacobsen JR. Intrauterine supraventricular tachycardia. *Acta Obstet Gynecol Scand* 1978; **57**: 407–10.

173 Newburger JW, Keane JF. Intrauterine supraventricular tachycardia. *J Pediat* 1979; **95**: 780–6.
174 Lingman G, Ohrlander S, Ohlin P. Intrauterine digoxin treatment of fetal paroxysmal tachycardia. *Br J Obstet Gynaecol* 1980; **87**: 340–2.
175 Kerenyi TD, Gleicher N, Meller J, Brown E, Steinfeld L, Chitkara U. Transplacental cardioversion of intrauterine supraventricular tachycardia with digitalis. *Lancet* 1980; **ii**: 393–4.
176 Harrigan JT, Kangos JJ, Sikka A, Spisso KR, Natarajan N, Rosenfeld D. Successful treatment of fetal congestive heart failure secondary to tachycardia. *N Engl J Med* 1981; **304**: 1527–9.
177 Heaton FC, Vaughan R. Intrauterine supraventricular tachycardia: cardioversion with maternal digoxin. *Obstet Gynecol* 1982; **60**: 749–52.
178 Gembruch U, Venn HJ, Redel DA, Hansmann M. Wolff–Parkinson–White syndrome with paroxysmal supraventricular tachycardias of the fetus and the newborn. *Klin Pädiatr* 1982; **194**: 320–3.
179 King CR, Mattioli L, Goertz KK, Snodgrass W. Successful treatment of fetal supraventricular tachycardia with maternal digoxin therapy. *Chest* 1984; **85**: 573–5.
180 Allan LD, Crawford DC, Anderson RH, Tynan M. Evaluation and treatment of fetal arrhythmias. *Clin Cardiol* 1984; **7**: 467–73.
181 Kleinman CS, Copel JA, Weinstein EM, Santulli TV Jr, Hobbins JC. Treatment of fetal supraventricular tachyarrhythmias. *J Clin Ultrasound* 1985; **13**: 265–73.
182 Hicks JM, Brett EM. Falsely increased digoxin concentrations in samples from neonates and infants. *Ther Drug Monit* 1984; **6**: 461–4.
183 Schlebusch H, von Mende S, Grunn U, Gembruch U, Bald R, Hansmann M. Determination of digoxin in the blood of pregnant women, fetuses and neonates before and during anti-arrhythmic therapy, using four immunochemical methods. *Eur J Clin Chem Clin Biochem* 1991; **29**: 57–66.
184 Weaver JB, Pearson JF. Influence of digitalis on time of onset and duration of labour in women with cardiac disease. *BMJ* 1973; **iii**: 519–20.
185 Wolff F, Breuker KH, Schlensker KH, Bolte A. Prenatal diagnosis and therapy of fetal heart rate anomalies: with a contribution on the placental transfer of Verapamil. *J Perin Med* 1980; **8**: 203–8.
186 Lilja H, Karlsson K, Lindecrantz K, Sabel KG. Treatment of intrauterine supraventricular tachycardia with digoxin and verapamil. *J Perinat Med* 1984; **12**: 151–4.
187 Rey E, Duperron L, Gauthier R, Lemay M, Grignon A, LeLorier J. Transplacental treatment of tachycardia-induced fetal heart failure with verapamil and amiodarone: a case report. *Am J Obstet Gynecol* 1985; **153**: 311–2.
188 Truccone N, Mariona F. Intrauterine conversion of fetal supraventricular tachycardia with combination of digoxin and verapamil. *Pediatric Pharmacology* 1985; **5**: 149–53.
189 Owen J, Colvin EV, Davis RO. Fetal death after successful conversion of fetal supraventricular tachycardia with digoxin and verapamil. *Am J Obstet Gynecol* 1988; **158**: 1169–70.
190 Weiner CP, Thompson MIV. Direct treatment of fetal supraventricular tachycardia after failed transplacental therapy. *Am J Obstet Gynecol* 1988; **158**: 1169–70.
191 Klein V, Repke JT. Supraventricular tachycardia in pregnancy: cardioversion with verapamil. *Obstet Gynecol* 1984; **63**: 16S–18S.
192 Byerly WG, Hartmann A, Foster DE, Tannenbaum AK. Verapamil in the treatment of maternal paroxysmal supraventricular tachycardia. *Ann Emerg Med* 1991; **20**: 552–4.
193 Brittinger WD, Schwarzbeck A, Wittenmeier KW, *et al.* [Clinical experimental studies on the blood pressure reducing effect of verapamil]. *Dtsch Med Wochenschr* 1970; **95**: 1871–7.
194 Rodriguez-Escudero FJ, Aranguren G, Benito JA. Verapamil to inhibit the cardiovascular side effects of ritodrine. *Int J Gynaecol Obstet* 1981; **19**: 333–6.
195 Langer A, Hung CT, McA'nulty JA, Harrigan JT, Washington E. Adrenergic blockade: a new approach to hyperthyroidism during pregnancy. *Obstet Gynecol* 1974; **44**: 181–6.
196 Cottrill CM, McAllister RG Jr, Gettes L, Noonan JA. Propranolol therapy during pregnancy labor and delivery: evidence for transplacental drug transfer and impaired neonatal drug disposition. *J Pediatr* 1977; **91**: 812–4.
197 Teuscher A, Bossi E, Imhof P, Erb E, Stocker FP, Weber JW. Effect of propranolol on fetal tachycardia in diabetic pregnancy. *Am J Cardiol* 1978; **42**: 304–7.

279

198 Taylor EA, Turner P. Anti-hypertensive therapy with propranolol during pregnancy and lactation. *Postgrad Med J* 1981; **57**: 427–30.

199 Erkkola R, Lammintausta R, Liukko P, Anttila M. Transfer of propranolol and sotalol across the human placenta. *Acta Obstet Gynecol Scand* 1982; **61**: 31–4.

200 Eibschitz I, Abinader EG, Klein A, Sharf M. Intrauterine diagnosis and control of fetal ventricular arrhythmia during labor. *Am J Obstet Gynecol* 1975; **122**: 597–600.

201 Dumesic DA, Silverman NH, Tobias S, Golbus MS. Transplacental cardioversion of fetal supraventricular tachycardia with procainamide. *N Engl J Med* 1982; **307**: 1128–31.

202 Vintzileos AM, Campbell WA, Soberman SM, Nochimson DJ. Fetal atrial flutter and X-linked dominant vitamin D-resistant rickets. *Obstet Gynecol* 1985; **65**: 39S–44S.

203 Azancot-Benisty A, Jacqz-Aigrain E, Guirgis NM, Decrepy A, Oury JF. Clinical and pharmacologic study of fetal supraventricular tachyarrhythmias. *J Pediatr* 1992; **121**: 608–13.

204 Given BD, Phillippe M, Sanders SP, Dzau VJ. Procainamide cardioversion of fetal supraventricular tachyarrhythmia. *Am J Cardiol* 1984; **53**: 1460–1.

205 Hallak M, Neerhof MG, Perry R, Nazir M, Huhta JC. Fetal supraventricular tachycardia and hydrops fetalis: combined intensive, direct, and transplacental therapy. *Obstet Gynecol* 1991; **78**: 523–5.

206 Arnoux P, Seyral P, Llurens M, *et al.* Amiodarone and digoxin for refractory fetal tachycardia. *Am J Cardiol* 1987; **59**: 166–7.

207 Plomp TA, Vulsma T, de Vildjer JJM. Use of amiodarone during pregnancy. *Eur J Obstet Gynecol Reprod Biol* 1992; **43**: 201–7.

208 Wren C, Hunter S. Maternal administration of flecainide to terminate and suppress fetal tachycardia. *BMJ* 1988; **296**: 249.

209 Kofinas AD, Simon NV, Sagel H, Lyttle E, Smith N, King K. Treatment of fetal supraventricular tachycardia with flecainide acetate after digoxin failure. *Am J Obstet Gynecol* 1991; **165**: 630–1.

210 Perry JC, Ayres NA, Carpenter RJ Jr. Fetal supraventricular tachycardia treated with flecainide acetate. *J Pediatr* 1991; **118**: 303–5.

211 Vanderhal AL, Cocjin J, Santulli TV Jr, Carlson DE, Rosenthal P. Conjugated hyperbilirubinemia in a newborn infant after maternal (transplacental) treatment with flecainide acetate for fetal tachycardia and fetal hydrops. *J Pediatr* 1995; **126**: 988–90.

212 Smoleniec JS, Martin R, James DK. Intermittent fetal tachycardia and fetal hydrops. *Arch Dis Child* 1991; **66**: 1160–1.

213 van Engelen AD, Weijtens O, Brenner JI, Kleinman CS, Copel JA. Management outcome and follow-up of fetal tachycardia. *J Am Coll Cardiol* 1994; **24**: 1371–5.

214 Allan LD, Chita SK, Sharland GK, Maxwell D, Priestley K. Flecainide in the treatment of fetal tachycardias. *Br Heart J* 1991; **65**: 46–8.

215 Meden H, Neeb U. Transplacental cardioversion of fetal supraventricular tachycardia using sotalol. *Z Geburtshilfe Perinatol* 1990; **194**: 182–4.

216 De Catte L, De Wolf D, Smitz J, Bougatef A, de Schepper J, Foulon W. Hypothyroidism as a complication of amiodarone treatment for persistent fetal supraventricular tachycardia. *Prenat Diagn* 1994; **14**: 762–5.

217 Kohl T, Tercanli S, Kececioglu D, Holzgreve W. Direct fetal administration of adenosine for the termination of incessant supraventricular tachycardia. *Obstet Gynecol* 1995; **85**: 873–4.

218 Fernandez C, De Rosa GE, Guevara E, Velazquez H, Pueyrredon HR. Reversion by vagal reflex of a fetal paroxysmal atrial tachycardia detected by echocardiography. *Am J Obstet Gynecol* 1988; **159**: 860–1.

219 Martin CB Jr, Nijhuis JG, Weijer AA. Correction of fetal supraventricular tachycardia by compression of the umbilical cord: report of a case. *Am J Obstet Gynecol* 1984; **150**: 324–6.

220 Sherer DM, Sadovsky E, Menashe M, Mordel N, Rein AJ. Fetal ventricular tachycardia associated with nonimmunologic hydrops fetalis. *J Reprod Med* 1990; **35**: 292–4.

221 Stevens DC, Schreiner RL, Hurwitz RA, Gresham EL. Fetal and neonatal ventricular arrhythmia. *Pediatrics* 1979; **63**: 771–7.

222 Lingman G, Lundstrom NR, Marsal K. Clinical outcome and circulatory effects of fetal cardiac arrhythmia. *Acta Paediatr Scand* 1986; **329 (suppl)**: 120–6.

223 Lingman G, Lundstrom NR, Marsal K, Ohrlander S. Fetal cardiac arrhythmia. *Acta Obstet Gynecol Scand* 1986; **65**: 263–7.

224 Crawford D, Chapman M, Allan L. The assessment of persistent bradycardia in prenatal life. *Br J Obstet Gynaecol* 1985; **92**: 941–4.
225 Scott JS, Maddison PJ, Taylor PV, Esscher E, Scott O, Skinner RP. Connective-tissue disease, antibodies to ribonucleoprotein, and congenital heart block. *N Engl J Med* 1983; **309**: 209–12.
226 Buyon JP, Ben-Chetrit E, Karp S, *et al.* Acquired congenital heart block. *J Clin Invest* 1989; **84**: 627–34.
227 Buyon JP, Waltuck J, Kleinman C, Copel J. In utero identification and therapy of congenital heart block. *Lupus* 1995; **4**: 116–21.
228 Ishimaru S, Izaki S, Kitamura K, Morita Y. Neonatal lupus erythematosus: dissolution of atrioventricular block after administration of corticosteroid to the pregnant mother. *Dermatology* 1994; **189**: 92–4.
229 Chua S, Ostman-Smith I, Sellers S, Redman CW. Congenital heart block with hydrops fetalis treated with high-dose dexamethasone; a case report. *Eur J Obstet Gynecol Reprod Biol* 1991; **42**: 155–8.
230 Watson WJ, Katz VL. Steroid therapy for hydrops associated with antibody-mediated congenital heart block. *Am J Obstet Gynecol* 1991; **165**: 553–4.
231 Carpenter RJ Jr, Strasburger JF, Garson A Jr, Smith RT, Deter RL. Fetal ventricular pacing for hydrops secondary to complete atrioventricular block. *J Am Coll Cardiol* 1986; **8**: 1434–6.
232 Walkinshaw SA, Welch CR, McCormack J, Walsh K. In utero pacing for fetal congenital heart block. *Fetal Diagn Ther* 1994; **9**: 183–5.
233 Sholler GF, Walsh EP. Congenital complete heart block in patients without anatomical cardiac defects. *Am Heart J* 1989; **118**: 1193–8.
234 Julkunen H, Kaaja R, Wallgren E, Teramo K. Isolated congenital heart block: fetal and infant outcome and familial incidence of heart block. *Obstet Gynecol* 1993; **82**: 11–6.
235 McMillan TM, Bellet S. Ventricular paroxysmal tachycardia: report of a case in a pregnant girl of sixteen years with an apparently normal heart. *Am Heart J* 1931; 7: 70–8.
236 Peters CM, Penner SL. Orthostatic paroxysmal ventricular tachycardia. *Am Heart J* 1946; **32**: 645–52.
237 Hair TE, Eagen JT, Orgain ES. Paroxysmal ventricular tachycardia. *Am J Cardiol* 1962; **9**: 209–14.
238 Adams CW. Functional paroxysmal ventricular tachycardia. *Am J Cardiol* 1962; **9**: 215–22.
239 Rally CR, Walters MB. Paroxysmal ventricular tachycardia without evident heart disease. *Can Med Assoc J* 1962; **86**: 268–73.
240 Pine HL, Fox L, Shook DM. Paroxysmal ventricular tachycardia complicating pregnancy. *Am J Cardiol* 1965; **15**: 732–4.
241 Gettes LS, Surawicz B. Long-term prevention of paroxysmal arrhythmias with propranolol therapy. *Am J Med Sci* 1967; **254**: 257–65.
242 Russell RO. Paroxysmal ventricular tachycardia associated with pregnancy. *Alabama Journal of Medical Science* 1969; **6**: 111–20.
243 Reed RL, Cheney CB, Fearon RE, Hook R, Hehre FW. Propranolol therapy throughout pregnancy: a case report. *Anesth Analg* 1974; **53**: 214–18.
244 Timmis AD, Jackson G, Holt DW. Mexiletine for control of ventricular dysrhythmias in pregnancy. *Lancet* 1980; **2**: 647–8.
245 Alpert BS, Boineau J, Strong WB. Exercise-induced ventricular tachycardia. *Pediatr Cardiol* 1982; **2**: 21–55.
246 Menon KPS, Mahapatra RK. Paroxysmal ventricular tachycardia associated with Bell's palsy in a teenager at late pregnancy. *Angiology* 1984; **35**: 534–6.
247 Brodsky MA, Sato DA, Oster PD, Schmidt PS, Chesnie BM, Henry WL. Paroxysmal ventricular tachycardia with syncope during pregnancy. *Am J Cardiol* 1986; **58**: 563–4.
248 Vlay SC. Catecholamine-sensitive ventricular tachycardia. *Am Heart J* 1987; **114**: 455–61.
249 Connaughton M, Jenkins BS. Successful use of flecainide to treat new onset maternal ventricular tachycardia in pregnancy. *Br Heart J* 1994; **72**: 297.
250 Chandra NC, Gates EA, Thamer M. Conservative treatment of paroxysmal ventricular tachycardia during pregnancy. *Clin Cardiol* 1991; **14**: 347–50.

20: Pulmonary embolism

CELIA OAKLEY

After hypertension pulmonary thromboembolism is the leading cause of maternal death during pregnancy and the puerperium,[1] the death rate being between 2 and 4/100 000 vaginal deliveries and 18 to 36/100 000 caesarean sections.[2] Pregnancy results in both a hypercoagulable state[3] and venous stasis.[4] During the last trimester blood flow to the legs is reduced in the supine or sitting position because of compression of the abdominal aorta and inferior cava by the uterus.[6] Flow is additionally reduced after engagement of the fetal head. Hormonally induced reduction in venous tone causes venous dilatation and further slows the rate of blood flow from the legs.[7] The reported incidence of thromboembolic events has been as high as 1 in 70 pregnancies.[5,6]

Early papers suggested that 20% of non-pregnant patients with deep vein thrombosis went on to have pulmonary emboli if they were not treated with anticoagulants[8] and that untreated pulmonary embolism in pregnancy had a 13% mortality which could be reduced to 1% with treatment.[9] Unfortunately the diagnosis of pulmonary embolism is all too frequently missed. Although it should be high on the list of causes of dyspnoea and cardiovascular collapse, it may occur unexpectedly during pregnancy or more often postpartum. Pulmonary embolism is particularly likely in women treated by bed rest because of pre-eclampsia or following delivery by caesarean section and the incidence continues to be higher than during the pregnancy for the first six weeks after delivery. This risk has been estimated to be nearly 50 times higher during pregnancy and the puerperium than outside it in healthy women.[5,10]

Predisposing factors

Although there are good reasons for pulmonary embolism to complicate pregnancy or the puerperium, it is important to check whether patients also have an inherited or acquired coagulopathy in addition to that caused by the pregnancy. Deficiencies of antithrombin III, protein C, or protein S or the presence of antiphospholipid antibodies may have been responsible and should be identified.[3,11] Blood should be taken for this purpose before warfarin is started. Women with inherited coagulopathies are likely to have a family history of thromboembolic events (either venous or systemic) in young people particularly during pregnancy and if this is found the woman should remain on warfarin treatment for life. The child too should be tested in due course.

Clinical symptoms

The cardiovascular response to pulmonary embolism depends upon the extent to which the circulation through the lungs is obstructed, whether the patients had pre-existing cardiac or pulmonary disease, and probably also upon the release of platelet-derived vasoconstrictor agents from the emboli. It is usually marked by the sudden onset of dyspnoea and tachycardia which may be followed rapidly by collapse and death.[11–13] Chest pain is uncommon unless there is pulmonary infarction with pleurisy, but massive central pulmonary embolism may cause myocardial ischaemia from a combination of tachycardia, hypoxaemia, and hypotension.

Shortness of breath caused by pulmonary embolism may also develop more insidiously and be attributed mistakenly to the pregnancy or to panic. The patient may have had transient syncope or haemoptysis or pleuritic pain caused by infarction. Minor breathlessness may be caused by peripheral pulmonary embolism. The rapid passage of embolic material from the central pulmonary arteries to the periphery may result in syncope followed by recovery or the first embolus may be followed by massive pulmonary embolism causing collapse, right ventricular dilatation, and death or low output failure. Early studies showed that two thirds of fatal cases of pulmonary embolism died within an hour of the onset of symptoms.[14] Most deaths are caused by delay in establishing the diagnosis and in instituting effective treatment. There is no time to lose.

Massive pulmonary embolism

Tachypnoea is usually striking unless the patient is close to death. The venous pressure, although raised, may be difficult to observe because of the strenuous respiratory efforts or because the patient is supine on account of hypotension. A third heart sound gallop is prominent but the pulmonary closure sound is soft or absent (not accentuated as is usually stated) because the raised ventricular diastolic pressure usually equals the pulmonary artery diastolic pressure (Figure 20.1). More than two thirds of the lung circulation must be occluded to cause right ventricular failure in a previously healthy person. The embolic material may lodge in the central pulmonary arteries and a sudden loss of cardiac output follows inability of the right ventricle to pass blood beyond the obstruction. The unprepared right ventricle can rarely raise its systolic pressure higher than 50 or 60 mm Hg and its diastolic pressure may rise to 20 or 30 mm Hg with similar pressure in the right atrium and pulmonary artery. If the circulation fails the pulmonary artery pressure may not be even as high as this. The patient may collapse with no detectable output but the ECG often continues in sinus rhythm—electromechanical dissociation.

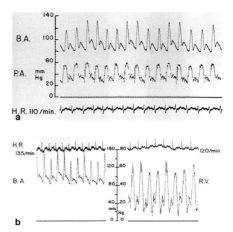

FIGURE 20.1—*(a) Simultaneously recorded brachial (BA) and pulmonary artery (PA) pressures from a patient with massive pulmonary embolism. The brachial pressure is well maintained at about 120/80 but is ill sustained with a narrow base indicating a low stroke volume and there is pulsus paradoxus from acute dilatation of the right heart chambers. The pulmonary artery pressure is raised at 55/30. (b) The "spiky" brachial artery (BA) pressure and the right ventricular (RV) pressure whose diastolic pressure is greatly raised and similar to that in the pulmonary artery.*

TABLE 20.1—*Massive pulmonary embolism: emergency measures to save life.*

- Elevate legs
- Give oxygen
- Chest compression (if patient unconscious)
- Full cardiopulmonary resuscitation (if respiratory efforts have ceased)
- Intravenous fluids
- Heparin
- Mechanical clot dispersion by catheter

The arterial pulse is rapid and transient (Figure 20.1). Intense vasoconstriction may maintain blood pressure, obscuring the low stroke volume, but the blood pressure may collapse if the patient is sat up. The increase in physiological dead space plus a vagal drive to breathe is responsible for the increased respiratory effort which results in alveolar hyperventilation and a reduced PCO_2. The lungs are strikingly clear to auscultation.

In subacute massive embolism the clinical presentation may be far from dramatic despite dyspnoea, a history of syncope, and right ventricular failure. It is still all too often missed.

The arterial blood gases in patients with massive or major pulmonary embolism show hypoxaemia with reduced PCO_2 and a normal pH. The ECG may appear "normal" immediately although comparison with later records after recovery may show a shift of the axis inferiorly and posteriorly with the well known "Q3T3" pattern, S waves as far as V7 and often an RSR in V1 all caused by right ventricular dilatation. T wave inversion in the right chest leads is often not apparent on the first ECG but may appear later as the patient recovers (Figure 20.2). Sinus rhythm is usually maintained. Sinus bradycardia is sometimes an agonal event. A chest radiograph may be unhelpful except by excluding tension pneumothorax or collapse of a lung because of often poor quality caused by exaggerated respiratory movement in patients too ill to be properly positioned for short distance antero-posterior films taken with portable sets. If a good film is obtained it will probably already show dilatation of the main pulmonary artery ("conus") and right atrium and the lung fields may show widespread oligemia contrasting with sparse well perfused segments. A "herald" infarct seen as a wedge-shaped peripheral opacity is a classic sign though rarely seen.

Echocardiography provides the quickest confirmation of pulmonary embolism as it immediately identifies the dilated and almost immobile right ventricle bulging towards a small vigorously contracting left ventricle.[15] The ventricular septum buckles towards the left ventricle in diastole (Figure 20.3). Continuous wave Doppler shows a peak velocity of the tricuspid regurgitant jet which is usually >2·5 m/sec, unless the patient is moribund when it may be less. It is rarely much higher in truly acute cases without previous emboli or pulmonary disease. Central pulmonary emboli may be seen on transoesophageal echocardiography but the indirect evidence given by the distended right ventricle shown on transthoracic echocardiography is sufficient for initiation of treatment. Rarely, coiled emboli, caught within the right atrium are seen swirling round and often entering the tricuspid valve as it opens only to be thrown back as it closes. Thrombi may also be visualised in the right ventricle or main pulmonary arteries. This is not an indication for immediate surgery but for immediate aggressive medical treatment, as these patients are particularly likely to die.

The life-threatening problem is caused by embolic material blocking the main pulmonary artery or its right and left branches. Once it moves on the immediate danger is past. Massive pulmonary embolism can kill immediately, or onward passage of embolic material from the central pulmonary arteries to the periphery can lead to almost as speedy clinical recovery (the faint on the way to the bathroom), followed by an "unexplained" pyrexia. Rapid action is essential to save life in massive pulmonary embolism that causes circulatory collapse. Emergency pulmonary embolectomy under primitive conditions carries a horrendous mortality[16] and patients who survive to be transferred to major cardiac surgery units have already selected themselves to be survivors. Infusion of streptokinase offers no immediate benefit and is not included in the emergency measures to save life.

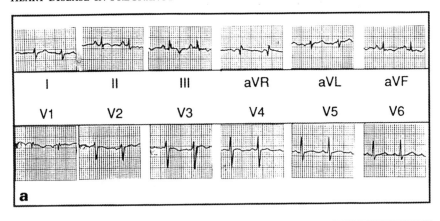

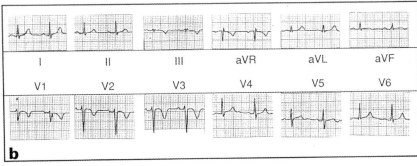

FIGURE 20.2—(a) Electrocardiogram from a young woman who had a massive pulmonary embolism during late pregnancy, showing sinus tachycardia, inferior axis, Q, and inverted T in lead III, and partial right bundle branch block with S to V7. The second record (b) shows a slower heart rate but there is now steep T wave inversion in leads to V1 to V3.

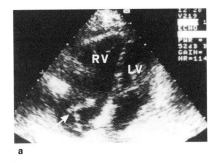
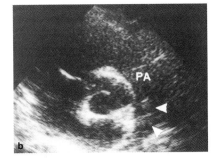

FIGURE 20.3—Dilated thin walled right ventricle with diastolic incursion towards the left ventricle can be identified immediately by echocardiography both after massive pulmonary embolism and in patients with much less dramatic features whose right ventricular dilatation may come as a surprise. The apical four chamber view shows the dilated right ventricle (RV) (a) and a long mobile thrombus in the right atrium (arrowed) (b). There is itrombas also in the main pulmonary artery (PA) (arrow heads) in (b).

Immediate relief of the obstructed right ventricle is needed to enable the patient to survive the first few hours. Heroic surgery achieves this only at great cost to life even if skilled surgical aid is available on site. Streptokinase may hasten resolution and reduce the small number of delayed deaths but this is uncertain.[17] Natural fibrinolysis in the lung is efficient. The embolic material is not adherent to the walls of the arteries and tends to break up and re-embolise down the lung, providing maximum exposure for lysis.

Emergency treatment of massive pulmonary embolism

The immediate emergency measures are to raise the patient's legs to increase venous return to the right ventricle, and to displace the uterus to one side if the pulmonary embolism is antepartum. Oxygen is given and if the patient is unconscious external cardiac massage will help to break up the embolic material and encourage its onward passage as well as to promote some circulation of blood. No drugs are helpful because the patient already has a maximum catecholamine surge, is intensely vasoconstricted, and the left ventricle, starved of blood, is maximally stimulated. A colloid or crystalline infusion helps to improve right ventricular filling pressure and output. The patient is taken immediately to the cardiac catheterisation laboratory or radiology department. As soon as possible a catheter is passed into the main pulmonary artery and contrast injected to identify the position of the pulmonary emboli. The catheter is advanced into the clot material and agitated vigorously. This fragments it so that it passes further down the pulmonary artery branches and can result in immediate unloading of the right ventricle with re-establishment of an effective circulation (Figure 20.4).[18-23] The cardiac output increases and blood pressure rises.

After mechanical clot dispersion small doses of streptokinase or tissue plasminogen activator can be injected selectively into pulmonary artery branches, but this is probably unnecessary. The embolised thrombus is soft and fragments easily having already been partially lysed in the peripheral veins from whence it came. With further intense endogenous fibrolytic activity in the lungs, the process of dissolution of the loose thrombus proceeds quickly. The catheter should be introduced through an arm or jugular vein to avoid passing it through and dislodging thrombus in iliac veins or inferior vena cava. If thrombolysis is planned the subclavian route should be avoided because the vein cannot be compressed adequately. Percutaneous catheter fragmentation is easy, can be life saving, and is not new but is still not widely known.[21-24]

Even in non-pregnant patients there are no convincing randomised trials to support the use of thrombolytic treatment of pulmonary embolism.[25] In the American urokinase pulmonary embolism trial 78 patients were randomly allocated to heparin treatment and 82 to urokinase followed by heparin. In the heparin group 31% died or had recurrent emboli compared with 23% in the urokinase-heparin group, but the study had insufficient

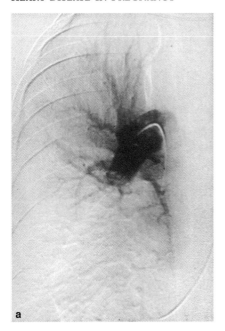 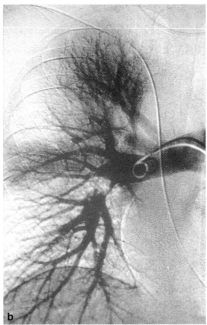

FIGURE 20.4—*Right pulmonary arteriogram from the same patient as in Fig. 2 (a) before and (b) after restoration of flow to the lower lobe by mechanical fragmentation of embolus. The pigtailed catheter is seen. There is still a large filling defect in the lower lobe artery but good peripheral perfusion around it.*

patients with massive pulmonary embolism and too few patients had long-term warfarin treatment.

Anticoagulant treatment must start with intravenous heparin. Large doses are required to attain a therapeutic activated partial thromboplastin time and frequent monitoring is needed until warfarin has become effective with an international normalised ratio of 2·0. Subsequent subcutaneous heparin may be preferred in women before delivery, to achieve an activated partial thromboplastin time of 1·5. Once daily low molecular weight heparin can also be used and the thromboplastin time does not then need to be measured.

Complete resolution is usual. Rarely patients develop chronic obstruction of a main pulmonary artery or of one or more major branches, sometimes but not always after an acute clinical episode and often associated with an inherited coagulopathy. Failure to resolve is suspected from continued shortness of breath and these rare patients may need elective pulmonary thrombectomy.

If the pulmonary embolism was antepartum anticoagulation should be maintained throughout the remainder of the pregnancy changing from warfarin (if this was chosen) to subcutaneous heparin two weeks before delivery. If caesarean delivery is planned for obstetric reasons warfarin can be continued and fresh frozen plasma given before operation. The condition is not analogous to that of artificial heart valves as the level of anticoagulation is lower and the fetal hazard therefore less. Anticoagulant treatment should be re-started postpartum and continued for at least three months. Postpartum pulmonary embolism is treated with intravenous heparin followed by oral anticoagulants for at least three months. Venography is not indicated. It does not influence management, is expensive, unpleasant, and not without hazard.

Venous stasis in the legs should be minimised by avoidance of the supine position and selection of a semi-prone posture for sleep. Placement of an intracaval filtration device is not recommended.[27,28] It is not necessary, is not free from complications, and if anticoagulation is stopped it does not always succeed in preventing recurrent embolism. Thirty years ago the inferior vena cava was ligated for antepartum pulmonary embolism[29] and various implanted devices designed to prevent passage of large thrombi have been popular in the USA and Europe but much less in the UK.

Perfusion lung scans (Figure 20.5) play no part in the diagnosis of massive pulmonary embolism in pregnancy because they are not instantly available and the patient is far too sick. It is inappropriate to do serial scans to follow the process of resolution until after the delivery. Echocardiographic Doppler examination can be carried out serially and provide immediate indirect information about resolution by showing restoration to normal of right ventricular function and pressure.

Lesser pulmonary embolism

Lesser pulmonary embolism in pregnancy may be marked by unexplained dyspnoea and this should never be taken lightly. The problem is one of diagnosis because shortness of breath is such a non-specific symptom and because of reluctance to use diagnostic methods which involve irradiation. The ECG may be normal or show T wave inversion in right sided leads which looks "borderline". A chest radiograph may also be normal but may show a prominent main pulmonary artery or a peripheral wedge-shaped shadow from previous infarction. Echocardiography should always be carried out promptly if pulmonary embolism is suspected. It may be normal but may surprise by showing right ventricular dilatation indicating a greater haemodynamic problem than had been suspected. A perfusion lung scan need not be carried out if echocardiography is diagnostic but should be done without hesitation if there is suspicion of pulmonary embolism but no other evidence in a patient with clear lungs on a chest radiograph and normal ECG and echocardiograph. Upon the results of echocardiography or the perfusion lung scan hangs the decision on whether to start anticoagulant treatment. It is unnecessary to do a ventilation lung scan and unnecessary to repeat the perfusion lung scan during the pregnancy. Once the diagnosis has been made heparin should be started followed by oral anticoagulant

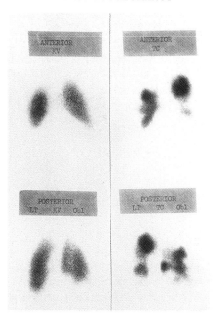

FIGURE 20.5—*Ventilation (on the left) and perfusion (on the right) lung scan after delivery in a patient who had subacute massive pulmonary embolism. The perfusion scan shows multiple defects.*

treatment for the rest of the pregnancy with a target international normalised ratio of 2.0.

Most patients do well. A pregnant haematologist with a bad obstetric history and no living children complained of new and increasing dyspnoea and consented to a perfusion lung scan, which confirmed that she had multiple pulmonary emboli. Intravenous heparin in hospital was followed by resolution of her dyspnoea but vaginal bleeding. She insisted that the heparin be stopped and refused warfarin. Fortunately with rapid mobilisation, the use of anti-embolism stockings, and other measures to avoid venous stasis, the rest of the pregnancy was uncomplicated and the outcome successful. Another woman was admitted to an obstetric hospital with dyspnoea and collapsed there. She was given intravenous streptokinase and rushed to Hammersmith by ambulance. Mechanical clot dispersion by catheter was immediately carried out (Figure 20.4) and followed by intravenous heparin until warfarin became effective. She took warfarin through the remainder of the pregnancy. Both mother and baby did well.

Pulmonary infarction may cause pleuritic pain, haemoptysis, or a haemorrhagic pleural effusion. Pulmonary embolism should be suspected in any pregnant or postpartum patient with these symptoms or with an unexplained pleural effusion. The main importance of pulmonary infarction, apart from causing pain and fever, is that it may presage fatal pulmonary embolism. Pulmonary infarction may also follow major or massive embolism through the process of resolution. This results from re-embolisation of fragmented autolysing emboli within the lungs, embolic material entering peripheral pulmonary branches during the process of lysis. If a small peripheral artery is completely blocked by such an embolus, infarction with pleurisy may follow. Such an event does not necessarily mean recurrence of pulmonary embolism from an extracardiac source. Recurrent pulmonary embolism is unusual in patients who are maintained on oral anticoagulant treatment and steps are taken to prevent venous stasis.

Ventilation perfusion lung scans should be used in the puerperium to follow the resolution of pulmonary embolism in any patient who has had pulmonary embolism in pregnancy or in the postpartum period (Figure 20.5). Resolution is sometimes complete within a month but full resolution may take up to a year. Rarely is it incomplete. When pulmonary embolism occurs during pregnancy a single perfusion scan suffices for diagnosis and no further scans are needed until postpartum when serial scans should be carried out until resolution becomes complete.

Pulmonary embolism may also be caused by fat, tumour, or amniotic fluid embolism.[30] Fat embolism may occur after major fractures. Tumour embolism may develop in chorioncarcinoma and can cause progressive pulmonary hypertension. Peripartum amniotic fluid embolism is rare and may mimic pulmonary thromboembolism. It is a common subclinical event but occasionally causes sudden circulatory embarrassment or collapse during or immediately after delivery particularly in multiparous patients and during surgical delivery.[26]

Summary

Pulmonary embolism in pregnancy or the puerperium is an emergency requiring immediate recognition and effective treatment. Most fatal cases die within an hour of the onset of symptoms. Echocardiography provides immediate confirmation of the diagnosis. Mechanical clot fragmentation by catheter is effective in cases of massive embolism and there is no justification for emergency pulmonary embolectomy. Elective embolectomy is needed for only rare patients with chronic obstruction of a main or major pulmonary artery. Minor pulmonary embolism is often overlooked, thereby missing the opportunity to prevent fatal embolism.

References

1 Department of Health and Social Security. *Report on Confidential Enquiries into Maternal Deaths in England and Wales.* 1985–7. *HMSO* 1991.
2 Moseley P, Kerstein MD. Pregnancy and thrombophlebitis. *Surg Gynecol Obstet* 1980; **150:** 593–9.
3 Shaper AG. The hypercoagulable states. *Ann Intern Med* 1985; **102:** 814–28.
4 Lees MM, Taylor SH, Scott DB, *et al.* A study of cardiac output at rest throughout pregnancy. *Journal of Obstetrics and Gynaecology of the British Commonwealth* 1967; **74:** 319–28.
5 Coon WW. Epidemiology of venous thromboembolism. *Ann Surg* 1977; **48:** 149–64.
6 Bolan JC. Thromboembolic complications of pregnancy. *Clin Obstet Gynecol* 1983; **26:** 913–22.

7 Goodrich SM, Wood JE. Peripheral venous distensibility and velocity of venous blood flow during pregnancy or during oral contraceptive therapy. *Am J Obstet Gynecol* 1964; **90**: 740–44.

8 Handin RI. Thromboembolic complications of pregnancy and oral contraceptives. *Prog Cardiovasc Dis* 1974; **16**: 395–405.

9 Aaro LA, Jeurgens JL. Thrombophlebitis associated with pregnancy. *Am J Obstet Gynecol* 1971; **109**: 1128–36.

10 Foster CS, Genton E, Henderson M, *et al*, eds. The epidemiology of venous thrombosis. *Milbank Memorial Fund Quarterly: Health and Society* 1972; **50**: 1–255.

11 Stein PD, Willis PW, DeMets DL. History and physical examination in acute pulmonary embolism without pre-existing cardiac or pulmonary disease. *Am J Cardiol* 1981; **47**: 218–23.

12 Bell WR, Simon TL. Current status of pulmonary thromboembolic disease: pathophysiology, diagnosis, prevention and treatment. *Am Heart J* 1982; **103**: 239–62.

13 Bell WR, Simon TL, Demets DL. The clinical features of submassive and massive pulmonary emboli. *Am J Med* 1977; **62**: 355–60.

14 Coon WW, Coller FA. Clinicopathologic correlation in thromboembolism. *Surg Gynecol Obstet* 1959; **109**: 259–69.

15 Cheriex EC, Sreeram N, Eussen YFJM, Pieters FAA, Wellens HJJ. Cross sectional Doppler echocardiography as the initial technique for the diagnosis of acute pulmonary embolism. *Br Heart J* 1991; **72**: 52–7.

16 Cohn LH, Shumway NE. Pulmonary embolectomy during pregnancy. *Arch Surg* 1973; **106**: 214–15.

17 Hall RJC, Young C, Sutton GC, Campbell S. Treatment of acute massive pulmonary embolism by streptokinase during labour and delivery. *BMJ* 1992; **30**: 647–9.

18 Brady AJB, Crake T, Oakley CM. Percutaneous catheter fragmentation and distal dispersion of proximal pulmonary embolus. *Lancet* 1991; **338**: 1186–9.

19 Essop MR, Middlemost S, Skoulangis J, Sareli P. Simultaneous mechanical clot fragmentation and pharmacologic thrombolysis in acute massive pulmonary embolism. *Am J Cardiol* 1992; **69**: 427–30.

20 Horstkotte D, Heintzen MP, Straner BF, Leschke M. Aggressive non-surgical management of massive pulmonary embolism with cardiogenic shock. *Eur Heart J* 1991; **12** (**suppl**): 52A.

21 Oakley CM. The diagnosis and management of pulmonary embolism. In: Tinker, Rapin HM, eds. *Care of the critically ill patient*. Amsterdam: Springer-Verlag, 1982: 223–5.

22 Oakley CM. The diagnosis and management of pulmonary embolism. Tinker, Zapol, eds. Care of the critically ill patient. 2nd ed. Amsterdam: Springer-Verlag, 1991: 307–14.

23 Allison DJ. Interventional radiology. In: Grainger RG, Allison DJ, eds. *Diagnostic radiology*. Edinburgh: Churchill Livingstone, 1986: 2121–65.

24 Feltrin G, Pramstraller C, Fiore D, Penizzi F. Fragmentation of pulmonary emboli. *Radiol Med* 1980; **66**: 793–8.

25 Goldhaber SZ. Thrombolysis for pulmonary embolism. *Prog Cardiovasc Dis* 1991; **39**: 113–34.

26 National Cooperative Study. The urokinase-pulmonary embolism trial. *Circulation* 1973; **47** (**suppl II**): 38–45.

27 Narayan H, Cullimore J, Krarup K, Thurston H, MacVicar J, Bolia A. Experience with the cardiac inferior vena cava filter as prophylaxis against pulmonary embolus in pregnant women with extensive deep vein thrombosis. *Br J Obstet Gynaecol* 1992; **99**: 637–40.

28 Aburahma AF, Basting DF, Tiley EH, Killmer SM, Boland JP. Management of DVT of the lower extremity in pregnancy. *West Virginia Medical Journal* 1993; **83**: 445–7.

29 Sauter RD, Fletcher FW, Lewis RF, Wentzel FJ. Inferior vena cava and ovarian vein ligation for antepartum pulmonary thromboembolization. *JAMA* 1966; **196**: 290–2.

30 Chuang AF, Merkatz IR. Survival following amniotic fluid embolism with early heparinization. *Obstet Gynecol* 1973; **42**: 809–14.

21: Hypertension and pre-eclamptic toxaemia

MICHAEL DE SWIET

Hypertension in pregnancy may have many different causes but by far the most important is pre-eclampsia. It is pre-eclampsia that makes hypertension the leading cause of maternal mortality in the United Kingdom.[1] Pre-eclampsia is responsible for about half of induced pre-term deliveries; and the need to detect pre-eclampsia as early as possible is a major reason for antenatal care. Although pre-eclampsia was formerly diagnosed on the basis of oedema, albuminuria, and raised blood pressure, it is now realised that the condition is caused by an unknown placental factor that affects the endothelium of blood vessels.[2] As every organ has a blood supply, pre-eclampsia has the potential to be a multisystem disease (Table 21.1). Therefore the management of pre-eclampsia involves far more than the treatment of hypertension alone.

The precise cause of pre-eclampsia is still unknown and largely because of this there is no specific marker that distinguishes patients who have pre-eclampsia from those who do not. There is no blood test which precisely diagnoses pre-eclampsia and even renal biopsy, formerly thought to be specific[3] has now been shown to yield false positive and false negative results.[4] However, it is generally accepted that pre-eclampsia is a condition most common in primigravidae in whom the blood pressure rises in the second half of pregnancy in association with proteinuria; that pre-eclampsia can result in eclamptic grand mal convulsions, and that it entirely remits after delivery. Patients may have hypertension before they are pregnant and then may or may not develop superadded pre-eclampsia.

In normal patients the blood pressure tends to fall in the first half of pregnancy, rising to pre-pregnancy levels or higher from about 30 weeks' gestation.[5] Any definition of pre-eclampsia based on blood pressure criteria must take account of these possibilities. The Redman and Jeffries definition is: a diastolic blood pressure below 90 mm Hg before 20 weeks; a rise in diastolic blood pressure after 20 weeks' gestation to above 90 mm Hg and by at least 25 mm Hg above the first blood pressure recorded in pregnancy.[6] This definition has a high probability to predict the subsequent development of proteinuria in primigravidae but for the reasons given above it is not

TABLE 21.1—*Clinical features of pre-eclampsia.*

- Central nervous system
  Eclamptic convulsions
  Cerebral haemorrhage, intraventricular or subarachnoid
  Cerebral infarction: microinfarction or macroinfarction (for example, cortical blindness caused by infarction of occipital cortex)

- Coagulation system
  Thrombocytopaenia
  Microhaemangiopathic haemolysis
  HELLP syndrome
  (Haemolysis, Elevated Liver enzymes, Low Platelets)
  Disseminated intravascular coagulation

- Eyes
  Retinal detachment
  Retinal oedema

- Kidney
  Acute tubular necrosis
  Acute cortical necrosis
  Unspecified renal failure

- Liver
  Rupture
  Infarction
  Jaundice
  Decreased synthesis of soluble clotting substances
  HELLP syndrome

- Respiratory system
  Laryngeal oedema
  Pulmonary oedema
  Adult respiratory distress syndrome

infallible. Some patients meeting these criteria will not have other features of pre-eclampsia and other patients will appear to have pre-eclampsia without meeting these blood pressure criteria. Because we do not have a specific marker for pre-eclampsia no definition based on blood pressure alone is precise.

Pre-eclampsia is therefore recognised in patients who have the clinical features listed above (Table 21.1) and who also have abnormalities that may be found on investigation (Table 21.2).

Hypertension is a common problem in pregnancy, affecting perhaps 10% of all pregnant women, depending on its definition. However, cardiologists are usually only involved in the severe cases or in other unusual circumstances, for example secondary hypertension from coarctation of the aorta. Most cardiologists therefore have little experience in the management of hypertension in pregnancy. This may be a particular problem in pre-pregnancy counselling for women with hypertension, either concerning the general advisability of pregnancy or the specific problems of individual antihypertensive drugs. This chapter will discuss these issues.

TABLE 21.2—*Features of pre-eclampsia found on investigation.*

- The maternal syndrome
  Abnormal liver function tests*
  Haemolysis*
  Hyperuricaemia*
  Hypocalcaemia
  Increased packed cell volume*
  Proteinuria*
  Raised antithrombin III in plasma
  Raised fibronectin in plasma
  Raised von Willebrand factor in plasma
  Thrombocytopenia*

- The fetal syndrome
  Intrauterine growth retardation—ultrasound*
  Intrauterine hypoxia—cardiotochography*

* Tests commonly used in the United Kingdom.

Blood pressure measurement

All the well known problems of conventional sphygmomanometry such as cuff size, observer error and bias, and blood pressure variability apply to blood pressure measurement in pregnancy. However, in pregnancy there are specific problems relating to the position of the patient. The blood pressure is lower in the second half of pregnancy in patients lying supine. This is because the gravid uterus obstructs the venous return from the lower limbs and reduces pre-load. Therefore blood pressure should be measured in the left lateral or sitting position. Because of difficulties in maintaining the sphygmomanometer cuff at the level of the heart in the left lateral position, sitting is the preferred position.[7]

In the UK (though not in the USA) K_4 rather than K_5 has been recommended for the measurement of diastolic blood pressure. This is because of concern that K_5 may be audible at zero cuff pressure. In practice this is a rare problem. It was not found in 250 patients recently studied at Queen Charlotte's Hospital in whom the diastolic blood pressure was always greater than 50 mm Hg.[8] K_5 is nearer to intra-arterial diastolic blood pressure than is K_4; and most importantly even trained observers have great difficulty in consistently recognising K_4.[8] For these reasons it is likely that K_5 will be recommended for measurement of diastolic blood pressure in pregnancy in the UK and that other international organisations such as the WHO and the International Society for the Study of Hypertension in Pregnancy will change their recommendation in line with current American practice which is also to use K_5.

"White coat hypertension" in which the blood pressure is excessively high because of arousal due to the clinical environment is as much of a problem in pregnancy as in other conditions, if not more. Its impact is minimised by devices which allow blood pressure to be measured frequently and outside the hospital, such as 24 hour ambulatory monitoring.[9]

Automatic blood pressure devices, either ambulatory or static for use in intensive care patients, need to be calibrated specifically for pregnancy and specifically for pre-eclampsia. Many of the machines in current use have not been validated. In pre-eclampsia in particular, the physical characteristics of blood vessels are altered. The pattern of pressure changes between systole and diastole analysed by oscillometric machines is altered and the algorithm used to calculate diastolic pressure is no longer accurate. In severe pre-eclampsia, machines that rely on oscillometric measurement may under-estimate diastolic blood pressure by 15 mm Hg compared with conventional sphygmomanometry. Even machines using a microphone to detect Korotkoff sounds are not immune from this problem. We recommend the SpaceLabs 90207 and the SpaceLabs Scout as the only automatic blood pressure machines that have been shown to be reasonably accurate in severe pre-eclampsia so far.

Pre-eclampsia (usually presenting after 30 weeks' gestation)

There are two important differences between the management of hypertension from pre-eclampsia and the management of hypertension outside pregnancy. Most cases of non-pregnant hypertension are idiopathic or "essential" and the major purpose of their treatment is to prevent the long term complications of stroke and myocardial infarction. A few patients present outside pregnancy with acute severe hypertension that must be treated immediately because of the risk of hypertensive encephalopathy, but this is now uncommon. It is realised that acute lowering of blood pressure in the non-pregnant state has major risks.

However, pregnancy and pre-eclampsia do not last for long enough to justify or need treatment of hypertension to prevent long term complications; the long term risks do not exist. But there are major acute risks of eclampsia and cerebral haemorrhage; the latter is the dominant cause of the increase in maternal mortality seen in pre-eclampsia and by contrast with the condition outside pregnancy is the most important reason for treatment.[1] Acute lowering of blood pressure is commonly necessary in severe pre-eclampsia.

Secondly, hypertension is only one aspect of pre-eclampsia. It is variable in its expression and may even be absent in patients who otherwise have severe manifestations of the condition. Pre-eclampsia is a multisystem disease affecting the endothelium of all blood vessels. Other features must be looked for and managed appropriately (Table 21.1). The presence of these features is variable and different aspects of the pre-eclamptic process may progress at different speeds. Progression is, however, relentless and no intervention has been shown to stop this progression except delivery.

Management

Patients who have a rise in blood pressure suggestive of pre-eclampsia, but have no symptoms and whose blood pressure remains less than 150 mm Hg systolic and less than 100 mm Hg diastolic can be managed as outpatients, particularly if there are day-care facilities available. All other patients should be managed in hospital, not because hospital admission affects the progression of pre-eclampsia but because it allows more intensive monitoring of mother and fetus, both of whom are at risk. As the only intervention that affects the progression of pre-eclampsia is delivery, the purpose of monitoring is to detect deterioration in maternal or fetal condition that demands delivery. Other ancillary measures that may help are giving the mother glucocorticoids that cross the placenta (dexamethasone, betamethasone), which aid fetal lung maturation; and treatment of maternal hypertension to allow the pregnancy to continue for long enough to allow glucocorticoids to take effect. In general, once pre-eclampsia has caused the blood pressure to rise to the level that demands antihypertensive treatment (more than 170 systolic or more than 110 diastolic) it is unlikely that the pregnancy will be able to continue for more than a few days: one of the fetal or maternal features noted in Table 21.1 will necessitate delivery.

Antihypertensive treatment

The reason for using antihypertensive drugs is to reduce the risk of the cerebral complications of pre-eclampsia. It is generally believed that blood pressures in excess of 170 systolic or 110 diastolic in pre-eclampsia, carry a distinct risk of cerebral haemorrhage and eclampsia (though the latter may occur at lower blood pressures). For this reason clinicians think that antihypertensive treatment is mandatory once the blood pressure reaches these levels. The target blood pressure should be about 140/90. Blood pressures reduced to below this put the fetus and maternal brain at risk from impaired perfusion in the maternal circulation. This practice has never been subjected to clinical trial and almost certainly never will be for obvious reasons. However, a blood pressure of 170/110 is just below the level of blood pressure (180–190/120–130 mm Hg) at which cerebral autoregulation fails.[11]

By contrast the Cochrane database meta-analysis of all trials of antihypertensive drugs for mild to moderate hypertension suggested that treatment of lower degrees of blood pressure (where there is no acute maternal risk) does not improve the fetal outcome.[12] It only reduces the incidence of severe hypertension. The position is clear in patients presenting with hypertension after 30 weeks' gestation. However, patients with hypertension before pregnancy are likely to be receiving anti-hypertensives at the beginning of pregnancy and have been excluded from most of the trials in the Cochrane database and there is evidence to support the use of methyldopa for fetal reasons in early pregnancy (see below); so in patients presenting with hypertension before 30 weeks and in those treated before pregnancy, the position is not so clear and there may be a case for treating mild to moderate hypertension.

Antihypertensive drugs to lower blood pressure acutely

Hydralazine

Hydralazine is the drug that is used most commonly for blood pressure control in acute severe hypertension. Intravenous boluses will lower the blood pressure to a safe level in most acute episodes of pre-eclampsia.[13] The drug may also be given intramuscularly or by intravenous infusion. The patient should be managed in an intensive care unit. As indicated above, once the blood pressure has risen to levels greater than 170/110 because of pre-eclampsia, the patient is likely to require delivery soon, so long term blood pressure control is not relevant.

Labetalol

Labetalol is a combined alpha- and beta-adrenergic blocking agent. It may also be given by intravenous infusion for acute control of blood pressure.[14] Patients with a history of asthma should not be given labetalol because of its beta-blocking component. No formal comparisons of labetalol and hydalazine have been made. Clinicians tend to use the drug that they are most familiar with for emergency control of blood pressure.

Nifedipine

The calcium antagonist nifedipine is effective for oral control of acute severe hypertension even though it has not been licensed for this purpose in the United Kingdom.[15] It has been suggested that nifedipine should not be given in conjunction with magnesium (for control of seizures) because magnesium potentiates its hypotensive effect.[16] This risk has probably been exaggerated.

Anticonvulsant drugs

If a patient has an eclamptic fit most obstetricians in the UK would formerly have used intravenous diazepam to control the seizure.[17,18] A few would have substituted parenteral phenytoin. Once the patient's condition is stable with regard to blood pressure and when other acute problems such as thrombocytopenia have been controlled, she would be delivered if the fit occurred antenatally.

In the USA parenteral magnesium sulphate has long been used for seizure control.[14]

In 1995 the Eclampsia Trial Collaborative Group reported an important multicentre international trial comparing magnesium and diazepam and magnesium and phenytoin in patients with eclampsia.[20] Magnesium was clearly superior to either phenytoin or diazepam in preventing further seizures (relative risks 52% by comparison with diazepam and 67% by comparison with phenytoin). There were also insignificant trends towards better maternal and fetal outcomes. Therefore all concerned with the management of eclampsia must become familiar with the use of magnesium sulphate. Concern about respiratory paralysis has not been justified and theoretical objections that magnesium sulphate is not an anticonvulsant do not seem relevant: the drug is either working as a selective cerebral vasodilator or has some less specific metabolic neuroprotective mechanism. The recommended regimen is that used in the collaborative trial: a loading dose of 4 g intravenously over 5 minutes followed by intravenous infusion of 1 g/hour for 24 hours. Alternatively intramuscular magnesium sulphate may be used 5 g in each buttock every four hours, but it is painful. Providing the respiratory rate is greater than 16/minute, the urine output is greater than 25 ml/hour and knee jerks are present, there is no need for estimation of magnesium concentrations in the blood. They were not measured in the collaborative trial. Measurement of magnesium concentrations in women who have signs suggesting a risk of magnesium toxicity requires further evaluation.

The question of anticonvulsant prophylaxis in patients with fulminant pre-eclampsia who have not yet had a seizure is more difficult.[21] From the data of the collaborative trial, magnesium would be the drug to use if anticonvulsant prophylaxis is indicated. Lucas et al showed that magnesium was considerably better than phenytoin for seizure prophylaxis.[22] 2138 women with pre-eclampsia as defined by systolic blood pressure greater than 140 mm Hg and diastolic blood pressure (K_5) greater than 90 mm Hg were randomised to receive phenytoin or magnesium. The trial was stopped prematurely when ten of the women receiving phenytoin had seizures compared with none of those receiving magnesium. However 2128 women had no seizures at all. The mortality of eclampsia is about 2%.[23] Thus it has been estimated that 5000 women would have to be treated prophylactically with magnesium to prevent one maternal death.[24] It is by no means clear which women with pre-eclampsia are at risk of eclamptic seizures. In a recent UK survey of all 383 cases of eclampsia occurring in 1992, 11% had neither proteinuria nor significant hypertension at the time of the first fit and 43% did not have the combination of these abnormalities that many would demand before instituting seizure prophylaxis.[23] The American study did not address the issue of blood pressure control in preventing seizures.[22] There is urgent need of a placebo controlled trial of magnesium sulphate for prophylaxis of seizures in patients with adequately controlled blood pressure. Until such a trial has been done, clinicians will have to use their judgement, perhaps reserving magnesium for those patients who have blood pressures that are particularly hard to treat, or where there seems to be substantial cerebral irritability.

Other very important features of the management of fulminating pre-eclampsia such as fluid balance, the correction of coagulopathy, and the timing and route of delivery are beyond the scope of this chapter.

Hypertension presenting before 30 weeks

Pre-eclampsia can occur at gestations between 20 and 30 weeks and if it does, it is severe. In the average UK hospital no more than five women per thousand have pre-eclampsia presenting before 30 weeks. The earlier hypertension presents, the more likely is it that non-toxaemic hypertension is the cause or is the major contributing factor. The reason for choosing a "water shed" of 30 weeks is that there are clinical trial data to support improved fetal survival from long term antihypertensive therapy, particularly with methyldopa, when compared with placebo in patients presenting before 30 weeks' gestation.[25,26] In Redman's trial of methyldopa compared with placebo there was a significant reduction in the perinatal loss rate from 6% to 1% in 106 women treated with methyldopa compared with 107 women treated with placebo.[25] Entry criteria were blood pressures persistently greater than 95 mm Hg diastolic before 30 weeks' gestation but not so high as to demand antihypertensive therapy for maternal safety. What is uncertain is why the methyldopa group did better, as the improvement could not be correlated with the antihypertensive effect. It was not clear to what extent there was any improvement in fetal outcome in women who had pre-eclampsia as opposed to non-toxaemic hypertension.[25]

The choice of 30 weeks was arbitrary. Meta-analysis of all trials of antihypertensive drugs for mild to moderate hypertension irrespective of gestational age and presentation does not indicate fetal benefit, which is shown only in severe maternal hypertension. Therefore if treatment in early pregnancy is beneficial, there is likely to be increasing benefit the earlier treatment is instituted, rather than an absolute difference between those presenting before or after 30 weeks.

Non-toxaemic hypertension

As indicated, the earlier in pregnancy that hypertension presents, the more likely is it to be non-toxaemic. As in the non-pregnant state, most cases of non-toxaemic hypertension in pregnancy have no obvious cause (essential hypertension) and in less than 5% can a cause be found. However, some forms of secondary hypertension have specific problems which must be considered.

Phaeochromocytoma

Nearly every maternal mortality report has a death from phaeo-chromocytoma. The condition can mimic all the features of pre-eclampsia[27] and undiagnosed it has a mortality of 50%.[28] As in the non-pregnant state most cases lack the typical features so all patients with severe hypertension in pregnancy should be screened for phaeochromocytoma by whatever method is used locally. Because methyldopa interferes with many biochemical screens for phaeochromocytoma and as methyldopa is the preferred long term treatment for hypertension in pregnancy the need to screen for phaeochromocytoma must be considered before starting treatment. If the tests suggest phaeochromocytoma, treatment should be started immediately with alpha and beta-adrenergic blockade. I prefer phenoxybenzamine and propranolol notwithstanding any concern about the use of beta-blocking agents in pregnancy. Once effective alpha and beta-blockade have been established the maternal risk should be eliminated.[29] The tumour may be localised antenatally by ultrasound or magnetic resonance imaging which is considered safe in pregnancy. If the tumour has been localised with confidence, then it may be removed by a combined approach at the time of delivery[29] or subsequently.[30] If the tumour has not been localised before delivery (which is more likely with lesions outside the adrenal glands) delivery is safe under combined alpha and beta-adrenergic blockade. The tumour can be localised and removed after delivery.

Coarctation of the aorta

Most patients with substantial coarctation have the lesion repaired before pregnancy. If this has not been done, the risk is of dissection of the aorta because of the increased cardiac output of pregnancy.[31] Patients who have any degree of coarctation should have their blood pressure scrupulously controlled by beta-adrenergic blockade notwithstanding any possible risks to the fetus. Beta-blockade is preferred because it reduces cardiac contractility and therefore the shear stress on the aorta (Chapter 5).

Renal disease

Renovascular hypertension has no specific problems in pregnancy but renal parenchymal disease does: hypertension and renal impairment interact in a way that is not understood to increase the risks of superadded pre-eclampsia and acute and chronic fetal distress. For example in renal disease the presence of hypertension increases the incidence of intrauterine growth retardation from 2% to 16% and of pre-term delivery from 11% to 20%.[32]

Essential hypertension

This is the diagnosis in most women presenting before 20 weeks. It is now realised that essential hypertension per se does not put the fetus at risk. The only risk is of developing superadded pre-eclampsia; in women with essential hypertension requiring treatment before pregnancy, the risk of developing pre-eclampsia is probably about 20%, compared with 10% in those without hypertension. The management of patients with essential hypertension early in pregnancy therefore depends on stopping them developing pre-eclampsia or life threatening hypertension.

Severe hypertension early in pregnancy may persuade doctors that the pregnancy should be terminated because continuing the pregnancy will put the mother's life at extra risk. In practice this does not happen: women with severe hypertension do not often get pregnant; the blood pressure can usually be controlled more easily in early pregnancy; and if it cannot, the conceptus usually dies and the pregnancy terminates itself.

Chronic antihypertensive therapy

Methyldopa

There are no good data that indicate that treatment with antihypertensive drugs reduces the risk of pre-eclampsia but, as indicated above, the Redman trial did show that fetal outcome was improved when women were given methyldopa rather than placebo;[25] and there are long term follow-up data at seven years which show no detriment to the offspring in the methyldopa-treated group.[33] It is for these reasons that methyldopa is the drug most commonly used for long term control of blood pressure in pregnancy. The usual dose range is 250 mg to 1 g three times a day. At high doses the sedative effects are marked but these patients often require admission for monitoring so sedation is not much of a problem. Methyldopa should not be used if there is a substantial risk of maternal depression and for this reason I change treatment in all patients to a beta-blocking agent, calcium antagonist, or converting enzyme inhibitor after delivery.

Although there is almost uniform agreement about methyldopa as the first drug for long term treatment of hypertension, there is no consensus about alternative or additional drugs, largely because of a lack of adequate clinical trials.

Beta-blocking drugs

Oxprenolol has been compared with methyldopa[34,35] using the same entry criteria as in the methyldopa versus placebo trial.[25] Initial reports that the use of oxprenolol was associated with larger babies[34] were not supported in a subsequent study.[35] Atenolol has been compared with placebo; although there was no difference in fetal outcome, the authors found less proteinuric pre-eclampsia (a remarkable outcome) and fewer hospital admissions, hardly surprising as the blood pressures were lower.[36] But worryingly, the same authors in another placebo-controlled trial of atenolol in early pregnancy, found a high incidence of severe growth retardation in the atenolol group.[37] For this reason atenolol should not be used in the first half of pregnancy. It is not clear whether the risk of growth retardation is specific to atenolol or general to all beta-blocking drugs. As atenolol does not have intrinsic sympathomimetic activity (unlike oxprenolol) the drug's pharmacological profile may be important. However, until the matter is cleared up, I do not use beta-blocking drugs to control blood pressure in the first half of pregnancy unless there is some specific reason such as coarctation of the aorta. Nevertheless beta-blocking drugs do not need to be stopped before conception and nor does any other antihypertensive drug.

Hydralazine

Hydralazine can be used as an adjunct to methyldopa. The side effects of tachycardia and headache are usually not a problem if methyldopa is being taken as well. Treatment in pregnancy does not last long enough for the development of lupus to be a problem. Tachyphylaxis limits the use of hydralazine to late pregnancy.

Labetalol

Like hydralazine, labetalol has been used for long term as well as acute control of pressure. Comparative trials of labetalol and methyldopa have not been large enough to exclude important differences in outcome. There has been a trend towards an increased risk of growth retardation with labetalol.

Nifedipine

Nifedipine is the only calcium antagonist for which there is any extensive experience in pregnancy, and this is anecdotal rather than in the context of a clinical trial.[15,38] At least in part this is because of the lack of a product licence for its use in hypertension in pregnancy in the United Kingdom. The most extensive report of its long term use showed a poor fetal outcome, but the study was conducted in a particularly high risk group of pregnancies.[38] At present nifedipine is my preferred additional or alternative drug for long term use in pregnancy when methyldopa is either ineffective or contraindicated.

Diuretics

Diuretics were formally used extensively for the "treatment" or prevention of pre-eclampsia. Meta-analysis has shown that they reduce oedema but have no impact on perinatal survival.[39] Diuretics are theoretically contraindicated as the circulating blood volume is already contracted in severe pre-eclampsia and any further reduction might impair placental perfusion. Diuretics also raise the concentration of serum urate which is used to monitor the progress of pre-eclampsia (Table 21.2). For these reasons, and because they are not very effective hypotensive agents, diuretics are not used to control blood pressure in pregnancy.

Angiotensin converting enzyme inhibitors

These drugs should not be used after the first trimester. They cause renal failure in the fetus which is shown before delivery as oligohydramnios and after delivery as oliguria, and anuria.[40] The condition can be fatal for the fetus; both captopril and enalapril have been implicated.

303

Prevention of pre-eclampsia

Because of the importance of pre-eclampsia and as no treatment will cure the condition except delivery, the possibility of prevention of pre-eclampsia is particularly important. There are two main groups of women at risk: those who have had it before and those who have some underlying condition such as hypertension or renal disease that predisposes patients to the condition. Early trials with antiplatelet agents, in particular low dose aspirin 60 to 150 mg/day were encouraging, suggesting a 70% reduction in risk.[41,42] By contrast recent large trials such as CLASP (Collaborative Low-dose Aspirin Study in Pregnancy) showed no overall reduction in risk and meta-analysis indicates no more than a 12% reduction of risk.[43] However further analysis of the CLASP data did suggest that early onset pre-eclampsia might be reduced by as much as 50%[43] and early onset pre-eclampsia (before 34 weeks) is the most severe form of the disease. If a patient has early onset pre-eclampsia in the second trimester, the risk of recurrence of some form of pre-eclampsia is between 20% and 40% depending on the population studied.[44] There is a 10% recurrence risk of recurrent early onset pre-eclampsia.[44] Other risk factors for early onset pre-eclampsia are pre-existing renal disease[45] and pre-existing hypertension, though how severe the hypertension has to be is uncertain.

My practice is to advise aspirin 75 mg a day from 12 weeks' gestation for the following patients: women who have had a fetal loss because of pre-eclampsia or unexplained intrauterine growth retardation (similar placental lesions): women who have had pre-eclampsia before 34 weeks, who have documented impaired renal function, and women who have been treated with antihypertensive drugs before pregnancy. The CLASP trial showed that aspirin given in this way is safe for mother and child.[43]

Management of hypertension before pregnancy and in early pregnancy

Patients should be investigated for hypertension in the usual way and treatment should be instigated and optimised with regard to blood pressure control. There are no levels of blood pressure above which pregnancy cannot be countenanced. Patients should be counselled about the risks of pre-eclampsia and the possible benefits of antiplatelet therapy.

No antihypertensive drugs have shown to be teratogenic, and none are likely to be harmful in the first weeks of pregnancy. Therefore the choice of drugs to be used before pregnancy may be made irrespective of any consideration of a future pregnancy. Once the patient becomes pregnant, her blood pressure is likely to fall because of the marked vasodilatation that occurs in early pregnancy. (Indeed if this does not occur it is an ominous sign for the success of the pregnancy.) As soon as the patient knows she is pregnant, it should be possible to withdraw antihypertensive drugs or substitute methyldopa, depending on the amount of antihypertensive therapy necessary before pregnancy.

References

1 Department of Health, Welsh Office, Scottish Office and Health Department, Department of Health and Social Security, Northern Ireland. *Report on Confidential Enquiries into Maternal Deaths in the United Kingdom 1988–1990*. London: HMSO, 1994.
2 Roberts JM, Taylor RN, Musci TJ, *et al*. Pre-eclampsia: an endothelial cell disorder. *Am J Obstet Gynecol* 1989; **161**: 1200–4.
3 Spargo B, McCartney CP, Winemiller R. Glomerular capillary endotheliosis in toxemia of pregnancy. *Archives of Pathology* 1959; **68**: 593–9.
4 Fisher ER, Pardo V, Paul R, Hayrashi TT. Ultrastructural studies in hypertension. IV. Toxemia in pregnancy. *Am J Pathol* 1969; **55**: 109–31.
5 MacGillivray I, Rose GA, Rowe B. Blood pressure survey in pregnancy. *Clin Sci* 1969; **37**: 395–407.
6 Redman CWG, Jeffries M. Revised definition of pre-eclampsia. *Lancet* 1988; **ii**: 809–812.
7 National High Blood Pressure Education Programme. National High Blood Pressure Education Programme Working Group Report on High Blood Pressure in Pregnancy. *Am J Obstet Gynecol* 1990; **163**: 1691–1712.
8 Shennan AH, Gupta M, Halligan A, Taylor D, de Swiet M. Korotkoff phase IV in pregnancy cannot be reliably reproduced using mercury sphygmomanometry. *Lancet* 1996; **343**: 139–42.
9 Shennan AH, Kissane J, de Swiet M. Validation of the Spacelabs 90207. *Br J Obstet Gynaecol* 1993; **100**: 904–8.
10 Matthews DD. A randomised controlled trial of bed rest and sedation of normal activity and non-sedation in the management of non-albuminuric hypertension in late pregnancy. *Br J Obstet Gynaecol* 1977; **84**: 108–14.
11 Redman CWG. Hypertension in pregnancy. In: de Swiet M, ed. *Medical disorders in obstetric practice*. 3rd ed. Oxford: Blackwell, 1995: 200.
12 Collins R, Duley L. Any antihypertensive therapy for pregnancy. *The Cochrane Pregnancy and Childbirth Database* Issue 1; 1995.
13 Paterson-Brown S, Robson SC, Redfern N, *et al*. Hydralazine boluses for the treatment of severe hypertension. *Br J Obstet Gynaecol* 1994; **101**: 409–13.
14 Garden A, Davey DA, Dommisse J. Intravenous labetalol and intravenous dihydralazine in severe hypertension in pregnancy. *Clin Exp Hypertens* 1982; **1(B)**: 371–83.
15 Walters BNJ, Redman CWG. Treatment of severe pregnancy-associated hypertension with the calcium antagonist nifedipine. *Br J Obstet Gynaecol* 1984; **91**: 330–6.
16 Waisman CD, Mayorga LM, Camera MI, *et al*. Magnesium plus nifedipine: potentiation of hypotensive effect in pre-eclampsia? *Am J Obstet Gynecol* 1988; **159**: 308–9.
17 Chamberlain GVP, Lewis PJ, de Swiet M, *et al*. How obstetricians manage hypertension in pregnancy. *BMJ* 1978; **i**: 626–7.
18 Hutton JD, James DK, Stirrat GM, *et al*. Management of severe pre-eclampsia and eclampsia by UK consultants. *Br J Obstet Gynaecol* 1992; **99**: 554–6.
19 Pritchard JA, Cunningham FG, Pritchard SA. The Parkland Memorial Hospital protocol for treatment of eclampsia: evaluation of 245 cases. *Am J Obstet Gynecol* 1984; **148**: 951–63.
20 The Eclampsia Trial Collaborative Group. Which anticonvulsant for women with eclampsia? *Lancet* 1995; **345**: 1455–63.
21 Chua S, Redman CWG. Are prophylactic anticonvulsants required in severe pre-eclampsia? *Lancet* 1991; **337**: 250–1.
22 Lucas MJ, Leveno KJ, Cunningham FG. A comparison of magnesium sulphate with phenytoin for the prevention of eclampsia. *N Engl J Med* 1995; **332**: 201–5.
23 Douglas KA, Redman CWG. Eclampsia in the United Kingdom. *BMJ* 1994; **309**: 1395–1400.
24 Saunders K, Hammersley B. Magnesium for eclampsia. *Lancet* 1995; **34**: 788–9.
25 Redman CWG, Beilin LJ, Bonnar J, *et al*. Fetal outcome in trial of antihypertensive treatment in pregnancy. *Lancet* 1976; **ii**: 753–6.
26 Leather HM, Humphreys DM, Baker P. A controlled trial of hypotensive agents in hypertension in pregnancy. *Lancet* 1968; **i**: 488–90.
27 Lamming GD, Symonds EM, Rubin PC. Phaeochromocytoma in pregnancy: still a cause of maternal death. *Clin Exp Hypertens* 1990; **9**: 57–68.
28 Blair RG. Phaeochromocytoma and pregnancy. *Journal of Obstetrics and Gynaecology of the British Commonwealth* 1963; **70**: 110–19.

29 Harper MA, Murnaghan GA, Kennedy L, *et al.* Phaeochromocytoma in pregnancy. Five cases and a review of the literature. *Br J Obstet Gynaecol* 1989; **96**: 594–606.
30 Schenker JG, Chowers I. Phaeochromocytoma and pregnancy. *Obstet Gynaecol Surv* 1971; **26**: 739–47.
31 Deal K, Wooley CF. Coarctation of the aorta and pregnancy. *Ann Intern Med* 1973; **78**: 706–10.
32 Surian M, Ibascia E, *et al.* Glomerular disease and pregnancy: a study of 123 pregnancies in patients with primary and secondary glomerular disease. *Nephrol* 1984; **36**: 101–5.
33 Redman CWG, Ounsted MK. Safety for the child of drug treatment for hypertension in pregnancy. *Lancet* 1982; **i**: 1237.
34 Gallery EDM, Saunders DM, Hunyor SN, *et al.* Randomised comparison of methyldopa and oxprenolol for treatment of hypertension in pregnancy. *BMJ* 1979; **i**: 1591–4.
35 Fidler J, Smith V, de Swiet M. Randomised controlled comparative study of methyldopa and oxprenolol for the treatment of hypertension in pregnancy. *BMJ* 1983; **286**: 1927–30.
36 Rubin PC, Butters L, *et al.* Placebo-controlled trial of atenolol treatment of pregnancy-associated hypertension. *Lancet* 1983; **i**: 431–4.
37 Butters L, Kennedy S, Rubin PC. Atenolol in essential hypertension during pregnancy. *BMJ* 1990; **301**: 587–9.
38 Constantine G, Beevers DG, Reynolds AC. Nifedipine as a second line antihypertensive drug in pregnancy. *Br J Obstet Gynaecol* 1987; **94**: 1136–42.
39 Collins R, Yusuf S, Peto R. Overview of randomised trials of diuretics in pregnancy. *BMJ* 1985; **290**: 17–23.
40 Rosa FW, Bosco LA, Graham CF. Neonatal anuria with maternal angiotensin-converting enzyme inhibition. *Obstet Gynecol* 1989; **74**: 371–4.
41 Beaufils M, Uzan S, Donsimoni R, *et al.* Prevention of eclampsia by early platelet therapy. *Lancet* 1985; **i**: 840–2.
42 Wallenburg HCS, Dekker GA, Makovitz JW, *et al.* Low-dose aspirin prevents pregnancy-induced hypertension and pre-eclampsia in angiotensin-sensitive primigravidae. *Lancet* 1986; **i**: 1–3.
43 CLASP (Collaborative Low-dose Aspirin Study in Pregnancy) Collaborative Group. CLASP: a randomised trial of low-dose aspirin for the prevention and treatment of pre-eclampsia among 9364 pregnant women. *Lancet* 1994; **343**: 619–29.
44 Sibai BM, Mercer B, Sarinoglu C. Severe pre-eclampsia in the second trimester: recurrent risk and long-term prognosis. *Am J Obstet Gynecol* 1991; **165**: 1408–1512.
45 Ihle BU, Long P, Oats J. Early onset pre-eclampsia: recognition of underlying renal disease. *BMJ* 1987; **294**: 79–81.

Cardiovascular drugs:

22: Anticoagulants

ELIZABETH A LETSKY

Physiological adjustments in the haemostatic and fibrinolytic mechanisms during normal pregnancy help to combat the hazard of haemorrhage at delivery but convert pregnancy into a hypercoagulable state (Chapter 3). Venous thromboembolism is one of the most serious complications that can arise in healthy pregnant women and the diagnosis and management present special problems.

In addition there are small numbers of women at increased risk of arterial thromboembolic phenomena during pregnancy, particularly those with cardiac disease and synthetic heart valve replacements. These women are often maintained on oral anticoagulants long term before conception and require effective continuing prophylaxis which will not adversely affect the fetus during gestation.

The place of oral anticoagulant therapy in pregnancy has become increasingly controversial during recent years. The reported hazards vary from country to country. Heparin, which carries virtually no risk for the fetus or neonate and few for the mother, has largely replaced the necessity to consider coumarins during pregnancy in many centres. The recent introduction of aspirin as prophylaxis against both venous and arterial thromboembolism has further blurred an already confused picture.

Management of thromboembolism arising de novo in pregnancy

Management of the acute phase may involve surgery, thrombolytic therapy, and heparin. Chronic phase treatment involves the anticoagulants heparin and warfarin. Nearly 30 years ago maternal mortality associated with pulmonary embolism (PE) in deep vein thrombosis (DVT) was reduced from 13% to 1% in an uncontrolled study.[1] The only published controlled study of anticoagulation compared with placebo had to be abandoned because of the high death rate in the placebo group.[2] It is now generally accepted that anticoagulant treatment should be instituted promptly for pulmonary embolism. A search of the literature showed a mortality of less than 1% (1/113 patients) in anticoagulated patients with pulmonary embolism in pregnancy.[3]

Acute phase treatment

Thrombolytic therapy

Thrombolytic therapy has been advocated in pregnancy complicated by ileofemoral venous thrombosis or by major PE followed by shock or pulmonary hypotension. There is evidence that patients who have thrombolytic therapy for DVT are much less likely to develop post-phlebitic leg symptoms. It has been suggested that the risk of massive PE is minimised in patients with extensive ileo-femoral thrombosis treated with strepto-kinase.

After pulmonary embolism one study showed that the pulmonary capillary volume and pulmonary diffusing capacity were normal in patients treated with thrombolytic therapy whereas they usually remained abnormal in patients treated with heparin and warfarin on follow up one year later, even if they were asymptomatic.[4]

Streptokinase

Streptokinase, the most commonly used agent, does not cross the placenta and so should not harm the fetus directly, but there is concern about the effects of maternal fibrinolysis on the placental bed.[5] In addition severe uterine bleeding would be expected if thrombolytic drugs were used postpartum. Nevertheless there have been anecdotal reports of successful treatment.[6]

Tissue plasminogen activator

There is little published experience of recombinant tissue plasminogen activator in pregnancy but it has been used with success as an alternative to streptokinase in one or two cases.[7,8] Without objective evidence of its benefits and risks, thrombolytic therapy cannot be recommended in pregnancy, except perhaps as a life-saving procedure in a shocked patient with massive pulmonary embolism (Chapter 20).

Anticoagulants

Both oral anticoagulants and heparin are avoided during pregnancy whenever possible because of their hazards to both mother and fetus. Nevertheless there are times when they have to be used, particularly if the diagnosis of thromboembolism is made during the antenatal period. In the acute phase the major problem is how to prevent thrombus extension,

308

embolism, or recurrent thrombosis without causing bleeding in either the infant or the mother. Heparin is the anticoagulant drug of choice in the acute phase.

Heparin

Most patients with venous thromboembolism are treated initially with heparin, which has particular advantages in pregnancy. Because it is strongly polar and non-lipid soluble it does not cross the placenta. It can be easily and rapidly reversed by protamine sulphate which immediately neutralises the effect of heparin so that emergency surgery can be carried out or bleeding from over dosage dealt with promptly. In addition its short circulating half-life (about 60 minutes) means that withholding treatment rapidly restores coagulation and haemostasis to normal. However this short half-life together with the fact that heparin must be administered parenterally is its main disadvantage even in the acute phase.

Acute-phase treatment   The object of heparin therapy in the initial phase is to prevent further, possibly fatal, episodes. To treat an established thrombus in a pregnant woman larger doses than usual are required because of increased plasma volume and activation of procoagulant factors. It should be administered by continuous infusion starting with 40 000 IU daily.

Although up to 40 000 IU/day have been given subcutaneously this is not usually practical because of bruising and irregular absorption.[9] Given in large doses heparin has a powerful antithrombin effect. The amount of heparin required to achieve therapeutic levels varies with the size of the thrombus. Larger doses are required for pulmonary emboli or massive ileofemoral thromboses than for a small DVT in the calf.

Laboratory control of therapeutic heparin   The aim is to achieve a level of heparin between 0·2 and 0·6 IU/ml by prolongation of the activated partial thromboplastin line (APTT). The results may be expressed in seconds or as a ratio compared with normal control plasma. For most reagents, ratios of 1:5 to 2:5 cover the therapeutic range. Laboratory control of heparin therapy is difficult generally because of wide variability in the sensitivity of APTT reagents for monitoring dosage.[10] There is also considerable individual variability in response to standard doses which further complicates in vitro standardisation and quality control. During pregnancy, haemostatic and plasma volume changes alter the sensitivity to heparin of the common tests that are used to monitor its anticoagulant effect and to adjust the dose.

Clinicians should be aware that there is substantial variability in laboratory assays which may be diurnal with higher values at night[11] even in patients on continuing intravenous infusion of heparin. The only side effect of therapeutic heparin administration in the acute phase of thromboembolism is bleeding but the preservative chlorbutal may cause hypotension.[12] Because of the risk of haematoma formation in patients who are fully anticoagulated other parenteral drugs such as antibiotics should be given intravenously rather than intramuscularly.

If it is necessary to reverse heparin therapy, cessation of infusion will be enough in most patients because of its short half-life. If the need is more urgent protamine sulphate 1 mg for every 100 units of administered heparin may be given.

Acute phase high dose heparin is given continuously intravenously for an arbitrary period of 3–7 days, depending on the severity of the initial episode and whether there is any evidence of recurrence.

Chronic phase treatment

After the acute phase the therapeutic options involve two main classes of anticoagulant drugs:

- The orally administered coumarin derivatives and indanediones.
- Heparin and heparinoids which have to be given parenterally. Before the introduction of self administered subcutaneous injections for small-dose prophylaxis heparin was used only over the short term.

Outside pregnancy long term prophylaxis for thrombophilia and chronic phase treatment of acute thromboembolism is achieved almost exclusively by using the coumarin derivative, warfarin—but during pregnancy the use of warfarin carries hazards for the mother, fetus and neonate throughout gestation and in the immediate postpartum period.

Warfarin

An important advantage of warfarin is that it can be taken by mouth but it has many disadvantages during pregnancy. It crosses the placenta and has adverse effects on the fetus throughout the ante-natal period including teratogenicity in the first trimester and an increasing haemorrhagic tendency, maximal during labour and delivery. A woman who is adequately anticoagulated on warfarin can bleed disastrously if an obstetric complication such as premature placental separation occurs or if urgent caesarean section or instrumental delivery is undertaken. Warfarin has a prolonged effect and the action cannot easily or rapidly be reversed. Administration of vitamin K achieves reversal within 24 hours but if warfarinisation is required after the emergency is over restabilisation after the administration of vitamin K is difficult as vitamin K may result in rebound hypercoagulability.

The only rapid method of reversing the effect of warfarin is by infusion of fresh frozen plasma, with all its hazards, to restore the depleted haemostatic factors. Another disadvantage is that because of the elevated coagulation factors and increasing blood volume in normal pregnancy the requirements during pregnancy are changing constantly and much more frequent monitoring and control of dosage is necessary than in the non-pregnant state. Drugs that interact with warfarin make its control more difficult and may increase the risk of bleeding in the mother and fetus. In particular antibiotics used in the treatment of urinary tract infection, a relatively common complication, alter the requirements of warfarin dramatically. Either dangerously low levels of haemostatic factors or inadequate anticoagulation may result if the laboratory control tests are not undertaken appropriately and the dose altered as necessary.[13,14]

Laboratory control of warfarin

The purpose of laboratory control in the chronic phase of treatment is to achieve and maintain a level of hypocoagulability which is effective in preventing thrombosis but is not sufficient to make the risk of spontaneous haemorrhage appreciable. It is not realistic or possible to induce a derangement of normal haemostatic mechanism without accepting some risk of bleeding.[15]

Prothrombin time The one stage prothrombin time of Quick is the most popular test in the United Kingdom for control of warfarin therapy.[15] The most important variable is the thromboplastin used in the test. Thromboplastins from animal sources, in particular rabbit, have been used and, in the past, from human brain but this is now precluded because of the danger of transmission of viral infections. There are a number of commercial rabbit-brain thromboplastins available. These various thromboplastins give different prolongations of prothrombin time with the same test plasma so it is not possible to define the therapeutic range unless the thromboplastin used is also specified. It is possible to use a reference thromboplastin to assess the sensitivity of the thromboplastin used in individual laboratories. These reference thromboplastins have all been calibrated in terms of a primary WHO human brain thromboplastin. The relative potency of each is defined by an international sensitivity index (ISI). In the anticoagulant clinic the measured prothrombin time is converted to a prothrombin ratio by comparing it with the mean of a number of normal plasma prothrombin times. If the sensitivity index of the thromboplastin used in the laboratory is known then each patient's ratio can be converted into an international normalised ratio (INR). The optimal therapeutic ratio for the INR is in general within the range of 2·0 to 4·0.[16] This is valid for all thromboplastins which have been standardised against the international reference thromboplastins supplied by the WHO.

A survey before these stringent measures were taken showed that to achieve a laboratory prothrombin ratio of between 2·0 and 4·0 there were wide differences in the dosage of warfarin given from centre to centre.[17] In particular much larger daily doses of warfarin were being given to women in the United States and Canada than in the United Kingdom. It seems that the difference in responsiveness of the various thromboplastins (and difficulties in conforming to international standardisations) still has an effect on prothrombin time reporting in North America and exposes patients to erratic dosing.[18,19] This has important implications in the reported incidence of adverse effects of warfarin.

Effects of warfarin on the fetus

The effects on the conceptus resulting from transplacental passage of oral anticoagulant drugs include a characteristic embryopathy, central nervous system abnormalities, and fetal bleeding.[20] There also seems to be an increased risk of abortion or prematurity thought to be caused by maternal and fetal haemostatic defects resulting in placental bleeding and early placental separation.[21] There is a definite but variable incidence of teratogenesis associated with the use of warfarin in the first trimester of pregnancy.[22,23]

Chondrodysplasia punctata, characterised by abnormal cartilage and bone formation, is the most common syndrome though warfarin is not the only cause of this malformation.[24,25] Coumarin induced embryopathy in the human fetus comprises nasal hypoplasia, hypertelorism and stippled epiphyses on radiographs. Stippled epiphyses occur in vertebrae, carpals, femur, and calcanei during infancy and early childhood but disappear with age.[26] Other skeletal abnormalities include brachydactyly, hypoplasia of terminal phalanges, radial deviation of fingers, skull abnormalities, and kyphoscoliosis. These abnormalities have been described after in utero exposure to oral anticoagulants only during the first trimester of pregnancy.[20] The skeletal abnormalities may be associated with optic atrophy, microcephaly, and mental retardation in some infants, but it is not clear whether these associations are a result of microhaemorrhages into cerebral tissue in the second and third trimesters rather than a first trimester effect.[27] Other congenital malformations such as polydactyly, corneal leukoma,[22] and asplenia[28] have been described, but it is not possible to be certain whether these were chance associations or not.

Other reported anomalies include intrauterine growth retardation, development delay, seizures, transient hypotonia, persistent truncus arteriosus, occipital meningomyelocele, hydrocephaly, and Dandy-Walker malformation.[29] The prospective and much-quoted study of Iturbe-Alessio *et al* reported an incidence of embryopathy of 28·6%.[30] The embryopathy consisted of chondrodysplasia punctata only and there were no central nervous system abnormalities. It has also been recognised for many years that the use of warfarin during late pregnancy (after 36 weeks' gestation) is associated with serious retroplacental and fetal bleeding—an important hazard to the fetus being intracerebral haemorrhage. With the development of prenatal ultrasound techniques reports are beginning to appear of large fetal intracranial haemorrhages associated with warfarin therapy in the second and third trimesters. This usually occurs only when maternal warfarin control is unsatisfactory but was observed in one case without apparent overanticoagulation.[31] These hazards can be explained by warfarin crossing the placenta together with the fact that the fetus has low concentrations of the clotting factors synthesised in the liver even without the influence of warfarin, because of the liver's functional immaturity.[32,33] For these reasons Hirsh *et al* recommended that, after an initial period of heparinisation in the acute attack, prophylactic heparin should continue to be used in the first trimester followed by warfarin between 13 and 36 weeks, reverting to small dose prophylactic heparin for the last weeks of pregnancy.[34] These recommendations were widely followed in the past and are still followed in some centres in the UK.[35,36]

However, Sherman and Hall described a case of microcephaly in the newborn infant of a patient who had taken warfarin for the last six months of pregnancy only.[37] This stimulated further correspondence culminating in a report in which a further five cases of microcephaly occurring in California were cited and the largely American literature on the hazards of warfarin was reviewed.[38] The reported incidence of complications in the fetus was enormously high, nearly 28% of those exposed were either abnormal at birth or died in utero. Holzgreve *et al* also made the point that there should be long term follow up of the fetus exposed to warfarin as their reported case was apparently normal at birth but subsequently shown to have central nervous system developmental abnormality.[38] At Queen Charlotte's Hospital we conducted a follow up of 22 children for a mean of 4 years (22–67 months) who were exposed to warfarin in utero—two in the first trimester and 20 in which the mother had taken warfarin after 14 weeks' gestation. The children were drawn from a total of 45 women who took warfarin in pregnancy between 1974 and 1978. All the offspring had achieved normal developmental parameters. Although the fetal wastage was high (8·7%) our results suggested that the risk of permanent damage is low if the fetus survives.[39] An earlier study reported the outcome of 42 pregnancies in which the mothers had taken warfarin in the mid trimester. In twenty-two of them warfarin had been taken in the first trimester also. Although the spontaneous abortion rate was high there were no cases of chondrodysplasia punctata or microcephaly.[40]

A more recent report studied the fetal and neonatal outcome of women with prosthetic heart valves exposed to warfarin or heparin or both for prophylaxis of thromboembolism during pregnancy in the period between 1978–89.[41] During the period September to December 1990, all live born children were called back for examination by a paediatrician blind to the type and duration of anticoagulant exposure. There were 18 children whose mothers were maintained on warfarin only throughout pregnancy. The ages at follow up ranged from 0·5–11·3 years (mean 5·2 years). There were no cases of chondrodysplasia punctata either during the neonatal period or at follow up. Neither were there any central nervous system malformations. There was however, a high incidence of nasal hypoplasia (12 cases—66%) and hypertelorism (11 cases—61%). Of the 11 children exposed to both

313

warfarin and heparin whose ages were between 1·8 and 8·2 years at follow up, four had nasal hypoplasia and two had hypertelorism, but again none had evidence of stippled epiphyses either in the neonatal period or at follow up. There appears to be an increased fetal wastage in women taking warfarin in terms of abortion and still birth but the risk of significant damaging embryopathy or central nervous system malformation is not high.

The prospective study showed that the 28·6% risk of embryopathy from warfarin exposure in Mexico was confined to the period between the 6th and 12th week of gestation.[30] In contrast a report from Pavankumar et al in New Delhi gave details of ten years experience of pregnancy in patients with cardiac valve replacements, 37 of whom had 47 pregnancies.[42] They were managed before and throughout pregnancy on a strictly monitored coumarin regimen through to the last week when they were switched to heparin 5000 six hourly until delivery. Although fetal wastage was high (8·5%) none of the neonates had any congenital abnormalities and they were developmentally normal on discharge although there was no long term follow up.

Why are there such gross discrepancies between reports from various centres of the hazards of warfarin for the fetus? One simple explanation is that it may be a dosage phenomenon. The reports of high incidences of both chondrodysplasia punctata and mid-trimester central nervous system developmental effects come mainly from North America where much higher mean daily doses were being given than in the United Kingdom.[17] This was thought to be the result in part of the different laboratory reagents and the failure to submit the insensitive thromboplastins used to international standardisation. The central nervous system abnormalities seemed to occur in the offspring of those women on higher doses of warfarin.[43] Certainly in the United Kingdom it is difficult to find a clinically obvious case of microcephaly, central nervous system abnormality or chondrodysplasia punctata, and over the past years many women with cardiac abnormalities have taken warfarin throughout the first trimester. This must be encouraging for physicians who have to manage pregnant women with artificial heart valves in the United Kingdom, because small dose heparin is not a safe alternative to warfarin for prevention of thromboembolism in these cases.

Patients may continue to breast feed while they are taking warfarin as there is no detectable secretion of warfarin in breast milk.[44,45] Infants who are breast fed while their mothers are taking warfarin are not at any increased risk of abnormal bleeding. This does not apply to phenindione as maternal therapy has caused severe haemorrhage in a breast fed infant.[46]

Heparin

Heparin seems to be the drug of choice at least during the antenatal period as it does not cross the placenta. Its main disadvantage is that it has to be given parenterally. Bonnar pioneered the use of self-administered subcutaneous heparin for the treatment and prophylaxis of thromboembolism in pregnancy.[9] Its efficiency depends on the fact that in doses too small to have a direct effect on thrombin in the circulation, heparin inhibits the activation of factor X to factor Xa, an action almost identical with and potentiated by the naturally occurring anticoagulant antithrombin III. Low-dose prophylactic subcutaneous heparin, when given to cover surgery, does not require monitoring if hepatic and renal function are normal. A standard dose is 5000 IU eight hourly. During pregnancy, however, treatment continues for much longer and requirements are greater particularly in the weeks approaching full term.[47] The half-life of heparin injected subcutaneously is about 18 hours compared with intravenous heparin which has a half-life of 1·5 hours. The small doses of heparin do not lower the concentration of coagulation factors in the plasma and therefore the effect cannot be measured by using the crude tests of coagulation bioactivity such as the activated partial thromboplastin time or prothrombin time. The introduction of a more specific assay method based on the ability of heparin to accelerate the neutralisation of factor Xa has allowed these low concentrations of heparin in the plasma to be measured. There are now a number of commercial kits available using chromogenic substrates, and most district general hospitals can offer this investigation if required. Because of variations in renal function it has been suggested that frequent monitoring should be undertaken so that dangerous or inadequate anticoagulation can be avoided. Experience suggests that a plasma heparin concentration of 0·02 to 0·2 IU/ml provides adequate prophylaxis against venous thromboembolism without the hazard of bleeding. At Queen Charlotte's Hospital we use 10 000 IU 12-hourly throughout the antenatal period, altering the dose only by reducing it if concentrations of more than 0·2 IU/ml are found. We take samples for heparin assay at each antenatal clinic visit. A rapid method to check that there is not over anticoagulation is to perform coagulation screening tests, particularly the thrombin time, which should be within the normal range.

Although patients often show initial reluctance most can be taught to give themselves subcutaneous heparin and therefore can be discharged home after acute phase treatment. In the UK no difference has been found in bruising between sodium and calcium heparin.[48] Possible injection sites are the thighs or abdominal wall.

Because of the high incidence of thromboembolism in the days following labour and delivery and the increased risk following operative delivery, subcutaneous heparin is continued throughout labour and delivery whether it be normal vaginal, instrumental, or by caesarean section. The heparin assay is checked in the week preceding delivery. A small controlled trial of prophylactic subcutaneous heparin therapy showed no excess of antenatal or postnatal bleeding associated with small dose heparin.[49]

The question of low-dose heparin prophylaxis and epidural anaesthesia remains controversial. Provided that the heparin assay is within the prophylactic range or there is no significant prolongation of coagulation screening tests (activated partial thromboplastin time and particularly thrombin time, which is peculiarly sensitive to therapeutic levels of heparin), it is quite safe to give epidural analgesia during heparin prophylaxis in my opinion. Given in appropriate low dosage, heparin does not interfere with activation of haemostatic mechanisms at the site of injury. The debate is well set out in a published report.[50]

Postpartum the dose of heparin is empirically reduced to 7500 units twice daily because of reduction in circulating blood volume and the fact that the concentration of clotting factors returns to normal during the puerperium. The option of switching to warfarin postpartum after 3–5 days, when the risk of secondary postpartum haemorrhage is much less, is largely a question of patient convenience. Neither anticoagulant prevents the mother breast-feeding. Heparin has the disadvantage of daily injections but does not require laboratory control, whereas warfarin, though taken by mouth, needs repeated prothrombin time estimations to control the dosage and the mother has to make frequent hospital visits for blood to be taken for laboratory testing. Self monitoring of the INR (and APTT) soon to be available in the UK will greatly reduce the inconvenience as well as improving anticoagulant control (as has blood sugar monitoring in diabetes).

Complications of long term heparin therapy

Thrombocytopenia

This is a well recognised complication of heparin treatment with a reported incidence of 1–30%. The pathophysiology is not well understood and remains controversial. A prospective study found that patients could be divided into two groups on clinical grounds.[51] One group had mild asymptomatic thrombocytopenia of early onset, the platelet count being above $65 \times 10^9/l$. The cause of this type of thrombocytopenia seemed to be a direct effect of heparin on the platelets. The second group had severe delayed onset thrombocytopenia associated with a heparin-dependent IgG antibody and a high incidence of thromboembolic complications with some fatalities. The nature and mechanism of action of the antibody has recently been defined.[52] Different approaches are needed in the management of these two types of heparin-induced thrombocytopenia. Patients with mild early onset thrombocytopenia need no active treatment, but those with severe thrombocytopenia ($<50 \times 10^9/l$) of delayed onset should be given oral anticoagulants with or without antiplatelet drugs and the heparin stopped immediately. There continue to be sporadic reports of heparin associated thrombocytopenia[53] but in our own experience and that of others in the United Kingdom, thrombocytopenia does not appear to be a significant problem. It is thought that the lack of this complication may be due to the source of heparin which is generally used in the United Kingdom.

Osteopenia

The most important hazard of heparin treatment is a form of bone demineralisation known as osteopenia. The cause is unknown although it has been attributed to a deficiency of 1,25-dihydrotachysterol.[54]

A retrospective follow up study of 20 women treated during and after pregnancy with subcutaneous heparin suggested that even those patients who are asymptomatic may have some degree of bone demineralisation as assessed by tomography of the small bones of the hand.[55] The data suggested that treatment with 20 000 units a day for more than 20 weeks is associated with bone demineralisation—that it is not an idiosyncratic response, but may occur in all patients if treated long enough. This is particularly worrying as bone demineralisation, like osteoporosis, does not seem to be reversible and because women treated with heparin for long periods in pregnancy will suffer further demineralisation and increased risk of fractures following menopause.

A more recent report questioned our findings.[56,58] The spine and hip radiographs of 70 women who had received therepeutic or prophylactic heparin for variable periods during pregnancy were examined. There were 12 (17%) with obvious osteopenia including two with multiple fractures of the spine. Re-examination 6–12 months postpartum showed that changes were reversible in most cases. The changes did not appear to be related to either the duration of therapy or the daily dosage in this study.

Low molecular weight heparins (LMWH)

Low molecular weight heparins (LMWH) are prepared from standard unfractionated heparin by enzymatic degradation, chemical degradation, or gel infiltration. Some few preparations have been available for clinical use on an experimental basis for some years. Their advantage in terms of prophylaxis of venous thrombosis is their alleged enhanced antithrombotic properties (anti-Xa activity) and reduced haemorrhagic hazard (antithrombin effect). It is well known that the antithrombin activity of heparin is critically dependent on molecular size. There is an inverse correlation between the anticoagulant activity of heparin in terms of anti-Xa activity and molecular size. Although LMWH are commonly referred to in a generic sense, they are not completely interchangeable in terms of efficacy and safety. The biological half-life of anti-Xa activity of LMWH is approximately twice as long as that of unfractionated heparin and it is well absorbed from subcutaneous injection sites. This means that one injection daily is sufficient to achieve safe prophylaxis. The size of the molecule also influences its interaction with platelets and if the heparin molecules are reduced to less than 5000 to 8000 daltons the possible reaction with platelets is blocked and therefore the incidence of heparin associated thrombocytopenia is reduced.[57] Most clinical trials have been devoted to finding a safe but effective dose.

Another problem has been the in vitro monitoring of dosage. The assessment of the correct dose of LMWH has been made even more difficult by the lack of guidance by in vitro assays because the LMWH have been calibrated against unfractionated heparin, which has been shown to be inappropriate. However, it seems that the haemorrhagic hazard can be controlled by factor Xa in vitro assays with appropriate standardisation of the assay using LMWH as the baseline. LMWH have now been licensed for clinical use in a variety of conditions but not, as yet, for pregnancy. A few centres are using LMWH to treat and prevent recurrence of thromboembolism in the antenatal period. The obvious practical advantage for the woman is the reduction in the number of self-administered long term injections. The correct dose has yet to be found for safe and effective prophylaxis in pregnancy but one daily injection is sufficient. More importantly perhaps it is hoped that a reduction in the total dosage should reduce the risk of the serious complication of osteopenia.

However, preliminary studies in patients[58] and in animals[59] show that LMWH is associated with bone demineralisation although severe demineralisation appears to be less with LMWH than with heparin.[60] It is encouraging that there is no evidence to suggest that LMWH cross the placenta at any stage of pregnancy.[61,62]

Anecdotal reports of the use of LMWH and our own reported experience[64] of thromboprophylaxis in 18 patients have been favourable.[63-65] There were no episodes of thromboembolism, and no prenatal losses. Mean heparin concentrations (anti-Xa assay) two to four hours after injection were $0\cdot134 \pm 0\cdot122$ μ/ml and no thrombocytopenia were observed. Three out of six dual x ray absorbitometry (DEXA) scans performed one to nine months after cessation of heparin showed low bone density in spine or hip compared to age and sex matched controls. Effects on bone demineralisation require further investigation.

Heparin remains the drug of choice for long term management of venous thromboembolism during pregnancy, but whether or not prophylaxis should be instituted in women entering pregnancy with a history of previous thromboembolism or with other high risk factors is a matter for debate, given the high rate of maternal bone demineralisation.

Prophylaxis of thromboembolism

There are three groups of patients in whom prophylaxis should be considered:

- Those who are at high risk because of age, parity, obesity, or operative delivery
- Those who have had thromboembolism in the past
- Those with cardiac disease.

In regard to the first group it is generally thought but not proved that the risk of thromboembolism is greatest in the postnatal period so that any prophylaxis need be used only to cover labour and the peurperium. It would seem reasonable to use some form of prophylaxis for all patients over 30 years of age having an emergency caesarean section and also in women over 35 years old even if they have a normal vaginal delivery. Although in the past we used intravenous dextran to cover labour and caesarean section so that an epidural anaesthetic could be administered, we now give intrapartum prophylactic subcutaneous heparin whether an epidural analgesic is being given or not and we do not believe that prophylactic heparin is a contraindication to epidural anaesthesia. In fact dextran affects platelet function, reducing adhesiveness and aggregation, and this may be more likely to increase the hazard of bleeding in the epidural space than prophylactic heparin. It has been suggested that the bleeding problems using dextran 40 can approach the frequency of those encountered with oral anticoagulants. Although there has been no systemic evaluation of efficacy and risks of dextran in pregnancy, Bergqvist et al found no cases of deep venous thrombosis in 19 patients given dextran during caesarean section, whereas there were three venous thromboses in 150 patients undergoing caesarean section who did not receive dextran.[66]

There are several other drawbacks to dextran. It interferes with blood compatibility testing and therefore blood must be taken for crossmatching before the infusion is started in case transfusion should be required.

Dextran should be avoided in any obstetric patient with cardiac or renal impairment or with a history of allergic reactions as dextran can cause anaphylaxis with acute fetal distress[66a]. The incidence of this possible but rare complication is said to vary between 1/400[67] and 1/1400.[68]

The second group of patients who may require prophylaxis are those who enter pregnancy with a history of previous thromboembolism. These are considered to be at risk throughout pregnancy but the need for prophylactic anticoagulation during the total antenatal period as well as intrapartum and postpartum—once widely accepted—is now under challenge.

The practice was largely based on a retrospective survey which found that previous thromboembolism carried a 12% risk of recurrent thromboembolism in pregnancy.[69] This study was subject to diagnostic bias without objective confirmation. It appears that the risk of recurrent antenatal thromboembolism has been over-estimated and may be of the order of 2% or less.[43]

It is difficult to argue for routine antenatal prophylaxis in women with a history of simple thromboembolism and no extra risk factors, given the risks of warfarin administration and the substantial risk of bone demineralisation when heparin is given long term.

An alternative is to use low-dose aspirin which has been shown in recent years to have a prophylactic effect not only in arterial but also in venous thromboembolism.[70] The safety of aspirin during pregnancy is controversial.[71] There are anxieties regarding adverse effects during pregnancy, parturition, and the puerperium and these have been reviewed.[72] However, in the recently published results of the Collaborative Low-dose Aspirin Study[73] for the prevention and treatment of pre-eclampsia, it became clear that there was little risk of bleeding in over 4000 women receiving aspirin and that low-dose aspirin was generally safe for the fetus and newborn infant with no evidence of increased bleeding or developmental particularly cardiovascular, abnormality. As a consequence, our group at Queen Charlotte's has recently introduced a regimen of low dose aspirin prophylaxis (75 mg daily) for those women with low risk of recurrence in the antenatal period, who would otherwise have had no anticoagulant treatment until onset of labour or delivery by elective caesarean section.

Our present approach is to counsel patients with a history of thromboembolism about the relative risks of prophylactic drugs and recurrence of thromboembolism in the antenatal period. All women should have been screened after the initial episode to exclude genetic risk factors such as deficiencies of protein C, protein S and antithrombin III, Activated Protein C (APC) resistance (Factor V Leiden) or dysfibrinogenaemia, all of which may require long term prophylaxis apart from pregnancy. The lupus anticoagulant and anticardiolipin syndrome should also be excluded as all of these conditions require special management in pregnancy.

Antenatal subcutaneous heparin is recommended only in those patients who are at particular risk having had more than one episode in the past, a family history, or who have inherited abnormalities of the haemostatic mechanisms leading to thrombophilia. Subcutaneous heparin is also used antenatally in those patients who are particularly concerned about recurrence. This is an uneasy compromise but only a large study with multicentre cooperation would answer the question of relative risks and benefits of antenatal prophylaxis of thromboembolism because the numbers at risk in any one centre are too small.

Prevention of thromboembolism in pregnancy in women with cardiac problems

The one condition for which warfarin should still be recommended in pregnancy is in the prevention of *arterial* thromboembolism in patients with prosthetic heart valves, mitral valve disease, and atrial fibrillation. Unless full anticoagulation is maintained in patients with artificial heart valves there is the risk of valve thrombosis or of systemic embolism.[74-85] The risk of systemic embolism is high if the patient receives no prophylaxis at all.[85] There is a similar hazard with mitral valve disease.[86] There is no acceptable substitute for adequate oral anticoagulant drugs in patients with prosthetic heart valves. Despite improvements in valve design and materials systemic embolism and valve thrombosis remain the major causes of late morbidity and mortality. Inadequate anticoagulation increases the risk of thrombo-embolism two to six times.[87] Although adding dipyridamole or aspirin to warfarin further reduces the risk of systemic embolism after valve replacement[88] there is good evidence that antiplatelet drugs alone are ineffective.[89] In one large series of 68 pregnancies coumarins were replaced by antiplatelet drugs (aspirin or dipyridamole or both) which resulted in three fatal valve thromboses and a 20% incidence of systemic embolism.[90] The use of small dose heparin alone has been associated with disastrous and fatal thrombosis of the prosthesis.[91] There has been reported failure of therapeutic heparin prophylaxis.[92,93] Effective anticoagulation must be continued whenever women become pregnant after valve replacement. The only exceptions are those with biovalves whose anticoagulants can be stopped three months after surgery except when mitral valve replacement is accompanied by atrial fibrillation or major left atrial enlargement.

In the past it was thought that the intensity of anticoagulant therapy should be maintained to give an INR of about 3·0 in all patients with artificial heart valves to provide adequate protection. There have now been three studies which have shown that a regimen of moderate intensity (INR 2·0–3·0) is just as effective as higher intensity anticoagulation.[94–96] High intensity anticoagulation was associated with significantly more bleeding.

An analysis of published reports suggests that fetal embryopathy and mid-trimester effects of warfarin are dose related. It is encouraging to know that less intense regimens are as protective as the higher dose regimen. It may also explain the relative lack of reported adverse fetal effects associated with maternal warfarin in the UK.

Another suggestion has been to use fixed minidose warfarin which has been shown to prevent thromboembolism in certain conditions which carry the risk of venous thromboembolism, such as after major surgery.[97] There has been one anecdotal report of fixed minidose warfarin during pregnancy in a woman with ATIII deficiency.[98] She had a subclavian vein thrombosis at 18 weeks' gestation which was treated with heparin intravenously and resulted in clinical resolution of the thrombosis. She was unable to tolerate the prophylactic heparin regimen which followed, and was therefore managed with 1 mg of warfarin daily from 32 weeks' gestation and for six weeks postpartum. This regimen did not reduce the concentration of clotting factors II, VII, IX, or X. Fetal cord blood samples were obtained at 33, 36 and 38 weeks and coagulation factor assays were within reference range. There were no further thromboses through pregnancy or postpartum.

This anecdotal report is interesting and lower doses of warfarin for anticoagulation during pregnancy deserve further investigation but it is unlikely that fixed minidose warfarin will ever have a place in prophylaxis of thromboembolism associated with heart disease although a lower therapeutic regimen is now generally accepted as being effective.

It has been suggested that it would be preferable to replace all diseased valves with biovalves in women in the reproductive years, so avoiding the hazards of full anticoagulant treatment during pregnancy, however this is achieved. Unfortunately, evidence is accumulating that there is no ideal prosthesis for women during their reproductive years. The prosthesis should be durable, non-thrombogenic, and haemodynamically satisfactory. Biological prostheses have been shown to have altered durability in the second and third decade of life. Pregnancy has a profound effect on the maternal cardiovascular system, thus altering the stress on biological prostheses. Altered calcium metabolism during pregnancy may also be an important factor leading to calcification and early valve degeneration.[99] Although bioprostheses afford the opportunity of uncomplicated pregnancy without the need for anticoagulation and continue to be recommended, the accelerated rate of deterioration observed during and after pregnancy and the need for reoperation, sometimes in the presence of haemodynamic deterioration, counteract their desirability.[100]

The extensive recent literature on this subject has revealed several facts. The danger of chondrodysplasia punctata is confined to the period of gestation between six and nine weeks and this embryopathy occurs only in fetuses who are exposed to warfarin during this period of gestation.[30] We also know that the embryopathy and the central nervous system malformations may well be dose-related[17] and that incidence of these complications have perhaps been over emphasised in the past.[26,38] Our follow up study[39] and the reports from Hong Kong[40,41] suggest that the risks in terms of significant development abnormality to the fetus exposed to warfarin at any time in gestation are small. Even if the fetus is exposed to warfarin during the sixth to the 12th week of gestation the risk of chondrodysplasia punctata is small if the dose of warfarin is not excessive and laboratory control of the INR conforms to international standards.[41,42] Javares et al[101] wrote that the use of minimum doses of warfarin, resulting in a low prothrombin ratio may reduce the teratogenic and abortion risks. In the series of Iturbe-Alessio[30] two women whose treatment was changed to subcutaneous heparin in the early weeks (seven to 12 weeks) of pregnancy thrombosed their valves.[83] However, they were managed on a small dose of heparin (10 000 twice daily IU) and this is ineffective for the prophylaxis of arterial thromboembolism.[93]

A prospective study from Naples looked at the outcome of medium to low dose warfarin during pregnancy in 20 women with mechanical heart valve prostheses, aged between 23 and 31 years.[102] The mean (SD) prothrombin ratio (INR) measured weekly was 2·06 (0·45) and the mean daily warfarin dosage 4·1 mg (1·63). The women conceived while taking warfarin and were maintained on warfarin throughout the first and second trimesters to the 37th week of pregnancy. Caesarean section was electively carried out in 19 of the 20 women at 38 weeks' gestation, the warfarin being discontinued 48 hours before. There were no thromboembolic or haemorrhagic complications and no spontaneous abortions, stillbirths, or deaths. No evidence of embryopathy was found on cardiac, neurological, radiological, or echocardiographic examination. It is true that these women were preselected as requiring medium to low doses of warfarin for adequate low intensity prophylaxis before pregnancy was embarked upon, but the study emphasises again the dose-related nature of the fetal abnormalities.

322

In contrast, another prospective study looked at 60 pregnancies in 49 patients with prosthetic heart valves, in 40 of whom oral anticoagulation was used at some time during the antenatal period and came up with very different findings.[103] Three infants had a warfarin embryopathy. Spontaneous abortions and stillbirths occurred only in the warfarin treated group and there was an increased incidence of low birth weight and prematurity in the offspring of women taking warfarin. However, there was a significant association between prematurity and the mother's New York Heart Association (NYHA) functional class. This study came from Brazil and the warfarin control was much less strict than in the report of Cotrufo et al.[102] The INR was not used to report the prothrombin time and the assay was every three weeks rather than weekly. This is yet another example of the differing experience in Europe compared with the Americas.

The most striking report in this respect, however, is that of Sbarouni and Oakley.[104] This was a retrospective study of 214 pregnancies in 182 women with prosthetic heart valves from major cardiac centres in Europe. Most of the women were in NYHA class I or II in sinus rhythm. There were 151 pregnancies with mechanical heart valves and 63 pregnancies in those with bioprostheses. Eighty-three per cent of the pregnancies with bioprostheses and 73% of those with mechanical heart valves resulted in healthy babies, term or preterm, with no adverse sequelae. The events that were reported included spontaneous abortions as well as therapeutic terminations. The incidence of still births and spontaneous abortions did not differ in the two groups. Fifty-three per cent of the women with mechanical heart valves had taken warfarin at some time during pregnancy, 40% during the first trimester, but no embryopathies were reported. There were 13 valve thromboses (four fatal), eight embolic events (two fatal) and seven severe bleeds in women with mechanical heart valves. Most complications occurred in association with heparin treatment but one fatal aortic thrombosis occurred in a woman with a mechanical valve who refused anticoagulant treatment. The authors stated that their study showed that warfarin therapy is safe and effective and not associated with embryopathy. Their conclusions have been strongly criticised on the grounds that they were drawn from a retrospective survey, susceptible to selection recall and reporting biases and that their conclusions need to be interpreted in the context of other published reports.[105] However, warfarin's really bad press stems from a letter to the Lancet in 1976 concerning one case report and a retrospective analysis of the American literature.[38] The number of cases reviewed is much smaller than in the European report.

Nobody would argue that, in high dosage, warfarin causes chondro-dysplasia punctata and more importantly central nervous system developmental defects. In most European studies, however, these complications have been shown to be dose-related and most babies born to European women on a well-controlled warfarin regimen do not seem to have any serious disabling consequences if they survive the first trimester. Is nasal hypoplasia in her baby an unacceptable consequence for a woman motivated to have a successful pregnancy if the alternative is fatal maternal thromboembolism or potentially crippling osteopenia as a result of long term therapeutic doses of heparin?

Two other points have been raised following Ginsberg and Barron's commentary.[105] Intravenous long lines which may be in place for weeks during therapeutic heparin administration provide a site for entry of bacteria which may infect prosthetic heart valves notwithstanding meticulous aseptic procedures.[106] The accelerated rate of deterioration of bioprostheses in young women, particularly during pregnancy which was challenged by Ginsberg and Barron was reaffirmed by reference to appropriate published data.[100]

There is no ideal solution to this problem but the incidence of side-effects in the United Kingdom appears to be low. This, together with the fact that subcutaneous prophylactic heparin is ineffective in preventing thromboembolism in this situation has led us to adopt a policy of continuing warfarin from the 12th to the 36th week of pregnancy when the risk of fetal (and maternal) bleeding is overwhelming. The patient is admitted to hospital and given continuous intravenous infusion of heparin to achieve a concentration of 0·4 to 0·6 U/ml as measured by heparin assay. It is believed that the clotting system of the fetus returns to normal after warfarin has been withheld for 7 to 9 days. At that time the dose of heparin should be reduced to give a concentration of less than 0·2 U/ml and labour should be induced. If the patient goes into labour while on warfarin then fresh frozen plasma will correct her coagulopathy. Some recommend giving vitamin K to the mother to reverse the action of warfarin in the fetus but this is hazardous because of a rebound hypercoagulable effect in the mother and problems in reestablishing warfarin therapy after delivery. In extreme cases vitamin K has been given to the fetus in utero by transamniotic injection.[107] After delivery the patient should recommence warfarin but should continue to receive intravenous heparin, to give a concentration of 0·4 to 0·6 U/ml until effective warfarin anticoagulation is reestablished.

Personal conclusions

Anticoagulant treatment of patients with prosthetic heart valves during pregnancy remains controversial. Bioprostheses which do not require anticoagulant cover are liable to deteriorate rapidly in young people, especially under the stress of pregnancy. The combination of artificial heart valve prosthesis, pregnancy, and anticoagulation creates a high risk pregnancy which is very difficult to manage. Long term therapeutic heparin is difficult to monitor and carries the hazard of bone demineralisation and systemic infection. Strongly motivated women in a stable cardiac state have a reasonable chance of successful outcome if adequately and appropriately anticoagulated with warfarin, which can be avoided between six and 12 weeks' gestation and stopped two weeks before planned delivery. The use of warfarin should be strictly controlled with the INR, aiming to keep the prothrombin ratio around 2·0 to 2·5 using low to medium dosage. Long term therapeutic heparin is not ideal and should be used only when it is thought wise to interrupt warfarin treatment. It carries the hazard of bone demineralisation and systemic infection, and laboratory control is difficult. There is no haemostatic hazard for the breast-fed infant whose mother is taking warfarin.

Women with prosthetic heart valves in the reproductive years need intensive and explicit education about the potential dangers of pregnancy for themselves and their infants.

The importance of reporting suspected pregnancy early should be emphasised so that the switch from warfarin to therapeutic heparin can be made, if necessary before six weeks' gestation, should the woman and her physician so desire. It is impractical, inappropriate, and hazardous for a woman to change to therapeutic heparin before pregnancy while trying to conceive.

References

1 Villasanta U. Thromboembolic disease in pregnancy. *Am J Obstet Gynecol* 1965; **93**: 142–60.

2 Barritt DW, Jordan SC. Anticoagulant drugs in the treatment of pulmonary embolism: a controlled trial. *Lancet* 1960; **i**: 1309–12.

3 Moseley P, Kerstein MD. Pregnancy and thrombophlebitis. *Surg Gynecol Obstet* 1980; **150**: 593–7.

4 Sharma GVRK, Burlesco VA, Sasahara AA. Effect of thrombolytic therapy on pulmonary-capillary blood volume in patients with pulmonary embolism. *N Engl J Med* 1980; **303**: 842–5.

5 Meissner AJ, Misiak A, Ziemski JM, *et al.* Hazards of thrombolytic therapy in deep vein thrombosis. *Br J Surg* 1987; **74**: 991–3.

6 Delclos GL, Davila F. Thrombolytic therapy for pulmonary embolism in pregnancy: a case report. *Am J Obstet Gynecol* 1986; **155**: 375–6.

7 Baudo F, Caimi TM, Redaelli R, *et al.* Emergency treatment with recombinant tissue plasminogen activator of pulmonary embolism in a pregnant woman with antithrombin III deficiency. *Am J Obstet Gynecol* 1990; **163**: 1274–5.

8 Seifried E, Gabelmann A, Ellbruck D, Schmidt A. Thrombolytic therapy of pulmonary artery embolism in early pregnancy with recombinant tissue-type plasminogen activator. *Geburtshilfe Frauenheilkd* 1991; **51**: 655–8.

9 Bonnar J. Long term self-administered heparin therapy for prevention and treatment of thromboembolic complication in pregnancy. In: Kakkar VV, Thomas DP, eds. *Heparin chemistry and clinical usage*. London: Academic Press, 1976.

10 Kitchen S, Jennings I, Woods TAL, Preston FE, on behalf of the Steering Committee of the UK National Quality Assessment Scheme for Blood Coagulation. Wide variability in the sensitivity of APTT reagents for monitoring of heparin dosage. *J Clin Pathol* 1996; **49**: 10–14.

11 Decousus HA, Croze M, Levi FA, *et al.* Circadian changes in anticoagulant effect of heparin infused at a constant rate. *BMJ* 1985; **290**: 341–4.

12 Bowler GMR, Galloway DW, Meiklejohn BH, Macintyre CCA. Sharp fall in blood pressure after injection of heparin containing chlorbutol. *Lancet* 1986; **i**: 848–9.

13 Hirsh J. Oral anticoagulant drugs. *N Engl J Med* 1991; **324**: 1865–75.

14 Hirsh, J, Fuster V. Guide to anticoagulant therapy part 2: Oral anticoagulants. *Circulation – AHA Medical/Scientific Statement – Special Report* 1994; **89**: 1469–80.

15 Dacie JV, Lewis SM. Laboratory control of anticoagulant, thrombolytic and anti-platelet therapy. *Practical haematology*. 8th ed. Edinburgh: Churchill Livingstone, 1995.

16 Poller L. Laboratory control of anticoagulant therapy. *Semin Thromb Hemost* 1986; **12**: 13–19.

17 Poller L, Taberner DA. Dosage and control of oral anticoagulants: an international collaborative survey. *Br J Haematol* 1982; **51**: 479–85.

18 Hirsh J. Is the dose of warfarin prescribed by American physicians unnecessarily high? *Arch Intern Med* 1987; **147**: 769–71.

19 Bussey HI, Force RW, Bianco TM, Leonard AD. Reliance on prothrombin time ratios causes significant errors in anticoagulation therapy. *Arch Intern Med* 1992; **152**: 278–82.

20 Hall JG, Pauli RM, Wilson KM. Maternal and fetal sequelae of anticoagulation during pregnancy. *Am J Med* 1980; **68**: 122–40.

21 Gallus AS. Anticoagulants in the prevention and treatment of thromboembolic problems in pregnancy including cardiac problems. In: Greer IA, Turpie AGG, Forbes CD, eds *Haemostasis and thrombosis*. London: Chapman & Hall Medical, 1992.

22 Ginsberg JS, Hirsh J, Turner DC, Levine MN, Burrows R. Risks to the fetus of anticoagulant therapy during pregnancy. *Thromb Haemost* 1989; **61**: 197–203.

23 Pineo GF, Hull RD. Adverse effects of coumarin anticoagulants. *Drug Saf.* 1993; **9**: 263–71.

24 Sheffield LJ, Danks DM, Mayne KV, Hutchinson LA. Chondrodysplasia punctata – 23 cases of a mild and relatively common variety. *J Pediatr* 1976; **89**: 916–23.

25 Curry CJR, Magenis RE, Brown M, *et al.* Inherited chondrodysplasia punctata due to a deletion of the terminal short arm of an X chromosome. *N Engl J Med* 1984; **311**: 1010–15.

26 Shaul WL, Hall JG. Multiple congenital anomalies associated with oral anticoagulants. *Am J Obstet Gynecol* 1988; **127**: 191–8.

27 De Vries TW, Van der Veer E, Heijmans HSA. Warfarin embryopathy: patient, possibility, pathogenesis and prognosis. *Br J Obstet Gynaecol* 1993; **100**: 869–71.

28 Cox DR, Martin L, Hall BD. Asplenia syndrome after fetal exposure to warfarin. *Lancet* 1977; **ii**: 1134.

29 Kaplan LC. Congenital Dandy Walker malformation associated with first trimester warfarin – a case report and literature review. *Teratology* 1985; **32**: 333–7.

30 Iturbe-Alessio I, del Carmen Fonseca M, Mutchinik O, Santos MA, Zajarias A, Salazar E. Risks of anticoagulant therapy in pregnant women with artificial heart valves. *N Engl J Med* 1986; **315**: 1390–3.

31 Ville Y, Jenkins E, Shearer MJ, *et al.* Fetal intraventricular haemorrhage and maternal warfarin. *Lancet* 1993; **341**: 1211.

32 Andrew M, Paes B, Milner R, *et al.* Development of the human coagulation system in the full term infant. *Blood* 1987; **70**: 165–72.

33 Andrew M, Paes B, Milner R, *et al.* Development of the human coagulation system in the healthy premature infant. *Blood* 1988; **72**: 1651–7.

34 Hirsh J, Cade JF, O'Sullivan EF. Clinical experience with anticoagulant therapy during pregnancy. *BMJ* 1970; **i**: 270–3.

35 Anonymous. Venous thromboembolism and anticoagulants in pregnancy. *BMJ* 1975; **ii**: 421–2.

36 De Swiet M, Fidler J, Howell R, Letsky EA. Thromboembolism in pregnancy. In: Jewell DP, ed. *Advanced medicine*. London: Pitman Medical, 1981.

37 Sherman S, Hall BD. Warfarin and fetal abnormality. *Lancet* 1976; **i**: 692.

38 Holzgreve W, Carey JC, Hall BD. Warfarin-induced fetal abnormalities. *Lancet* 1976; **ii**: 914–15.

39 Chong MKB, Harvey D, de Swiet M. Follow-up study of children whose mothers were treated with warfarin during pregnancy. *Br J Obstet Gynaecol* 1984; **91**: 1070–3.

40 Chen WWC, Chan CS, Lee PK, Wang RY, Wong VC. Pregnancy in patients with prosthetic heart valves: an experience with 45 pregnancies. *QJM* 1982; **51**: 358–65.

41 Wong V, Cheng CH, Chan KC. Fetal and neonatal outcome of exposure to anticoagulants during pregnancy. *Am J Med Genet* 1993; **45**: 17–21.

42 Pavankumar P, Venugopal P, Kaul U, *et al.* Pregnancy in patients with prosthetic cardiac valve. A 10-year experience. *Scand J Thorac Cardiovasc Surg* 1988; **22**: 19–22.

43 De Swiet M. Thromboembolism. In: de Swiet M, ed. *Medical disorders in obstetric practice*, 3rd ed. Oxford: Blackwell Scientific Publications, 1995.

44 Orme M L'e, Lewis M, de Swiet M, *et al.* May mothers given warfarin breast-feed their infants? *BMJ* 1977; **i**: 1564–5.

45 McKenna R, Cale ER, Vasan U. Is warfarin sodium contraindicated in the lactating mother? *J Pediatr* 1983; **103**: 325–7.
46 Eckstein H, Jack B. Breast feeding and anticoagulant therapy. *Lancet* 1970; **i**: 672–3.
47 Whitfield LR, Lele AS, Levy G. Effect of pregnancy on the relationship between concentration and anticoagulant action of heparin. *Clin Pharmacol Ther* 1983; **34**: 23–8.
48 Walker MG, Shaw JW, Thomson GJL, Cummings JGR, Leathomas M. Subcutaneous calcium heparin versus intravenous sodium heparin in treatment of established acute deep vein thrombosis of the legs; a multicentre prospective randomised trial. *BMJ* 1987; **294**: 1189–92.
49 Howell R, Fidler J, Letsky E, de Swiet M. The risks of antenatal subcutaneous heparin prophylaxis: a controlled trial. *Br J Obstet Gynaecol* 1983; **90**: 1124–8.
50 Thorburn J, Letsky E. Epidural anaesthesia is contraindicated in mothers on low-dose heparin. In: Morgan B, ed. *Controversies in obstetric anaesthesia*. London: Edward Arnold, 1990.
51 Chong BH, Pitney WR, Castaldi PA. Heparin-induced thrombocytopenia: association of thrombotic complications with heparin-dependent IgG antibody that induces thromboxane synthesis and platelet aggregation. *Lancet* 1982; **ii**: 1246–8.
52 Aster RH. Heparin-induced thrombocytopenia and thrombosis. *N Engl J Med* 1995; **332**: 1374–6.
53 Cines DB, Tomaski A, Tannenbaum S. Immune endothelial cell injury in heparin-associated thrombocytopenia. *N Engl J Med* 1987; **316**: 581–9.
54 Aarskog D, Aksnes L, Markestad T, Ulstein M, Sagen N. Heparin-induced inhibition of 1,25-dihydroxyvitamin D formation. *Am J Obstet Gynecol* 1984; **148**: 1141–2.
55 De Swiet M, Dorrington Ward P, Fidler J, *et al*. Prolonged heparin therapy in pregnancy causes bone demineralization (heparin-induced osteopenia). *Br J Obstet Gynaecol* 1983; **90**: 1129–34.
56 Dahlman T, Lindvall N, Hellgren M. Osteopenia in pregnancy during long-term heparin treatment: a radiological study post-partum. *Br J Obstet Gynaecol* 1990; **97**: 221–8.
57 Warkentin TE, Levine MN, Hirsh J, *et al*. Heparin-induced thrombocytopenia in patients treated with low-molecular-weight heparin or unfractionated heparin. *N Engl J Med* 1995; **332**: 1330–6.
58 Monreal M, Olive A, Lafoz E. Heparins, coumarin, and bone density. *Lancet* 1991; **338**: 706.
59 Matzsc T, Bergqvist D, Hedner U, Nilsson B, Ostergaard P. Induction of osteoporosis in rats by standard heparin and low molecular weight heparin. *Thromb Haemost* 1987; **58**: 36.
60 Shefras J, Farquharharson RG. Bone density studies in pregnant women receiving heparin. *Eur J Obstet Gynecol Reprod Biol* 1996; **65**: 171–4.
61 Forestier F, Daffos F, Rainaut M, Toulemonde F. Low molecular weight heparin (CY216) does not cross the placenta during the third trimester of pregnancy. *Thromb Haemost* 1987; **57**: 234.
62 Omri A, Delaloye JF, Andersen H, Bachmann F. Low molecular weight heparin Novo (LHN-1) does not cross the placenta during the second trimester of pregnancy. *Thromb Haemost* 1989; **61**: 55–6.
63 Priollet P, Roncato M, Aiach M, Housset E, Poissonnier MH, Chavinie J. Low-molecular-weight heparin in venous thrombosis during pregnancy. *Br J Haematol* 1986; **63**: 605–6.
64 Melissari E, Parker CJ, Wilson NV, *et al*. Use of low molecular weight heparin in pregnancy. *Thromb Haemost* 1992; **68**: 652–6.
65 Sturridge F, Letsky EA, de Swiet M. The use of low molecular weight heparin for thromboprophylaxis. *Br J Obstet Gynaecol* 1994; **101**: 69–71.
66 Bergqvist A, Bergqvist D, Hallbrook T. Acute deep vein thrombosis after caesarean section. *Acta Obstet Gynecol Scand* 1979; **58**: 473–6.
66aBarbier P, Jonville AP, Autret E, Coureau C. Fetal risks with Dextrans during delivery. *Drug Safety* 1992; 7: 71–3.
67 Paull JA. A prospective study of dextran-induced anaphylactoid reactions in 5745 patients. *Anaesth Intensive Care* 1987; **15**: 163–7.
68 Ring J, Messmer K. Incidence and severity of anaphylactoid reactions to colloid volume substitutes. *Lancet* 1977; **i**: 466–9.
68 Badaracco MA, Vessey M. Recurrence of venous thromboembolic disease and use of oral contraceptives. *BMJ* 1974; **i**: 215–17.

70 Antiplatelet Trialists' Collaboration. Collaborative overview of randomised trials of antiplatelet therapy III: reduction in venous thrombosis and pulmonary embolism by antiplatelet prophylaxis among surgical and medical patients. *BMJ* 1994; **308**: 235–46.

71 Ginsberg JS, Hirsh J, Marder VJ. Thrombotic and hemorrhagic complications in the obstetric patient. In: Colman RW, Hirsh J, Marder VJ, Salzman EW, eds. *Hemostasis and thrombosis: basic principles and clinical practice.* 3rd ed. Philadelphia: JB Lippincott, 1994.

72 De Swiet M, Fryers G. The use of aspirin in pregnancy. Possible adverse effects during pregnancy parturition and the puerperium? *J Obstet Gynaecol* 1990; **110**: 467–82.

73 Collaborative Low-dose Aspirin Study in Pregnancy: Collaborative Group. CLASP: a randomised trial of low-dose aspirin for the prevention and treatment of pre-eclampsia among 9364 pregnant women. *Lancet* 1994; **343**: 619–29.

74 Bjork VO, Henze A. Management of thromboembolism after aortic valve replacement with the Bjork-Shiley tilting disc valve. *Scand J Thorac Cardiovasc Surg* 1975; **9**: 183–91.

75 Ibarra-Perez C, Arevalo-Toledo N, Alvarez-De La Cadena O, Noriega-Guerra L. The course of pregnancy in patients with artificial heart valves. *Am J Med* 1976; **61**: 504–12.

76 Oakley C, Doherty P. Pregnancy in patients after valve replacement. *Br Heart J* 1976; **38**: 1140–8.

77 Limet R, Grondin CM. Cardiac valve prosthesis, anticoagulation and pregnancy. *Ann Thoracic Surg* 1977; **23**: 337–41.

78 Lutz DJ, Noller KL, Spittell JA, Danielson GK, Fish CR. Pregnancy and its complications following cardiac valve prosthesis. *Am J Obstet Gynecol* 1978; **131**: 460–8.

79 Larrea JL, Nunez L, Reque JA, Gil-Aguado M, Matarros R, Minguez JA. Pregnancy and mechanical valve prostheses: a high-risk situation for the mother and the fetus. *Ann Thorac Surg* 1983; **36**: 459–63.

80 Oakley, CM. Pregnancy in patients with prosthetic heart valves. *Br Heart J* 1983; **286**: 1680–2.

81 Ben Ismail M, Abid F, Trabelsi S, Taktak M, Fekih M. Cardiac valve prosthesis anticoagulation and pregnancy. *Br Heart J* 1986; **55**: 101–5.

82 Lee PK, Wang RYC, Chow JSF, Cheung KL, Wong VC, Chan TK. Combined use of warfarin and adjusted subcutaneous heparin during pregnancy in patients with an artificial heart valve. *J Am Coll Cardiol* 1986; **8**: 221–4.

83 Iturbe-Alessio I, Salazar E. Anticoagulation in pregnant women with artificial heart valves. *N Engl J Med* 1987; **316**: 1663–4.

84 Stein PD, Kantrowitz A. Antithrombotic therapy in mechanical and biological prosthetic heart valves and saphenous vein bypass grafts. *Chest* 1989; **95**: 107S–17S.

85 Letsky EA, de Swiet M. Maternal hemostasis: coagulation problems of pregnancy. In: Schafer AI, Loscalzo J, eds. *Thrombosis and hemorrhage.* Cambridge, MA, USA: Blackwell Scientific Publications, 1994.

86 Levine HJ, Pauker SC, Salzman EW. Antithrombotic therapy in valvular heart disease. *Chest* 1989; **95**: 98S–106S.

87 Edmund LH. Thrombotic and bleeding complications of prosthetic heart valves. *Ann Thorac Surg* 1987; **44**: 430–45.

88 Turpie AGG, Gent M, Laupacis A, *et al.* Reduction in mortality by adding acetylsalicyclic acid (100 mg) to oral anticoagulants in patients with heart valve replacement. *Can J Cardiol* 1991; **7**: 95A.

89 Brott WH, Zajtchuk R, Bowen TE, Davia J, Green DC. Dipyridamole-aspirin as thromboembolic prophylaxis in patients with aortic valve prosthesis. Prospective study with the Model 2320 Starr-Edwards prosthesis. *J Thorac Cardiovasc Surg* 1981; **81**: 623–35.

90 Salazar E, Zajarias A, Gutierrez N, Iturbe I. The problem of cardiac valve prostheses, anticoagulants and pregnancy. *Circulation* 1984; **70**: 1169–77.

91 Tapanaainen J, Ikäheimo M, Jouppila P, Kortelainen ML, Salmela P. Thrombosis in a mechanical aortic valve prosthesis during subcutaneous heparin therapy in pregnancy; a case report. *Eur J Obstet Gynecol Reprod Biol* 1990; **36**: 175–7.

92 Bennett GG, Oakley CM. Pregnancy in a patient with a mitral valve prosthesis. *Lancet* 1968; **i**: 616–19.

93 Golby AJ, Bush EC, DeRook FA, Albers GW. Failure of high-dose heparin to prevent recurrent cardioembolic strokes in a pregnant patient with a mechanical heart valve. *Neurology* 1992; **42**: 2204–6.

94 Turpie AGG, Gunstensen J, Hirsh J, Nelson H, Gent M. Randomized comparison of two intensities of oral anticoagulant therapy after tissue heart valve replacement. *Lancet* 1988; **i**: 1242.
95 Saour JN, Sieck JO, Mamo LAR, Gallus AS. Trial of different intensities of anticoagulation in patients with prosthetic heart valves. *N Engl J Med* 1990; **322**: 428.
96 Altman R, Rouvier J, Gurfinkel E, *et al*. Comparison of two levels of anticoagulant therapy in patients with substitute heart valves. *J Thorac Cardiovasc Surg* 1991; **101**: 427–31.
97 Poller L, McKernan A, Thomson JM, Elstein M, Hirsch PJ, Jones JB. Fixed minidose warfarin; a new approach to prophylaxis against venous thrombosis after major surgery. *BMJ* 1987; **295**: 1309–12.
98 Porreco RP, McDuffie RS, Peck SD. Fixed mini-dose warfarin for prophylaxis of thromboembolic disease in pregnancy: a safe alternative for the fetus? *Obstet Gynecol* 1993; **81**: 806–7.
99 Badduke BR, Jamieson WRE, Miyagishima RT, *et al*. Pregnancy and childbearing in a population with biologic valvular prostheses. *J Thorac Cardiovasc Surg* 1991; **102**: 179–86.
100 Antretter H, Bonatti J. Pregnancy and prosthetic heart valves. *Lancet* 1994; **344**: 1643–4.
101 Javares T, Coto EO, Maiques V, Rincon A, Such M, Caffarena JM. Pregnancy after heart valve replacement. *Int J Cardiol* 1984; **5**: 731–9.
102 Cotrufo M, de Luca TSL, Calabro R, Mastrogiovanni G, Lama D. Coumarin anticoagulation during pregnancy in patients with mechanical valve prostheses. *Eur J Cardiothorac Surg* 1991; **5**: 300–5.
103 Born D, Martinez EE, Almeida PAM, *et al*. Pregnancy in patients with prosthetic heart valves: the effects of anticoagulation on mother, fetus, and neonate. *Am Heart J* 1992; **124**: 413–17.
104 Sbarouni E, Oakley CM. Outcomes of pregnancy in women with valve prostheses. *Br Heart J* 1994; **71**: 196–201.
105 Ginsberg JS, Barron WM. Pregnancy and prosthetic heart valves. *Lancet* 1994; **344**: 1170–1.
106 Bignardi GE, Barrett S, Foale R, Spyrou N. Pregnancy and prosthetic heart valves. *Lancet* 1994; **344**: 1643–4.
107 Larsen JF, Jacobsen B, Holm HH, Pedersen JF, Mantoni M. Intrauterine injection of vitamin K before the delivery during anticoagulant treatment of the mother. *Acta Obstet Gynecol Scand* 1978; **57**: 227–30.

Cardiovascular drugs:

23: Antihypertensive drugs

CELIA OAKLEY, MICHAEL DE SWIET

This chapter is complementary to chapter 21 and deals with the drugs used for the treatment of raised blood pressure in pregnancy.

Ever since the thalidomide disaster there has quite properly been extreme reluctance to introduce any new drugs in pregnancy. The repertoire of antihypertensive agents to be used in pregnancy is therefore restricted. Even among drugs with which there is experience, the track record of the drug tends to be anecdotal rather than based on trial evidence.

When drugs are used concern is not only about possible teratogenic effects which may operate during the period of organogenesis in the first trimester, but also about the effect of the drug on later fetal development and function. If the drug is continued until delivery and through labour it is necessary to consider possible effects on uterine activity and then whether the drug is excreted in any quantity in breast milk. Adverse effects on the fetus caused by the mode of action or true side effects of the hypotensive agents have to be separated from the deleterious effects both of untreated maternal hypertension and of the drop in placental perfusion which may follow reduction in perfusion pressure.

Reliance has traditionally been placed on bedrest for pre-existing non-gestational hypertension in late pregnancy as this protects both mother and fetus by lowering blood pressure and improving placental perfusion[1,2] but there is no evidence that bedrest influences the development of pre-eclampsia. Reduction in utero-placental perfusion following reduction in blood pressure by pharmacological means is likely to be an inescapable effect of anti-hypertensive agents with different modes of action. This may be why treatment of high blood pressure in pregnancy reduces maternal mortality and morbidity but benefit to the fetus has been less easy to demonstrate. The main risk to the fetus is from superimposed pre-eclamptic toxaemia which also threatens the mother's life, and the high risk of this complication is likely to be reduced by good blood pressure control in early pregnancy and indeed before conception.[3,4]

Alpha-methyldopa

Methyldopa is a centrally acting drug whose antihypertensive effect is related to alpha-agonist action within the brain with resultant peripheral sympathetic inhibition. It reduces both cardiac output and peripheral vascular resistance.[5] It has been used extensively for many years as the antihypertensive agent of choice for the treatment of essential hypertension during pregnancy[6] and has been shown to improve fetal outcome,[3,7] although one study showed that infants whose mothers had received methyldopa between the 16th and 20th week of gestation had smaller heads than infants of mothers not so treated.[8] However this had no effect on the infants' cognitive abilities. Since methyldopa is not a beta-blocking drug it is safe in asthmatic women but may need to be combined with other agents for adequate blood pressure control in those with severe hypertension. Like beta-blockers, methyldopa crosses the placenta.

Methyldopa causes drowsiness and may cause depression, nasal stuffiness, orthostatic hypotension, and fluid retention. Toxic effects include a positive direct Coomb's test in up to 20% of patients and, rarely, actual haemolytic anaemia, abnormal liver function tests, or the lupus syndrome. The newborn may also have a positive Coomb's test but haemolytic anaemia has not been reported.

Hydralazine

Hydralazine is a direct vasodilator which has also been used extensively in hypertensive pregnancies and shown to be safe but as long term therapy it is relatively ineffective on its own and produces side effects of headache and fluid retention through stimulation of the renin angiotensin system causing salt and water retention.[9–11] Its main use is for control of severe acute hypertension when it is given by intravenous infusion or intramuscularly. Optimal maternal haemodynamic monitoring in an intensive care environment is required so as to maintain pregnancy for a further 48 hours while steroids are given to mature the fetal lungs and reduce the risk of respiratory distress.

Diuretics

Like low sodium diets, diuretics are not used for the treatment of gestational hypertension because the blood volume is already depleted in these patients.[12,13] They are rarely necessary either in the long term treatment of essential hypertension in pregnancy even though agents such as methyldopa, hydralazine, and nifedipine tend to promote fluid retention and leg oedema. A thiazide may be used if gross oedema is causing discomfort. Frusemide is used for pulmonary oedema which is a rare complication of hypertension in pregnancy and is more likely to be caused by misguided, over enthusiastic fluid infusion than by left ventricular failure.

Beta-adrenergic blocking drugs

Beta-adrenergic blocking drugs are effective antihypertensive agents in pregnancy.[14,15] They do not have any teratogenic effects but their use remains slightly controversial because of concern that they may adversely affect fetal growth as well as the baby's condition at birth. Beta-adrenergic tone affects umbilical blood flow.[16] Beta-blocking drugs reduce umbilical blood flow in pregnant sheep[17] and may also impair the response to fetal distress. Low Apgar scores with bradycardia, apnoea, and hypoglycaemia have been the main worries.[18-21] Polycythemia[22] and hyperbilirubinaemia[23] have also been reported but others have noticed no such effects.[4,15] No consistent effect on the duration of labour has been observed. A difficulty in establishing whether beta-blocking drugs exert adverse effects on the fetus when used long term in pregnancy is that hypertension itself adversely affects fetal growth and development and is associated with increased risk of abortion, prematurity, stillbirth, and small-for-dates babies. Reports of such effects may have more to do with the maternal disorder for which the drug was prescribed rather than a direct effect of the beta-blocking drug.

A wide range of beta-blocking drugs with differing features is available. It is not known whether these are important in regard to side effects. Choice can be made between beta-1 selective agents such as atenolol and metoprolol and non-selective drugs such as propranolol and oxprenolol. Partial agonist activity is possessed by pindolol, oxprenolol and acebutalol but not by propranolol, atenolol, and metoprolol. Water soluble beta-blockers such as atenolol are less likely than lipid soluble ones such as oxprenolol to enter the brain and cause hallucinations and they are excreted by the kidneys. Beta-blocking drugs with vasodilator properties include labetalol, which is non-selective and has been available for years; celiprolol and carvedilol were introduced more recently for the treatment of hypertension but are not yet among the limited number of drugs of which there is experience in pregnancy.

In assessing the outcome of pregnancy in patients receiving beta-blocking drugs the effects of long term use in patients with pre-existing hypertension have to be separated from those of acute use in patients with pre-eclampsia in whom there is no concern about possible effects on fetal growth and to compare methyldopa, the universal first choice because of its excellent track record, with beta-adrenergic blocking drugs in the different categories. Data are limited. Oxprenolol has been compared with methyldopa in two randomised trials[23-25] which produced opposite results concerning the effects of oxprenolol on birth weight.[23-25] In one study,[23,24] oxprenolol was associated with an increase in birth weight; in the other[25] it was not. Atenolol has been compared with placebo[26,27] but not with methyldopa. The authors suggested that atenolol causes growth retardation when given in the first half of pregnancy, but this might have been the result of reduction of the blood pressure. It is unclear whether intrinsic sympathomimetic activity possessed by oxprenolol but not by metoprolol is relevant. Metoprolol is a beta-1 selective agent without partial agonist activity and was studied in a trial in which metoprolol alone or together with hydralazine and a diuretic was compared with hydralazine.[28] Perinatal mortality and fetal growth retardation were less in the metoprolol treated group than in the group receiving hydralazine. Some reports have referred only to short term use of beta-blocking agents.

Labetolol is a non-selective beta-blocker which also has alpha-adrenergic-blocking activity and a direct vasodilator action. It is safe in pregnancy and has been compared with methyldopa in small trials in which it was found to be effective in reducing blood pressure and to have no adverse effects on the fetus.[29-32] It is also used for acute blood pressure reduction and may be given by intravenous infusion.

To differentiate the possible ill effect of a beta-blocking drug on fetal growth from a similar effect of the hypertension itself it is relevant to compare experience with the use of beta-blocking drugs throughout pregnancy in patients with hypertrophic cardiomyopathy with outcomes in patients with pre-existing hypertension similarly treated. The good experience with propranolol and subsequently with atenolol in patients with hypertrophic cardiomyopathy treated throughout pregnancy[33] suggests that fetal growth retardation observed in hypertensive patients may either be directly attributable to the hypertension or to ill-effects of blood pressure reduction or of beta-adrenergic blockade on the utero-placental circulation, which are confined to the hypertensive patient and are not specific drug effects. The outcome of pregnancy is worse in patients with severe hypertension and they receive more drugs. Other possible adverse influences in hypertensive patients include smoking, which has a powerful adverse effect on cardiovascular risk in hypertensive subjects, and excess alcohol intake which may also influence fetal growth during pregnancy.

The many available beta-blockers are equally effective in reducing blood pressure. Differences in safety in relation to their different categories when used in pregnancy have not been defined. The importance of partial agonist activity—the ability to stimulate as well as block—is uncertain but these drugs cause less bradycardia. Beta-blockers which are "cardio-selective" have less effect on beta-2 receptors so they cause less peripheral vasoconstriction but are not cardiospecific. They are contraindicated in asthmatic patients but are preferred in those who are diabetic because they interfere less with awareness of hypoglycaemia.

In general it is wise to confine the long term use of beta-blockers in pregnancy to those with which there is greatest experience. One should prefer propranolol, oxprenolol, metoprolol, or labetalol (and thus a mix of categories). The high doses that used to be used are unnecessary and may have contributed to adverse effects. It is better to combine a lower dose of beta-blocker with methyldopa or hydralazine than to use higher doses. Good control of maternal blood pressure is paramount and methyldopa alone may be inadequate or cause excessive sedation. Uncontrolled hypertension in mid or late pregnancy carries a bad fetal prognosis whatever drugs are used. The best treatment of pregnancy induced hypertension, pre-eclampsia, is delivery of the baby whose main risk is prematurity. Beta-blocking drugs are safe and effective when used to protect the mother and gain some fetal maturity in the third trimester.

Calcium channel blocking drugs

No calcium antagonist is licensed for use in the treatment of hypertension during pregnancy but the use of nifedipine has crept in over the years and it seems to be safe.[34] Like other vasodilating drugs, it is unsatisfactory for use on its own because it produces headache and fluid retention but works well in combination with methyldopa or a beta-adrenergic blocking drug. Nifedipine is commonly used for the treatment of acute hypertension in pre-eclamptic patients.[35,36]

Angiotensin-converting-enzyme inhibitors

These drugs should not be used during pregnancy because they cause fetal renal failure with oligohydramnios before delivery and oliguria or anuria in the neonate, with potentially fatal consequences.[37,38]

References

1 Matthews DD. A randomised controlled trial of bed rest and sedation of normal activity and non-sedation in the management of non-albuminuric hypertension in late pregnancy. *Br J Obstet Gynaecol* 1977; **84**: 108–14.
2 Curet LB, Olson RW. Evaluation of a program of bed rest in the treatment of chronic hypertension in pregnancy. *Obstet Gynecol* 1979; **53**: 336–40.
3 Redman CWG, Beilin LJ, Bonnar J, *et al.* Fetal outcome in trial of antihypertensive treatment in pregnancy. *Lancet* 1976; **ii**: 753–6.
4 Redman CWG, Ounsted MK. Safety for the child of drug treatment for hypertension in pregnancy. *Lancet* 1982; **i**: 1237.
5 Van Zwieten PA. Pharmacology of centrally acting hypotensive drugs. *Br J Clin Pharmacol* 1980; **10**: 13S–20S.
6 Lewis PJ, Bulpitt CJ, Zuspan FP. A comparison of current British and American practice in the management of hypertension in pregnancy. *J Obstet Gynaecol* 1980; **1**: 78–82.
7 Leather HM, Humphries DM, Baker P, Chadd MA. A controlled trial of hypotensive agents in hypertension in pregnancy. *Lancet* 1968; **ii**: 488–90.
8 Jones HMR, Cummings AJ, Setchell KDR, Lawson AM. A study of the disposition of α-methyldopa in newborn infants following its administration to the mother for the treatment of hypertension during pregnancy. *Br J Clin Pharmacol* 1979; **8**: 433–40.
9 Lamminatausta R. The renin-aldosterone system in dihydralazine therapy during hypertensive pregnancy. *Int J Clin Pharmacol* 1978; **16**: 581–4.
10 Vink GJ, Moodley J, Philpott RH. Effect of dihydralazine on the fetus in the treatment of maternal hypertension. *Obstet Gynecol* 1980; **55**: 519–22.
11 Berkowitz RC. Antihypertensive drugs in the pregnant patient. *Obstet Gynecol Surv* 1980; **35**: 191–204.
12 Palomaki JF, Lindheimer MD. Sodium depletion simulating deterioration in a toxemic pregnancy. *N Engl J Med* 1970; **282**: 88–9.
13 Macleon AB, Doig JR, Aickin DR. Hypovolemia, pre-eclampsia and diuretics. *Br J Obstet Gynaecol* 1978; **85**: 597–603.
14 Eliahou HE, Silverberg DS, Reisin E, Roman I, Mashiach S, Serr DM. Propranolol for the treatment of hypertension in pregnancy. *Br J Obstet Gynaecol* 1978; **85**: 431–6.

15 Rubin PC. Beta-blockers in pregnancy. *N Engl J Med* 1981; **305**: 1323–6.

16 Ladner E, Brinkman CR, Weston P, Assali NS. Dynamics of uterine circulation in pregnant and non-pregnant sheep. *Am J Physiol* 1970; **218**: 257–63.

17 Oakes GK, Walker AD, Ehrenkranz RA, Chez RA. Effect of propranolol infusion on the umbilical and uterine circulations of pregnant sheep. *Am J Obstet Gynecol* 1976; **125**: 1038–42.

18 Joelson I, Barton MD. The effect of blockade of the beta-receptors of the sympathetic nervous system of the fetus. *Acta Obstet Gynecol Scand* 1969; **48** (**3 suppl**): 75–9.

19 Turnstall MB. The effect of propranolol on the onset of breathing at birth. *Br J Anaesthesiol* 1969; **41**: 792.

20 Habib A, McCarthy JS. Effects on the neonate of propranolol administered during pregnancy. *J Pediatr* 1977; **91**: 808–11.

21 Pruyn SC, Phelan JP, Buchanan CG. Long-term propranolol therapy in pregnancy: maternal and foetal outcome. *Am J Obstet Gynecol* 1979; **135**: 485–9.

22 Gladstone GR, Hordof A, Gersong WM. Propranolol administration during pregnancy: effects on the fetus. *J Pediatr* 1975; **86**: 962–4.

23 Gallery EDM, Saunders DM, Hunyor SN, et al. Randomised comparison of methyldopa and oxprenolol for treatment of hypertension in pregnancy. *BMJ* 1979; **i**: 1591–4.

24 Gallery EDM, Ross MR, Gyory AZ. Antihypertensive treatment in pregnancy: analysis of different responses to oxprenolol and methyldopa. *BMJ* **291**: 563–6.

25 Fidler J, Smith V, de Swiet M. Randomised controlled comparative study of methyldopa and oxprenolol for the treatment of hypertension in pregnancy. *BMJ* 1983; **286**: 1927–30.

26 Rubin PC, Butters L, Clark DL, et al. Placebo-controlled trial of atenolol in treatment of pregnancy-associated hypertension. *Lancet* 1983; **i**: 431–4.

27 Butters L, Kennedy S, Rubin PC. Atenolol in essential hypertension during pregnancy. *BMJ* 1990; **301**: 587–9.

28 Sandstrom B. Antihypertensive treatment with the adrenergic beta-receptor blocker metoprolol during pregnancy. *Gynecol Obstet Invest* 1978; **9**: 195–204.

29 Michael CA. Use of labetalol in the treatment of severe hypertension during pregnancy. *Br J Clin Pharmacol* 1979; **8** (**suppl 2**): 211S–15S.

30 Lamming GD, Symonds EB. Use of labetalol and methyldopa in pregnancy-induced hypertension. *Br J Clin Pharmacol* 1979; **8** (**suppl 2**): 217S–22S.

31 Lamming GD, Pipkin FB, Symonds EM. Comparison of the alpha and beta blocking drug, labetalol and methyldopa in the treatment of moderate and severe pregnancy-induced hypertension. *Clin Exp Hypertens* **2**: 865–95.

32 Plokin PF, Breart G, Maillard F, et al. Comparison of antihypertensive efficacy and prenatal safety of labetalol and methyldopa in the treatment of hypertension in pregnancy: a randomised controlled trial. *Br J Obstet Gynaecol* 1988; **95**: 868.

33 Oakley GDG, McGarry K, Limb DG, Oakley CM. Management of pregnancy in patients with hypertrophic cardiomyopathy. *BMJ* 1979; **i**: 1749–50.

34 Constantine G, Beevers DG, Reynolds AL, et al. Nifedipine as a second line anti-hypertensive drug in pregnancy. *Br J Obstet Gynaecol* 1987; **94**: 1136–42.

35 Walters BNJ, Redman CWG. Treatment of severe pregnancy-associated hypertension with the calcium antagonist nifedipine. *Br J Obstet Gynaecol* 1984; **91**: 330–6.

36 Seabe SJ, Moodley J, Becker P. Nifedipine in acute hypertensive emergencies in pregnancy. *S Afr Med J* 1989; **76**: 248.

37 Rosa FW, Bosco LA, Graham CF, et al. Neonatal anuria with maternal angiotensin converting enzyme inhibition. *Obstet Gynecol* 1989; **74**: 371.

38 Anon (editorial). Are ACE inhibitors safe in pregnancy? *Lancet* 1989; **2**: 482.

24: Antiarrhythmic drugs

MARK H ANDERSON

Antiarrhythmic drugs in common with all other drugs should be avoided during pregnancy wherever possible. In patients with a previous history of frequent symptomatic arrhythmias definitive treatment such as radio-frequency ablation should be considered before the patient becomes pregnant. Nevertheless some patients with arrhythmias are first seen during pregnancy and others who have had few symptoms may have a resurgence requiring pharmacological control. In patients who are already taking antiarrhythmic drugs and who intend to become pregnant consideration should be given to whether the drugs should be stopped for the duration of pregnancy. If this is not possible it is advisable, well before conception, to switch to a drug with which there is some experience in pregnancy.

The choice of antiarrhythmic drug should be based on a correct diagnosis of the arrhythmia and a thorough knowledge of the maternal pharma-cokinetics, potential teratogenicity, and toxic effects of the drug in the newborn and during breast feeding. Unfortunately most of the data on antiarrhythmic drugs during pregnancy come from isolated case reports. In this chapter I will review the data on the safety and efficacy of the most commonly used antiarrhythmic drugs. The selection of antiarrhythmic drugs for specific arrhythmias is considered further in chapter 19.

Drug disposition and pregnancy

Aside from any teratogenic potential of antiarrhythmic drugs pregnancy has complex effects on the pharmacokinetics of these agents in the mother and the dynamics of placental transfer affect fetal exposure and the direct pharmacological effect on the fetus.

Maternal factors

Absorption: delayed gastric emptying may reduce drug absorption because drugs are destroyed in the stomach, while slower intestinal transit may result in increased absorption of agents which pass through the stomach intact. Antacids, commonly prescribed for reflux symptoms during pregnancy may also interfere with drug absorption. Procainamide absorption may be affected in this way.[1]

Haemodynamic factors: cardiac output rises by around 40% during pregnancy, resulting in increased renal blood flow and increased passive renal excretion. Circulating volume and total body water are increased by over 50% resulting in an increased volume of distribution, and possibly needing increased loading doses of water soluble drugs.

Protein binding: serum albumin concentration falls steadily during pregnancy giving rise to an increase in the non-protein-bound fraction of drugs such as phenytoin.[2,3] While total concentrations of alpha[1]-acid glycoprotein do not change, the binding of basic drugs (such as lignocaine) to this protein appears to be reduced.[4] Thus while total plasma drug concentrations may be unchanged the increased free fraction may give rise to an increased effect.

Hepatic metabolism: alteration in protein binding may result in altered hepatic metabolism which, depending on the kinetics of drug excretion, may result in increased, decreased, or stable drug levels. Peak–trough concentration ratios of drugs may also change. Alterations in hepatic enzyme activity may also affect drug levels.

Renal excretion: increased blood flow and alteration in protein binding may increase removal of drugs that are predominantly excreted by this route.

The fetoplacental unit

Transfer of drugs across the placenta depends on the lipid solubility of the drug, the pH of maternal and fetal fluids, maternal and fetal protein binding, the ionisation constant (pKa) of the drug, and its molecular weight. Drugs with high lipid solubility and lower molecular weight penetrate more readily than hydrophilic ionised drugs.[5] Transfer of weak acids and bases is also affected by the acid-base milieu. Fetal plasma is usually more acidic than maternal, the pH being 0·1 lower. Weakly basic drugs become more ionised after crossing the placenta and therefore become "trapped" in the more acidic fetal circulation. Amniotic fluid similarly has a lower pH and basic drugs may accumulate in it. The placenta contains enzymes capable of metabolising many pharmacologically active substances and these enzymes may affect the amount of drug crossing the placenta.

Overall, the complexity of the changes in maternal drug absorption, distribution, metabolism, and excretion, in combination with placental transfer and fetal metabolism make prediction of the precise behaviour of any individual drug during pregnancy difficult.

Classification of antiarrhythmic drugs

Considerable time and effort have been expended in various attempts to classify antiarrhythmic drugs. The most enduring has been the Vaughan

Williams classification, originally described in 1970,[6] and modified to take account of the development of newer compounds, particularly in Class 1 (Table 24.1).[7,8] Simple guidelines for the choice of antiarrhythmic drugs for individual arrhythmias can be deduced from this classification (Table 24.2).[9] It is, however, inadequate to enable a choice of antiarrhythmic drug to be made under all circumstances. The conventional Vaughan Williams classification also excludes many antiarrhythmic drugs such as digoxin and adenosine. A fully informed decision can be made only with detailed knowledge of the mechanism of the clinical arrhythmia, the mechanism of action of the antiarrhythmic drug, and the way in which this action may be modified by conditions in the subject, such as ischaemia. Recognition of these problems led to the development of the Sicilian Gambit, an approach to the classification of antiarrhythmic drugs based on their action on arrhythmogenic mechanisms.[10] Essentially this classification identifies drugs by their ability to interact with one or more ion channels, ion pumps, and receptors.

TABLE 24.1—*Vaughan Williams classification of antiarrhythmic drugs.*[6]

Class	Action
I	Drugs with direct membrane action (sodium channel blockade) (a) Depress phase 0, slow conduction, prolong repolarisation (b) Depress phase 0 (abnormal fibres only), shorten repolarisation (c) Appreciably depress phase 0, extremely slow conduction, slight effect on repolarisation
II	Sympatholytic drugs
III	Drugs that prolong repolarisation
IV	Calcium channel blockers

TABLE 24.2—*Selection of antiarrhythmic drug type based on the Vaughan Williams classification.*[9] D = digoxin; A = adenosine.

Arrhythmia	Prevention/termination	Control of ventricular rate
Atrial tachycardias	Ia, Ic, II, III	II, III, IV, D
Atrial flutter/fibrillation	Ia, Ic, II, III	II, III, IV, D
AV junctional tachycardia	II, III, IV, D, A	
Atrioventricular tachycardia	Ia, Ic, II, III, IV, D, A	
Ventricular tachycardia	Ia, Ib, Ic, II, III, (IV)	

Arrhythmias are classified by their mechanism at a cellular or tissue level to identify vulnerable parameters, alteration of which may result in their termination. The appropriate drug to modify these vulnerable regions may then be chosen. While this approach is more complex than the Vaughan Williams classification it has the advantage of including all antiarrhythmic drugs, and being capable of adapting to new information on existing drugs and the development of new agents. The drugs discussed in this chapter are ranked in accordance with this system and their Vaughan Williams class is given in parallel.

Individual antiarrhythmic drugs

Sodium channel blockers

Lignocaine (Vaughan Williams Type 1b)

There is extensive experience with lignocaine during pregnancy because of its widespread use as a local anaesthetic agent at the time of labour and delivery. When used as an antiarrhythmic drug lignocaine is usually given as a 100 mg bolus followed by an infusion of between 1 and 4 mg/minute. After an intravenous bolus dose the plasma lignocaine concentration declines rapidly as a result of extensive redistribution in body tissues, followed by a slower elimination phase from metabolism and redistribution into skeletal muscle and fat. At therapeutic concentrations about 60% to 70% of the drug is bound to plasma proteins, particularly alpha$_1$-acid glycoprotein. About 90% of a parenteral dose is metabolised in the liver by deethylation to monoethylglycinexylidide and glycinexylidide. Less than 10% of the drug is excreted unchanged in the urine. The therapeutic range of lignocaine is 2–4 µg/ml although control of ventricular ectopic beats may be achieved at lower concentrations.[11]

Lignocaine given intravenously rapidly crosses the placenta to the fetus. Shnider and Way gave lignocaine 2 mg/kg intravenously to 16 healthy full-term women 30 seconds to 43 minutes before vaginal delivery and detected the drug in the umbilical vein within 2 to 3 minutes.[12] Within 6 minutes the maternal arterial:fetal umbilical vein concentration ratio remained constant, umbilical vein concentrations being around 55% of those in the mother. This was also the case in 9 mothers who received a higher loading dose. Subsequent elimination half-lives were similar in mother and baby. Similar ratios have been reported after epidural anaesthesia.[13] The lower fetal concentrations probably reflect lower alpha$_1$-acid glycoprotein concentrations in the fetus.[14] Because lignocaine is a mildly basic drug, levels in the fetus increase during fetal acidosis as a result of ion trapping.[15]

High serum concentrations of lignocaine may produce central nervous system depression in the newborn. Of 42 infants with umbilical vein lignocaine concentrations of less than 2·5 µg/ml only one had an Apgar score at one minute of less than 7.[13] In the 8 infants with lignocaine concentrations of 2·5 µg/ml or greater 4 had Apgar scores of less than 7, although all responded rapidly to oxygen and resuscitative measures.

There are isolated reports of lignocaine use during pregnancy for arrhythmia control with satisfactory maternal and fetal outcome.[16] The Collaborative Perinatal Project monitored 50 282 mother–child pairs, of whom 293 had been exposed to lignocaine during the first trimester.[17]

There was no evidence of a teratogenic effect. Greater than expected number of respiratory tract anomalies (3), tumours (2) and inguinal hernias (8) were found but the significance of these findings is unknown. Lignocaine use at some time during pregnancy was recorded in 947 mother–child pairs without evidence of harm.

In summary, while lignocaine crosses the placenta with ease there is considerable evidence of its safety during pregnancy. When given close to the time of delivery attention should be paid to minimising the dose and the potential for fetal depression should be considered. Because lignocaine as an antiarrhythmic drug is usually administered to patients at high risk the benefits of its use appear to outweigh any minor risks involved.

Breast feeding A woman who developed acute onset ventricular tachycardia whilst nursing a 10-month old infant received 125 mg in boluses plus an infusion of 2 mg/minute.[18] Seven hours later the lignocaine concentration in breast milk was 0·8 μg/ml (40% of maternal serum concentration). The American Academy of Pediatrics considers lignocaine treatment to be compatible with continued breast feeding.[19]

Mexiletine (Vaughan Williams type 1b)

Mexiletine is a local anaesthetic agent, structurally similar to lignocaine and active when given orally. It is a lipid soluble drug and crosses the placenta freely, giving similar maternal and cord blood concentrations.[20,21] At doses up to those which cause maternal toxicity the drug dose is not teratogenic in mice, rats, and rabbits.[22-24]

There are four reports in the literature of maternal use of mexiletine during pregnancy. An uneventful pregnancy, delivery, and subsequent child development ensued in a 26-year-old primigravida who was treated throughout pregnancy with mexiletine 200 mg three times daily and atenolol 50 mg/day for ventricular tachycardia.[25] Another patient with mitral valve prolapse received mexiletine throughout pregnancy without adverse effect on mother or fetus.[21] A healthy infant was delivered to a 30-year-old woman treated with mexiletine 600 mg/day and propranolol 60 mg/day from the 14th week of pregnancy for ventricular extrasystoles and ventricular tachycardia.[26] Finally, a 34-year-old woman with paroxysmal ventricular tachycardia was treated with mexiletine 200 mg three times daily, and propranolol 40 mg three times daily from 32 weeks' gestation onwards.[20] A normal male infant was delivered at 39 weeks' gestation. Mild bradycardia, probably related to the propranolol, was noted in the first 6 hours after birth.

In summary there is little experience of mexiletine during pregnancy but no adverse effects have been reported. Its use is justified only for life-threatening arrhythmias, when other agents with a better documented safety profile have failed.

Breast feeding There are three reports in the literature of mothers who breast fed whilst taking mexiletine. One patient, taking 600 mg/day in divided doses had milk and plasma samples taken at two days and six weeks postpartum.[20] The milk:plasma ratios were 2·0 and 1·1, respectively. No mexiletine could be detected in the infant's serum on either occasion. A second woman gave 12 matched milk and serum samples between 2 and 5 days postpartum.[26] The mean milk:plasma ratio was 1·45 (range 0·78–1·89). A third woman taking mexiletine 600 mg/day and atenolol 50 mg/day breast fed for 17 days before discontinuing because of a decline in infant weight from 2600 g at birth to 2155 g.[25] Subsequent outcome was unremarkable. The American Academy of Pediatrics considers mexiletine treatment to be compatible with continued breast feeding.

Tocainide (Vaughan Williams type 1b)

Because of the risk of bone marrow depression with this drug (which may exceed 1:300) it is rarely used for management of ventricular tachycardias. There is little experience of its use during pregnancy.

Breast feeding No data are available.

Phenytoin (Vaughan Williams type 1b)

Although primarily an anticonvulsant, phenytoin has been used in the treatment of supraventricular and ventricular arrhythmias, particularly when they are associated with digoxin toxicity.[27,28] Most of the pharmacokinetic and safety data on its use have been obtained from pregnant patients with epilepsy. It may be administered orally or intravenously and is well absorbed. It is metabolised in the liver and less than 5% appears unchanged in the urine. Antiarrhythmic plasma concentrations are 10–18 µg/ml and when used in an emergency intravenous doses of 100 mg are given at five minute intervals until the arrhythmia is abolished or adverse effects appear (hypotension, bradycardia, or ataxia). The total dose should not exceed 1000 mg/24 hours. Maintenance doses need to be individually adjusted by measurement of plasma drug concentrations because the drug follows non-linear kinetics at higher plasma drug concentrations.

Phenytoin readily crosses the placenta and maternal and fetal concentrations are similar at birth.[29] The teratogenic effects of phenytoin were first recognised in 1964[30] and subsequently a distinct pattern of abnormalities, described as the fetal hydantoin syndrome has been recognised.[31-34] Phenytoin also behaves as a transplacental carcinogen and has been reported to be associated with neuroblastoma,[35-37] ganglioneuroblastoma,[38] neuro-ectodermal tumours,[39] extrarenal Wilms tumour,[40] mesenchymoma,[41] lymphangioma,[42] and ependymoblastoma.[43] The teratogenic effects of phenytoin may be related to accumulation of epoxide metabolites in patients who are slow metabolisers.[44]

341

Because of these problems phenytoin should not be used as an antiarrhythmic drug during pregnancy except in patients with digoxin toxicity who have failed to respond to other agents.

Breast feeding Concentrations of phenytoin in breast milk range from 18% to 45% of maternal plasma levels[45-47] and the total dose absorbed by a breast feeding infant is small. With the exception of one case of methaemoglobinaemia and drowsiness[48] no adverse effects have been reported. The American Academy of Pediatrics considers that phenytoin is compatible with continued breast feeding.[19]

Procainamide (Vaughan Williams type 1a)

This drug is an activated state blocker of sodium channels with a medium speed time constant for recovery. It is used both for control of ventricular tachyarrhythmias and for prevention of atrial flutter and fibrillation. It may be given orally or parenterally and is usually well absorbed. Absorption may be delayed by altered motility or pH changes from antacids.[1] The drug is acetylated in the liver to an active metabolite, N-acetylprocainamide, at a rate related to genetic phenotype. Both drug and metabolite are excreted by active renal tubular secretion and glomerular filtration, and therefore tend to accumulate in patients with heart failure or renal failure. Data on maternal-fetal distribution is sparse but in three cases fetal:maternal procainamide blood concentration ratios of 0·28, 0·91, and 1·1 were reported; the N-acetylprocainamide ratios were 0·86 and 0·9.[49-51] In these patients procainamide treatment started at 24 weeks in two cases and 30 weeks in the third. Procainamide use earlier in pregnancy has not been associated with teratogenicity.[17,52] Nonetheless experience is limited and procainamide should be used in pregnancy only for life-threatening ventricular arrhythmias. It should not be used for supraventricular arrhythmias.

Breast feeding There is a single report of the concentration of procainamide and N-acetylprocainamide in breast milk.[53] Samples were taken postpartum every three hours for 15 hours in a patient who had taken 500 mg four times daily for the week before delivery. Mean serum concentrations of procainamide and N-acetylprocainamide were 1·1 µg/ml and 1·6 µg/ml respectively, compared with 5·4 and 3·5 µg/ml in the milk. Mean milk:serum ratios for procainamide and its metabolite were 4·3 (range 1·0–7·3) and 3·8 (range 1·0–6·2). Even at these concentrations the authors concluded that the infant received less than 65 mg of active drug each day, which was thought unlikely to yield clinically significant serum concentrations. The American Academy of Pediatrics considers procainamide to be compatible with continued breast feeding.[19] However, the effects of long term exposure of the infant have not been assessed.

Disopyramide (Vaughan Williams type 1a)

This drug has a similar action to procainamide and may be used in the treatment of supraventricular and ventricular arrhythmias. The drug is well absorbed and there is limited tissue binding. About 50% of the drug is excreted unchanged in the urine and a further 20% is excreted as the mono-N-alkylated metabolite.[54] The elimination half-life averages 6·5 hours and is prolonged in renal and hepatic failure. The drug crosses the placenta and fetal:maternal plasma ratios range from 0·26 to 0·78.[55-57]

There are a few reports of the use of disopyramide during pregnancy all with uneventful maternal and fetal outcome.[56-58] Following a report of early initiation of labour when disopyramide was given at 32 weeks of gestation[59] a study of the oxytocic effects of the drug was made in 10 women at term.[60] The women received 150 mg disopyramide 6 hourly for 48 hours. Eight delivered within 48 hours compared with none in a control group of 10 women.

Opinions on the safety of disopyramide during pregnancy differ[61-63] but although it appears safe the limited experience with the drug means it should be prescribed only for serious arrhythmias.

Breast feeding Disopyramide is excreted in breast milk and in four published cases milk:maternal serum concentration ratios varied from 0·4 to 6·2 depending on the time between the last dose and sampling.[56,58,64,65] In two cases infant plasma was analysed and the drug was undetectable (below the minimum sensitivity of the test). No adverse effects from breast feeding whilst taking disopyramide have been described and the American Academy of Pediatrics considers disopyramide treatment to be compatible with continued breast feeding.[19]

Quinidine (Vaughan Williams type 1a)

Like procainamide and disopyramide quinidine is an activated sodium channel blocker with a medium rate time constant for recovery from block. When given orally 70%–80% of the drug is absorbed and about 80% is protein bound in plasma. The elimination half-life is 6–8 hours and over 80% of the drug is hydroxylated in the liver, the remainder being excreted unchanged in the urine.[66] Quinidine crosses the placenta and fetal serum concentrations are similar to those in the mother.[67-69]

Quinidine has been used as an antiarrhythmic drug in pregnancy since the 1920s.[70,71] There are no reports of congenital abnormalities from quinidine use during pregnancy and in a series of 17 newborns exposed to quinidine during pregnancy there was no increase in the incidence of major birth defects.[71a] Rarely quinidine can stimulate uterine contractions at normal doses[72] whilst toxic doses may lead to abortion.[73] Quinidine inhibits pseudocholinesterase[74] and has the potential for toxicity when succinylcholine or ester-type local anaesthetics such as cocaine are used. A mother treated with quinidine for fetal supraventricular tachycardia developed signs of quinidine toxicity with normal serum quinidine concentrations (1·4–3·3 µg/ml) but high concentrations of the active metabolite 3-hydroxyquinidine.[67] It is unclear whether this was an idiosyncratic effect or related to alterations in metabolism during pregnancy. Fetal growth retardation occurred during one pregnancy in which a combination of metoprolol and quinidine was used to control maternal ventricular tachycardia.[75]

In adult cardiology quinidine is generally restricted to use as a second-line agent for prevention of atrial fibrillation. Caution has been advised in its use because a meta-analysis confirmed its effectiveness in preventing recurrence of atrial fibrillation, but suggested a 3-fold increase in mortality in the drug treated group.[76] Quinidine has been used in combination with digoxin to treat fetal supraventricular tachycardias[77,78] and alone for fetal ventricular tachycardia.[79]

Overall there is a moderate amount of experience of the use of quinidine during pregnancy and it appears relatively safe. However, caution should be exercised and it should be prescribed only for serious or life-threatening arrhythmias.

Breast feeding Concentrations of quinidine in breast milk are similar to or lower than those in serum[80] and the American Academy of Pediatrics considers breast feeding while taking quinidine to be safe.[19]

Flecainide (Vaughan Williams type 1c)

Flecainide is a sodium channel blocker with a slow time-constant for channel recovery. Flecainide, at doses four times the usual human dose may show teratogenicity and embryotoxicity in some breeds of rabbits and rats.[81] Reports of flecainide use throughout pregnancy are sparse but in one patient flecainide 100 mg twice daily was used in combination with sotalol for treatment of ventricular tachycardia.[82] Fetal development and postnatal development were normal. Flecainide has been most widely used from 30 weeks of pregnancy onwards for the treatment of fetal arrhythmias associated with hydrops fetalis. In 17 women treated with between 100 and 400 mg of flecainide/day in divided doses maternal fetal serum drug ratios ranged between 0·5 and 0·86.[82–85] In fifteen of these cases the fetus reverted to sinus rhythm shortly after flecainide administration. There was one intrauterine death after three days of flecainide but cordocentesis had been done within the previous 24 hours and may have been responsible.[85] In the same series one infant died suddenly aged 4 months although no longer receiving treatment with flecainide. In the remaining infants the perinatal course was uneventful, apart from additional treatment required for hydrops and the requirement for continuing postnatal antiarrhythmic drugs in some. Flecainide appears to accumulate at high concentrations in amniotic fluid but this does not appear to be of consequence.[86]

There is little experience of the use of flecainide for treatment of maternal arrhythmias throughout pregnancy and its use cannot therefore be recommended. However, there is quite extensive experience with its use late in pregnancy and it is justified for the control of serious fetal arrhythmias associated with hydrops fetalis.

Breast feeding Flecainide is concentrated in breast milk when compared with plasma.[82] A detailed study was performed in eleven healthy volunteers who elected not to breast feed.[87] They received 100 mg twice daily for five days. Peak milk levels of flecainide occurred 3–6 hours after administration, and mean milk:plasma ratios on days 2, 3, 4, and 5 were 3·7, 3·2, 3·5, and 2·6, respectively. The authors estimated the average fetal daily dose as 0·27 mg/kg or 4·28 mg per m^2. Thus the likelihood of toxic levels of flecainide accumulating in the fetus is low. Flecainide metabolites are of low efficacy and lipid solubility and therefore unlikely to cause problems either. The American Academy of Pediatrics considers flecainide to be compatible with breast feeding[19] although there are no reports of breast fed infants whose mothers were receiving flecainide.

Propafenone (Vaughan Williams type 1c)

This drug has a similar mechanism of action to flecainide with a faster recovery from receptor blockade. The drug is metabolised to an active metabolite, 5-hydroxypropafenone. The drug and its metabolite have a high affinity for $alpha_1$-acid glycoprotein.[88] There are few data on its use during pregnancy. It has been shown to be embryotoxic in some animal studies when given at 10 to 40 times the normal human dosage.[89] Cord to maternal plasma concentration ratios were measured in a single patient.[90] For the parent drug the ratio was 0·14 and for the metabolite 0·42. Free drug concentrations are similar in cord and maternal plasma while free metabolite levels are higher (0·25 ng/ml compared with 0·17 ng/ml) in cord plasma.

There are three reports of propafenone use during pregnancy. One patient received 300 mg three times daily from the 19th week of pregnancy until a normal infant was delivered by caesarean section at 36 weeks.[91] Fetal: maternal plasma ratios of drug and metabolite were 0·29 and 0·45 respectively. In a second case the drug was started at 26 weeks for paroxysmal supraventricular and ventricular tachycardias and continued throughout pregnancy until the spontaneous delivery of a normal infant at 36 weeks.[90] A third patient received a short course of treatment with 850 mg daily for fetal supraventricular tachycardia.[92] In this patient propafenone and a number of other drugs proved ineffective and direct fetal administration of amiodarone was eventually used.

In the absence of data on the teratogenicity of propafenone in early pregnancy its use cannot be recommended.

345

Breast feeding   There are no reports on the effect of breast feeding on the infant in mothers taking propafenone. Milk to maternal plasma ratios have been measured at 0·20 for the drug and 0·50 for the metabolite.[90] Total dosage to the infant when corrected for body weight is around 3% of that to the mother. Breast feeding is likely to be safe therefore.

Encainide (Vaughan Williams type 1c)

Encainide is another sodium channel blocker with a slow time constant for recovery from channel blockade. The drug is metabolised to active metabolites 0-demethyl encainide and 3-methoxy-o-demethyl encainide. There is little experience of this drug in pregnancy and only a single report of its use for control of fetal arrhythmia.[71] Animal experiments suggest that it crosses into breast milk.[71]

Calcium channel blockers

Verapamil (Vaughan Williams type 4)

This calcium-channel blocking drug is widely used for the acute and chronic control of supraventricular arrhythmias, for hypertension, and in the treatment of angina. It is rapidly absorbed but has high first-pass metabolism with only a small proportion being excreted unchanged in the urine. It is about 90% plasma protein bound with a half-life of 3–7 hours.[93] Fetal:maternal plasma ratios range from 0·17 after a single dose to 0·44 after an infusion of 2 µg/kg/minute for 60–110 minutes.[94]

There are no reports of congenital defects in association with verapamil. In 76 patients exposed to verapamil during the first trimester in the Michigan Medicaid study one birth defect was seen against three expected (F Rosa, personal communication). Verapamil boluses up to 10 mg may be given acutely to terminate supraventricular arrhythmias without adverse effect on fetal heart rate.[95,96] Rapid bolus administration may be associated with hypotension so the drug should be given in this way only where close maternal monitoring is possible. Although verapamil is widely used for the prophylaxis of recurrent supraventricular arrhythmias there are few reports of its use during pregnancy. This is perhaps because the drug is withdrawn once pregnancy is discovered, because the generally benign nature of this group of arrhythmias does not justify prophylactic drug therapy throughout pregnancy. Verapamil has been widely used for control of fetal supraventricular arrhythmias, usually in combination with digoxin or other antiarrhythmic drugs.[97–101] In most cases the drug has been well tolerated but there is a single report of fetal death after 4 weeks' treatment with verapamil 120 mg three times daily and digoxin.[101] No necropsy was done but the authors speculated that complete heart block related to the drug combination might have been responsible. Verapamil has also been used without adverse effect for control of severe pregnancy induced hypertension[102] and to limit the adverse effect of sympathomimetic drugs used for tocolysis.[103]

The acute administration of verapamil during pregnancy appears to be safe. There is little information about chronic administration throughout pregnancy and although the drug does not appear to be teratogenic caution must be advised in its use.

Breast feeding In three studies the concentration of verapamil in breast milk was found to be between 23% and 64% of that in maternal plasma. In infants it was either low or undetectable; the breast fed child receives less than 1% of the maternal dose.[104-106] The American Academy of Pediatrics does not consider verapamil therapy contraindicated during breast feeding.[19]

Potassium channel blockers

Amiodarone (Vaughan Williams type 3 and others)

Amiodarone is a benzofuran derivative containing 37·5% iodine by weight. Oral absorption is erratic, bioavailability ranging between 22% and 86%. The drug is highly lipophilic and accumulates in large amounts in fat and muscle during prolonged treatment. The concentration in the myocardium is 10–50 times that in plasma. The drug is largely eliminated by metabolism, less than 1% being excreted unchanged in the urine. Its major metabolite desethylamiodarone (DEA) contributes substantially to its antiarrhythmic efficacy.[107,108] The plasma half-life after a single dose is 3·2–80 hours but on withdrawal of long term treatment may exceed 100 days.[109]

Amiodarone's predominant action as a potassium channel blocker is to prolong ventricular depolarisation and hence refractoriness, but it has a number of other actions. It shows use-dependent blockade of sodium channels, has alpha- and beta-blocking actions, and has calcium channel blocking activity.

Amiodarone has been widely used as an antiarrhythmic agent for serious or life-threatening arrhythmias, its use being limited mainly by the potential for thyroid, hepatic, and pulmonary dysfunction with prolonged treatment. For this reason there is considerable documentation of its use during pregnancy.

Both amiodarone and desethylamiodarone cross the placenta in considerable quantities (Table 24.3) and concentrations of desethyl-amiodarone tend to be higher.

Animal studies using doses of 5–200 mg/kg in rats, rabbits, and mice have failed to show any increase in minor or major abnormalities. One study showed increased perinatal and postnatal mortality, reduced birth weight and reduced growth rate in survivors at a dose of 90 mg/kg/day.[110] Fetal outcome has been reported in a total of 43 pregnancies with

TABLE 24.3—*Fetal/maternal plasma ratios of amiodarone and desethylamiodarone (DEA) at term.*[169-175]

First author	Maintenance amiodarone dose (mg/day)	Duration of treatment (weeks)	Amiodarone fetal/maternal ratio	DEA fetal/ maternal ratio
Plomp[169]	200	Entire	0·61	0·63
	200	pregnancy	0·15	0·29
	200		0·17	0·30
Penn[170]	200	23	0·35	N/A
McKenna[171]	400	7	0·13	0·29
Pitcher[172]	600 for 1 week	3	0·1	0·25
	400 for 1 week			
	200 for 1 week			
Robson[173]	200	Entire pregnancy	0·1	0·19
	400 mg→600 mg for last 3 weeks	17	0·145	0·22
Arnoux[174]	800	6	0·125	0·196*
Strunge[175]	200→400 at 18 weeks	Entire pregnancy	0·27	0·55

*For fetal arrhythmia.

amiodarone exposure (Table 24.4). Overall most pregnancies had a successful outcome without any adverse effect attributable to the amiodarone. However there were more "small for dates" babies than expected suggesting amiodarone may adversely affect fetal growth.

Potentially the most serious adverse effect is hypothyroidism in the newborn. In most cases described in Table 24.4 thyroid function in the neonate was measured and found to be normal but in eight cases abnormalities were noted. Case 4 had an elevated cord blood T4 (209 nmol/l) but TSH remained within the reference range and the infant was clinically normal. Severe hypothyroidism at birth with goitre, hypotonia, bradycardia, and macroglossia occurred in case 8. Cord blood thyroid function tests showed a TSH concentration >100 mU/l (normal 10–20 mU/l) and a T4 of 35·9 µg/l (normal 60–170 µg/l). Thyroxine was given immediately after birth but despite rapid return of thyroid function to normal his bone age at 20 months was estimated to be only 12 months and psychomotor development was retarded. In a third case (case 11) in which 800 mg/day of amiodarone was used to control fetal arrhythmia for 6 weeks before birth the free T3 index and free T4 index were reduced at birth and the TSH and total T4 levels were raised. With the exception of the T4 level all these results had returned to normal by one month. Clinical development was normal.

In case 14, again after high doses of amiodarone (600 mg/day) there was a goitre and the infant had an elevated TSH and reduced free T4. Thyroxine was administered for the first three months when thyroid function had

TABLE 24.4—Outcome of 43 pregnancies with exposure to amiodarone.

Case No	First author	Amiodarone dose (mg/day)	Gestational week amio started	Delivery week	Other drugs	Birth weight (g) (centile)	Adverse effects/comments
1	McKenna[171]	400	34	41	Quinidine	3220 (35)	Bradycardia during first 48 hours post delivery
2	Penn[170]	200	16	39	None	2660 (<10)	Prolonged QT interval
3	Pitcher[172]	400 (see Table 24.1)	37	39	Propranolol, digoxin, verapamil	Not stated	None
4	Robson[173]	200	BP	37	Mod., warf., verapamil	3500 (80)	Elevated T4, normal TSH None
5		400→600	22	39	Metoprolol	2900 (20)	
6	Rey[176]	228	BP	?	Propranolol	2670 (—)	None
7	Strunge[175]	200→400	BP	40	None	3650 (60)	
8	De Wolfe[177]	200	13	38	None	2450 (<10)	Congenital hypothyroidism with persistent growth retardation
9	Widerhorn[178]	400→200	BP	38	None	2500 (<10)	None
10		200	BP	35	None	2960 (50)	None
11	Arnoux[174]	800	32	38	Digoxin	Not stated	Abnormal TFT at birth (see text). Amiodarone given for fetal arrhythmia
12	Rey[179]	400	28	33	Verapamil	2700 (80)	Amiodarone & verapamil given for fetal arrhythmia
13	Wladimiroff[180]	?	25	31	Digoxin, verapamil Procainamide Propranolol	Not stated	For fetal arrhythmia. Infant died day 2 post delivery

TABLE 24.4—*Outcome of 43 pregnancies with exposure to amiodarone—cont.*

Case No	First author	Amiodarone dose (mg/day)	Gestational week amio started	Delivery week	Other drugs	Birth weight (g) (centile)	Adverse effects/ comments
14	Laurent[181]	600	32	35	Digoxin	2960	Amiodarone for fetal arrhythmia. Congenital hypothyroidism at birth with complete recovery by 3 months
15	Gembruch[182]	◇	32	37	Verapamil disopyramide quinidine propafenone	2400 (<10)	Amiodarone for fetal arrhythmia
16	Magee[183]	400	BP	92% at >37 weeks	Acebutolol	1925 (<10)	Hyperthyroid, fetal brady
17		200	BP		Prop., Digoxin	2242 (<5)	
18		228	BP		Prop., Quin.	2670 (<10)	
19		228	BP		Prop.	2298 (<10)	Fetal/neonatal brady
20		286	BP		Sotalol	2790 (10–25)	
21		286	BP		Metop.	2812 (10–25)	
22		600→400	20		Aten.	3700 (50–75)	
23		286	25			3740 (75–90)	
24		400	25		Aten., Digoxin Metop.	2380 (<10) 3160 (50)	
25		428	32				
26		600	15			2800 (10–25)	Fetal bradycardia
27	Plomp[169]	200	BP	34	None	1535 (10)	Impaired fetal growth

28		200	34	40	Metop.	2880 (10)	Hypothyroidism developed postnatally
29							
30		200	BP	40	None	3320 (5)	None
31		200	BP	41	None	3930 (90)	None
		200	BP	40	None	3380 (50)	None
32	De Catte[112]	◇	26	32	Digoxin, Propaf.	2940 (>95)	Fetal hypothyroidism treated in utero
33	Valensise[184]	400→200	8	38	None	3450	None
34		200	BP	38	None	3680	None
35	Matsumura[185]	200	◆	40	None	3100	
36		200	◆	40	None	2480	
37		200	BP	40	None	3100	
38		200	◆	40	None	3170	Low T4/raised TSH at birth
39		200	◆	40	None	3070	
40		200	BP	29	None	1700	
41		200	◆	41	None	3640	Hypoglycaemia after caesarean section
42		200	◆	Not stated	None	3230	None
43		200	◆	Not stated	None	3100	None

◇ Amiodarone given by direct injection into umbilical vein.
◆ Exact time not given. Between 20 and 32 weeks.
Mod.: Moduretic (Hydrochlorotriazide + amiloride)
Warf.: Warfarin
Prop.: Propranolol
Aten.: Atenolol
Metop.: Metoprolol
Propaf.: Propafenone

returned to normal. Subsequent physical and mental development was normal. One infant (case 28, Table 24.4) developed hypothyroidism in the postnatal period with continued amiodarone administration during breast feeding. Amiodarone had been given only during the last 6 weeks of pregnancy and metoprolol had been given throughout. The infant had delayed motor development and impaired speech performance at 5 years of age. In case 32 cordocentesis was used to monitor fetal thyroid function. A markedly raised TSH was found at 28 weeks but reverted to normal after intramniotic L-thyroxine treatment. Postnatal development was unremarkable. Finally, in case 38 a low T4 and raised TSH were noted at birth but had returned to normal by one month.

In summary, there is a substantial risk of neonatal hypothyroidism resulting from maternal amiodarone exposure during pregnancy and even short periods of exposure at relatively high doses can cause this. Amiodarone and desethylamiodarone concentrations fall steadily in the neonate over the first few months. While the neonate's thyroid function returns to normal psychomotor development may show permanent impairment. Therefore amiodarone during pregnancy should be reserved for life-threatening arrhythmias in mother or fetus. In patients who do receive amiodarone during pregnancy estimation of fetal thyroid function by cordocentesis or amniocentesis is advisable.[111] Intramniotic injection of T4 may reverse the fetal thyroid abnormalities[112] and reduce the size of the fetal goitre.[113]

Breast feeding A study in suckling rats has shown no influence on neonatal weight gain. Both amiodarone and DEA accumulated in neonatal lung, and livers.

Amiodarone and DEA are excreted in human breast milk. A woman treated with 400 mg daily had amiodarone and DEA concentrations in milk and plasma measured between nine days and nine weeks after delivery.[171] The concentrations were highly variable over a 24 hour period and milk:plasma ratios of amiodarone ranged from 2·3 to 9·1 and of DEA from 0·8–3·8. Calculated intakes of the nursing infant were 1·4–1·5 mg/kg/day of amiodarone and 0·5–0·7 mg/kg/day of DEA. Plasma concentrations of amiodarone in the infant remained at 0·4 μg/ml (about 25% of maternal levels) from birth to 9 weeks. Similarly variable drug and metabolite concentrations were observed in four other mothers who breast fed their infants and no adverse effects were reported in any of these infants.[169,175] Nevertheless significant amounts of amiodarone and DEA are transferred to the neonate and the effect of this chronic exposure is unknown. The one neonate with documented chronic exposure showed no evidence of drug accumulation but the pharmacokinetics of amiodarone and DEA in neonates are unknown.[171] Therefore breast feeding is not recommended if the mother is taking amiodarone or has taken it over the long term within the last 3–6 months.

Sotalol (Vaughan Williams type 2 and 3)

Sotalol combines conventional beta-blockade with potent potassium channel blockade and like amiodarone it prolongs the action potential, extending refractoriness. The drug is a racemic mixture of d- and l-sotalol. The beta-blocking activity resides in the l-isomer whilst the potassium channel blocking activity is present in both isomers. The drug is well absorbed after oral administration and bioavailability exceeds 90% in the pregnant and non-pregnant states. Protein binding is negligible and the drug is mainly excreted unchanged in the urine.[114] Because of increased renal perfusion in pregnancy the elimination half-time of the drug is reduced by about 30% and dosing regimens may have to be adjusted accordingly.

Placental transfer of sotalol has been measured in 12 hypertensive pregnant women who were receiving an average of 433 mg/day of sotalol. The mean fetal:maternal drug ratio was 0·95 (cord plasma concentration = (0·79 × maternal) + 0·28) and amniotic fluid concentrations were 4·1 times higher than cord plasma concentrations.[115] Eight women scheduled for caesarean section were given a single dose of 80 mg sotalol 3 hours before operation. Fetal:maternal plasma ratio was 0·47.[116] In a single woman in whom caesarean section was performed 11 hours after the last dose of regular sotalol 80 mg twice daily fetal:maternal plasma concentration ratio was 1·42.[82] A ratio of 0·84 was recorded at delivery in another woman treated with 80 mg three times daily throughout gestation.[117]

In rabbits sotalol is not teratogenic in doses up to 100 times the maximum recommended human dose.[71] Human experience with exposure to the drug during the first trimester is limited to the one case in which sotalol 80 mg twice daily and flecainide 100 mg twice daily were continued throughout pregnancy for the suppression of ventricular tachycardia.[82] A normal infant was delivered at 37 weeks' gestation and subsequent development was normal. In the study of 12 hypertensive women the drug was started at between 18 and 31 weeks of gestation and all infants were liveborn.[115] Two infants had substantial congenital abnormalities resulting in neonatal death but sotalol was not implicated in either case, having been started at 21 and 28 weeks, respectively. Four infants were below the tenth centile for birth weight and six had transient neonatal bradycardia that did not require intervention.

While beta-blockers are generally well tolerated during pregnancy experience with sotalol is limited, particularly during the first trimester. It should therefore be used only for life-threatening arrhythmias when the benefits will outweigh the poorly quantified risk of its use.

Breast feeding Twenty paired samples of breast milk and maternal blood were obtained from five breast feeding mothers in the hypertension study described above.[115] The precise timing of collection and dosage details were not given. The mean milk:plasma ratio was 5·4 (range 2·2–8·8). No adverse effects were noted in the neonate but their plasma concentrations were not measured. A pre-feed milk:plasma ratio of 5·64 was recorded five days after delivery in a single patient receiving 80 mg three times daily.[117] The dose was subsequently reduced to 80 mg twice daily and at 105 days the ratio was 2·43. The authors calculated that the neonate received 20%–23% of the maternal dose by weight. No adverse effects on the neonate were observed. The American Academy of Pediatrics regards sotalol therapy as compatible with breast feeding.[19]

Muscarinic (M2)-receptor blockers

Atropine

Atropine has a number of uses in proprietary medicines and in anaesthetic practice, but its main antiarrhythmic use is in the emergency treatment of bradycardias of vagal origin and of cardiac arrest with asystole.[118] Atropine is well absorbed orally but for the treatment of bradycardias is normally given intravenously. About 50% is excreted unchanged in the urine. After intravenous injection concentrations fall to less than 5% of peak within 10 minutes.

Atropine rapidly crosses the placenta and fetal levels approach 50% of maternal within 3 minutes.[119] Atropine causes tachycardia and loss of beat-to-beat variation in the fetus and this was once used as a test of placental transfer function.[120] Other studies have suggested that atropine has a minimal effect on fetal heart rate and the progress of labour.[121]

Exposure to atropine occurs in over 1% of pregnancies. The Collaborative Perinatal Project monitored 1198 exposures to atropine during pregnancy without any evidence of increased incidence of fetal malformations.[17] Exposure of 381 infants of Michigan Medicaid mothers in the first trimester was not associated with any substantial increase in congenital abnormalities (F Rosa, personal communication).

Breast feeding It is unlikely that appreciable amounts of atropine appear in breast milk after single intravenous doses and the American Academy of Pediatrics considers its use safe during lactation.[19]

Cardiac glycosides

Digoxin

Digoxin is the most widely used of the cardiac glycosides for control of arrhythmias. Digoxin binds to and inhibits the membrane-bound cation transport enzyme, magnesium-dependent sodium and potassium-linked adenosine triphosphate, causing increased intracellular sodium levels. About two thirds of the administered dose is absorbed when the drug is given in tablet form. Only 20% of the drug is protein bound, but it is widely distributed to all body tissues. The plasma half-life is about 40 hours and excretion is predominantly renal, 80% being recovered unchanged in the urine. In pregnancy plasma digoxin levels may be overestimated as a result of the production of endogenous digoxin-like substances by the placenta or fetus.[122,123]

Digoxin passes rapidly across the placenta[124-127] and umbilical vein concentrations reach a plateau within 30 minutes of a maternal intravenous dose. Cord blood concentrations range between 50% and 100% of maternal levels.[124,126-128] In adults digoxin is strongly bound to cardiac tissue and concentrations reach 40–60 times those in plasma.[129] While the highest concentrations in the fetus are found in the heart, relative concentrations are much lower.[127]

The lack of reports of teratogenicity associated with digoxin is reassuring in view of its long history of availability and relatively common use. There are many reports of the use of digoxin for control of fetal arrhythmias without adverse effects.[130-132] There are fewer reports of exposure throughout pregnancy, but first trimester exposure has not been associated with increased congenital abnormalities[133] and in the Michigan Medicaid study one birth defect (not cardiac) was noted in 34 recipients (1·5 defects expected). In patients taking digoxin mean gestation was reduced from 39·9 weeks in a control group to 38·5 weeks, and the mean duration of labour was reduced from 8 to 4 hours, possibly as a result of a stimulant effect of the drug on the myometrium.[134]

There seems to be no important effect of maternal digoxin treatment in neonates but not surprisingly maternal digoxin toxicity has been associated with miscarriage and neonatal death.[135,136]

In summary, there are no reports of adverse effects on the fetus or neonate following digoxin usage at any stage of pregnancy. In view of the long history of use of digitalis glycosides it seems unlikely that a substantial teratogenic effect has been overlooked although no formal large scale studies of safety in pregnancy have been conducted.

Breast feeding   Digoxin is excreted into breast milk with milk:plasma concentration ratios of 0·6–0·9.[128,137-139] However, the total amount excreted is only 1–2 µg/day and after 10 days of breast feeding no digoxin could be detected in neonatal plasma.[139] The American Academy of Pediatrics regards digoxin therapy as compatible with breast feeding.[19]

Adenosine

Adenosine is an endogenous, purine-based nucleotide found in all cells. It is widely used for the termination of sustained supraventricular arrhythmias and has become popular because of its short duration of action and lack of a negative inotropic effect. There are no data on the placental transfer of adenosine but there appears to be no effect on fetal heart rate following maternal injection[140-142] although direct fetal injection produces a dramatic transient impairment of atrioventricular conduction.[143]

The cellular ubiquity of adenosine makes it an unlikely teratogenic agent and limited animal studies have confirmed its safety.[144] In pregnant ewes neither continuous infusion nor bolus administration of adenosine had any effect on fetal blood gases, heart rate, or arterial pressure.[145]

There are now five reports of the successful use of 6 or 12 mg boluses of adenosine to terminate maternal supraventricular tachycardias.[140–142,146,147] In no case was an adverse effect observed in the infant.

As with any relatively untried agent caution should be advised in its use during pregnancy. However, the biological ubiquity, efficacy, and short duration of action of adenosine all favour its safety. Its use in pregnancy may be permitted subject to systematic recording of adverse events.

Breast feeding   There are no data available.

Beta-blockers (Vaughan Williams type 2)

There are many different beta-blockers available all of which have similar antiarrhythmic efficacy but propranolol remains the beta-blocker most widely used for its antiarrhythmic effect. Beta-blockers exert a non-specific effect on arrhythmias which are dependent on sympathetic drive and may be used to treat supraventricular and ventricular arrhythmias alone, or in combination with other antiarrhythmic agents.

Propranolol is almost completely absorbed from the gastrointestinal tract and is widely distributed through the body tissues. The drug is a weak base and is strongly bound to $alpha_1$-acid glycoprotein. Excretion is almost totally by hepatic metabolism, and only small amounts of unchanged drug are excreted in the urine. The elimination half-life is between four and six hours during prolonged administration. The pharmacokinetics do not change significantly during pregnancy.[148]

Propranolol crosses the placenta and fetal:maternal plasma ratios between 0·19 and 1·27 have been reported.[149,151–153] There are only isolated case reports of the pharmacokinetics of propranolol in the neonate. One report suggested that the drug is cleared to undetectable levels within one hour of birth[152] whilst in another a considerable rise in drug concentration was reported over the same period.[150]

Among 402 Michigan Medicaid women exposed to propranolol during the first trimester 22 major birth defects were observed (18 expected).[71a] The occurrence of sporadic reported abnormalities[154–156] does not suggest that the drug is particularly teratogenic.

Not surprisingly propranolol may give rise to fetal bradycardia and a reduced heart rate response to external stimuli has been reported.[157] A range of fetal adverse effects have been described in association with propranolol, although some may be related to the maternal disease being treated or to coincident treatment with other drugs. Briggs[71a] reviewed 23 reports of the outcome of 167 liveborn infants and described the commonest complications associated with prolonged propranolol treatment in utero

(Table 24.5). The connection between propranolol and these effects is not clear, although higher doses do seem to produce adverse effects more commonly. A potential mechanism for intrauterine growth retardation has been suggested by experiments in pregnant ewes which showed a reduction in umbilical vein flow in response to maternal or fetal infusion of beta-blockers.[158] While retrospective studies have suggested a high incidence of intrauterine growth retardation,[159] a number of prospective studies of propranolol[160–163] and other beta-blocking agents[164–166] have not confirmed these findings. Hypoglycaemia and bradycardia are well recognised complications of propranolol use in adults and their occurrence in the neonate is not surprising.

TABLE 24.5—*Incidence of neonatal adverse effects in 167 reported cases of propranolol use in pregnancy.*[71a]

Adverse effect	No (%) Cases
Intrauterine growth retardation	23 (14)
Hypoglycaemia	16 (10)
Bradycardia	12 (7)
Respiratory depression at birth	6 (4)
Hyperbilirubinaemia	6 (4)
Small placenta	4 (2)
Polycythemia	2 (1)

Summary

There is far greater experience with the use of propranolol and other beta-blocking agents during pregnancy than with other antiarrhythmic drugs. While these agents are not entirely free from adverse effects the incidence is relatively low and they can be used in pregnancy for control of important arrhythmias where the benefits outweigh the risks.

Breast feeding   Propranolol is excreted in breast milk with milk:maternal plasma ratios of 0·2–1·5.[152,167,168] Drug concentrations in the breast feeding infant are likely to be low and there are no reports of bradycardia or hypoglycaemia in nursing infants. The American Academy of Pediatrics considers beta-blocker therapy to be compatible with breast feeding.[19]

Conclusion

Choice of an antiarrhythmic drug for a pregnant patient remains difficult because of the lack of systematic studies of the pharmacology and safety of antiarrhythmic agents during pregnancy. The low prevalence of serious arrhythmias in women of child-bearing age contributes to the difficulty in conducting such research. Some large-scale studies such as the Michigan Medicaid study have been conducted but have yet to be published. In selecting an antiarrhythmic agent the physician must be guided by data from published case reports. There are insufficient data to consider any antiarrhythmic drug to be completely safe during pregnancy and therefore a drug should be prescribed only after precise diagnosis of the arrhythmia and identification of risk in leaving the arrhythmia untreated. The greatest volume of data exists for lignocaine, verapamil, propranolol, amiodarone, atropine and digoxin.

With the exception of amiodarone these drugs seem to have few side effects and no serious teratogenic effects. Amiodarone is associated with low birth weight, and hypothyroidism occurs in 20% of pregnancies in which it is used. Fetal hypothyroidism from amiodarone may be associated with subsequent delayed neurological development and should be sought in utero. Amiodarone should therefore be reserved for potentially life-threatening arrhythmias. The same is true for most antiarrhythmic drugs for which there are insufficient data to comment on their safety. It seems likely that a large number of cases of antiarrhythmic drug exposure during pregnancy go unreported. The development of a registry to record pregnancy-related antiarrhythmic drug exposure is required if a more scientific approach to drug choice is to be adopted.

References

1 Bigger JT, Giardina EGV. Drug interactions in antiarrhythmic therapy. *Ann NY Acad Sci* 1984; **427**: 140–62.

2 Chen S, Perucca E, Lee J, Richens A. Serum protein binding and free concentration of phenytoin and phenobarbitone in pregnancy. *Br J Clin Pharmacol* 1982; **13**: 547–52.

3 Dean M, Stock B, Patterson J, Levy G. Serum protein binding of drugs during and after pregnancy in humans. *Clin Pharmacol Ther* 1980; **28**: 253–61.

4 Wood M, Wood AJJ. Changes in plasma drug binding and alpha₁-acid glycoprotein in mother and newborn infant. *Clin Pharmacol Ther* 1981; **29**: 522–6.

5 Schanker LS. Passage of drugs across body membranes. *Pharmacol Rev* 1962; **14**: 501–30.

6 Vaughan Williams EM. Classification of antiarrhythmic drugs. In: Sandoe E, Flensted-Jensen E, Olesen KH, eds. *Symposium on cardiac arrhythmias*. Sodertalje: Ab Astra, 1970: 449–72.

7 Harrison DC, Winkle RA, Sami M, Mason JW. Encainide: a new and potent antiarrhythmic agent. In: Harrison DC, ed. *Cardiac arrhythmias—a decade of progress*. Boston: K Hall, 1981: 315–30.

8 Vaughan Williams EM. A classification of antiarrhythmic actions reassessed after a decade of new antiarrhythmic drugs. *J Clin Pharmacol* 1984; **24**: 129.

9 Cobbe SM. Clinical usefulness of the Vaughan Williams classification system. *Eur Heart J* 1987; **8 (suppl A)**: 65–9.

10 Anonymous. The 'Sicilian Gambit'. *Eur Heart J* 1991; **12**: 1112–31.

11 Benowitz NL, Meister W. Clinical pharmacokinetics of lignocaine. *Clin Pharmacokinet* 1978; **3**: 77–101.

12 Shnider SM, Way EL. The kinetics of transfer of lidocaine (Xylocaine) across the human placenta. *Anesthesiology* 1968; **29**: 944–50.

13 Shnider SM, Way EL. Plasma levels of lidocaine (Xylocaine) in mother and newborn following obstetrical conduction anaesthesia. *Anesthesiology* 1968; **29**: 951–8.

14 Wood M, Wood AJJ. Changes in plasma drug binding and alpha₁-acid glycoprotein in mother and newborn infant. *Clin Pharmacol Ther* 1981; **29**: 522–6.

15 Brown WE Jr, Bell GC, Alper MH. Acidosis, local anaesthetics and the newborn. *Obstet Gynecol* 1976; **48**: 27–30.

16 Stokes IM, Evans J, Stone M. Myocardial infarction and cardiac arrest in the second trimester followed by assisted vaginal delivery under epidural analgesia at 38 weeks gestation. *Br J Obstet Gynaecol* 1984; **91**: 197–8.

17 Heinonen OP, Slone D, Shapiro S. *Birth defects and drugs in pregnancy.* Littleton, MA: PSG Pub Inc, 1977.
18 Zeisler JA, Gaarder TD, De Mesquita SA. Lidocaine excretion in breast milk. *Drug Intelligence and Clinical Pharmacology* 1986; **20**: 691–3.
19 Committee on Drugs, American Academy of Pediatrics. The transfer of drugs and other chemicals into human milk. *Pediatrics* 1994; **93**: 137–50.
20 Timmis AD, Jackson G, Holt DW. Mexiletine for control of ventricular dysrhythmias in pregnancy. *Lancet* 1980; **ii**: 647–8.
21 Gregg AR, Tomich PG. Mexiletine use in pregnancy. *J Perinatol* 1988; **8**: 33–5.
22 Matsuo A, Kast A, Tsunenari Y. Reproduction studies of mexiletine hydrochloride by oral administration. *Iyakuhin Kenkyu* 1983; **14**: 527–49.
23 Nishimura M, Kast A, Tsunenari Y. Reproduction studies of mexiletine hydrochloride by intravenous administration. *Ikakuhin Kenkyu* 1983; **14**: 550–70.
24 Product information. *Mexitel.* Boehringer Ingelheim, 1992.
25 Lownes HE, Ives TJ. Mexiletine use in pregnancy and lactation. *Am J Obstet Gynecol* 1987; **157**: 446–7.
26 Lewis AM, Patel L, Johnston A, Turner P. Mexiletine in human blood and breast milk. *Postgrad Med J* 1981; **57**: 546–7.
27 Atkinson AJ Jr, Davison R. Diphenylhydantoin as an antiarrhythmic drug. *Annu Rev Med* 1974; **25**: 99–113.
28 Rotmensch HH, Graf E, Ayzenberg O, Amir C, Laniado S. Self poisoning with digitalis glycosides: successful treatment of three cases. *Isr J Med Sci* 1977; **13**: 1109–13.
29 Shapiro S, Hortz SC, Siskind V, *et al.* Anticonvulsants and prenatal epilepsy in the development of birth defects. *Lancet* 1976; **i**: 272–5.
30 Janz D, Fuchs S. Are anti-epileptic drugs harmful when given during pregnancy? *German Medical Monographs* 1964; **9**: 20–3.
31 Meadow SR. Anticonvulsant drugs and congenital abnormalities. *Lancet* 1968; **ii**: 1296.
32 Loughnan PM, Gold H, Vance JC. Phenytoin teratogenicity in man. *Lancet* 1973; **i**: 70–2.
33 Janz D. Antiepileptic drugs and pregnancy: altered utilization patterns and teratogenesis. *Epilepsia* 1982; **23 (suppl 1)**: S53–63.
34 Hanson JW, Myrianthopoulos NC, Harvey MAS. Risks of offspring of women treated with hydantoin anticonvulsant and emphasis on fetal hydantoin syndrome. *J Pediatr* 1976; **89**: 662–8.
35 Allen RW, Jr, Ogden B, Bentley FL, Jung AL. Fetal hydantoin syndrome, neuroblastoma, and hemorrhagic disease in a neonate. *JAMA* 1979; **244**: 1464–5.
36 Pendergrass TW, Hanson JW. Fetal hydantoin syndrome and neuroblastoma. *Lancet* 1976; **ii**: 150.
37 Ehrenbard LT, Chagantirs K. Cancer in the fetal hydantoin syndrome. *Lancet* 1981; **ii**: 97.
38 Seeler RA, Israel JN, Royal JE, Kaye CI, Rao S, Abulaban M. Ganglioneuroblastoma and fetal hydantoin–alcohol syndromes. *Pediatrics* 1979; **63**: 524–7.
39 Jimenez JF, Seibert RW, Char F, Brown RE, Seibert JJ. Melanotic neuroectodermal tumour of infancy and fetal hydantoin syndrome. *Am J Pediatr Hematol Oncol* 1981; **3**: 9–15.
40 Taylor WF, Myers M, Taylor WR. Extrarenal Wilms' tumour in an infant exposed to intrauterine phenytoin. *Lancet* 1980; **ii**: 481–2.
41 Blattner WA, Hanson DE, Young EC, Fraumeni JF. Malignant mesenchymoma and birth defects. *JAMA* 1977; **238**: 334–5.
42 Kousseff BG. Subcutaneous vascular abnormalities in fetal hydantoin syndrome. *Birth Defects* 1982; **18**: 51–4.
43 Lipson A, Bale P. Ependymoblastoma associated with prenatal exposure to diphenylhydantoin and methylphenobarbitone. *Cancer* 1985; **55**: 1859–62.
44 Buehler BA, Delimont D, Van Waes M, Finnell RH. Prenatal prediction of risk of the fetal hydantoin syndrome. *N Engl J Med* 1990; **322**: 1567–72.
45 Mirkin BL. Placental transfer and neonatal elimination of diphenylhydantoin. *Am J Obstet Gynecol* 1971; **109**: 930–3.
46 Rane A. Urinary excretion of diphenylhydantoin metabolites in newborn infants. *J Pediatr* 1974; **85**: 543–5.
47 Kaneko S, Suzuki K, Sato T, Ogawa Y, Nomura Y. The problem of antiepileptic medication at the neonatal period: is breast feeding advisable? In: Janz D, Dam M, Richens A, Bossi L, Helge H. eds. *Epilepsy, Pregnancy and the Child.* New York: Raven Press, 1981.

48 Finch E, Lorber J. Methaemoglobinaemia in the newborn: probably due to phenytoin excreted in human milk. *Journal of Obstetrics and Gynaecology of the British Empire* 1954; **61**: 833.

49 Dumesic DA, Silverman NH, Tobias S, Golbus MS. Transplacental cardioversion of fetal supraventricular tachycardia with procainamide. *N Engl J Med* 1982; **307**: 1128–31.

50 Weiner CP, Thompson MIB. Direct treatment of fetal supraventricular tachycardia after failed transplacental therapy. *Am J Obstet Gynecol* 1988; **158**: 570–3.

51 Allen NM, Page RL. Procainamide administration during pregnancy. *Clinical Pharmacy* 1993; **12**: 58–60.

52 Merx W, Effert S, Heinrich KW. Heart disease in pregnancy, intra- and postpartum. *Z Geburtshilfe Perinatol* 1974; **178**: 317–36.

53 Pittard WB III, Glazier H. Procainamide excretion in human milk. *J Pediatr* 1983; **102**: 631–3.

54 Keefe DLD, Kates RE, Harrison DC. New antiarrhythmic drugs: their place in therapy. *Drugs* 1981; **22**: 363–400.

55 Tadmor OP, Keren A, Rosenak D, *et al.* The effect of disopyramide on uterine contractions during pregnancy. *Am J Obstet Gynecol* 1990; **162**: 482–6.

56 Ellsworth AJ, Horn JR, Raisys VA, Miyagawa LA, Bell JL. Disopyramide and N-monodesalkyl disopyramide in serum and breast milk. *Drug Intelligence and Clinical Pharmacy* 1989; **23**: 56–7.

57 Shaxted EJ, Milton PJ. Disopyramide in pregnancy: a case report. *Curr Med Res Opin* 1979; **6**: 70–2.

58 MacKintosh D, Buchanan N. Excretion of disopyramide in human breast milk. *Br J Clin Pharmacol* 1985; **19**: 856–7.

59 Leonard RF, Braun TE, Levy AM. Initiation of uterine contractions by disopyramide during pregnancy. *N Engl J Med* 1978; **299**: 84–5.

60 Tadmor OP, Keren A, Rosenak D, *et al.* The effect of disopyramide on uterine contractions during pregnancy. *Am J Obstet Gynecol* 1990; **162**: 482–6.

61 Rotmensch HH, Rotmensch S, Elkayam U. Management of cardiac arrhythmias during pregnancy: current concepts. *Drugs* 1987; **33**: 623–63.

62 Rotmensch HH, Elkayam U, Frishman W. Antiarrhythmic drug therapy during pregnancy. *Ann Intern Med* 1983; **98**: 487–97.

63 Tamari I, Eldar M, Rabinowitz B, Neufeld HN. Medical treatment of cardiovascular disorders during pregnancy. *Am Heart J* 1982; **104**: 1357–63.

64 Barnett DB, Hudson SA, McBurney A. Disopyramide and its N-monodesalkyl metabolite in breast milk. *Br J Clin Pharmacol* 1982; **14**: 310–12.

65 Hoppu K, Neuvonen PJ, Korte T. Disopyramide and breast feeding. *Br J Clin Pharmacol* 1986; **21**: 553.

66 Winkle RA, Glantz SA, Harrison DC. Pharmacological therapy of ventricular arrhythmias. *Am J Cardiol* 1975; **36**: 629–47.

67 Killeen AA, Bowers LD. Foetal supraventricular tachycardia treated with high-dose quinidine: toxicity associated with marked elevation of the metabolite, ˙3(S)-3-hydroxyquinidine. *Obstet Gynecol* 1987; **70**: 445–9.

68 Hill LM, Malkasian GD Jr. The use of quinidine sulfate throughout pregnancy. *Obstet Gynecol* 1984; **64**: 730–5.

69 Guntheroth WG, Cyr DR, Mack LA, Benedetti T, Lenke RR, Petty CN. Hydrops from reciprocating atrioventricular tachycardia in a 27-week foetus requiring quinidine for conversion. *Obstet Gynecol* 1985; **66** (**suppl**): 29S–33S.

70 Meyer J, Lackner JE, Schochet SS. Paroxysmal tachycardia in pregnancy. *JAMA* 1930; **94**: 1901–4.

71 McMillan TM, Bellet S. Ventricular paroxysmal tachycardia: report of a case in a pregnancy girl of sixteen years with an apparently normal heart. *Am Heart J* 1931; 7: 70–8.

71a Briggs CJ, Freeman RK, Yaffe SJ. Drugs in pregnancy and lactation—a reference guide to fetal and neonatal risk. Baltimore, MA: Williams and Wilkins, 1994.

72 Meyer J, Lackner JE, Schochet SS. Paroxysmal tachycardia in pregnancy. *JAMA* 1930; **94**: 1901–4.

73 Merx W. Herzrhythmusstorungen in der schwangerschaft. *Dtsch Med Wochensch* 1972; **97**: 1987–8.

74 Kamban JR, Frans JJ, Smith BE. Inhibitory effect of quinidine on plasma pseudocholinesterase activity in pregnant women. *Am J Obstet Gynecol* 1987; **157**: 897–9.

75 Braverman AC, Franks JJ, Smith BE. New onset ventricular tachycardia during pregnancy. *Int J Cardiol* 1991; **33**: 409–12.

76 Coplen SE, Antman EM, Berlin JA, Hewitt P, Chalmers TC. Efficacy and safety of quinidine therapy for maintenance of sinus rhythm after cardioversion. A meta-analysis of randomized controlled trials. *Circulation* 1990; **82**: 1106–16.

77 Spinnato JA, Shaver DC, Flinn GS, Sibai BM, Watson DL, Marin-Garcia J. Fetal supraventricular tachycardia: in utero therapy with digoxin and quinidine. *Obstet Gynecol* 1984; **64**: 730–5.

78 Guntheroth WG, Cyr DR, Mack LA, Benedetti T, Lenke RR, Petty CN. Hydrops from reciprocating atrioventricular tachycardia in a 27-week foetus requiring quinidine for conversion. *Obstet Gynecol* 1985; **66** (**suppl**): 29S–33S.

79 Shere DM, Sadovsky E, Menase M, Mordel N, Rein AJJT. Fetal ventricular tachycardia associated with nonimmunologic hydrops fetalis: a case report. *J Reprod Med* 1990; **35**: 292–4.

80 Hill LM, Malkasian GD Jr. The use of quinidine sulfate throughout pregnancy. *Obstet Gynecol* 1979; **54**: 366–8.

81 Product information, *Tambocor*. 3M Pharmaceuticals, 1993.

82 Wagner X, Jouglard J, Moulin M, Miller AM, Petitjean J, Pisapia A. Coadministration of flecainide acetate and sotalol during pregnancy: lack of teratogenic effects, passage across the placenta, and excretion in human breast milk. *Am Heart J* 1990; **119**: 700–2.

83 Wren C, Hunter S. Maternal administration of flecainide to terminate and suppress fetal tachycardia. *BMJ* 1988; **296**: 249.

84 Kofinas AD, Simon NV, Sagel H, Lyttle E, Smith N, King K. Treatment of fetal supraventricular tachycardia with flecainide acetate after digoxin failure. *Am J Obstet Gynecol* 1991; **165**: 630–1.

85 Allan LD, Chita SK, Sharland GK, Maxwell D, Priestley K. Flecainide in the treatment of fetal tachycardias. *Br Heart J* 1991; **65**: 46–8.

86 Bourget P, Pons JC, Delouis C, Fermont L, Frydman R. Flecainide distribution, transplacental passage, and accumulation in the amniotic fluid during the third trimester of pregnancy. *Ann Pharmacother* 1994; **28**: 1031–4.

87 McQuinn RL, Pisani A, Wafa S, *et al.* Flecainide excretion in human breast milk. *Clin Pharmacol Ther* 1990; **48**: 262–7.

88 Gillie AM, Yee YG, Kates RE. Binding of antiarrhythmic drugs to purified human alpha 1-acid glycoprotein. *Biochem Pharmacol* 1985; **34**: 4279–82.

89 Product information. *Rhythmol*. Knoll Pharmaceuticals, 1993.

90 Libardoni M, Piovan D, Busato E, Padrini R. Transfer of propafenone and 5-OH-propafenone to foetal plasma and maternal milk. *Br J Clin Pharmacol* 1991; **32**: 527–8.

91 Brunozzi LT, Meniconi L, Chiocchi P, Liberatir R, Zuanetti G, Latini R. Propafenone in the treatment of chronic ventricular arrhythmias in a pregnant patient. *Br J Clin Pharmacol* 1988; **26**: 489–90.

92 Gembruch U, Manz M, Bald R, *et al.* Repeated intravascular treatment with amiodarone in a fetus with refractory supraventricular tachycardia and hydrops fetalis. *Am Heart J* 1989; **118**: 1335–8.

93 Spiegelhalder B, Eichelbaum M. Determination of verapamil in human plasma by mass fragmentography using stable isotope labelled verapamil as internal standard. *Arzneimittelforschung* 1977; **27**: 1–7.

94 Strigl R, Gastroph G, Hege HG, Düoring P, Mehring W. Nachweis von Verapamil in Mutterlichen und fetalen Blut des Menschen. *Geburtshilfe Frauenheilkd* 1980; **40**: 496–9.

95 Klein V, Repke JT. Supraventricular tachycardia in pregnancy: cardioversion with verapamil. *Obstet Gynecol* 1984; **63**: 16S–18S.

96 Byerly WG, Hartmann A, Foster DE, Tannenbaum AK. Verapamil in the treatment of maternal paroxysmal supraventricular tachycardia. *Ann Emerg Med* 1991; **20**: 552–4.

97 Lilja H, Karlsson K, Lindecrantz K, Sabel KG. Treatment of intrauterine supraventricular tachycardia with digoxin and verapamil. *J Perinat Med* 1984; **12**: 151–4.

98 Rey E, Duperron L, Gauthier R, Lemay M, Grignon A, LeLorier J. Transplacental treatment of tachycardia-induced fetal heart failure with verapamil and amiodarone: a case report. *Am J Obstet Gynecol* 1985; **153**: 311–12.

99 Maxwell DJ, Crawford DC, Curry PVM, Tynan MJ, Allan LD. Obstetric importance, diagnosis, and management of fetal tachycardias. *BMJ* 1988; **297**: 107–10.

100 Weiner CP, Thompson MIV. Direct treatment of fetal supraventricular tachycardia after failed transplacental therapy. *Am J Obstet Gynecol* 1988; **158**: 570–3.

101 Owen J, Colvin EV, Davis RO. Fetal death after successful conversion of fetal supraventricular tachycardia with digoxin and verapamil. *Am J Obstet Gynecol* 1988; **158**: 1169–70.

102 Brittinger WD, Schwarzbeck A, Wittenmeier KW, *et al.* Linisch-Experimentelle Untersuchungen uber die Blutdruckendende Wirkung von Verapamil. *Dtsch Med Wochenschr* 1970; **95**: 1871–7.

103 Rodriguez-Escudero FJ, Aranguren G, Benito JA. Verapamil to inhibit the cardiovascular side effects of ritodrine. *Int J Gynaecol Obstet* 1981; **19**: 333–6.

104 Andersen HJ. Excretion of verapamil in human milk. *Eur J Clin Pharmacol* 1983; **25**: 279–80.

105 Anderson P, Bondesson U, Mattiasson I, Johansson BW. Verapamil and norverapamil in plasma and breast milk during breast feeding. *Eur J Clin Pharmacol* 1987; **31**: 625–7.

106 Miller MR, Wither R, Bhamra R, Holt DW. Verapamil and breast-feeding. *Eur J Clin Pharm* 1986; **30**: 125–6.

107 Nattel S, Davies M, Quantz M. The antiarrhythmic efficacy of amiodarone and desethylamiodarone alone and in combination, in dogs with acute myocardial infarction. *Circulation* 1988; **77**: 200–8.

108 Kato R, Venkatesh N, Namiya K, Yabek S, Kannan R, Singh BN. Electrophysiological effects of desethylamiodarone, an active metabolite of amiodarone: comparison with amiodarone during chronic administration in rabbits. *Am Heart J* 1988; **115**: 351–9.

109 Latini R, Tognoni G, Kates RE. Clinical pharmacokinetics of amiodarone. *Clin Pharmacokinet* 1984; **9**: 136–56.

110 Barchewitz G, Harris L, Mazue G. Toxicology. In: Harris L, Roncucci, eds. *Amiodarone.* Paris: Médecine et Sciences Internationales 1986: 195–6.

111 Perelman AH, Johnson RL, Clemons RD, Finberg HJ, Clewell WH, Trujillo L. Intrauterine diagnosis and treatment of fetal goitrous hypothyroidism. *J Clin Endocrinol Metab* 1990; **71**: 618–21.

112 De Catte L, De Wolf D, Smitz J, *et al.* Hypothyroidism as a complication of amiodarone treatment for persistent fetal supraventricular tachycardia. *Prenatal Diagnosis* 1994; **14**: 762–5.

113 Alfonso-Fischbach AL, Guegan C, Saura R, Maugey-Laulom B, Sandler B. Prenatal diagnosis and treatment of fetal hypothyroid goiter. *Journal de Gynecologie, Obstetrique et Biologie de la Reproduction* 1994; **23**: 888–91.

114 O'Hare MF, Leahey W, Murnaghan GA, McDevitt DG. Pharmacokinetics of sotalol during pregnancy. *Eur J Clin Pharmacol* 1983; **24**: 521–4.

115 O'Hare MF, Murnaghan GA, Russell CJ, Leahey WJ, Varma MP, McDevitt DG. Sotalol as a hypotensive agent in pregnancy. *Br J Obstet Gynaecol* 1980; **87**: 814–20.

116 Erkkola R, Lammintausta R, Liukko P, Anttila M. Transfer of propranolol and sotalol across the human placenta. Their effect on maternal and fetal plasma renin activity. *Acta Obstet Gynecol Scand* 1982; **61**: 31–4.

117 Hackett LP, Wojnar-Horton RE, Dusci LJ, Ilett KF, Roberts MJ. Excretion of sotalol in breast milk. *Am Heart J* 1990; **119**: 700–2.

118 Advanced Life Support Group. *Advanced cardiac life support—the practical approach.* London: Chapman & Hall, 1983.

119 Kivalo I, Saarikoski S. Placental transmission of atropine at full-term pregnancy. *Br J Anaesth* 1977; **49**: 1017–21.

120 Hellman LM, Fillisti LP. Analysis of the atropine test for placental transfer in gravidas with toxemia and diabetes. *Am J Obstet Gynecol* 1965; **91**: 797–805.

121 Aboud T, Raya J, Sadri S, Grobler N, Stine L, Miller F. Fetal and maternal cardiovascular effects of atropine and glycopyrrolate. *Anesth Analg* 1983; **62**: 426–30.

122 Hicks JM, Brett EM. Falsely increased digoxin concentrations in samples from neonates and infants. *Ther Drug Mon* 1984; **6**: 461–4.

123 Schlebusch H, von Mende S, Grunn U, Gembruch U, Bald R, Hansmann M. Determination of digoxin in the blood of pregnant women, fetuses and neonates before and during anti-arrhythmic therapy, using four immunochemical methods. *Eur J Clin Chem Clin Biochem* 1991; **29**: 57–66.

124 Rogers MC, Willserson JT, Goldblatt A, Smith TW. Serum digoxin concentration in the human fetus, neonate and infant. *N Engl J Med* 1972; **287**: 1010–3.

125 Soyka LF. Digoxin: placental transfer, effects on the fetus, and therapeutics use in the new born. *Clin Perinatol* 1975; **2**: 23–35.

126 Allonen H, Kanto J, Lisalo E. The foeto–maternal distribution of digoxin in early human pregnancy. *Acta Pharmacologica and Toxicologica* 1976; **39**: 477–80.

127 Saarikoski S. Placental transfer and fetal uptake of ₃H-digoxin in humans. *Br J Obstet Gynaecol* 1976; **83**: 879–84.

128 Chan V, Tse TF, Wong V. Transfer of digoxin across the placenta and into breast milk. *Br J Obstet Gynaecol* 1978; **85**: 605–9.

129 Thompson AJ, Hargis J, Murphy ML, Doherty JE. Tritiated digoxin. Tissue distribution in experimental myocardial infarction. *Am Heart J* 1974; **88**: 319–24.

130 Lingman G, Ohrlander S, Ohlin P. Intrauterine digoxin treatment of fetal paroxysmal tachycardia: case report. *Br J Obstet Gynaecol* 1980; **87**: 340–2.

131 Kerenyi TD, Gleicher N, Meller J, *et al.* Transplacental cardioversion of intrauterine supraventricular tachycardia with digitalis. *Lancet* 1980; **ii**: 393–4.

132 Heaton FC, Vaughan R. Intrauterine supraventricular tachycardia: cardioversion with maternal digoxin. *Obstet Gynecol* 1982; **60**: 749–52.

133 Bortolotti U, Milano A, Mazzucco A, *et al.* Pregnancy in patients with a porcine valve bioprosthesis. *Am J Cardiol* 1982; **50**: 1051–4.

134 Weaver JB, Pearson JF. Influence of digitalis on time of onset and duration of labour in women with cardiac disease. *BMJ* 1973; **iii**: 519–20.

135 Potondi A. Congenital rhabdomyoma of the heart and intrauterine digitalis poisoning. *J Forensic Sci* 1967; **11**: 81–8.

136 Sherman JL, Locke RV. Transplacental neonatal digitalis intoxication. *Am J Cardiol* 1960; **6**: 834–7.

137 Finley JP, Waxman MB, Wong PY, Lickrish GM. Digoxin excretion in human milk. *J Pediatr* 1979; **94**: 339–40.

138 Levy M, Granit L, Laufer N. Excretion of drugs in human milk. *N Engl J Med* 1977; **297**: 789.

139 Loughnan PM. Digoxin excretion in human breast milk. *J Pediatr* 1978; **92**: 1019–20.

140 Harrison JK, Greenfield RA, Wharton JM. Acute termination of supraventricular tachycardia by adenosine during pregnancy. *Am Heart J* 1992; **123**: 1386–8.

141 Mason BA, Ricci-Goodman J, Koos BJ. Adenosine in the treatment of maternal paroxysmal supraventricular tachycardia. *Obstet Gynecol* 1992; **80**: 478–80.

142 Leffler S, Johnson DR. Adenosine use in pregnancy: lack of effect on fetal heart rate. *Am J Emerg Med* 1992; **10**: 548–9.

143 Kohl T, Tercanli S, Kececioglu D, Holzgreve W. Direct fetal administration of adenosine for the termination of incessant supraventricular tachycardia. *Obstet Gynecol* 1995; **85**: 873–4.

144 Shepard TH. *Catalog of teratogenic agents.* 6th ed. Baltimore: Johns Hopkins University Press, 1989; **40**: 566.

145 Mason BA, Ogunyemi D, Punla O, Koos BJ. Maternal and fetal cardiorespiratory responses to adenosine in sheep. *Am J Obstet Gynecol* 1993; **168**: 1558–61.

146 Afridi I, Moise KJ Jr, Rokey R. Termination of supraventricular tachycardia with intravenous adenosine in a pregnant woman with Wolff–Parkinson–White syndrome. *Obstet Gynecol* 1992; **80**: 481–3.

147 Podolsky SM, Varon J. Adenosine use during pregnancy. *Ann Emerg Med* 1991; **20**: 1027–8.

148 O'Hare MF, Kinney CD, Murnaghan GA, McDevitt DG. Pharmacokinetics of propranolol during pregnancy. *Eur J Clin Pharmacol* 1984; **27**: 583–7.

149 Langer A, Hung CT, McA'nulty JA, Harrigan JT, Washington E. Adrenergic blockade: a new approach to hyperthyroidism during pregnancy. *Obstet Gynecol* 1974; **44**: 181–6.

150 Cottrill CM, McAllister RG Jr, Gettes L, Noonan JA. Propranolol therapy during pregnancy labor and delivery: evidence for transplacental drug transfer and impaired neonatal drug disposition. *J Pediatr* 1977; **91**: 812–4.

151 Teuscher A, Bossi E, Imhof P, Erb E, Stocker FP, Weber JW. Effect of propranolol on fetal tachycardia in diabetic pregnancy. *Am J Cardiol* 1978; **42**: 304–7.

152 Taylor EA, Turner P. Anti-hypertensive therapy with propranolol during pregnancy and lactation. *Postgrad Med J* 1981; **57**: 427–30.

153 Erkkola R, Lammintausta R, Liukko P, Anttila M. Transfer of propranolol and sotalol across the human placenta. *Acta Obstet Gynecol Scand* 1982; **61**: 31–4.

154 Bott-Kanner G, Schweitzer A, Schoenfeld A, Joel-Cohen J, Rosenfeld JB. Treatment with propranolol and hydralazine throughout pregnancy in a hypertensive patient: a case report. *Isr J Med Sci* 1978; **14**: 466–8.

155 O'Connor PC, Jick H, Hunter JR, Stergachis A, Madsen S. Propranolol and pregnancy outcome. *Lancet* 1981; **ii**: 1168.

156 Duminy PC, Burger P du T. Fetal abnormality associated with the use of captopril during pregnancy. *S Afr Med J* 1981; **60**: 805.

157 Jenson OH. Fetal heart rate response to a controlled sound stimulus after propranolol administration to the mother. *Acta Obstet Gynecol Scand* 1984; **63**: 199–202.

158 Oakes GK, Walker AD, Ehrenkranz RA, Chez RA. Effect of propranolol infusion on the umbilical and uterine circulation of pregnant sheep. *Am J Obstet Gynaecol* 1976; **126**: 1038–42.

159 Pruyn SC, Phelan JP, Buchanan GC. Long-term propranolol therapy in pregnancy: maternal and fetal outcome. *Am J Obstet Gynaecol* 1979; **135**: 485–9.

160 Eliahou HE, Silverburg DS, Reisin E, Romem I, Mashiach S, Serr DM. Propranolol for the treatment of hypertension in pregnancy. *Br J Obstet Gynaecol* 1978; **85**: 431–6.

161 Tcherdakoff PH, Colliard M, Berrard E, Kreft C, Dupay A, Bernaille JM. Propranolol in hypertension during pregnancy. *BMJ* 1978; **ii**: 670.

162 Bott-Kanner G, Schweitzer A, Reisner SH, Joel-Cohen SJ, Rosenfeld JB. Propranolol and hydrallazine in the management of essential hypertension in pregnancy. *Br J Obstet Gynaecol* 1980; **87**: 110–4.

163 Oakley CDG, McGarry K, Limb DG, Oakley CM. Management of pregnancy in patients with hypertrophic cardiomyopathy. *BMJ* 1979; **1**: 1749–50.

164 Rubin PC, Butters L, Low RA, Reid JL. Atenolol in the treatment of essential hypertension during pregnancy. *Br J Clin Pharm* 1982; **37**: 688–92.

165 Galler ED, Ross MR, Gyory AZ. Antihypertensive treatment in pregnancy: analysis of different responses to oxprenolol and methyldopa. *BMJ* 1985; **291**: 563–6.

166 Ellenbogen A, Jaschevatsky O, Davidson A, Anderman S, Grunstein S. Management of pregnancy induced hypertension with pindolol: comparative study with methyldopa. *Int J Gynaecol Obstet* 1986; **24**: 3–7.

167 Levitan AA, Manion JC. Propranolol therapy during pregnancy and lactation. *Am J Cardiol* 1973; **32**: 247.

168 Bauer JH, Pape B, Zajicek J, Groshong T. Propranolol in human plasma and breast milk. *Am J Cardiol* 1979; **43**: 860–2.

169 Plomp TA, Vulsma T, de Vildjer JJM. Use of amiodarone during pregnancy. *Eur J Obstet Gynecol Reprod Biol* 1992; **43**: 201–7.

170 Penn IM, Barrett PA, Pannikote V, Barnaby PF, Campbell JB, Lyons NR. Amiodarone in pregnancy. *Am J Cardiol* 1985; **56**: 196–7.

171 McKenna WJ, Harris L, Rowland E, Whitelaw A, Storey G, Holt D. Amiodarone therapy during pregnancy. *Am J Cardiol* 1983; **51**: 1231–3.

172 Pitcher D, Leather HM, Storey GAC, Holt DW. Amiodarone in pregnancy. *Lancet* 1983; **i**: 597–8.

173 Robson DJ, Jeeva Raj MV, Storey GC, Holt DW. Use of amiodarone during pregnancy. *Postgrad Med J* 1985; **61**: 75–7.

174 Arnoux P, Seyral P, Lurens M, *et al.* Amiodarone and digoxin for refractory fetal tachycardia. *Am J Cardiol* 1987; **59**: 166–7.

175 Strunge P, Frandsen J, Andreasen F. Amiodarone during pregnancy. *Eur Heart J* 1988; **9**: 106–9.

176 Rey E, Bachrach LK, Buttow GN. Effects of amiodarone during pregnancy. *Can Med Assoc J* 1987; **136**: 959–60.

177 De Wolf D, De Schepper J, Verhaaren H, Deneyer M, Smitz J, Sacre-Smits L. Congenital thyroid goitre and amiodarone. *Acta Paediatr Scand* 1988; **77**: 616–8.

178 Widerhorn J, Bhandari AK, Bughi S, Rahimtoola SH, Elkayam U. Fetal and neonatal adverse effects profile of amiodarone treatment during pregnancy. *Am Heart J* 1991; **122**: 1162–6.

179 Rey E, Duperron L, Gauthier R, Lemay M, Grignon A, LeLorier J. Transplacental treatment of tachycardia-induced fetal heart failure with verapamil and amiodarone: a case report. *Am J Obstet Gynecol* 1985; **153**: 311–12.

180 Wladimiroff JW, Stewart PA. Treatment of fetal cardiac arrhythmias. *Br J Hosp Med* 1985; **34**: 134–40.

181 Laurent M, Betremieux P, Biron Y, LeHelloco A. Neonatal hypothyroidism after treatment by amiodarone during pregnancy [letter]. *Am J Cardiol* 1987; **60**: 942.

182 Gembruch U, Manz M, Bald R, *et al.* Repeated intravascular treatment with amiodarone in a fetus with refractory supraventricular tachycardia and hydrops fetalis. *Am Heart J* 1989; **118**: 1335–8.

183 Magee LA, Downar E, Sermer M, Boulton BC, Allen LC, Koren G. Pregnancy outcome after gestational exposure to amiodarone in Canada. *Am J Obstet Gynecol* 1995; **172**: 1307–11.

184 Valensise H, Civitella C, Garzetti GG, Romanini C. Amiodarone treatment in pregnancy for dilatative cardiomyopathy with ventricular malignant extrasystole and normal maternal and neonatal outcome. *Prenatal Diagnosis* 1992; **12**: 705–8.

185 Matsumura LK, Born D, Kunii IS, Franco DB, Maciel RM. Outcome of thyroid function in newborns from mothers treated with amiodarone. *Thyroid* 1992; **2**: 279–81.

25: Antimicrobial therapy

ROBERT G FELDMAN

Antimicrobials are the commonest group of drugs prescribed during pregnancy and some of these drugs therefore have a considerable safety record.[1,2] Knowledge of potential risks to the mother and fetus of antimicrobial therapy is, however, far from complete and it is particularly important to balance the risk-benefit implications before embarking on treatment. The multitude of metabolic, physiological and physical changes that occur during pregnancy require that special attention be paid to the kind of antimicrobial agents that are given and their dosage. During pregnancy special care should be taken when choosing drugs for any infection but this chapter will focus on treatment of cardiac infections.

Changes during pregnancy that are relevant to the administration of antimicrobials

Many of the changes that occur during pregnancy are dynamic and often become more pronounced in the later stages of gestation. The placenta, fetus, and amniotic fluid are three extra compartments, which complicate the pharmacokinetics of all drugs. Although active placental transport mechanisms exist, all major antimicrobial drugs cross the placenta by passive diffusion and as the feto-maternal barrier becomes thinner during pregnancy the rate of diffusion increases. The increasing bulk of the uterus leads to reduced gastrointestinal mobility which in turn may lead to delayed gastric emptying and increased intestinal transit times. This can reduce the bioavailability of orally administered drugs because of the increased time that they are exposed to gastric acid and because of reduced uptake.[3]

Pregnancy results in a radical alteration in the intravascular volume which can increase by up to 50% by the eighth month of gestation, and this in turn leads to a reduced plasma protein concentration. It is not uncommon for the serum albumin concentration to fall 25% by the end of pregnancy.[4] The increased volume of distribution results in lower serum concentrations compared with the non-pregnant state while the lower serum protein concentration alters the ratio of bound to free drug which often increases the tissue to serum ratio and decreases serum levels as well as increasing the rate of excretion. These adaptations are accompanied by an augmented hepatic metabolism, and an increased renal blood flow and glomerular filtration rate, all of which further enhance the elimination of antimicrobial agents.

Pregnancy is also accompanied by an alteration in immunological response which, in general leads to a mild degree of immunosuppression. The immune system of the host is an important factor in the response to antimicrobial chemotherapy and the reduced responsiveness of the immune system may be relevant when treating difficult infections.[5]

Potential risk during pregnancy

There are a number of adverse reactions which are particular to pregnancy, in addition to those normally associated with the non-pregnant state. However, the overall incidence of adverse effects is not increased during pregnancy.[6] Apart from adverse reactions in the mother, the risk of causing abnormalities in the developing fetus is of paramount concern when giving any drug during pregnancy. The active drug or its metabolites may be teratogenic or cause unwanted biochemical changes in the fetus. Pregnant women who have renal dysfunction, including pyelonephritis, develop fatty necrosis of the liver and renal failure when they are given tetracycline.[7] In addition, erythromycin estolate is contraindicated in pregnancy as it causes reversible hepatitis in 10% to 15% of women in late pregnancy.[8] Tetracycline is also contraindicated during pregnancy as fetal exposure during the last two trimesters is associated with tooth discoloration and dysplasia and inhibition of bone growth.[9] Limb abnormalities and cataracts have also been described in infants born to mothers treated with large doses of tetracycline in the first trimester.[10]

Pharmacokinetic characteristics of antimicrobials which are relevant to treatment

Cardiac infections, particularly endocarditis, are particularly challenging to treat because although many of the causative organisms are extremely sensitive to a wide range of antimicrobials, the deep seated nature of the infection requires prolonged treatment often with a combination of agents. In vitro tests on the causative organisms and the therapeutic agents used to treat them can aid the choice of treatment but cannot readily predict outcome.[5] However, it is essential that antibiotics should be chosen which are known to be active against the infecting organism. Additional factors, described below, relating to the pharmacokinetics of antimicrobials also have an important part to play and should be considered when choosing drugs for endocarditis.

Protein binding

The in vivo interaction between free drug and molecular binding sites, especially serum proteins, is complex to a degree that the clinical implications of protein binding remain controversial. What is certain is that protein bound antimicrobial agents are not active but act as a pool of active drug. The extent of protein binding has no direct effect on efficacy but it is important to ensure that sufficient free drug is available to kill any target organism. In pregnancy, in which the concentration of serum proteins including albumin decreases, the pharmacokinetics of any protein bound drug are altered. In addition, bioassays of antimicrobials using standard human serum as a control diluent may give false results.

Method of metabolism and excretion

Most antimicrobial agents are excreted in the urine, at least to some degree. As stated above, the elimination of a drug is often considerably altered during pregnancy. Usually this means that drug concentrations are lower than in the non-pregnant state and in certain cases dosage and time between doses have to be altered accordingly. The route of excretion together with the distribution and protein binding of the drug determines the availability and half-life.

Tissue penetration

Penetration into vegetations is irregular and occurs in three distinct patterns, which have been shown by following the fate of ^{14}C-labelled antimicrobial agents.[11] The glycopeptides remain in the outer areas of the vegetation and do not penetrate into the centre. Beta-lactams produce a concentration gradient so that they do penetrate to the centre of vegetations but at a lower concentration than the periphery. The gradient is more pronounced for ceftriaxone than for penicillin. Finally some agents diffuse homogeneously and these include the fluoroquinolones and tobramycin.

Postantibiotic effect

The postantibiotic effect is the ability to inhibit bacterial growth after the removal of an antibiotic. The aminoglycosides and fluoroquinolones have a postantibiotic effect so with these drugs it is not necessary to maintain constant levels above the inhibitory concentration of the target organism. Conversely, beta-lactams and glycopeptides have no postantibiotic effect so it is prudent to maintain levels continuously above the inhibitory concentration.

Kill curves

The speed with which antimicrobials and combinations of antimicrobials kill organisms has been correlated with successful outcome.[5] Kill times for streptococci treated with glycopeptides can be prolonged whereas kill times are usually short for aminoglycosides, fluoroquinolones, and rifampicin. Combinations can further enhance killing, for example amoxycillin and gentamicin show synergy when treating enterococci and streptococci.

Antimicrobial agents

Beta-lactam antibiotics

This large group of antibiotics inhibit cell wall synthesis by binding to one or more bacterial penicillin binding proteins. The group as a whole has an exceptionally broad spectrum and is the mainstay of most anti-infective treatment. Penicillins have the best safety record of any group of antimicrobial drugs.[10,12] The only contraindication is allergy which is no more common during pregnancy. The cephalosporins are a closely related group of drugs with similar actions and pharmacokinetic profiles and while they do not have the same proven safety record, there have been no reported cases of teratogenicity. Amoxycillin combined with the beta-lactamase inhibitor, clavulanic acid, has also been given during pregnancy without adverse effect.[13] Maternal serum levels vary widely but are less than in non-pregnant women primarily as a result of increased renal clearance. However, with most antimicrobials in this group serum concentrations remain well above the MIC of most organisms which are being treated. In difficult cases in which the organism being treated is only intermediately sensitive, careful consideration should be given to dosage which may have to be increased. Serum concentrations of the antibiotic may also help in the management of these cases.

Penicillin desensitisation has been described during pregnancy, which may be justified for difficult infections when there are no other reasonable alternatives. In one study fifteen pregnant women, including one with endocarditis, were successfully desensitised.[14]

Aminoglycosides

This group of antibiotics bind to the 30S ribosomal subunit and inhibit protein synthesis by causing miscoding. These antibiotics are particularly used because they are rapidly cidal, have a prolonged postantibiotic effect, and often act synergistically with beta-lactam antibiotics. They are, however, relatively toxic and may cause nephrotoxicity and ototoxicity so it is essential that serum concentrations are monitored regularly. The aminoglycosides are active against a broad range of gram-negative and gram-positive bacteria but they are not active against anaerobic organisms. Most streptococci are resistant to aminoglycosides but there is often a synergistic effect when aminoglycosides are given with beta-lactam antibiotics. Aminoglycosides are eliminated exclusively by the renal route so, as would be expected, concentrations in pregnant women are consistently lower than in non-pregnant patients.[2] However, the clearance seems to decrease towards the end of pregnancy, at least for tobramycin.[15] There is also a concentration of aminoglycoside in the renal tissue of the fetus which raises the possibility that these antibiotics may harm the fetus. There are no confirmed reports of renal toxicity in infants born to mothers treated with aminoglycosides but ototoxicity has been reported in infants whose mothers were treated with streptomycin for tuberculosis.[16] Vestibular and cochlear abnormalities have not been reported after other aminoglycosides but these are difficult to measure in early infancy. In addition, animal studies suggest that pups born to pregnant guinea-pigs treated with kanamycin are more susceptible to ototoxicity when subsequently exposed to the drug for a second time.[17] No teratogenic effects have been reported for any of the aminoglycosides.

A reappraisal of the dosing schedules of aminoglycosides has taken place over the last few years. It has become clear that infrequent high peak levels are effective and potentially less toxic than the conventional three times daily dosage regimens.[15,18] In an animal model of streptococcal endocarditis, once daily tobramycin in combination with penicillin was as effective as a three times daily dosage.[19] However, in another animal study of enterococcal endocarditis, high dose three times daily netilmicin, also in combination with penicillin, was more effective than lower doses or less frequent doses.[20]

Fluoroquinolones

While these antimicrobials, which inhibit bacterial DNA gyrase, are of great potential use in treating cardiac infections because of their ability to kill at low concentration and penetrate tissues well, there has been little experience of using them in pregnancy or endocarditis. In addition, animal experiments suggest that the fluoroquinolones may not be entirely safe during pregnancy so it is advisable to avoid them during pregnancy unless there is no alternative. One study of 38 pregnant women treated with quinolone drugs, mostly in the first trimester, showed that there was a significant increase in fetal distress compared with a control group, but no increased incidence of fetal cartilaginous abnormalities.[21] In a study in Macaca monkeys high doses (70 mg/kg/day) were associated with fetal death but no fetal abnormalities were observed.[22] This study also showed that there were no major pharmacokinetic differences between non-pregnant and pregnant subjects suggesting that dosages do not need to be altered. Cartilaginous lesions have been described in infant rats and dogs treated with large doses of fluoroquinolones and these data also suggest caution before using these drugs during pregnancy.[23]

Lincosamides

Clindamycin, which binds to the 50S ribosomal subunit and inhibits protein synthesis, is a useful alternative to beta-lactam antibiotics for the treatment of streptococci and staphylococci but unfortunately there have been few studies of this drug during pregnancy.[9] It is also active against

Mycoplasma hominis and many anaerobic bacteria. There are no reported cases of adverse effects in pregnancy but it should be remembered that clindamycin predisposes patients to pseudomembranous colitis. The pharmacokinetics of clindamycin are similar to those in the non-pregnant state and the dose should therefore not be altered.[24]

Sulphonamides

Sulphonamides, which inhibit bacterial uptake of para-aminobenzoic acid and thus inhibit bacterial folate synthesis, have only rarely been associated with adverse effects in pregnancy. Many of their drawbacks during pregnancy are theoretical. Fetal glucose-6-phosphate dehydrogenase and glutathione concentrations are low and therefore administration of sulphonamides could theoretically lead to fetal haemolysis. Also, sulphonamides compete with bilirubin for albumin binding sites so sulphonamides, particularly those with a long half-life, should be avoided in the last trimester as they may induce hyperbilirubinaemia and kernicterus.[2] Adverse reactions to sulphonamides are relatively common compared to other antimicrobials. It is usually unnecessary to prescribe sulphonamides during pregnancy as a penicillin or cephalosporin can almost always be used instead.

Trimethoprim

Trimethoprim, which is a bacterial dihydrofolate reductase inhibitor and therefore also interferes with folate synthesis, should be avoided during pregnancy, especially in the first trimester. The safety of trimethoprim during pregnancy has not been well documented especially as it is often given in combination with sulphamethoxazole (as co-trimoxazole).[25] Co-trimoxazole has been reported to cause cleft-palates in rats and megaloblastic anaemia.[26] However, trimethoprim alone has been used in a number of studies during pregnancy without adverse effect.[27-29]

Glycopeptides

The glycopeptides, and vancomycin in particular, are the mainstay of treatment of serious infections caused by coagulase negative staphylococcal infections as these organisms are commonly resistant to beta-lactam antibiotics. These antibiotics act by inhibiting cell wall synthesis but act on a different target from the beta-lactams. They are active exclusively against gram-positive bacteria. Their main adverse effects are renal toxicity and ototoxicity and serum concentrations (especially the trough concentration) should be strictly monitored.[30] Vancomycin is excreted in the urine so increased clearance during pregnancy may lead to a dosage requirement considerably higher than normal: one report describes a woman who required a dose of 1·25 g three times daily to achieve a peak serum concentration of 25·8 µg/ml and a trough concentration of 11·6 µg/ml.[31] Vancomycin should be given slowly by infusion over 100 minutes as described by the manufacturer to avoid "the red-man" syndrome. One reported case highlights the dangers of rapid administration: a pregnant woman in labour received a dose of vancomycin over a three minute period which precipitated hypotension in the mother and an episode of fetal bradycardia.[32]

No teratogenic effects of vancomycin have been reported. Animal models, whilst demonstrating the nephrotoxic potential of vancomycin at high doses, have not shown any teratogenic effects either.[33] There are few data on whether administration of vancomycin during pregnancy causes nephrotoxicity or ototoxicity but the available reports suggest that it does not. There are several case reports of single subjects who have received vancomycin with no ill effects in their infants.[31,32,34] Also, a more rigorous study of 10 women who received vancomycin during the second and third trimester showed no evidence of nephrotoxicity or ototoxicity, as assessed by auditory evoked responses, in the infants.[35]

Rifampicin

Rifampicin, which is an inhibitor of bacterial RNA polymerase, undoubtedly causes unwanted effects in the fetus. It is however a potentially useful antibiotic in difficult cardiac infections as it kills rapidly, penetrates tissues well and is usually active against staphylococci and streptococci. It should however not be given alone as spontaneous mutations which lead to bacterial resistance are common. Rifampicin is also active against *Mycobacterium tuberculosis* and the cases describing the use of this antibiotic in pregnancy are exclusively when it was used for the treatment of tuberculosis. This complicates the evaluation of the toxicity of rifampicin as tuberculosis itself may be deleterious to the fetus and other drugs given concomitantly are also known to have adverse effects on the fetus. However, animal studies in which the drug could be given alone suggested that rifampicin is teratogenic. Pregnant rats given 15 times the normal dosage gave birth to pups with malformations which were usually neurological in nature.[36] Rabbits receiving 20 times the normal dose were unaffected but mice receiving a similar dose produced litters with a 19% malformation rate.[36] There is no definitive evidence confirming or refuting teratogenicity in humans.[36,37] In addition to the possible teratogenic effects, rifampicin can induce hypoprothombinaemia and haemorrhage presumably by interfering with fetal hepatic metabolism: of 229 pregnant women receiving anti-tuberculous therapy including rifampicin, 10 delivered infants with haemorrhagic tendencies.[36,37]

Anti-fungal agents

As cardiac fungal infections are rare there is little experience with any anti-fungal agent in pregnancy. In 21 published cases amphotericin B was no more toxic than in non-pregnant patients and no teratogenic or other fetal abnormalities were noted.[38] Flucytosine is known to be teratogenic and is therefore contraindicated in pregnancy.[39] Fluconazole and the newer imidazoles have proven useful for treating systemic candidaemias but there is virtually no evidence regarding safety during pregnancy. There is one reported case of congenital malformations following administration of fluconazole during pregnancy.[40]

Conclusions

Beta-lactam antibiotics should remain the first choice for treating all cardiac infections in pregnancy where possible. In the case of penicillin or amoxycillin allergy, cephalosporins are worth trying before prescribing other agents. A good history should be obtained. Combination therapy is often required when treating endocarditis and an aminoglycoside such as gentamicin is the best choice in combination with a beta-lactam agent. More resistant gram-positive organisms such as coagulase negative staphylococci and some enterococci should be treated with vancomycin. However, the penetration of vancomycin into vegetations is poor, it has no postantibiotic effect and it often has prolonged kill curves, so a second agent should be considered. All other agents are potentially harmful to the fetus so the possibility of increased efficacy should be balanced against the possible harmful effects. Secondary agents to consider include rifampicin, clindamycin, sulphonamides and trimethoprim. Resistant gram-negative organisms should be treated with a fluoroquinolone such as ciprofloxacin only if there is no suitable beta-lactam drug. Fungal infections should be treated with amphotericin B.

Prophylaxis for endocarditis, when required, should be restricted to amoxycillin if possible. It is justifiable to use single doses of vancomycin and aminoglycosides if necessary.

References

1 Friese K. Antibiotic therapy in pregnancy. *Immun Infekt* 1993; **21**: 111–14.
2 Chow AW, Jewesson PJ. Pharmacokinetics and safety of antimicrobial agents during pregnancy. *Reviews of Infectious Diseases* 1985; 7: 287–313.
3 Krauer B, Krauer F. Drug kinetics in pregnancy. *Clin Pharmacokinet* 1977; **2**: 167–81.
4 Mendenhall NW. Serum protein concentrations in pregnancy. I. Concentrations in maternal serum. *Am J Obstet Gynecol* 1970; **106**: 388–99.
5 Stratton CW. *In vitro* testing: correlations between bacterial susceptibility, body fluid levels and effectiveness of antibacterial therapy. In: Lorain V, ed. *Antibiotics in laboratory medicine.* Baltimore: Williams & Wilkins, 1991: 849–79.
6 Caldwell JR, Cluff L. Adverse reactions to antimicrobial agents. *JAMA* 1974; **230**: 77–80.
7 Whalley JP, Adams RH, Combes B. Tetracycline toxicity in pregnancy. *JAMA* 1964; **189**: 357–62.
8 McCormack WM, George H, Donnar A, *et al.* Hepatotoxicity of erythromycin estolate during pregnancy. *Antimicrob Agents Chemother* 1977; **12**: 630–5.
9 Landers DV, Green JR, Sweet RL. Antibiotic use during pregnancy and the postpartum period. *Clin Obstet Gynecol* 1983; **26**: 391–406.
10 Schwarz RH. Consideration of antibiotic therapy during pregnancy. *Obstet Gynecol* 1981; **58**: 95S–9S.
11 Carbon C, Cremieux AC, Fantin B. Pharmacokinetic and pharmacodynamic aspects of therapy of experimental endocarditis. *Infect Dis Clin North Am* 1993; 7: 37–51.

12 Ledger WJ. Antibiotics in pregnancy. *Clin Obstet Gynecol* 1977; **20**: 411–21.

13 Pedler SJ, Bint AJ. Comparative study of amoxicillin-clavulanic acid and cephalexin in the treatment of bacteriuria during pregnancy. *Antimicrob Agents Chemother* 1985; **27**: 508–10.

14 Wendel GD Jr, Stark BJ, Jamison RB, Molina RD, Sullivan TJ. Penicillin allergy and desensitization in serious infections during pregnancy. *N Engl J Med* 1985; **312**: 1229–32.

15 Bourget P, Fernandez H, Delouis C, Taburet AM. Pharmacokinetics of tobramycin in pregnant women. Safety and efficacy of a once-daily dose regimen. *J Clin Pharm Ther* 1991; **16**: 167–76.

16 Robinson GC, Cambon KG. Hearing loss in infants of tuberculous mothers treated with streptomycin during pregnancy. *N Engl J Med* 1964; **271**: 949–51.

17 Wang Z, Liou L. Auditory effect of kanamycin given to newborn guinea pigs whose mothers received kanamycin during pregnancy. *Ann Otol Rhinol Laryngol* 1994; **103**: 983–5.

18 MacGowan AP, Bedford KA, Blundell E, *et al.* The pharmacokinetics of once daily gentamicin in neutropenic adults with haematological malignancy. *J Antimicrob Chemother* 1994; **34**: 809–12.

19 Saleh Mghir A, Cremieux AC, Vallois JM, Muffat Joly M, Devine C, Carbon C. Optimal aminoglycoside dosing regimen for penicillin-tobramycin synergism in experimental streptococcus adjacens endocarditis. *Antimicrob Agents Chemother* 1992; **36**: 2403–7.

20 Fantin B, Carbon C. Importance of the aminoglycoside dosing regimen in the penicillin-netilmicin combination for treatment of enterococcus faecalis-induced experimental endocarditis. *Antimicrob Agents Chemother* 1990; **34**: 2387–91.

21 Berkovitch M, Pastuszak A, Gazarian M, Lewis M, Koren G. Safety of the new quinolones in pregnancy. *Obstet Gynecol* 1994; **84**: 535–8.

22 Hummler H, Richter WF, Hendrickx AG. Developmental toxicity of fleroxacin and comparative pharmacokinetics of four fluoroquinolones in the cynomolgus macaque (Macaca fascicularis). *Toxicol Appl Pharmacol* 1993; **122**: 34–45.

23 Keller H. Comparison of the adverse effect profile of different substances such as penicillins, tetracyclines, sulfonamides and quinolones. *Infection* 1991; **19 (suppl 1)**: S19–24.

24 Philipson A, Sabath LD, Charles D. Erythromycin and clindamycin absorption and elimination in pregnant women. *Clin Pharmacol Ther* 1976; **19**: 68–77.

25 Gleckman R, Blagg N, Joubert DW. Trimethoprim: mechanisms of action, antimicrobial activity, bacterial resistance, pharmacokinetics, adverse reactions, and therapeutic indications. *Pharmacotherapy* 1981; **1**: 14–20.

26 Lawson DH, Paice BJ. Adverse reactions to trimethoprim-sulfamethoxazole. *Reviews of Infectious Diseases* 1982; **4**: 429–33.

27 Cruikshank DP, Warenski JC. First-trimester maternal listeria monocytogenes sepsis and chorioamnionitis with normal neonatal outcome. *Obstet Gynecol* 1989; **73**: 469–71.

28 Soper DE, Merrill Nach S. Successful therapy of penicillinase-producing neisseria gonorrhoeae pharyngeal infection during pregnancy. *Obstet Gynecol* 1986; **68**: 290–1.

29 Bailey RR, Peddie BA, Bishop V. Comparison of single dose with a five-day course of trimethoprim for asymptomatic (covert) bacteriuria of pregnancy. *NZ Med J* 1986; **99**: 501–3.

30 Saunders NJ. Why monitor peak vancomycin concentrations? *Lancet* 1994; **344**: 1748–50.

31 Salzman C, Weingold AB, Simon GL. Increased dose requirements of vancomycin in a pregnant patient with endocarditis. *J Infect Dis* 1987; **156**: 409.

32 Hill LM. Fetal distress secondary to vancomycin-induced maternal hypotension. *Am J Obstet Gynecol* 1985; **153**: 74–5.

33 Byrd RA, Gries CL, Buening MK. Developmental toxicology studies of vancomycin hydrochloride administered intravenously to rats and rabbits. *Fundam Appl Toxicol* 1994; **23**: 590–7.

34 MacCulloch D. Vancomycin in pregnancy. *N Z Med J* 1981; **93**: 93–4.

35 Reyes MP, Ostrea EM, Jr, Cabinian AE, Schmitt C, Rintelmann W. Vancomycin during pregnancy: does it cause hearing loss or nephrotoxicity in the infant? *Am J Obstet Gynecol* 1989; **161**: 977–81.

36 Steen JS, Stainton Ellis DM. Rifampicin in pregnancy. *Lancet* 1977; **ii**: 604–5.

37 Snider DE Jr, Layde PM, Johnson MW, Lyle MA. Treatment of tuberculosis during pregnancy. *Am Rev Respir Dis* 1980; **122**: 65–79.

38 Ismail MA, Lerner SA. Disseminated blastomycosis in a pregnant woman – review of amphotericin B usage during pregnancy. *Am Rev Respir Dis* 1982; **126**: 350–3.

39 Bennett JE. Flucytosine. *Ann Intern Med* 1977; **86**: 319–22.

40 Lee BE, Feinberg M, Abraham JJ, Murthy AR. Congenital malformations in an infant born to a woman treated with fluconazole. *Pediatr Infect Dis J* 1992; **11**: 1062–4.

26: Management of labour and delivery in the high risk patient

CELIA OAKLEY

In patients with few or no symptoms of cardiovascular disease and who can call upon cardiovascular reserve the conduct of labour and delivery does not differ from that which is dictated by obstetric indications. High risk patients are those who are unable to increase cardiac output, have coarctation or aortic wall disease, congenital heart disease with right to left shunts, pulmonary hypertension, raised left atrial pressures, or left ventricular outflow tract obstruction.

Normal labour involves intermittent surges in cardiac output and blood pressure which may be potentially dangerous for patients at risk of aortic dissection due to coarctation, the Marfan or Ehlers–Danlos syndrome, or Takayasu aortitis. Elective caesarean section under epidural anaesthesia is preferable for many such patients to prevent swings in blood pressure and always if there is obstetric concern that labour may be prolonged. If normal delivery is chosen the second stage should be expedited and beta-adrenergic blockade should be continued throughout labour to minimise stress on the aortic wall. These drugs do not alter the duration of labour and propranolol has been used therapeutically in dysfunctional labour.[1]

Patients with a raised left atrial pressure are at risk of a further rise in pressure during the physical stresses of labour and particularly in the third stage when 500 ml or more of blood from the uterus and placenta may be returned into the circulation if there is little blood loss. In such patients frusemide 20 mg or 40 mg should be given intravenously at the start of labour and the patient should be sat up immediately after delivery. Oxytocic agents should be given as indicated to avoid uncontrolled blood loss in the third stage. Syntocinon is not a vasoconstrictor so minimises the increase in venous return to the thorax and therefore any rise in left atrial pressure. Swan–Ganz monitoring of pulmonary artery and wedged pulmonary capillary pressures is only occasionally needed. If there is real concern, planned caesarean section is preferable, to avoid maternal physical stress and expedite delivery. Patients with mitral stenosis or hypertrophic cardiomyopathy should continue beta-adrenergic blocking treatment to avoid tachycardia. In mitral stenosis the left atrial pressure is directly related to heart rate and in hypertrophic cardiomyopathy coronary flow and left ventricular filling both require optimal diastolic time.

Patients with cyanotic or potentially cyanotic congenital heart disease increase right to left shunting during normal labour which if chosen should be expedited to avoid prolonged fetal hypoxaemia. Vaginal delivery may be suitable for patients with only potential or mild cyanosis in tetralogy of Fallot or Ebstein's anomaly. Patients with more serious arterial desaturation nearly always deliver prematurely and planned caesarean section is safest to avoid physical stress with consequent increase in maternal and fetal hypoxaemia.

Although patients with cyanotic congenital heart disease have a paradoxical increase in the risk of both thrombosis and of bleeding the haemorrhagic risk is to some extent obviated during pregnancy. This is because the hazard is caused by a reduced circulating plasma volume with reduction in available plasma clotting factors as well as abnormal platelet behaviour. In pregnancy the plasma volume expands despite increase in packed cell volume caused by greater right to left shunting, and platelet activity increases. Low dose heparin reduces the heightened thrombo-embolic risk which cyanosed patients face because of their relative immobility while in hospital despite encouragement of postural manoeuvres to avoid caval compression and the use of anti-embolism stockings. Inhaled oxygen with maximal delivery through nasal cannulae improves oximetry readings which should be recorded both at rest and after walking.

Women with Eisenmenger syndrome are at high risk (Chapter 6) and should not undergo normal labour which increases the risks to a premature and dysmature fetus as well as to the mother. Fetal growth needs meticulous monitoring. Caesarean section should be planned and performed as soon as fetal growth slows or stops and every effort should be made to maintain a stable maternal cardiovascular state with maximal oxygenation and generous hydration during and after operation. Our experience has been that abdominal delivery under general anaesthesia secures the least cardio-vascular stress and metabolic need, minimises right to left shunting by removing physical effort and maintains best possible fetal condition before and during delivery.[2] These patients tolerate general anaesthesia well and do not present the risks that have been suggested on theoretical grounds.[3]

Low dose heparin should be given up to the time of delivery and re-started postpartum. The patient should be returned to intensive care where close observation and oximetry can be continued. Mobilisation should be slow and heparin maintained until the patient leaves the hospital which should be at least ten days after delivery because risk persists for some time postpartum.

In a recent report 13 pregnancies in 12 women with Eisenmenger syndrome were associated with three maternal deaths (23%), two during gestation and one postpartum.[3] This is the largest personal series published and the relatively good outcome was attributed to bed rest after the second trimester, oxygen therapy, heparin prophylaxis, and planned caesarean section under general anaesthesia. Seven pregnancies were successful. One of the babies had a ventricular septal defect.

The same policy has been our practice at Hammersmith both for women with the Eisenmenger syndrome and those with primary pulmonary hypertension. None of our patients has died during pregnancy or parturition. All the babies born to the women with the Eisenmenger syndrome were both premature and small for dates but all the babies who reached at least 31 weeks' gestation survived. The maternal deaths all occurred some days after delivery and not in direct relation to it. As in the review by Gleicher et al,[4] the highest mortality was amongst women with the Eisenmenger complex (ventricular septal defect) but in contrast to that paper necropsy showed no cause for the deaths and none of our patients died from thromboembolism or heart failure. A recent patient with the Eisenmenger complex monitored in hospital showed progressive bradycardia with a simultaneous fall in arterial saturation on oximetry, followed by cardiac arrest. Others who had been observed seemed to die in the same way with a "vaso-vagal" attack associated with systemic vasodepression, maintenance or a rise in the high pulmonary vascular resistance and consequent preferential ejection from the right ventricle directly into the aorta, bypassing the lungs. Resuscitation was unsuccessful in each case. Patients with Eisenmenger syndrome associated with patent ductus or atrial septal defect did better as did four patients with pulmonary hypertension without congenital septal defects, all of whom survived. A fifth patient who had had a ventricular septal defect closed at age six developed falling arterial saturation and cardiac output after uncomplicated caesarean delivery and died on day five. This was apparently the result of a progressive shut down in the pulmonary microvasculature which was totally resistant to oxygen, nitric oxide, and prostacycline.

Epidural analgesia and anaesthesia are popular with obstetric anaesthetists. Vasodilatation is minimal with epidural analgesia for normal delivery and is anyway well tolerated by patients able to increase their stroke volume and benefits patients with regurgitant valve disease or left to right shunts. Regurgitant volume and left atrial pressure are minimised in patients with mitral or aortic regurgitation and left to right shunting is reduced in atrial septal defect. Regional anaesthesia is also suitable for patients with aortic wall disease.

Epidural anaesthesia for caesarean section is less advisable in patients with limited stroke volume or congenital heart disease with right to left shunts. Patients with primary type pulmonary hypertension in whom right ventricular output cannot be increased are at risk from hypotension and patients with the Eisenmenger syndrome may have profound increase in hypoxaemia. Patients with aortic or mitral stenosis may not be able to increase stroke volume if the stenosis is severe and are at risk from a fall in blood pressure though potentially benefitted by redistribution of blood volume away from the thorax which keeps the left atrial pressure down.

Patients with hypertrophic cardiomyopathy need a sufficient left ventricular filling pressure to maintain stroke volume because of the diastolic fault and severe cases are at risk of developing pulmonary congestion or oedema. Vasodilatation on the other hand may result in cardiogenic shock by reducing venous return, lowering left atrial pressure, and critically reducing left ventricular volume. Severely compromised patients may be best managed if pulmonary artery and wedge pressures are monitored by a Swan–Ganz catheter. Beta-blockade should be maintained to avoid tachycardia.

Epidural anaesthesia for caesarean section is associated with unpredictable hypotension reported in 25% to 45% even of normal subjects and caused by a fall in cardiac output as a result of a reduction in venous return, although this can be counteracted by preliminary infusion of Ringer-lactate solution.[5] The technique also has the disadvantages of a conscious and therefore apprehensive patient. Even with fluid loading the opiate infusion usually given for sedation causes further venous dilatation and further reduction in venous return to the thorax. This, coupled with systemic arterial vasodilatation, can lead to loss of blood pressure in cardiac patients with limited stroke output which can only be regained by further volume replacement. The use of vasoconstrictors such as ephedrine to regain lost blood pressure causes tachycardia. Fragile patients are rendered vulnerable to any sudden blood loss as may occur during operative delivery and there is the added problem of more restricted surgical access in a conscious patient without muscle relaxation. Although the technique is well tolerated in normal subjects this may not be the case in patients with heart disease when cardiac output is relatively fixed as in mitral stenosis or pulmonary hypertension.[5]

Caesarean section in cardiac patients has usually been restricted to obstetric indications but surgical delivery is preferable in patients with marginal cardiovascular reserve to avoid the physical stress of labour. General anaesthesia minimises maternal metabolic need, providing complete rest with optimal oxygenation. Blood pressure, heart rate, volaemia, and the distribution of blood volume can be controlled. It allows patients who are taking warfarin to be delivered expeditiously without transfer to heparin two weeks earlier and with the minimal period unprotected by effective anticoagulation (Chapter 10). Moreover, surgical delivery is the safest method of delivery for the children of mothers whose heart disease is likely to get worse rather than better and for whom the current pregnancy may be the only one.

The postpartum period is a time of high risk. Patients with potentially high left atrial pressure should be sat up as soon as possible after delivery. The circulatory changes of pregnancy decline rapidly during the first postpartum week but may take up to four weeks to resolve completely particularly in patients who have had minimal blood loss. Pulmonary congestion or sudden pulmonary oedema remains a risk in the puerperium and diuretic treatment may be needed.

Antibiotic prophylaxis should be given to susceptible patients to cover prolonged or surgical deliveries but is discretionary for normal deliveries. It will be chosen for patients with prosthetic valves or previous endocarditis (Chapter 11).

References

1 Mitrani A, Oettinger M, Abinader EG. Use of propranolol in dysfunctional labour. *Br J Obstet Gynaecol* 1975; **82**: 651–5.
2 Lumley J, Whitwam JG, Morgan M. General anaesthesia in the presence of Eisenmenger's syndrome. *Journal of Anaesthesia and Analgesia Current Researches* 1977; **56**: 543–7.
3 Avila WS, Grinberg M, Snitcowsky R, *et al.* Maternal and fetal outcome in pregnant women with Eisenmenger's syndrome. *Eur Heart J* 1995; **16**: 460–4.
4 Gleicher N, Midwall J, Hochberger D, Jaffin H. Eisenmenger syndrome in pregnancy. *Obstet Gynecol Surv* 1979; **34**: 721–41.
5 Robson S, Hunter S, Boys R, Dunlop W, Bryson M. Changes in cardiac output during epidural anaesthesia for caesarian section. *Anaesthesia* 1989; **44**: 475–9.

27: Anaesthesia for the pregnant cardiac patient

DAVID ZIDEMAN, JULIE WATTS

Cardiovascular disease is a major cause of maternal morbidity and mortality although it occurs in only 2% of the obstetric population.[1] It is the third most common cause of maternal death in the UK after thromboembolism and hypertensive disorders.[2]

Improved medical and surgical care and the increasing age of the obstetric population has changed the incidence and type of heart disease encountered in pregnant women. Increasing numbers of women with fully or partly corrected congenital heart disease are surviving to reproductive life. Congenital heart disease accounted for half the maternal deaths from cardiac disease during the years 1988–1990. Ischemic heart disease is becoming more common as a result of the increasing age of conception and smoking habits. There are also women who have undergone previous cardiac transplantation and are now surviving to go through a successful pregnancy.

This population is unique as administration of anaesthesia demands simultaneous care of the mother and the fetus, whose needs may conflict. The anaesthetist may become involved with several medical management problems in pregnant women with cardiac disease.

- Analgesia and anaesthesia for labour and delivery.
- Anaesthesia for caesarean section as an elective or emergency procedure.
- Anaesthesia of pregnant women for non-cardiac surgery
  Termination of pregnancy
  Incidental surgery such as appendicectomy and cholecystectomy
- Anaesthesia for cardiac surgery
  a. Minor, such as DC cardioversion and insertion of pacemaker
  b. Major, including valve replacement and coronary artery bypass grafting
- Postoperative analgesia
- Peripartum care and monitoring of critically ill obstetric patients with coincidental cardiovascular disease

Cardiovascular physiology in pregnancy and labour

The physiological changes of pregnancy place considerable demands on the normal heart and peripheral circulation. The changes become apparent from early in the first trimester and persist into the puerperium. Consideration of pregnant women with cardiovascular disease presents problems in detection of deterioration and prediction of cardiac reserve.

Resting cardiac output and intravascular volume increase by 50% by the 20th week of pregnancy. A fall in systemic and pulmonary vascular resistance is mediated by hormonally induced vasodilatation and the creation of a low resistance circulation in the uteroplacental unit. During the latter half of pregnancy aortocaval compression occurs by the large intra-abdominal uterus, and the cardiac output is increasingly affected by maternal position as a result of changes in venous return.[3] Cardiac output is the product of heart rate and stroke volume and therefore changes in either may have profound physiological effects. The resting heart rate increases by up to 20 beats/min throughout pregnancy and stroke volume also increases by 20%–25% but is dependent on the maintenance of venous return to the heart.

During labour and delivery there are further substantial changes in cardiovascular function. As labour begins, the cardiac output increases as a result of tachycardia secondary to pain and increased circulating catecholamines, so that at cervical dilatation of 8 cm catecholamine concentrations are 12% to 15% above pre-labour values.[4,5] Uterine contractions may increase cardiac output by a further 10% to 25% from the extrusion of about 500 ml into the circulation with each contraction. So with each contraction, there may be a total increase in cardiac output of 20% to 40%.[6,7] During the second stage of labour the cardiac output may be 45% to 50% above pre-labour values.

Following vaginal delivery cardiac output can increase by as much as 80% over pre-labour values as a result of autotransfusion from the placenta and relief of inferior vena cava compression. By one hour after delivery cardiac output has returned to pre-labour values.[4] This is a time of greatly increased risk in women with cardiac disease. The increase in cardiac output is reduced by approximately 50% following caesarean section whether under epidural or general anaesthesia.

Anaesthetic considerations

Pregnant women who have cardiovascular disease should be evaluated early in pregnancy by a multidisciplinary medical team. High risk patients must be identified by obstetricians, cardiologists, and anaesthetists. Anaesthetists need an understanding of the type, severity, and progression of their cardiac disease in the context of the normal adaptations to pregnancy. The overall aim must be the safe delivery of a baby with minimal deterioration in the mother's condition.

There should be continual evaluation and frequent, honest, and sympathetic discussion with the patient and her partner. An agreed plan for the management of labour and delivery should be written in the mother's notes. The general trend is for a carefully monitored pregnancy and a planned induction of labour.[8] Optimal analgesia should be maintained throughout labour and delivery. The management of the second stage of labour is influenced by the degree of cardiac impairment, but assisted vaginal delivery with minimal maternal effort is sensible. Caesarean section is indicated for obstetric reasons or acute deterioration in the mother's condition. The clinical management depends on the indication and urgency for delivery. One advantage of a planned induction is, for example, the manipulation of anticoagulant drugs to allow clotting variables to approach normal values and so allow regional anaesthesia.

Many problems are those shared with pregnant women without heart disease.[9] Surgery and anaesthesia in the first trimester should be avoided if possible because of increased rates of spontaneous abortion and potential teratogenic effects of anaesthetic agents. In general, drugs used in general anaesthesia are lipid soluble and readily cross the placenta. Human data are lacking to ensure the safety of these agents in early pregnancy. However, large retrospective studies including nearly 8000 women who underwent surgery during gestation failed to show any increased incidence of congenital malformations.[10,11] There is no evidence that any specific anaesthetic technique including the use of nitrous oxide is contraindicated if surgery is necessary during the first 16 weeks of gestation. Propofol is not licensed for use in pregnancy although teratology studies in animals showed no teratogenic effects.

After 20 weeks' gestation there is increased risk of problems associated with the aspiration of gastric contents. It is therefore recommended that routine antacid prophylaxis such as ranitidine 50 mg orally eight hourly should be taken, with clear fluids only throughout labour.

To maintain optimal venous return and cardiac output labouring women should be nursed in the full left lateral position and receive supplementary oxygen. Nevertheless many mothers to be who have cardiac disease may prefer to find their own position which is most comfortable to them without compromising the baby.

Cardiovascular monitoring

The extent of monitoring during labour and the resultant clinical intervention depends on the degree of impaired cardiac function. Women with high risk cardiac disease should be nursed in high dependency areas. Staff must be familiar with invasive monitoring techniques and be able to interpret and respond rapidly, accurately, and appropriately to changes. It is important to continue cardiovascular monitoring and treatment in women with severe cardiac impairment into the puerperium as this is the time when many maternal deaths occur. This period extends for three to five days after delivery.

All women in labour should have adequate intravenous access established with two large bore (14G or 16G) peripheral cannulas. Cardiotocography to assess uterine tone and fetal well being is routine.

Other monitoring for women with cardiac disease should include continuous electrocardiographic monitoring using leads II and V_5. This facilitates the detection of arrhythmias and myocardial ischaemia and allows prompt intervention. Pulse oximetry is useful especially in women with cyanotic congenital heart disease. A fall in oxygen saturation gives an early indication of reduction of pulmonary blood flow and changes in flows through intracardiac shunts.

For women with more severe cardiac disease direct intravascular pressure recording may be necessary for their optimal management. The risk:benefit ratio of such invasive techniques must be assessed for each woman.[12] Intra-arterial cannulae allow direct and continuous monitoring of arterial blood pressure and allows for multiple sampling of blood for measurement of arterial blood gases and acid base status. Central venous catheters allow direct right atrial pressure monitoring and venous access for infusion of fluids or vasoactive drugs. This may be the technique of choice in patients with less severe myocardial dysfunction where left ventricular filling is reflected by right sided pressure changes and also for patients with congenital heart disease and intracardiac shunts, particularly those with right to left shunts associated with pulmonary hypertension.

The use of pulmonary artery catheters in pregnant women with cardiac disease is controversial and is much less common in the United Kingdom than in North American practice.[12,13]

The pulmonary artery catheter allows measurement of pulmonary artery pressures and pulmonary wedge pressures which reflect left atrial pressure and thus left ventricular filling pressure. This may be specifically helpful in patients with left ventricular dysfunction from cardiomyopathy or following myocardial infarction. They may also be indicated when the maintenance of left ventricular filling is critical to cardiac output, as in mitral or aortic stenosis and hypertrophic obstructive cardiomyopathy. There may be problems with arrhythmias on insertion and, in patients with intracardiac shunts, they may provide limited information with unacceptable risks. There has been a death reported during removal of a pulmonary artery catheter in a patient with the Eisenmenger syndrome four days after delivery, which was thought to be the result of dislodging a thrombosis into the coronary or cerebral circulation.[14] In patients with the Eisenmenger syndrome and ventricular septal or aorto-pulmonary defects pressure is in any case immutably linked to the systemic pressure so such catheterisation provides no useful information.

With all intravascular catheters meticulous care should be taken to avoid introduction of air or debris into the circulation. There is a risk of paradoxical embolism through established intracardiac shunts or even during transient opening of a patent foramen ovale during Valsalva manoeuvres in labour. Catheters must be removed as soon as possible or when they are no longer providing useful information, thus reducing the risk of thrombosis or infection.

Finally the elective use of echocardiography and other such non-invasive techniques allows the accurate assessment of myocardial function during pregnancy and labour. The examination should be made by a single experienced operator who can recognise any change in myocardial functional impairment in relation to previous examinations.

Anaesthetic management of labour and delivery

The management of any woman with cardiac disease must depend on the specific disease involved, but general principles can be followed. Many of the anaesthetic publications in this field are based on anecdotal case reports and small uncontrolled series.

The potentially adverse haemodynamic changes during labour can be considerably influenced by the form of analgesia administered. Effective analgesia following an epidural block decreases pain and apprehension and can eliminate the associated changes in heart rate and blood pressure. It can attenuate the progressive rise in cardiac output throughout labour.[6,7] Minimal cardiovascular changes occur if there is careful attention to fluid preloading, positioning patients in the full lateral position and careful incremental epidural dosage. A sensory block to T10 level is required for adequate analgesia during the first stage of labour. In general, low concentrations of local anaesthetics combined with opiates administered by the epidural route provide good analgesia and minimal sympathetic blockade.[8] For example bupivacaine 0·25% without adrenaline in 2 to 3 ml increments plus fentanyl 50 µg may be used. During labour the use of epidural infusions of bupivacaine 0·0625 to 0·1% combined with fentanyl 2 µg/ml at infusion rates of 8 to 12 ml/hr will maintain good analgesia without the risk of sudden cardiovascular changes which can occur during epidural top ups using bolus drug administration techniques.

The reduction in sympathetic blockade may be particularly beneficial in patients with intracardiac shunts or some degree of left ventricular outflow obstruction, in whom sudden falls in systemic vascular resistance may produce catastrophic changes in blood pressure or cardiac output.

If hypotension does occur then vasopressors may be used cautiously after an assessment of the adequacy of fluid replacement. Ephedrine is usually the first line vasopressor in obstetric practice. In animal studies it maintained uteroplacental blood flow better than other vasopressors.[15] It has mixed alpha- and beta-adrenergic agonist effects and may produce unacceptable tachycardia. The clinical use of pure alpha-adrenergic agonists, like methoxamine or phenylephrine to treat hypotension resulting from epidural anaesthesia have failed to show any deleterious effects to the baby.[16,17]

Their lack of chronotropic activity may make them useful in obstetric patients with pre-existing cardiac disease.

The management of the second stage of labour depends on the degree of cardiac impairment and fetal well being. Assisted vaginal delivery of the fetus reduces myocardial work, oxygen consumption, and the rise in cardiac output.

Epidural analgesia does not alleviate the peak postpartum rise in cardiac output which is still a period of high risk in this group of patients. If oxytocics are required then an infusion of oxytocin is recommended to avoid the cardiovascular changes associated with bolus dosing, which include peripheral vasodilatation and hypotension, together with reflex tachycardia.[18] Bolus doses of oxytocin have also been associated with acute pulmonary hypertension.[19]

For patients who refuse or in whom epidural analgesia is contraindicated, the pain of labour can be managed by intravenous opiates with a patient-controlled analgesia device. A pudendal block or perineal infiltration is necessary for assisted vaginal delivery.

Anaesthetic management of caesarean section

In general, no one anaesthetic technique is exclusively indicated or contraindicated.[8] The anaesthetic management depends on the indication and urgency for delivery and the pathophysiology of the maternal cardio-vascular disease.

For elective or semi-urgent caesarean section there is almost always time to establish an adequate epidural block to the level of the T4 dermatome with careful incremental epidural dosing, meticulous management of fluids and posture, and close monitoring of the woman's cardiovascular variables.

In patients with less severe cardiac disease and good ventricular function who require emergency caesarean section spinal anaesthesia may be a suitable alternative despite the rapid onset of block, provided that postural hypotension is avoided.

The use of general anaesthesia presents the problem of hypertension and tachycardia on induction and emergence, and sudden changes in cardiac output. A technique using high dose opiates and low concentration of volatile agents can alleviate haemodynamic changes and minimise myocardial depression. It may increase the risk of maternal aspiration and neonatal respiratory depression.

The most difficult patients are those with an obstructed left ventricular outflow, such as aortic stenosis and hypertrophic obstructive cardio-myopathy, and those with cyanotic congenital heart disease with a right to left intracardiac shunt. Both groups are at risk of acute decompensation if they undergo a sudden and significant decrease in their systemic vascular resistance. Both epidural and general anaesthesia may cause these changes, and both have been used successfully with extreme caution, meticulous monitoring, and careful management by an experienced team.

Specific cardiovascular diseases

Aortic valve disease

Significant aortic stenosis has traditionally been considered a contraindication to pregnancy the quoted maternal mortality being 17%.[20]

Aortic stenosis leads to left ventricular hypertrophy. Stroke volume is fixed and the cardiac output is heart rate dependent. Diastolic blood pressure must be maintained to allow coronary perfusion to the non-compliant hypertrophied left ventricle with high left ventricular end diastolic pressures. Left ventricular filling is severely compromised by tachycardia, arrhythmias, and reduced venous return.

It is the conventional view that epidural analgesia or anaesthesia is contraindicated in these patients as a fall in systemic vascular resistance may produce severe hypotension, myocardial ischaemia and compromise, and reduction in cardiac output which is irreversible.[8,21]

Epidural anaesthesia has been used successfully for both labour and caesarean section.[22-25] Two case reports support the use of epidurals with careful incremental dosing with local anaesthetics and opiates with an effective block established over 30–40 minutes for caesarean section.[24,25] Invasive monitoring was used to ensure meticulous fluid management and maintenance of adequate left ventricular end diastolic filling.

A recent paper retrospectively reviewed 13 Canadian patients with congenital aortic stenosis who had 25 pregnancies with a generally satisfactory outcome.[22] All were functionally New York Heart Association class I or II before pregnancy. Three had severe stenosis and only four had substantial functional deterioration during pregnancy. Five pregnancies were terminated. Of the 20 pregnancies that went to term, 14 had spontaneous or assisted vaginal deliveries and six caesarean sections. All the caesarean sections were performed under epidural anaesthesia, and all women were offered epidural analgesia for labour. There were apparently no complications although the authors gave no details of the anaesthetic management. There were no maternal deaths.

If general anaesthesia is required for caesarean section then alfentanil in high dose (35 µg/kg) has been used to minimise the haemodynamic response to intubation and surgery in a patient with severe aortic stenosis.[26]

Theoretically epidural analgesia in the presence of aortic incompetence may be beneficial as it causes a reduction in regurgitation flow as a result of a moderate drop in blood pressure and maintenance of the heart rate. Cautious incremental dosing of the epidural together with careful fluid management and appropriate monitoring is advised. There has been a death reported in a patient with aortic incompetence and cardiac failure who required caesarean section but whose epidural block was established with a single dose of 0·5% bupivacaine resulting in catastrophic and irreversible hypotension.[27]

Hypertrophic obstructive cardiomyopathy

Hypertrophic obstructive cardiomyopathy in its more severe forms is uncommon. Septal hypertrophy or more generalised left ventricular hypertrophy encroaches upon the left ventricular cavity and stroke volume is restricted. Any increase in myocardial contractility or reduction in left ventricular filling pressure causes further increase in the left ventricular outflow tract gradient. The noncompliant left ventricle is critically dependent on an adequate pre-load and a slow sinus rhythm to optimise ventricular filling and coronary blood flow. These patients are usually taking beta-adrenergic blockers.

Most of these patients tolerate pregnancy well despite deterioration in their symptoms, but severe disease is a strong indication for invasive vascular monitoring. A pulmonary artery catheter allows optimal fluid management and the maintenance of high left ventricular filling pressures on which their stroke output depends, but they are also highly susceptible to pulmonary oedema.[28]

Many young women with mild hypertrophic cardiomyopathy are haemodynamically robust and epidural analgesia has been used successfully for labour and vaginal delivery, using both opiates alone and in combination with local anaesthetics.[30] It is important to maintain pre-load with fluids and to avoid aortocaval compression and tachycardia. If vasopressors are required then pure alpha-adrenergic agonists are indicated. Surges in sympathetic activity during labour have been counteracted with short acting intravenous beta-adrenergic blocking drugs, such as esmolol.[29]

If caesarean section is required then epidural anaesthesia may be appropriate using a careful incremental dosing technique. General anaesthesia is usually well tolerated.[31] Halothane is the ideal volatile agent to maintain anaesthesia as it produces a decrease in myocardial contractility with minimal reduction in systemic vascular resistance.

Mitral valve disease

Worldwide, mitral valve stenosis following rheumatic fever is probably still the most common cardiac problem in pregnant women. In developed countries it is relatively rare. The stenotic valve results in a relatively fixed cardiac output and increased left atrial pressure. The left atrium enlarges and pulmonary congestion develops. Pregnancy often results in deterioration. Pulmonary oedema may be precipitated by sinus tachycardia and especially if atrial tachyarrhythmias develop.

It is important to maintain cardiac output by avoiding tachycardia to allow for effective ventricular filling and left atrial emptying. In severe disease invasive haemodynamic monitoring facilitates careful manipulation of the pre-load.[32] Epidural analgesia has been used successfully in labour to provide good analgesia and pre-load reduction but the mainstay of management is prevention of sinus tachycardia by judicious use of beta-adrenergic blockade to counteract catecholamine driven sinus tachycardia.

Prosthetic heart valves

In general the main anaesthetic problems in women with prosthetic heart valves relate to the associated use of anticoagulants and thus the timing of regional anaesthesia.[33] Assuming optimal prosthetic valve function, women with an aortic valve prosthesis usually maintain a normal cardiac output during pregnancy, whilst those with a mitral valve prosthesis still have a relatively fixed cardiac output. Any patient who has had previous valvular surgery must be considered to have some degree of cardiac impairment and be closely monitored throughout pregnancy and delivery but only a minority have greatly reduced cardiovascular reserve. Most young women with prosthetic valves are in sinus rhythm and have been in New York Heart Association class I or II before pregnancy. They tolerate the haemodynamic changes without difficulty.

Planned induction of labour allows controlled manipulation of anticoagulant therapy. Heparin should replace warfarin at 36 to 38 weeks' gestation. The short-half life of intravenous heparin allows controlled manipulation of anticoagulant therapy and its anticoagulant effects rapidly decline or may be quickly reversed by protamine. This facilitates the use of regional anaesthetic techniques for anaesthesia and analgesia.

An alternative plan is elective caesarean section at 38 weeks' gestation in a mother who has continued to take warfarin. The delivery is covered by administration of fresh frozen plasma with a return to warfarin as soon as possible postpartum. Interim cover is provided by subcutaneous heparin. This technique minimises the maternal risk of suboptimal anticoagulation and allows for the safe delivery of an anticoagulated baby who will need vitamin K after delivery. General anaesthesia is well tolerated.

Women should be warned of the risk of epidural haematoma.[34] This is a rare but devastating complication and a high index of suspicion must be maintained. Prophylactic antibiotics should be given to all mothers with prosthetic valves.

Congenital heart disease

Regardless of the structural lesion involved cyanotic heart disease is associated with a higher maternal and fetal morbidity and mortality than non-cyanotic disease.[35-37] Increasing numbers of women are presenting in pregnancy with congenital heart disease following previous palliative or corrective surgery. Patients with non-cyanotic heart disease and those with left to right intracardiac shunts generally tolerate pregnancy and delivery with minimal problems.

Patients with cyanotic heart disease with a right to left shunt have one of the following lesions:

● Fallot's tetralogy with an obstruction to pulmonary outflow. This is amenable to surgical correction which is recommended before pregnancy.

- Common mixing chambers—single ventricles usually associated with transposition of the great vessels.
- The Eisenmenger syndrome. This comprises irreversible pulmonary hypertension associated with a right to left intracardiac shunt through an atrial or ventricular septal defect or persistent ductus arteriosus. The condition is not amenable to surgery except for consideration for heart lung transplantation.

The Eisenmenger syndrome

The major hazard to the mother with the Eisenmenger syndrome during pregnancy is increased right to left shunting as the cardiac output rises and systemic vascular resistance falls, resulting in worsening hypoxaemia. Death can occur at any time during pregnancy but is most common during labour or in the postpartum period.[38–40]

Management of these cases is best undertaken in an obstetric unit which is intimately attached to a hospital with rapid availability of cardiac investigative procedures, open heart surgery, and full intensive care facilities.

These women should be admitted to hospital during the latter half of pregnancy to optimise medical management.[41,42] They are at high risk of venous thromboembolism and therefore compression stockings and subcutaneous heparin should be prescribed. Supplemental oxygen is administered to increase arterial oxygen content and fetal growth may also thereby be improved. Regular platelet counts should be done as thrombocytopenia may develop.

Generally an assisted vaginal delivery is advised.[8,39] Planned induction rather than spontaneous labour allows for adequately supervised anaesthetic involvement. Regional anaesthesia is theoretically contraindicated in these patients because of the risk of increased right to left shunting following sympathetic blockade with increasing hypoxaemia, right ventricular failure, and a fall in cardiac output. A recent review of the obstetric anaesthetic management of five women with the Eisenmenger syndrome reported the successful use of epidural analgesia with bupivacaine 0·25% with or without additional fentanyl for assisted vaginal delivery.[41] All women were monitored with pulse oximetry, ECG, and direct arterial and central venous pressures. There was one death in a woman admitted as an emergency who died shortly after caesarean section under general anaesthesia, done to save the baby. A further case was reported to show no change in shunt fraction during a caesarean section under epidural anaesthesia.[43]

Historically, maternal mortality in women who sustain a viable pregnancy to delivery is quoted as 30%. Caesarean section in a woman with the Eisenmenger syndrome has been alleged to increase maternal mortality to 50% to 70% but this was a case report with a review of other case reports.[36]

A personal series from Brazil described 13 pregnancies in 12 women with the Eisenmenger syndrome.[42] There were two early maternal deaths and four spontaneous abortions. Of the seven patients who reached the end of the second trimester, all were kept in hospital until delivery, anticoagulated, and received oxygen therapy. Caesarean section was carried out in all patients because of deterioration in the maternal or fetal condition. All the women had general anaesthetics using etomidate, suxamethonium, and fentanyl but there was no detailed discussion of the anaesthetic technique or monitoring used. All the women survived to be discharged from hospital but one died on the 30th postpartum day. The overall maternal mortality was 23%. Other groups have reported that general anaesthesia is generally well tolerated using a variety of anaesthetic techniques.[44] The Brazilian paper is the largest personal experience yet reported and therefore of greater value than case reports and literature reviews.

Close monitoring is required throughout delivery and into the puerperium. This should include pulse oximetry, electrocardiography, and direct arterial and central venous pressure monitoring. Pulse oximetry is particularly useful in assessing changes in intracardiac shunts and reduction in pulmonary blood flow.

During labour, patients should be given supplemental oxygen and nursed in the full lateral position. They are extremely sensitive to changes in intravascular volume and venous return and careful fluid balance is essential with prompt replacement of any blood lost with crystalloid, colloid, or blood products as appropriate.

The pulmonary vasculature is exquisitely sensitive to hypoxia, hypercarbia, and acidosis and these conditions must be avoided. If it appears that there is increased right to left intracardiac shunting then the clinical management should be directed towards optimising venous return, reversing any pulmonary vasoconstriction, and perhaps systemic vasoconstriction.

The most potent selective pulmonary vasodilator is oxygen. Inhaled nitric oxide is also a potent pulmonary vasodilator which has been used successfully to improve pulmonary blood flow and oxygenation in patients with pulmonary hypertension from a variety of causes. Its use has not been described in pregnant women. Intravenous vasodilators such as prostacyclin, sodium nitroprusside, and glyceryl trinitrate all produce pulmonary vasodilatation, but may, even when administered directly into the pulmonary artery, produce unwanted systemic vasodilatation, systemic hypotension, and exacerbate hypoxemia. Nebulised prostacyclin avoids these systemic effects and looks promising.

The efficacy of all these agents depends heavily on the pulmonary blood flow. Myocardial contractility may be augmented by an inotropic agent such as dopamine. While this improves myocardial contractility it may cause pulmonary vasoconstriction but usually only when administered in doses greater than 10 µg/kg/min. If systemic vasoconstriction is required then an infusion of noradrenaline or phenylephedrine should be used and renal function must be closely monitored.

The use of vasodilators and vasoconstrictors is fraught with difficulty in patients with the Eisenmenger syndrome. Sudden swings in pulmonary or systemic vascular pressures must be avoided as these pharmacologically produced changes may be irreversible. So sensitive is the balance that a mechanical failure of a syringe pump or a change in drug infusion syringes could destabilise cardiovascular function.

Despite all efforts the mortality remains high in this condition.[38]

Ischaemic heart disease

Myocardial infarction in pregnancy is rare although the incidence of ischaemic heart disease may be increasing. The proportion of maternal deaths attributed to ischaemic heart disease in the United Kingdom was 30% to 39% of all cardiac related deaths in the period from 1985 to 1990. The highest incidence of myocardial infarction is in the third trimester. Most maternal deaths occur either at the time of infarction with an undeliverable baby or within two weeks of myocardial infarction. The overall mortality is 28% while peripartum myocardial infarction has a mortality of 30% to 40%.[45]

There are no clear guidelines as to the best method of delivery in pregnant patients following acute myocardial infarction or in those with severe coronary artery disease. Patients must be assessed for the degree of residual left ventricular dysfunction as decompensation may occur with the cardiovascular changes of pregnancy and labour. Efforts should be made to minimise cardiac workload and myocardial oxygen consumption. These patients are commonly treated with beta-adrenergic blocking drugs and low dose aspirin.

The degree of invasive monitoring for each patient should be decided individually after assessing the degree of myocardial dysfunction. There should be a minimal level of monitoring including electrocardiography, pulse oximetry, and noninvasive blood pressure measurement.

Epidural analgesia using a combination of local anaesthetic and opiates provides stable cardiovascular conditions in labouring women who have had a myocardial infarction.[45] One woman who had labour induced 12 days after a myocardial infarction and managed successfully with epidural analgesia has been reported.[46] She was monitored with intra-arterial and pulmonary artery catheters. After five hours there was no progress in labour and the pulmonary capillary wedge pressure had risen from 10 to 27 mm Hg despite an intravenous nitrate infusion. The epidural block was extended and a caesarean section done successfully.

If general anaesthesia is required it would be prudent to obviate the hypertensive and tachycardiac response to laryngoscopy and intubation with a short acting opiate such as alfentanil 20 to 35 µg/kg intravenously before induction. A skilled neonatal resuscitation team must be available at delivery as this dose of opiate may produce profound respiratory depression in the neonate. Oxytocin should be used cautiously as it may aggravate coronary artery spasm.

Any clinical signs of myocardial ischaemia must be treated aggressively with coronary vasodilators such as glyceryl trinitrate. The use of fibrinolytic or anticoagulant drugs, such as streptokinase or heparin, in the setting of acute ischaemia in the labouring woman is controversial as it may predispose to haemorrhage. If the mother continues to deteriorate despite treatment or the fetus appears compromised then caesarean section must be carried out.

Cardiac transplant recipients

There have been 13 successfully completed pregnancies reported in recipients of heart transplants since 1988.[47,48]

The transplanted heart is denervated and the cardiac output is preload dependent. In the absence of vagal tone the resting heart rate is higher (90 to 100 beats/minute) but it can increase over several minutes in response to increased circulating catecholamines. Contractility remains normal and the Frank Starling mechanism is intact so cardiac output may be augmented by increased venous return.

The response to drugs with primary cardiovascular actions may be altered. Bradycardia is uncommon, if it does occur isoprenaline and ephedrine can increase the heart rate by direct beta-adrenergic stimulation whilst anticholinergic drugs are ineffective.

The transplanted heart seems to adapt well to the physiological changes of pregnancy and labour.[49] There is a 30% incidence of pre-eclampsia during the pregnancies of patients with transplanted organs, compared with 3% in normal pregnant women. This may be spurious and related to the use of cyclosporin as an immunosuppressant drug. Side effects of cyclosporin include hypertension and proteinuria secondary to renal dysfunction. Nevertheless women should be managed as if they had pre-eclampsia. Coagulation status and liver function tests should be checked, blood pressure controlled, and renal function monitored.

All transplant recipients must be maintained on immunosuppressant therapy. Most of the anaesthetic implications of their use are related to the drugs' side effects. The only direct pharmacological effect is that of cyclosporin and azathiaprine on neuromuscular blockade. Azathiaprine increases the requirement for non-depolarising muscle relaxants by presynaptic inhibition of phosphodiesterase. Cyclosporin potentiates the action of non-depolarising muscle relaxants. Neither of these effects is usually clinically important, but in the labour ward, where magnesium may be given, there should be close monitoring of neuromuscular blockade if non-depolarising muscle relaxants are used.

Other side effects include the increased risk of infection in immuno-suppressed patients. There should be strict attention to aseptic technique if intravascular monitoring lines are required, and in carrying out regional blocks. Azathiaprine may cause thrombocytopenia, so the number of platelets should be counted before regional blockade. Cyclosporin is nephrotoxic and it is important to maintain renal perfusion and avoid hypotension, by adequate fluid management. Non-steroidal anti-inflammatory drugs should be avoided but additional steroid cover may be given.

In the reports of successful deliveries in cardiac transplant recipients there is information about the anaesthetic management in 11 cases. Women have delivered vaginally both with and without epidural anaesthesia. As cardiac output is preload dependent it is important to avoid aortocaval compression. Adequate intravascular volume and venous return can be maintained by generous fluid loading whilst establishing the block. In the presence of good ventricular function invasive monitoring is unnecessary.[50] Electrocardiographic monitoring is advised as atherosclerosis is accelerated in the transplanted heart and ischaemia is painless in a denervated heart.

The epidural block technique for caesarean section has been used without a problem. Spinal anaesthesia has been used successfully for a variety of surgical procedures in non-pregnant patients following heart transplantation but there are no reported cases in pregnant women.[51]

Anaesthesia for cardiac surgery

Open heart surgery is sometimes required during pregnancy if there has been severe deterioration in the maternal condition. The procedures that are needed are valve replacement for bacterial endocarditis and coronary artery bypass grafting.

Cardiopulmonary bypass during pregnancy was first described in 1958. In general maternal outcome has been satisfactory, mortality being less than 5%. Unfortunately fetal loss remains high at up to 30%. There are many reasons for high fetal mortality. Women who require cardiac surgery during pregnancy often have chronic maternal hypoxaemia and compromise of uteroplacental perfusion. Cardiopulmonary bypass introduces additional insults including hypotension, hypothermia, release of vasoactive substances, complement activation, and air and particulate embolism. All these factors may impede uteroplacental perfusion.

The optimal method to preserve fetal well being during cardiopulmonary bypass is unclear. There are general guidelines based on case reports and uncontrolled trials and surgery should be delayed if possible to the second trimester. There are no specific anaesthetic techniques recommended.[52-54]

Uterine activity and the fetal heart should be monitored. Baseline fetal heart rate and beat-to-beat variation often decrease during cardiopulmonary bypass. Prolonged slowing below 80 beats/minute is worrying and may respond to increased pump perfusion rates. It appears logical to use relatively high pulsatile flows of greater than $2L/min/M^2$ to maintain uteroplacental perfusion. The use of hypothermia remains controversial. There have been good fetal outcomes following the use of deep hypothermia and even circulatory arrest but in general moderate hypothermia at about 32°C or normothermia are recommended.

If caesarean section is required immediately before or during cardiopulmonary bypass then profuse bleeding from the placental site may occur because of full anticoagulation. The use of aprotinin, a potent inhibitor of fibrinolysis, has been described to control bleeding.[55]

Conclusion

The management of anaesthesia for pregnant patients requires extremely careful planning. An experienced team of a cardiologist, an obstetrician, a midwife, and an anaesthetist, plus all their supplementary staff, is essential to the process. Therefore these patients must be cared for in a fully equipped hospital providing obstetric, cardiac, and neonatal services. Carefully agreed plans must be written, tailored to the individual mother, and these must be followed without compromise. A successful outcome can be assured only if the mother and her fetus are cared for in optimal conditions.

References

1 De Swiet M. *Medical disorders in obstetric practice.* 3rd ed. Oxford: Blackwell Science, 1995.

2 *Report on Confidential Enquiries into Maternal Deaths in the United Kingdom. 1988–1990.* London: HMSO, 1991.

3 Clark SL, Cotton DB, Pivarnik JM, *et al.* Position changes and central haemodynamic profile during normal third-trimester pregnancy and post partum. *Am J Obstet Gynecol* 1991; **164**: 883–7.

4 Ronson SC, Dunlop W, Boys RJ, Hunter S. Cardiac output during labour. *BMJ* 1987; **295**: 1169–72.

5 Ueland K, Hansen JM. Maternal cardiovascular dynamics II. Posture and uterine contractions. *Am J Obstet Gynecol* 1969; **103**: 1–7.

6 Ueland K, Hansen JM. Maternal cardiovascular dynamics III. Labour and delivery under a local and caudal analgesia. *Am J Obstet Gynecol* 1969; **103**: 8–18.

7 Bonica JJ, Akamatsu TJ, Berges PU, Morikawa K, Kennedy WF Jr. Circulatory effects of peridural block: II. Effects of epinephrine. *Anesthesiol* 1971; **34**: 514–22.

8 Mangano DT. Anaesthesia for the pregnant cardiac patient. In: Shrider SM, Levinson G, eds. *Anesthesia for obstetrics.* 3rd ed. Baltimore: Williams and Wilkins, 1993.

9 Vincent RD. Anaesthesia for the pregnant patient. *Clin Obstet Gynaecol* 1994; **37**: 256–73.

10 Mazze RI, Kallen B. Reproductive outcome after anaesthesia and operation during pregnancy: a registry of 5405 cases. *Am J Obstet Gynecol* 1989; **161**: 1178–85.

11 Duncan PG, Pope WDB, Cohen MM, Greer N. Fetal risk of anesthesia and surgery during pregnancy. *Anesthesiol* 1986; **64**: 790–4.

12 Nolan TE, Wakefield ML, Devoe LD. Invasive haemodynamic monitoring in obstetrics. A critical review of its indications, benefits, complications and alternatives. *Chest* 1992; **101**: 1429–33.

13 Robinson S. Pulmonary artery catheters in Eisenmenger's syndrome: many risks, few benefits. Letter. *Anesthesiol* 1983; **58**: 588–9.

14 Devitt JH, Noble WH, Byrick RJ. A Swan–Ganz catheter related complication in a patient with Eisenmenger's syndrome. *Anesthesiol* 1982; **57**: 335–7.

15 Ralston DH, Schnider SM, DeLorimer AA. Effects of equipotent ephedrine, mephenteramine and methoxamine on uterine blood flow in the pregnant ewe. *Anesthesiol* 1974; **40**: 354–69.

16 Ramanathan S, Grant GJ. Vasopressor therapy for hypotension due to epidural anaesthesia for caesarian section. *Acta Anaesthesiol Scand* 1988; **32**: 559–65.

17 Wright PMC, Iftikhar M, Fitzpatrick KT, Moore J, Thompson W. Vasopressor therapy for hypotension during epidural anaesthesia for caesarian section: effects on maternal and fetal flow velocity ratios. *Anesth Analg* 1992; **75**: 56–63.

18 Weis FR Jr, Martello R, Mo B, Bochiechio P. Cardiovascular effects of oxytocin. *Obstet Gynecol* 1975; **46**: 211–4.

19 Secker NJ, Arnsbo P, Wallin L. Haemodynamic effects of oxytocin (Syntocinon R) and methyl ergometrine (Methergin) on the systemic and pulmonary circulation of pregnant anaesthetised women. *Acta Obstet Gynecol Scand* 1978; **57**: 97–103.

20 Arias F, Pineda J. Aortic stenosis and pregnancy. *J Reprod Med* 1978; **20**: 229–32.

21 Morgan M. Anaesthetic choice for the cardiac obstetric patient. *M E J Anaesth* 1990; **10**: 621–32.

22 Lao TT, Sermer M, MacGee L, Farine D, Colman JM. Congenital aortic stenosis and pregnancy—a reappraisal. *Am J Obstet Gynecol* 1993; **169**: 540–5.

23 Easterling TR, Chadwick HS, Otto CM, Benedetti TJ. Aortic stenosis in pregnancy. *Obstet Gynecol* 1988; **72**: 113–8.

24 Brain JE Jr, Seifan AB, Clark RB, Robertson DM, Quirk JG. Aortic stenosis, caesarean delivery, and epidural anaesthesia. *J Clin Anesth* 1993; **5**: 154–7.

25 Colclough GW, Ackerman WE, Walmsley PM, Hessel EA. Epidural anesthesia for a parturient with critical aortic stenosis. J Clin Anesth. 1995; 7: 264–5.

26 Redfern N, Bower S, Bullock RE, Hull CJ. Alfentanil for caesarean section complication by severe aortic stenosis: a case report. *Br J Anaesth* 1987; **59**: 1309–12.

27 Alderson JD. Cardiovascular collapse following epidural anaesthesia for caesarian section in a patient with aortic incompetence. *Anaesthesia* 1987; **42**: 643–5.

28 Tessler MJ, Hudson R, Naugler-Colville M, Biehl DR. Pulmonary oedema in two patients with hypertrophic obstructive cardiomyopathy (HOCM). *Can J Anaesth* 1990; **37**: 469–73.

29 Fairley CJ, Clarke JT. Use of esmolol in a parturient with hypertrophic obstructive cardiomyopathy. *Br J Anaesth* 1995; **75**: 801–4.

30 Minnich ME, Quirk JG, Clark RB. Epidural anesthesia for vaginal delivery in a patient with idiopathic hypertrophic subaortic stenosis. *Anesthesiol* 1987; **67**: 590–2.

31 Boccio RV, Chung JH, Harrison MD. Anesthetic management of caesarian section in a patient with idiopathic hypertrophic subaortic stenosis. *Anesthesiol* 1986; **65**: 663–5.

32 Clark SL, Phelan JP, Greenspoon J, Aldahl D, Horenstein J. Labour and delivery in the presence of mitral stenosis: central haemodynamic observations. *Am J Obstet Gynecol* 1985; **152**: 984–8.

33 McColgin SW, Martin JN, Morrison JC. Pregnant women with prosthetic heart valves. *Clin Obs Gynecol* 1989; **32**: 76–88.

34 Vandermeulen EP, Van Akentt, Vermylen J. Anticoagulants and spinal—epidural anesthesia. *Anesth Analg* 1994; **79**: 1165–77.

35 Weiss BM, Atanassoff PG. Cyanotic congenital heart disease and pregnancy: natural selection, pulmonary hypertension and anesthesia. *J Clin Anesth* 1993; **5**: 332–41.

36 Stoddart P, O'Sullivan G. Eisenmenger's syndrome in pregnancy: a case report and review. *International Journal of Obstetric Anesthesiology* 1993; **2**: 159–68.

37 Pitkin RM, Perloff JK, Koos BJ, Beatt MH. Pregnancy and congenital heart disease. *Am Intern Med* 1990; **112**: 445–54.

38 Roberts NV, Keast PJ. Pulmonary hypertension and pregnancy – a lethal combination. *Anaesth Intensive Care* 1990; **18**: 366–74.

39 Perloff JK. Congenital heart disease and pregnancy. A review. *Clin Cardiol* 1994; **17**: 579–87.

40 Shime J, Mocarski EJM, Hastings D, Webb GD, McLaughlin PR. Congenital heart disease in pregnancy: short and long term implications. *Am J Obstet Gynecol* 1987; **156**: 313–22.

41 Semdstad KG, Granlo R, Morison DH. Pulmonary hypertension and pregnancy: a series of eight cases. *Can J Anaesth* 1994; **41**: 502–12.

42 Avila WS, Grinberg M, Snitcowsky R, *et al.* Maternal and fetal outcome in pregnant women with Eisenmenger's syndrome. *Eur Heart J* 1995; **16**: 460–4.

43 Spinnato JA, Kraynack BJ, Cooper MW. Eisenmenger's syndrome in pregnancy: epidural anesthesia for elective cesarean section. *N Engl J Med* 1981; **304**: 1215–17.

44 Lumley J, Whitwam JG, Morgan M. General anaesthesia in the presence of Eisenmenger's syndrome. *Anesth Analg* 1977; **56**: 543–7.

45 Soderlin MK, Purhonen S, Haring P, Hietakorpi S, Koski E, Nuutinen LS. Myocardial infarction in a parturient. *Anaesthesia* 1994; **49**: 870–2.

46 Aglio LS, Johnson MD. Anaesthetic management of myocardial infarction in a parturient. *Br J Anaesth* 1990; **65**: 258–61.

47 Laiter SA, Yeagley CJ, Armitage JM. Pregnancy after cardiac transplantation. *Am J Perinatol* 1994; **11**: 217–19.

48 Baxi LV, Rho RB. Pregnancy after cardiac transplantation. *Am J Obstet Gynecol* 1992; **169**: 33–4.

49 Riley ET. Obstetric management of patients with transplants. *Int Anesthesiol Clin* 1995; **33**: 125–40.

50 Key TC, Resnik R, Dittrich HC, Reisner LS. Successful pregnancy after cardiac transplantation. *Am J Obstet Gynecol* 1989; **160**: 367–71.

51 Dash A. Anesthesia for patients with a previous heart transplant. *Int Anesthesiol Clin* 1995; **33**: 1–9.

52 Chambers CE, Clark SL. Cardiac surgery during pregnancy. *Clin Obstet Gynecol* 1994; **37**: 316–23.

53 Strickland RA, Oliver WC, Chantigan RC, Ney JA, Danielson GK. Anesthesia, cardiopulmonary bypass and the pregnant patient. *Mayo Clinic Proc* 1991; **66**: 411–29.

54 Becker RM. Intracardiac surgery in pregnant women. *Ann Thorac Surg* 1983; **36**: 453–8.

55 Lamarra M, Azzu AA, Kulatilake NP. Cardiopulmonary bypass in the early puerperium: a possible new role for aprotinin. *Ann Thorac Surg* 1992; **54**: 361–3.

28: Cardiac intervention and surgery during pregnancy

CELIA OAKLEY

Cardiac conditions that need surgery should have been diagnosed and usually operated upon before pregnancy, except for patients anticipating valve replacement who should if possible complete their pregnancies before this (Chapter 10). Heart surgery during pregnancy is therefore usually needed because the heart disease had previously been missed or underestimated or because of a sudden life-threatening complication. The indications for open heart surgery during pregnancy are related to failure of preconceptual diagnosis or advice because of late antenatal booking, iatrogenic complications of balloon aortic or mitral valvotomy causing catastrophic regurgitation, valve destruction from infective endocarditis (Chapter 11), aortic dissection, the occasional left atrial myxoma,[1,2] or thrombosis of a prosthetic cardiac valve. This may develop relatively acutely or be subacute. Thrombolysis should be attempted first but if it fails, valve re-replacement or débridement may be needed (Chapter 10).

Cardiac surgery during pregnancy does not usually carry greater risk to the mother's life than outside pregnancy but may jeopardise the fetus. Fetal wastage may reflect the severity of the maternal haemodynamic problem which should be optimised before the operation but this may not be possible in a deteriorating situation.

While closed cardiac surgery does not usually cause fetal hazard, operation under cardiopulmonary bypass is associated with high risk of fetal loss. Because of this, if the fetus is sufficiently mature it should be delivered by caesarean section immediately before the mother is placed on cardio-pulmonary bypass.[1]

Pericardiectomy was the first "cardiac" operation and has been practised for half a century, initially with high mortality because the patients had advanced tuberculous constriction with severe chronic congestion, and they died deeply jaundiced from liver failure. Nowadays the cause of constriction is usually unknown, the severity milder, and the surgery technically easier. Pericardiectomy in pregnancy is usually not needed but the condition may previously have been occult and only manifest in pregnancy because of the development of congestion caused by the increased blood volume and cardiac output. The operation can be carried out safely, preferably in mid-trimester without the need for cardiopulmonary bypass and with little risk to the fetus. However, it can also safely be left in most instances until after delivery at the expense only of some oedema and tachycardia. The risk is now likely to be substantially lower than the 2% to 4% for the mother and 7% to 9% for the fetus suggested in early reports (Chapter 17).[3]

Worldwide, mitral stenosis is the most common potentially lethal cardiac problem in pregnancy. Closed mitral valvotomy has been carried out safely for years with minimal risk to both mother and baby and with excellent results even in the 1950s.[4-6]

Open valvotomy is rarely necessary. Open mitral valvotomy or valve replacement carry a greater risk of fetal loss than closed valvotomy because of the need for cardiopulmonary bypass.

Young women have valves which are usually suitable for balloon mitral valvotomy ("valvuloplasty") and because of the growing experience with the technique (Chapter 8) closed mitral valvotomy has virtually disappeared from the surgical repertoire in the developed world. However, it remains a thoroughly satisfactory operation which is still carried out skilfully and with excellent results in parts of the world where mitral stenosis in the young is still prevalent and Inoue balloons are expensive (Chapter 8).[7,8]

Most patients needing intervention during pregnancy are in sinus rhythm. Despite this, because of the coagulopathy of pregnancy and stasis within the left atrium, there is a real risk of left atrial thrombus and subsequent embolism, so it is wise to carry out transthoracic and transoesophageal echocardiography immediately before the operation to check for the presence of thrombus or of spontaneous echo contrast ("smoke") indicating a risk of thrombosis. Anticoagulants should be given postoperatively until the patient is fully mobile. This is true whether the mitral valvotomy is going to be carried out by balloon dilatation or by closed or open surgical technique.

Balloon dilatation of the mitral[9,10] (or indeed of the pulmonary[11] or aortic[12,13]) valve can be carried out successfully in pregnancy without disturbing the fetus. The abrupt loss of blood pressure which accompanies balloon dilatation may not be well tolerated by the fetus if the balloon procedure is carried out during the first trimester and in any case procedures involving irradiation should be avoided if possible during the period of organogenesis. The second trimester is the best time and if a patient with mitral stenosis develops pulmonary congestion or oedema during the first trimester treatment with rest and control of heart rate with a beta-blocking drug will almost always get the patient out of trouble and allow intervention to be delayed until the middle trimester or indeed until after delivery.[14]

Coarctation of the aorta has been operated on successfully during pregnancy but is not advised unless life threatening complications such as aortic dissection have developed.[15] Most patients with unoperated coarctation do well in pregnancy and much better than in early reports.[16] Such patients are now seen much more rarely but even previously operated patients may present as emergencies from dissection or endocarditis (Chapter 5).

Aortic dissection in a patient with Marfan syndrome, a patient with previously undiagnosed coarctation of the aorta, or indeed in a previously healthy young pregnant woman should be suspected in the presence of severe chest pain with new aortic regurgitation or if the pain radiates through to the back or down into the abdomen or iliac fossae.[17,18] After confirmation of the diagnosis by transoesophageal echocardiography emergency aortic root replacement is needed for type A dissection. Localised dissections of the arch in a patient with coarctation or involving only the descending thoracic aorta should be treated conservatively with rest and beta-blocking drugs.

Myocardial infarction complicating pregnancy may need emergency coronary bypass if reperfusion is unsuccessful by catheterisation. Both thrombolysis and balloon coronary angioplasty have been used successfully in pregnancy and the insertion of a stent may improve the results of intervention for coronary artery dissection which is the most common cause of acute myocardial infarction in pregnancy and in the peripartum period.[19,20] If the threatened myocardial territory is considerable and coronary bypass is needed the infant if viable should be delivered first (Chapter 18).

Fortunately all of these dire cardiac emergencies are rare. Information on the risk of modern open heart surgery to the fetus is sparse. Early reports indicated that the fetal mortality rate was as high as 33%.[21,22] Little or no work has been done on the effects of cardiopulmonary bypass on utero-placental blood flow but improved fetal survival in more recent experience has been attributed to high blood flow perfusion and avoidance of hypothermia.[22] This may have reduced the fetal risk to about 20%.[23,24]

Much of the fetal risk relates to the maternal state. If this is precarious, the fetus faces high risk particularly during induction of anaesthesia before going on to cardiopulmonary bypass. The anaesthetist should try to minimise the induction time and to stabilise swings in heart rate and blood pressure which may occur during intubation. Cardiopulmonary bypass is far from physiological even with improved techniques. All open heart operations are necessarily carried out under full anticoagulation with heparin, which can lead to placental separation from retroplacental bleeding. In addition platelet aggregates cause micro-emboli and the risk to the fetus increases with longer duration of bypass. Changes in regional blood flow can jeopardise fetal safety if uteroplacental perfusion is compromised and this also depends on the mother's condition at the conclusion of the operation, her heart rate, blood pressure, output, and oxygenation (Chapter 27).

Continuous fetal monitoring is essential during induction, throughout the operation, and postoperatively. Fetal distress is indicated by slowing of the fetal heart and if this is noted prompt steps should be taken to try to improve the delivery and quality of blood to the fetus.

Antibiotics perioperatively or for the treatment of maternal endocarditis may damage the baby. Gentamicin can cause fetal deafness (Chapters 11 and 22).

In summary, the fetal risk during cardiopulmonary bypass depends on the maternal condition preoperatively and during induction, the duration of cardiopulmonary bypass, and the maternal condition postoperatively. Whenever possible surgery under cardiopulmonary bypass should be postponed until the fetus is viable and the fetus should always be delivered by caesarean section before the cardiac surgery to give the child the best chance of surviving, to relieve maternal circulatory stress, and to provide better operating conditions for the surgeon.

References

1 Trimakas AP, Maxwell KD, Berkay S, Gardener TJ, Achuff SC. Fetal monitoring during cardiopulmonary bypass for removal of a left atrial myxoma during pregnancy. *Johns Hopkins Medical Journal* 1979; **144**: 156–60.

2 Casarotto D, Bortolotti U, Russo R, Betti D, Schivazappa L, Thiene G. Surgical removal of a left myxoma during pregnancy. *Chest* 1979; **75**: 390–2.

3 Richardson PM, LeRoux BT, Rogers MA, Gotsman MS. Pericardiectomy in pregnancy. *Thorax* 1970; **25**: 627–30.

4 Brock RC. Valvulotomy in pregnancy. *Proc R Soc Med* 1952; **45**: 538–43.

5 Cooley DA, Chapman DW. Mitral commissurotomy during pregnancy. *JAMA* 1952; **150**: 1113–17.

6 Logan A, Turner RWD. Mitral valvulotomy in pregnancy. *Lancet* 1952; **i**: 1286–90.

7 El Maraghy M, Abou Senna I, El Tehwy F, Bassiouni M, Ayoub A, El-Sayed H. Mitral valvotomy in pregnancy. *Am J Obstet Gynecol* 1983; **145**: 708.

8 Goon MS, Raman S, Sinnathuray TA. Closed mitral valvotomy in pregnancy: a Malaysian experience. *Aust NZ J Obstet Gynaecol* 1987; **27**: 173.

9 Kalra GS, Arora R, Khan JA, Nigram M, Khalillulah M. Percutaneous mitral commissurotomy for severe mitral stenosis during pregnancy. *Cathet Cardiovasc Diagn* 1994; **33**: 28–30.

10 Patel JJ, Muclinger MJ, Mitha AS, Patel N. Percutaneous balloon dilatation of the mitral valve in critically ill young patients with intractable heart failure. *Br Heart J* 1995; **73**: 555–8.

11 Perloff JK. Congenital heart disease and pregnancy. *Clin Cardiol* 1994; **17**: 579–87.

12 Banning AP, Pearson JF, Hall RJC. Role of balloon dilatation of the aortic valve in pregnant patients with severe aortic stenosis. *Br Heart J* 1993; **70**: 544–5.

13 McIvor RA. Percutaneous balloon aortic valvuloplasty during pregnancy. *Int J Cardiol* 1991; **32**: 1–4.

14 Narasimhan C, Joseph G, Singh TC. Propranolol for pulmonary oedema in mitral stenosis. *Int J Cardiol* 1994; **44**: 178–9.

15 Waditel HL, Czarnicki SW. Coarctation of the aorta and pregnancy. *Am Heart J* 1966; **72**: 251–4.

16 Goodwin JF. Pregnancy and coarctation of the aorta. *Lancet* 1958; **i**: 16–20.

17 Mandel W, Evans EW, Walford RL. Dissecting aortic aneurysm during pregnancy. *N Engl J Med* 1954; **251**: 1059–61.

18 Hume M, Krosnick G. Dissecting aneurysm in pregnancy associated with aortic insufficiency. *N Engl J Med* 1961; **268**: 174–8.

19 Cowan NC, De Belder MA, Rothman MT. Coronary angioplasty in pregnancy. *Br Heart J* 1988; **59**: 588–92.

20 Hands ME, Johnson MD, Saltzman DH, Rutherford JD. The cardiac, obstetric and anaesthetic management of pregnancy complicated by acute myocardial infarction. *J Clin Anesth* 1990; **2**: 258–68.

21 Ueland K. Cardiac surgery and pregnancy. *Am J Obstet Gynecol* 1965; **92**: 148–62.

22 Zitnik RS, Brandenburg RO, Sheldon R, Wallace RB. Pregnancy and open heart surgery. *Circulation* 1969; **39(suppl1)**: 257–62.

23 Becker RM. Intracardiac surgery in pregnant women. *Ann Thorac Surg* 1983; **36**: 453–8.

24 Bernal JM, Miralles PJ. Cardiac surgery with cardiopulmonary bypass during pregnancy. *Obstet Gynecol Surv* 1986; **41**: 1–6.

29: Genetic counselling

SUSAN E HOLDER

This chapter is intended to act as a quick reference for doctors who are faced with a pregnant woman with heart disease who asks the question "What is the risk that my baby will have a heart problem?" In most cases, a risk figure is available, and appropriate investigations of the baby are suggested. However, genetic counselling is not just a case of providing a risk figure and arranging the necessary scans. One definition of genetic counselling is that it is: "An educational process that seeks to assist affected and/or at risk individuals to understand the nature of the genetic disorder, its transmission and the options open to them in management and family planning."[1] In other words, what do the family understand about the condition and what will they do with the risk figure they have been given? Do they perceive the risk as being high or low? If a problem is detected, is it amenable to surgery, and if so, when? Will special arrangements have to be made with regard to the delivery of the baby? Will the baby be affected to the same degree as the parent, or might it be more severely affected? If a severe problem is detected in the fetus, would they wish to consider having a termination of pregnancy? Figure 29.1 shows the appearance of the normal fetal heart at 18–20 weeks' gestation, using ultrasonography.

Some of these issues can be dealt with adequately by both the cardiologist and obstetrician involved in the case. Others may require referral to your local clinical genetics unit, especially if the family tree is complex or special investigations are required.

Risk calculation

In genetic counselling, it is standard practice to provide a figure for the risk of recurrence, usually expressed either as odds or percentages. There are a number of different types of risk estimation used in practice, but for the purposes of this chapter, the two main types are mendelian and empirical risks. Mendelian risks relate to those disorders known to be due to a single gene and with a clear mode of inheritance. Thus the offspring risk for those conditions known to be dominantly inherited, such as Marfan syndrome, is 50%. The offspring risk when a parent has an autosomal recessive disorder, such as Ellis–van Creveld syndrome, is likely to be negligible. This is because, in autosomal recessive conditions, the child, to be affected,

401

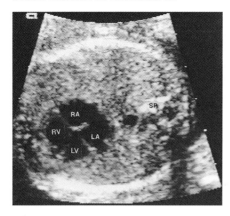

FIGURE 29.1—*Transverse section through the fetal chest at the level of the heart, showing a normal four chamber view. RA = right atrium, LA = left atrium, RV = right ventricle, LV = left ventricle. (Reproduced by permission of JS Carvalho, Royal Brompton Hospital, London, UK.)*

must receive an abnormal gene from both the mother and the father. The chance that the partner of an affected woman is also a carrier of a rare recessive gene is obviously small, unless the parents are consanguineous, in which case the risks to a child may be quite high.

Empirical risk figures are risks based on observed data, from family studies, rather than theoretical predictions based on an understanding of the mode of inheritance. This type of figure is used for most of the commoner non-mendelian disorders, such as neural tube defects, clefts of the lip and palate, and the majority of isolated congenital heart defects.

Mendelian disorders

The first task, when advising a mother with congenital heart disease about risks to her offspring, is to ensure that a mendelian disorder has been excluded, especially if she has other extracardiac abnormalities. Examples of some of the important single gene disorders that can be associated with congenital heart disease, along with their mode of inheritance, are given in Table 29.1, and described in greater detail in the appropriate section below.

Holt–Oram syndrome

The combination of skeletal abnormalities of the upper limb with congenital heart disease, usually secundum atrial septal defect (ASD), was first reported in 1960 by Holt and Oram.[2] It is an autosomal dominant condition with extremely variable expression in terms of both skeletal and cardiac defects.

Commonly the thumbs are involved and show either hypoplasia, triphalangism, or complete absence. The radius, ulna and humerus may be abnormal, and an inability to supinate and pronate the hand is common.

TABLE 29.1—*Mendelian disorders associated with heart disease.*

Disorder	Inheritance
Holt–Oram syndrome	Autosomal dominant
Noonan syndrome	Autosomal dominant
Marfan syndrome	Autosomal dominant
LEOPARD syndrome	Autosomal dominant
Long Q–T (Romano–Ward) syndrome	Autosomal dominant
Supravalvar aortic stenosis	Autosomal dominant
Ellis–van Creveld syndrome	Autosomal recessive
Jervell–Lange–Nielsen syndrome	Autosomal recessive
Kartagener's syndrome	?Autosomal recessive

Upper limb phocomelia occasionally occurs. The lower limbs are not affected.

ASD is the cardiac anomaly identified in over two thirds of cases. However, persistent ductus arteriosus, coarctation of the aorta, ventricular septal defect, transposition of the great vessels, and prolapsed mitral valve have all been reported in families in which other members have more typical features.[3]

Occasionally no congenital heart lesion is present, but arrhythmias or more minor ECG abnormalities are the only cardiac finding.

Mental retardation is not a feature of the Holt–Oram syndrome.

Detailed ultrasonography, including fetal echocardiography, should be offered at about 18–20 weeks of pregnancy, so that the extent of the limb abnormalities, if present, can be identified and their prognosis and management discussed. Secundum ASD, the commonest cardiac abnormality in Holt–Oram syndrome, is not detectable in the fetus, but other less common cardiac lesions should be excluded.

Recent genetic linkage studies have shown that a gene for Holt–Oram syndrome is located on chromosome 12.[4]

Noonan syndrome

This is a dysmorphic syndrome commonly associated with congenital heart disease, usually pulmonary stenosis. It can be dominantly inherited, although many cases are sporadic. The expression can be variable, so that a mildly affected mother can give birth to a more severely affected child, and diagnosis relies on recognition of the clinical phenotype.[5] Linkage studies in familial Noonan syndrome suggest that the gene is located on chromosome 12.[6]

The cardinal features of Noonan syndrome are short stature, a broad or webbed neck, and pectus excavatum or carinatum, associated with down-slanting palpebral fissures, ptosis, low-set posteriorly rotated ears, and a low posterior hairline. Cryptorchidism, commonly bilateral, occurs in 60% of affected boys, and may require corrective surgery. Affected girls do not have genital abnormalities. Mental retardation, usually mild, may be a feature of Noonan syndrome.

Congenital heart lesions occur in two thirds of patients. Pulmonary stenosis, atrial septal defects, and asymmetric septal hypertrophy have all been reported.

Detailed fetal echocardiography is indicated in any pregnancy when one or other parent has Noonan syndrome, or when parents have had a previous child with the condition.

Marfan syndrome

This connective tissue disorder has been described in detail in Chapter 12. It is inherited as an autosomal dominant, and so an affected parent has a 50% chance of passing it on to the offspring. The gene which causes Marfan syndrome has been isolated—the fibrillin gene on chromosome 15.[7] However, only a few families have identifiable mutations in their fibrillin gene, so accurate prenatal diagnosis is often not possible, unless several affected family members are available, in which case linkage can be used. Prenatal ultrasound, including fetal echocardiography, is not particularly helpful, as most of the clinical features of the condition are not necessarily present in the fetus or neonate. Affected parents who wish to discuss the possibility of prenatal diagnosis should be referred for genetic advice, preferably before starting their family, so that the feasibility of genetic tests can be considered and arranged.

LEOPARD syndrome

The name of this syndrome is an acronym for multiple Lentigines, ECG abnormalities, Ocular hypertelorism, Pulmonary stenosis, Abnormalities of the genitalia, Retardation of growth, and sensorineural Deafness. It is a diagnosis that should be considered in any patient with a combination of any of the above features with multiple lentigines. It is inherited as an autosomal dominant with variable expression, and mild mental retardation can be a feature.[8]

A variety of cardiac findings have been reported. ECG abnormalities may show axis deviations, unilateral or bilateral hypertrophy, or conduction abnormalities such as prolonged PR interval, hemiblock, bundle branch block, or complete heart block. Pulmonary stenosis may be either valvar or infundibular, and other cardiac defects such as aortic stenosis, mitral stenosis, and obstructive cardiomyopathy are less common.

Fetal echocardiography is indicated, to exclude a severe congenital heart lesion, if either parent has the LEOPARD syndrome.

404

Q–T (Romano–Ward) syndrome

This condition, in which syncopal attacks associated with a long QT interval (but not with deafness—see Jervell–Lange–Nielsen syndrome below) occur, is inherited in an autosomal dominant manner, with a 50% risk to offspring.[9] In theory, prenatal diagnosis is possible by fetal electrocardiography with enhanced resolution for T wave analysis. In practice, most affected families opt for diagnosis in the neonatal period by ECG and appropriate medical or surgical treatment. There is considerable genetic heterogeneity,[10,11] although causative genes are now being isolated.[12]

Supravalvar aortic stenosis

This anomaly can occur as a sporadic condition, but familial cases, in which it is inherited as an autosomal dominant with variable expression, have been reported.[13] Supravalvar pulmonary stenosis is a common associated finding. In view of its variability, even within families, offspring risks for an affected parent are difficult to assess, and may require cardiological assessment of other relatives to establish whether a case is truly sporadic or likely to be associated with a dominant gene. If other family members are known to be affected, then the offspring risk is likely to be 50%.

Prenatal diagnosis by fetal echocardiography is difficult, but it is worth excluding other congenital heart defects. Most cases can be diagnosed postnatally by appropriate investigations and are amenable to surgical correction.

Supravalvar aortic stenosis and peripheral pulmonary artery stenoses are both seen in Williams syndrome, a condition in which these heart defects are associated with mental retardation and characteristic facies. Most cases of Williams syndrome are now known to be the result of a submicroscopic deletion involving the elastin gene on the long arm of chromosome 7.[14] Similarly, familial cases of supravalvar aortic stenosis are associated with smaller deletions or other alterations in this same gene. It is therefore likely that precise genetic diagnosis may be available in the future.

Ellis–van Creveld syndrome

This condition is inherited as an autosomal recessive, and so offspring risks are generally low. However, it is important to recognise the typical combination of features, so that appropriate reassurance can be given about the risk to offspring.

Ellis–van Creveld syndrome is also known as chondroectodermal dysplasia. The characteristic features are postaxial polydactyly, short-limbed dwarfism, dysplastic nails, and a congenital heart defect, usually a large atrial septal defect.[15]

Jervell–Lange–Nielsen syndrome

The features of Jervell–Lange–Nielsen syndrome are a prolonged QT interval, leading to syncopal attacks, associated with congenital, or at least early onset, severe sensorineural deafness.[16] This latter feature permits differentiation from the Romano–Ward syndrome and, as the condition is autosomal recessive, offspring risks are low.

Kartagener syndrome

This condition is characterised by bronchiectasis, recurrent sinusitis, dextrocardia with or without other heart defects, and other evidence of partial or complete situs inversus. Diagnosis may require electron microscopic examination of cilia morphology, which consistently shows a reduced number of inner and outer dynein arms. Generally it is considered to be an autosomal recessive condition, with a low risk to offspring.[17]

Chromosomal abnormalities

Congenital heart disease is a fairly non-specific response to chromosomal imbalance. Any child or adult with a congenital heart lesion associated with dysmorphic features and mental retardation should have their karyotype checked to exclude a chromosome abnormality. Specific examples are the atrioventricular septal defect commonly identified in Down syndrome (trisomy 21) and coarctation of the aorta often found in girls with Turner syndrome (45XO).

Newer cytogenetic techniques have led to the identification of chromosome abnormalities previously beyond the limits of resolution of standard light microscopy. Specifically, the technique of fluorescence in situ hybridisation (FISH) allows the detection of submicroscopic chromosomal deletions. This technique is now available in most cytogenetic laboratories.

Two conditions in which congenital heart disease is associated with such microdeletions are Williams syndrome (discussed under supravalvar aortic stenosis), in which a microdeletion involving the elastin gene on the long arm of chromosome 7 has been identified using FISH, and velo-cardio-facial syndrome, in which a microdeletion on the long arm of chromosome 22 has been found.[18]

Velocardiofacial (VCF) syndrome can be considered to be part of a spectrum, with DiGeorge syndrome at the severe end of this spectrum and possibly some isolated congenital heart defects at the mild end. The term CATCH-22 is often used to describe this spectrum. This is an acronym for Cardiac abnormality, Abnormal facies, Thymic hypoplasia, Cleft palate and Hypocalcaemia as a result of a deletion on chromosome 22. Microscopically visible deletions of chromosome 22q have often been identified in DiGeorge syndrome, and it was this observation and the clinical overlap between the two conditions that led to the elucidation of the generally smaller deletions in VCF syndrome.

The characteristic features of VCF (or Shprintzen) syndrome are cleft palate or hypernasal speech, cardiac abnormalities such as ventricular septal defect or Fallot's tetralogy, and characteristic facies with a prominent nose. In most cases, VCF syndrome occurs as a sporadic condition, but it can be inherited as an autosomal dominant and the phenotype can be variable. For example, a mildly affected parent with just a cleft palate and ventricular septal defect, may have a child with mental retardation and severe congenital heart disease. Microdeletions involving chromosome 22q have also been found in occasional families with apparently dominant inheritance of isolated congenital heart lesions.[19]

Congenital heart disease

Congenital heart disease occurs in about 1% of births. Most cases (probably about 90%) are of unknown aetiology and are considered to result from multifactorial or "polygenic" inheritance. Only about 3% of cases follow simple mendelian inheritance. Chromosomal disorders and environmental causes account for the rest.

If environmental exposure is the cause of the maternal disease, then the risk to offspring is lower than when the disease is of unknown aetiology. An example is exposure to rubella, which is an unusual cause of persistent ductus arteriosus and other congenital heart lesions since the introduction of mass immunisation programmes, but may be a more prevalent cause in older age groups.

Genetic advice is most often requested by parents who have had one child with congenital heart disease. However, with improvements in management and surgery in recent years, many survivors are now reaching reproductive age and requesting genetic counselling with regard to risks to offspring. A number of studies have now been completed,[20-22] which provide information about offspring risks taking into account the sex of the affected parent as well as the precise anatomical lesion present in the parent. However, the number of subjects in these studies is generally small, and may not be representative, and the figures vary widely between studies. It would appear that the risks are higher for the offspring of affected women than of men, for reasons that are not understood. When a recurrence does occur, the lesion is identical to the affected parent in only about half the cases, which needs to be taken into account when counselling. Parents need to appreciate that a child may have a fatal or untreatable lesion as opposed to one that is amenable to surgery, and that prognosis should be discussed at the time of detection of the problem. Figure 29.2 shows an atrioventricular septal defect on fetal echocardiography.

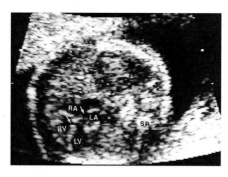

FIGURE 29.2—*Transverse section through the fetal chest at the level of the heart, which shows an atrioventricular septal defect with a common atrioventricular valve. The arrows point to the atrial and ventricular components of the defect. RA = right atrium, LA = left atrium, RV = right ventricle, LV = left ventricle. (Reproduced by permission of JS Carvalho, Royal Brompton Hospital, London, UK.)*

Table 29.2 gives general recurrence risks when the precise anatomical lesion is unknown, and Table 29.3 gives offspring risks, according to affected parent, for a number of the more common congenital heart defects. Both tables have been modified from those published in Peter Harper's textbook *Practical genetic counselling.*[23]

TABLE 29.2—*General recurrence risks in congenital heart disease.*

	Percentage risk
Population incidence	0·5–1
Sibling of isolated case	2–3
Half-sibling or second degree relative	1–2
Offspring of isolated case:	
Mother	5
Father	2–3
Two affected siblings (or sibling and parent)	10
More than two affected first degree relatives	50

Pulmonary hypertension

Primary pulmonary hypertension usually occurs as a sporadic condition, with a predominance of women, but occasional families showing autosomal dominant inheritance have been reported.[25]

Autoimmune disorders

Autoimmune disorders have been discussed in Chapter 13. Most of them are not inherited as single gene disorders, but often show familial aggregations. However, they may have a direct clinical effect on the fetus as, for example, in systemic lupus erythematosus (SLE). SLE is an

TABLE 29.3—*Offspring risks for specific congenital heart lesions.**

Lesion	Mother affected	Father affected
Ventricular septal defect	9·5	2·5
Atrial septal defect	6	1·5
Persistent ductus arteriosus	4	2
Fallot's tetralogy	2·5	1·5
Atrioventricular septal defect	14	1
Pulmonary stenosis	6·5	2
Aortic stenosis	18	5
Coarctation of aorta	4	2·5

* Based on multiple studies, collated by Nora et al.[24]

autoimmune disorder with a marked female predominance (M1:F8). The heart is involved in up to 25% of cases, in the form of pericarditis with or without a pericardial effusion. Cardiac symptoms do not necessarily predominate, the disease being a multisystem disorder, but affected women can have significant obstetric problems, including recurrent miscarriages, premature labour and an exacerbation of symptoms during pregnancy. Offspring of affected mothers may have complete heart block requiring supportive treatment in the neonatal period.

Cardiomyopathies

Hypertrophic cardiomyopathy is characterised by myocardial hypertrophy of unknown origin and uncertain prognosis. It shows considerable intrafamilial as well as interfamilial variability, making counselling difficult, but many families have been reported which show an autosomal dominant mode of inheritance. In a proportion of these families, disease-causing gene mutations have been identified, but the condition appears to be heterogeneous, making molecular analysis difficult. Three genes causing hypertrophic cardiomyopathy that have been isolated are the cardiac beta-myosin heavy chain gene, the cardiac troponin T gene, and the alpha-tropomyosin gene.[26,27]

Idiopathic dilated cardiomyopathy is also a heterogeneous group of disorders, and often shows a familial tendency. Most families are consistent with autosomal dominant inheritance, but occasional families with autosomal recessive inheritance and X-linked inheritance have been reported.[28,29] There is extreme variability of the clinical picture even within families, making risk estimation difficult. Review of the family history may help elucidate the inheritance pattern, but in small families it is often considered best to offer echocardiographic screening of all first degree relatives to detect occult disease. The marked heterogeneity of this condition has meant that genetic markers have not yet been identified.

Coronary artery disease and myocardial infarction

Coronary heart disease has numerous causes, both genetic and environmental. It is rarely cited as a cause for concern in terms of risk to offspring. However, familial hypercholesterolaemia is an autosomal dominant disorder that is considered to account for about 10–20% of early coronary heart disease and if this has been diagnosed in a parent, it is worth considering testing the children, so that early preventive measures can be introduced. Although the risk of inheriting the gene is 50% in such families, the risk of heart disease is considerably less than this, as a result of multiple confounding factors. The basic defect in familial hypercholesterolaemia is a low density lipoprotein receptor deficiency, and the gene is located on chromosome 19. Mutations have been identified in many cases, and provide an accurate means of screening in some families.[30]

References

1 Kelly TE. *Clinical genetics and genetic counselling.* Chicago: Year Book, 1986.
2 Holt M, Oram S. Familial heart disease with skeletal malformations. *Br Heart J* 1960; **22**: 236–42.
3 Hurst JA, Hall CM, Baraitser M. Syndrome of the month: the Holt–Oram syndrome. *J Med Genet* 1991; **28**: 406–10.
4 Terrett JA, Newbury-Ecob R, Cross GS, Fenton I, Raeburn JA, Brook JD. Holt–Oram syndrome is a genetically heterogeneous disease with one locus mapping to human chromosome 12q. *Nat Genet* 1994; **6**: 401–4.
5 Ranke MB, Heidemann P, Knupfer C, Enders H, Schmalz AA, Bierich JR. Noonan syndrome: growth and clinical manifestations in 144 cases. *Eur J Pediatr* 1988; **148**: 220–7.
6 Jamieson CR, van der Burgt I, Brady AF, *et al.* Mapping a gene for Noonan syndrome to the long arm of chromosome 12. *Nat Genet* 1994; **8**: 357–60.
7 Milewicz DM, Pyeritz R, Crawford ES, Byers PH. Marfan syndrome: defective secretion, synthesis and extracellular matrix formation of fibrillin by cultured dermal fibroblasts. *J Clin Invest* 1992; **89**: 79–86.
8 Gorlin RJ, Anderson RC, Blaw ME. Multiple lentigines syndrome: complex comprising multiple lentigines, electrocardiographic abnormalities, ocular hypertelorism, pulmonary stenosis, abnormalities of genitalia, retardation of growth, sensorineural deafness and autosomal dominant hereditary pattern. *Am J Dis Child* 1969; **117**: 652–62.
9 Ward OC. A new familial cardiac syndrome in children. *Journal of the Irish Medical Association* 1964; **54**: 103–6.
10 Curran M, Atkinson D, Timothy K, *et al.* Locus heterogeneity of autosomal dominant long QT syndrome. *J Clin Invest* 1993; **92**: 799–803.
11 Jiang C, Atkinson D, Towbin JA, *et al.* Two long QT syndrome loci map to chromosomes 3 and 7 with evidence of further heterogeneity. *Nat Genet* 1994; **8**: 141–7.
12 Wang Q, Curren ME, Splawski I, *et al.* Positional cloning of a novel potassium channel gene: KVLQT1 mutations cause cardiac arrhythmias. *Nat Genet* 1996; **12**: 17–23.
13 Schmidt MA, Ensing GJ, Michels VV, Carter GA, Hagler DJ, Feldt RH. Autosomal dominant supravalvular aortic stenosis: large three-generation family. *Am J Med Genet* 1989; **32**: 384–9.

14 Nickerson E, Greenberg F, Keating MT, McCaskill C, Shaffer LG. Deletions of the elastin gene at 7q11.23 occur in 90% of patients with Williams syndrome. *Am J Hum Genet* 1995; **56**: 1156–61.

15 Ellis RWB, Van Creveld S. A syndrome characterised by ectodermal dysplasia, polydactyly, chondro-dysplasia and congenital morbus cordis. *Arch Dis Child* 1940; **15**: 65–84.

16 Jervell A, Lange-Nielsen F. Congenital deaf-mutism, functional heart disease and prolongation of Q-T interval and sudden death. *Am Heart J* 1957; **54**: 59–68.

17 Kartagener M, Stucki P. Bronchiectasis with situs inversus. *Arch Pediatr* 1962; **79**: 193–207.

18 Scambler PJ, Kelly D, Lindsay E, *et al*. Velo-cardiofacial syndrome associated with chromosome 22 deletions encompassing the DiGeorge locus. *Lancet* 1992; **339**: 1138–9.

19 Wilson DI, Goodship JA, Burn J, Cross IE, Scambler PJ. Deletions within chromosome 22q11 in familial congenital heart disease. *Lancet* 1992; **340**: 573–5.

20 Dennis NR, Warren J. Risks to the offspring of patients with some common congenital heart defects. *J Med Genet* 1981; **18**: 8–16.

21 Emanuel R, Somerville J, Inns A, Withers R. Evidence of congenital heart disease in the offspring of parents with atrioventricular defects. *Br Heart J* 1983; **49**: 144–7.

22 Zellers TM, Driscoll DJ, Michels VV. Prevalence of significant congenital heart defects in children of parents with Fallot's Tetralogy. *Am J Cardiol* 1990; **65**: 523–6.

23 Harper PS. *Practical genetic counselling*. 4th ed. Oxford: Butterworth-Heinemann, 1993.

24 Nora JJ, Berg K, Nora AH. *Cardiovascular diseases. Genetics, epidemiology and prevention*. Oxford: Oxford University Press, 1991.

25 Thompson P, McRae C. Familial pulmonary hypertension: evidence of autosomal dominant inheritance. *Br Heart J* 1970; **32**: 758–60.

26 Geisterfer-Laurence AAT, Kass S, Tanigawa G, *et al*. A molecular basis for familial hypertrophic cardiomyopathy. *Cell* 1990; **62**: 999–1006.

27 Thierfelder L, Watkins H, MacRae C, *et al*. Alpha-tropomyosin and cardiac troponin T mutations cause familial hypertrophic cardiomyopathy. *Cell* 1994; **77**: 701–12.

28 Schmidt MA, Michels VV, Edwards WD, Miller FA. Familial dilated cardiomyopathy. *Am J Med Genet* 1988; **31**: 135–43.

29 Berko BA, Swift M. X-linked dilated cardiomyopathy. *N Engl J Med* 1987; **316**: 1186–91.

30 Goldstein JL, Hobbs HH, Brown MS. Familial hypercholesterolemia. In: Scriver CR, Beaudet AL, Sly WS, Valle D, eds. *The metabolic and molecular bases of inherited disease*. 7th ed. London: McGraw-Hill, 1995: 1981–2030.

411

30: Contraception for the cardiac patient

DENIS F HAWKINS

Contraception is a matter of primary importance for all patients with heart disease, for several reasons. They are concerned to use methods which will not cause deterioration in their heart condition. Planning pregnancy is of much greater importance than in the healthy woman. This may be because pregnancy should be fitted in, in relation to proposed operations. A patient with Fallot's tetralogy should certainly have her operation before she considers pregnancy. Patients with deteriorating conditions, particularly if they may need surgery, should be able to plan pregnancies in relation to the course of their disease. Mitral commissurotomy may be successful during pregnancy, but both the patient and the surgeon are happier if it is done between pregnancies. Women with progressive diseases such as Marfan's syndrome should undertake any proposed childbearing when they are young.

When procedures for preventing pregnancy are being considered with respect to patients who have a significant chance of dying of their heart disease within a few years, it is vital that it is the patient's values that are considered, not those of physicians or those of her family. All too often the patient is presented by one or both of these groups with views which either minimise potential hazards or exaggerate them. The excuse is that this is "in the patient's best interests". There is only one attitude which is in the best interests of the woman concerned, and that is to tell her the truth. She has a right to be presented with an accurate prognosis for both mother and baby when pregnancy is discussed, and to be given an accurate account of any potential hazards of procedures for contraception and sterilisation. The woman who is aware she may die within a few years may, at the extremes, have one of two diametrically opposed attitudes. One is that if she is going to die there is no way she would want to leave a young child on its own, in the care of others. The other extreme attitude is that she would have done a good job in producing a healthy baby, who if the mother dies, will live on, develop and be a credit to her memory.

For all these reasons, the concept of contraceptive counselling in women with heart disease has to be taken very seriously. The first step is to ensure that the physicians under whose care they are really understand a matter with which all obstetricians are familiar. That is, that all women aged between 12 and 48, regardless of their circumstances, can become pregnant. It is thus important that all women of reproductive age with any form of heart disease should receive appropriate contraceptive counselling, before they present with an unplanned pregnancy. The counselling must be given by someone who is prepared to secure and interpret detailed information about the heart condition concerned and its implications with respect to prognosis in general and prognosis for pregnancy in particular, and to consult with the patient's physician—preferably in that order. Perhaps the best person is an obstetrician and gynaecologist with a special interest in the management of heart disease in pregnancy. With any patient contemplating sterilisation an established requirement is that they be properly counselled in advance and that the information given to them is accurate, and this is particularly the case with women with heart disease.

Oral contraceptives

Combined oestrogen-progestagen oral preparations are probably the most effective and convenient readily available contraceptive procedure today. Claims have been made for "method failures" of less than 0·1 per 100 woman years, but everyday clinical experience is that the overall failure (pregnancy) rate is of the order of 1 to 3 per 100 woman years. Most of the pregnancies are probably due to "patient failures", missing taking pills according to the manufacturer's instructions, but the patient is just as pregnant! Some may be due to gastrointestinal upsets with intestinal hurry and decreased absorption, and coincident administration of certain other drugs such as rifampicin, phenytoin, phenobarbitone, phenylbutazone and certain antibiotics which reduce absorption of the synthetic sex hormones, but there is still doubt in most individual cases if this is responsible for a failure. Women with heart disease are a well motivated group, who generally read the instructions or are well instructed and their failures with "the pill" should be at the lower extreme of the range. Recovery of fertility after ceasing to take an oral contraceptive is a bit slower than after other methods of contraception, but 80% of women have had a baby within 18 months, and 95% within 3 years.[1]

There is then a good deal to be said for the use of combined oral contraceptives when reliability is considered, and this must be weighed in the balance when informed patients make a choice. The factors against the use of oral contraceptives in patients with heart disease are the risk of thromboembolic problems, including pulmonary embolism, biochemical changes predisposing to deterioration of atherosclerosis, hypertension, myocardial infarction in older women and haemodynamic changes consequent on fluid and electrolyte retention. These hazards have perhaps been overestimated in the past, due to overemphasis on isolated cases and to the fact that years ago the amounts of synthetic sex hormones in contraceptive pills were higher than they are today.

No form of hormone contraception conveys any protection against sexually transmitted diseases.

Thrombosis and embolism

There are considerable discrepancies in the literature as to whether or not oral contraceptives and their components affect a range of factors in the coagulation system, and if so, which factors they affect. The degree of conflict of evidence is such that coagulation factor studies do not provide good enough indications to say whether or not a particular patient is at risk, let alone whether or not oral contraceptives would be hazardous in this respect. Many of the studies were conducted with oral contraceptives containing more oestrogen and different progestagens from those used today.

To assess the risk it is therefore necessary to consider data from recent large scale studies of the incidence of thrombosis and embolism. In 1990 and 1991 the incidence of venous thrombosis or pulmonary embolism in over 540 000 women in the United Kingdom, not pregnant and not taking an oral contraceptive, was 1·1/10 000 woman years.[2] The incidence in over 100 000 women taking combined oral contraceptives with 30 or 35 µg of oestrogen was 3·0/10 000 woman years. This must be compared with the incidence in pregnant women—5·9/10 000 woman years.

Thus the risk of either a thrombosis or an embolism in the average woman taking a modern oestrogen-progestagen oral contraceptive is low, of the order of 1 in 3 300, but it is three times higher than in women not taking these preparations. On the other hand the comparable risk of thrombosis or embolism in a pregnancy that the contraceptive would have prevented is twice as high as in women taking a contraceptive pill. A reasonable conclusion is to advise any woman with a factor predisposing to thrombosis or embolism that she is exposing herself to a very small increased risk if she takes a combined oral contraceptive (see also Chapter 3).

These principles apply to patients with heart disease. If they have any history of thrombosis or embolism, any form of heart disease which predisposes to these conditions, or any other predisposing factor such as a family history of thrombosis, or varicose veins, then they should be advised against combined oral contraceptives.

What is by no means clear is the position with patients taking oral anticoagulants. On the one hand it can be argued that they are protected against the risk of thrombosis; on the other hand they are a high risk group by definition. If such a patient on prophylactic anticoagulants strongly desires oral contraception and has a strong case for really effective contraception, such as previous failures with other procedures, then the unknown nature of the risk must be explained before acceding to her wishes. Many doctors would deny oral contraceptives to a patient on full anticoagulation for a plastic heart valve, but the logic of such a view is difficult to see.

Biochemical changes and atherosclerosis

In the past, the balance of evidence was that the oestrogen components of a combined pill tended to increase high density lipoprotein cholesterol, which should reduce the risk of atherosclerosis, whilst progestagens appear to lower this cholesterol fraction and counterbalance the oestrogen effect.[3] Some progestagens also raise low density lipoprotein cholesterol, which might have deleterious effect. Possible interactions with cholesterol lowering agents like pravastatin have not been established. Triglyceride levels may be increased by oral contraception but the clinical significance of this is not clear.

The use of smaller doses of hormones in currently available preparations has minimised any biochemical effects on lipids; it is claimed that the progestagens used now are less likely to have any such effect, but the literature is conflicting.

If a patient considered to be at risk for atherosclerosis desires oral contraception then there is one safe way to approach the problem and that is to estimate plasma lipids on starting. If the levels are normal the estimation should be repeated after two months of taking the pill, and preferably every three months after.

Hypertension

There is little doubt that combined oral contraceptives cause hypertension in a small number of normotensive women. One estimate is that this occurs in less than 1% of women.[3,4] There is some evidence that women who are already hypertensive are more prone to the problem.

It is desirable to be cautious in this respect with women with heart disease. Those who are normotensive and wish to take an oral contraceptive should have their blood pressure checked one month after starting, again at three months, and thereafter when the prescription is renewed. Women with heart disease who are already hypertensive are best advised of the risk, albeit small, of their hypertension deteriorating. If they feel their reasons for taking an oral contraceptive outweigh this risk, then monthly checks on blood pressure are desirable.

Myocardial infarction

The pathology of arterial occlusion differs from that of venous thrombosis and embolism. The fast and variable blood flow through an artery makes it unlikely that occlusive thrombosis will occur, unless lesions of the arterial wall which reduce the flow already exist. This contrasts with the venous circulation, where increased coagulability or minor trauma may suffice to cause clot formation. Nonetheless, it was said years ago that older women taking a combined oral contraceptive had increased liability to myocardial infarction. It was said that in women over 40 the risk of myocardial infarction, albeit very small, was increased fivefold if they were taking an oral contraceptive. Apart from the fact that not all other studies confirmed this, the finding has to be viewed in perspective. The data were derived in the days when oral contraceptives contained considerably larger amounts of synthetic sex hormones than they do today. There was a tendency to study the age group 35 to 45, whilst the meaningful risk was in women over 40. Finally, several studies suggested that the risk was largely confined to women who smoked cigarettes, were obese or hyperlipidaemic or who were hypertensive.[4] This is all consistent with the problem being associated with pre-existing coronary artery disease.

As a result, women with heart disease aged 35 to 40 should be advised that there may be a small risk if they take an oral contraceptive, and those over 40 or with other predisposing factors should be strongly advised not to take combined oestrogen-progestagen oral contraceptives. Patients known to have coronary artery disease should be told that these preparations are absolutely contraindicated.

Fluid and electrolyte retention

Many women complain of fluid retention and abdominal bloating in the second half of the menstrual cycle or premenstrually. Often this forms part of a premenstrual syndrome. A number of studies on fluid retention have failed to confirm the claim. The reason is that these studies have failed to consider that women probably form a "multi-modal" population in this respect. That is, that a proportion get fluid retention, the majority do not. This may be a matter of the individual's balance between oestrogen and progesterone and their receptors. As a general principle, oestrogens tend to cause water and salt retention; progesterone is a diuretic. On average a combined oral contraceptive tends to relieve the symptoms of premenstrual tension, including fluid retention, perhaps because of supplementation of progesterone effects. Nonetheless, there is great individual variation in reaction to combined oestrogen-progestagen oral contraceptives. There is also variation in the tendency of oral contraceptives of different composition to produce fluid retention in a woman susceptible to this problem.

As a result, if a patient with a risk of or with controlled congestive heart failure wishes to take an oral contraceptive, there is only one way to determine her reaction in this respect, and that is to try her on a standard preparation and ask her to weigh herself daily for one cycle. If she does get related fluid retention, it is worth trying her on a pill of different composition, particularly with respect to the progestagen component.

Congenital heart disease

There are few patients with significant congenital heart disease in whom use of oestrogen-progestagen oral contraception has been recorded. In one study 13 patients took an oral contraceptive for an average of 5 years without attributable problems; one with an atrial septal defect developed pulmonary hypertension at the age of 38 after taking the pill for 6 years.[5]

Heart surgery

There is little information about the use of oral contraception after heart surgery. It is said that the drugs reduce the anticoagulant effects of phenindione or warfarin, so anticoagulated women may require adjustment of their dose.

Summary

In the past oral contraception has been condemned in cardiac patients. With currently available oral oestrogen-progestagen preparations, and appropriate precautions in specified cases, they may be a reasonable option for many women under the age of 40 with heart disease. Oral contraceptives are less likely to cause problems than is a pregnancy.

Other hormone contraceptives

Progestagen only oral contraceptives

There is little case for prescribing these in patients with heart disease. They are less reliable than combined oestrogen-progestagen preparations, with failure rates of 2 to 5/100 woman years. They require a high degree of patient reliability. As they usually do not prevent ovulation, but rely largely on short term effects on cervical mucus, missing a single pill can result in pregnancy. Problems with irregular bleeding and bouts of amenorrhoea, leading to suspicions of pregnancy, are common. As a result, discontinuation rates with the method are high—many women request an alternative after one to two years.

Apart from unreliability, progestagen only oral contraceptives seem to convey much the same risks for cardiac patients as combined preparations. In particular, thromboembolism rates are of the order of 3/10,000 woman-years,[12] much the same as with a combined pill, and there may be the same risk of hypertension developing.

Contraception postpartum may be particularly important to the cardiac patient, who may wish to postpone or prevent another pregnancy. It is common advice that breast feeding women should start a progestagen only oral contraceptive a very few weeks after delivery—breast feeding may often prevent ovulation but not always. The main reason for this advice is that combined oral contraceptives may reduce milk production in some women. The risk of any harm coming to the baby from the minuscule amounts of sex hormones in breast milk is minutely small, and secure contraception with a combined oestrogen-progestagen pill may be more appropriate for the breast feeding cardiac patient.

Vaginal rings releasing a progestagen proved unsatisfactory in practice. Subcutaneous implants releasing a progestagen are a relatively new development. They can cause the same bleeding problems as progestagen only pills, and problems with removal and replacement are being reported. They must be regarded as unsuitable for the cardiac patient until much more experience has been gained with their use.

Injectable progestagens, such as depot medroxyprogesterone, have been described as a contraceptive procedure which may be the one solution for the feckless and the irresponsible, as they have to be administered by a visiting nurse, and relieve the patient of the responsibility for her problems. Most cardiac patients are informed, responsible and motivated individuals who have enough problems with doctors, nurses and hospitals, without relying on them for contraception. The injectable progestagens convey the same metabolic risks and problems with bleeding and amenorrhoea as do progestagen only pills. Discontinuation rates after 1 and 2 years are very high, of the order of 25% and 50% respectively.[6]

The "once a month" injectable combined oestrogen-progestagen contraceptives have been the subject of large scale trials in recent years.[7] No untoward effects on coagulation profiles were detected, and plasma lipid levels fluctuated slightly in relation to the injections, but not to a degree likely to have clinical significance. Discontinuation rates were high, above 38% at 1 year, problems with menstruation being a prominent cause. There have been no reports of use in cardiac patients.

The "morning after pill" is intended to prevent implantation if taken within three days of unprotected intercourse. It consists of a total of 100 µg of ethinyloestradiol and 500 µg of levonorgestrel repeated after 12 hours. It is unwise to give a cardiac patient such a large dose of oestrogen even for a short time, and systemic upsets—nausea, vomiting, headaches and dizziness are common. The procedure is not so effective as insertion of an intra-uterine contraceptive device up to five days after unprotected intercourse, and this should be the preferred alternative.

Intra-uterine contraceptive devices

These devices have been described as the best available contraceptive for a proportion of parous women at certain times in their reproductive lives. They relieve a couple of taking responsibility for contraception, apart from verifying the presence of the device monthly, after menstruation, by palpating the strings in the cervix. Failure rates are probably higher than with oral contraceptives. Unwanted pregnancy rates with copper-bearing devices are claimed to be 1 to 3 per 100 woman years, and rather less with the latest versions. These must be viewed against the fact that follow up rates are seldom more than 90%, and it was shown with Lippes' loops that the pregnancy rate was twice as high in studies with 100% follow up as in studies with 90% follow up.[8]

There is in general no delay in return of fertility after removal of an intra-uterine contraceptive device. In 10 studies involving 3900 women between 72% and 96% of women conceived within one year of removal.[9] The exception is women who have had multiple sexual partners who have an increased risk of tubal infertility.

The principle problems with the devices are complications of insertion, which are uncommon, pelvic infection, menorrhagia and irregular bleeding, vaginal discharge, and spontaneous expulsion, which may pass unnoticed by the patient; and the problems of management of unwanted pregnancy when it occurs and of perforation of the uterus by the device, which is rare.

It was thought at one time that these complications are such that the use of the devices by cardiac patients was contraindicated, but recent studies have shown they can be used safely and effectively. In a recent study 170 women who had mitral commissurotomy or valve replacements had devices inserted with antibiotic cover and there were no cases of bacterial endocarditis.[10] Increased flow at, or duration of, menstruation was reported by 29% and 59% of women without and with anticoagulant treatment respectively, but the same problems were reported by 12 and 34% respectively of women who did not have intra-uterine devices after cardiac surgery. In only one woman did the device have to be removed because of severe bleeding.

Complications of insertion procedures

The "old wives' tale" of "cervical shock"—vasovagal syncope due to dilatation of the cervix without analgesia or anaesthesia—has been shown to occur during insertion of a device. Some 12% of anxious healthy women develop tachycardia during insertion, and 13% have bradycardia or develop a transient arrhythmia.[11,12] Rare cases of cardiac arrest have been reported. A cardiac patient should therefore be prepared for insertion of a device with a premedication including atropine, and insertion conducted under hospital conditions rather than in a family planning clinic.

The vagina and cervix always contain micro-organisms. The cervical glands and mucus plug present an anti-bacterial barrier to their ascent into the uterus. When they are introduced into the upper genital tract, some of these organisms are potentially pathogenic. The hazard can be much reduced by antiseptic cleansing of vagina and cervix before penetrating the cervix, and by good aseptic technique, but these areas are almost impossible to sterilise completely. Insertion of an intra-uterine contraceptive device is usually accompanied by introduction of a few micro-organisms into the uterine cavity. The insertion of a device nearly always causes some minor intra-uterine trauma, and it is likely that a transient bacteraemia can result,

419

much as with a dental extraction. Both these invasions are normally dealt with by natural defence mechanisms.

When intra-uterine devices were first used in cardiac patients there were a very few cases of bacterial endocarditis resulting, in patients with structural heart abnormalities, though there have been no recent reports, probably due to the use of antibiotic prophylaxis. Patients with organic heart disease should be given prophylaxis with a combination like co-amoxiclav and metronidazole to give some gram negative and anaerobic cover, for 24 hours. Perforation of the uterus when a device is inserted is rare, occurring in about 1 in 1000 insertions. A copper-bearing device which has perforated should be removed promptly to prevent bowel adhesions forming. The implications for a patient with heart disease are simply those of the laparoscopy or laparotomy that is likely to be necessary for removal. A basic rule for the prevention of perforation during insertion is to discontinue the attempt promptly if the patient is not fully relaxed or experiences significant pain.

Later complications

Problems with bleeding call for removal of the device and alternative contraception if they are a cause of concern to the patient or are contributing to anaemia.

Pelvic inflammatory disease or pelvic infection is twice as common in women with intra-uterine contraceptive devices as in the general population, but probably occurs in less than 5% of these women. Pelvic infection within the months after insertion may be reduced by the use of prophylactic antibiotics for insertion and with copper-bearing devices—one study reported a prevalence of less than 1% with these devices. On the other hand, women should be tactfully advised that intra-uterine devices do not provide the same protection against the acquisition of sexually transmitted diseases as do barrier methods of contraception. When pelvic infection occurs it should be treated promptly with antibiotics, and the device removed after 24 hours.

In the absence of pelvic infection, the uterine cavity becomes sterile within a month after insertion of an inert device, and probably sooner with a copper-bearing device. There should then therefore be no reason for antibiotics when removing a device by traction on the strings. If intra-uterine manipulations are required to remove the device, for example with missing strings, then patients with structural heart disease should have short term antibiotic cover.

Steroid containing intra-uterine contraceptive devices

When devices containing progesterone, intended to be released over a year were introduced, it was said that they added the side effects and complications of a "progestagen only" oral contraceptive to those of an intra-uterine device. There was no problem with menorrhagia but irregular and infrequent bleeding and amenorrhoea with its associated anxiety about unwanted pregnancy occurred. More recently, devices releasing levonor-gestrel have been introduced, and these would be expected to have less effect on plasma lipids than progesterone itself. Failure (pregnancy) rates as low as 0·5/100 woman years have been claimed. There have as yet been no studies orientated to patients with heart disease, but if the levonorgestrel devices are used in patients at risk of atherosclerosis, plasma lipids should be monitored at intervals.

"Emergency" contraception

Inserted within five days of unprotected intercourse a copper-bearing intra-uterine contraceptive device has a high degree of reliability in preventing implantation of a fertilised ovum. Cardiac patients presenting with this problem should be screened for sexually transmitted diseases and the same precautions taken, prophylactic antibiotics and, particularly if nulliparous, premedication in a hospital setting, as for other insertions.

Barrier contraception

Diaphragms and sheaths are undoubtedly the safest form of contraception for cardiac patients, from the point of view of lack of risk with respect to their heart disease. The main problem is failure rates due to failure to use them properly. The author of the best known study of diaphragm failures[13] called the process "WEUP—wilful exposure to unwanted pregnancy". All of the failures studied were due to failure to use the diaphragm at the mid-cycle, and all the women had an underlying desire for pregnancy, even though it was currently inconvenient. Similarly, most sheath failures are due to "risk-taking" and failure of the patient to ensure that the sheath is being used.

Cardiac patients are usually well motivated and well aware of the consequences of failure. With motivated couples in a stable relationship, failure rates with diaphragms used consistently with a contraceptive cream are as low as 2 to 3/100 woman years. Similarly with sheaths, failure rates are less than 5/100 woman years, of which three quarters are "patient failures", which can be avoided.

Some couples used the "belt and braces" approach, with a diaphragm used consistently and a sheath as well over the days of the mid-cycle. A few find that this reduces sexual intercourse to a mechanical process, and alternative contraception should be sought for them. It is a little surprising in how few couples this problem arises, and it may be compensated by an aspect of rubber fetishism.

421

Other contraceptive procedures

Prolonged breast feeding is a traditional and unreliable approach—many women ovulate sporadically whilst breast feeding, sometimes as early as five or six weeks after delivery. Coitus interruptus—withdrawal—is an unreliable process, which can give rise to the pelvic congestion syndrome in women. As Onan found, the consequences for men can also be undesirable.[14] Periodic abstinence—the safe period—and spermicides, most of which contain nonoxynol-9, both have significant failure rates. Postcoital douching is also unreliable and conveys the risk of air or fluid embolism.

None of these procedures convey both the safety and reliability required for cardiac patients.

Abortion

When abortion is considered by a cardiac patient with an unplanned pregnancy, it is not uncommon for the risks of continuing pregnancy either to be exaggerated or minimised by her cardiologist. It is essential in these cases the patient be given an accurate prognosis for herself and for the baby, and that she draws her own conclusions as to the desirability of abortion. Equally important is that she is not put under pressure by relatives, and at least one interview should be conducted with the patient on her own.

First trimester abortion in a cardiac patient has the same basic risks as any other surgical procedure and should be conducted in a hospital rather than an abortion clinic. The added risks in cardiac patients arise from general anaesthesia and from haemorrhage or infection. It is important in the prevention of these that retained products of conception are avoided. This involves the use of an adequate size suction catheter, even if this means dilating the cervix, and an ultrasound scan the following day to verify completion of the evacuation of the uterus. Patients with any anatomical cardiovascular lesion should have prophylactic antibiotics. Mifepristone can be used to induce abortion, but the risk of retained products is such that it should be followed by surgical evacuation of the uterus (rather than prostaglandins, which have cardiovascular effects), if the ultrasonographer is not confident the uterus is empty.

Second trimester abortion has greater risks of pelvic trauma, haemorrhage and infection, and these should be appraised against the risks of continuing the pregnancy. It is sometimes initiated with mifepristone, and a potent prostaglandin like vaginally administered gemeprost is used to produce the abortion. In addition to possible side effects of nausea, vomiting, diarrhoea and mild pyrexia, bradycardia or tachycardia, fall in blood pressure and reduced cardiac contractility can also occur. If gemeprost is used, the cardiac patient should be closely monitored. If untoward effects occur, an experienced gynaecologist may be needed to complete the abortion surgically. It should not be forgotten that a few gynaecologists had wide experience of performing legal abortions in the second trimester by evacuating the uterus vaginally, and had a safety record better than those achieved with prostaglandins.[15] Should such an individual be available, second trimester abortion by surgical evacuation of the uterus is a feasible alternative.

Tubal sterilisation

The advice so often given to cardiac patients "have your family while you are young and then get your tubes tied", is reasonable for all patients with heart disease, and with selected patients, for example those with Marfan's syndrome, should be put very strongly. With all women the decision for sterilisation must still be theirs, based on accurate information. With less relentlessly progressive heart conditions, and when there is a possibility of cardiac surgery improving prognosis, advice should be more circumspect. There are other factors to be considered, including not only the patient's social and marital circumstances, and the prognosis for these, but also the possible sequelae of sterilisation in younger women. These can include problems with menstruation. In various studies between 1% and 19% of women who had had tubal sterilisation these menstrual abnormalities eventually required hysterectomy. The problem is more prominent in women sterilised before the age of 30. There are cases of "defeminisation" in younger women who are sterilised, with loss of libido and related problems, but this is uncommon when the indication for the operation was medical. Sterilisation counselling in cardiac patients must be well informed and thorough.

Sterilisation is a considerably more effective procedure than any form of contraception, so much so that failures are usually expressed "per reproductive lifetime", instead of per 100 woman years. No operation for sterilisation yet devised is 100 per cent effective. There are over 55 cases in the literature of women who achieved a pregnancy, albeit ectopic, after hysterectomy.[16]

The commonest procedures for tubal sterilisation used today are the Pomeroy operation, in which a loop of each tube is ligated with catgut and excised through a small abdominal incision, and the application of metal clips or plastic rings to the tubes using a laparoscope. The "Oxford" modification of the Pomeroy operation involves resection of only a short length of tube and interposing the broad ligament between the two cut and ligated ends. Documented failure rates with the Pomeroy operation range from 0·1% to 0·8%.[17] With clips, failure rates range nil to 0·7%, and with rings nil to 2·7%. Failure rates are a bit higher if the operation is performed at the time of caesarean section or legal abortion. This has to be balanced by the inconvenience of re-admission to hospital and further anaesthesia, for "interval" sterilisation.

Sterilisation failure is usually a consequence of a surgical error, and it has been found that the incidence is inversely related to experience of the surgeon. Sometimes it is due to recanalisation or formation of a fistula bypassing the tubal obstruction. When pregnancy does occur after tubal sterilisation it is ectopic in between 4% and 64% in various studies.[17] This may sound alarming, but overall the incidence of ectopic pregnancy in women who have had tubal sterilisation in the previous two years is 0·15%, which is less than the overall risk of ectopic pregnancy in the general population of about 0·2 per hundred women of reproductive age per year.

Overall, it is probably safer for a woman with significant heart disease to have tubal sterilisation performed surgically by an experienced surgeon through a small laparotomy incision, under general anaesthesia. This takes less time than clip or ring sterilisation by laparoscopy, and cases of cardiac arrhythmia and cardiac arrest, and even isolated fatalities, have been reported during laparoscopy. It is not clear if these are due to the distension of the abdomen required alone or to the fact that it is distended with carbon dioxide. Full monitoring is required, and laparoscopy is generally regarded as contraindicated in patients with organic heart disease. Most gynaecologists feel that they can operate more efficiently and avoid emotional and physical reactions from a cardiac patient with general rather than local anaesthesia, but some anaesthetists may prefer spinal anaesthesia.

Vasectomy

In general this should be offered as an alternative to tubal sterilisation. Unless it is suggested or has been considered by the couple concerned, the procedure and its consequences is explained and the couple given time for consideration. Their conclusion may be motivated in a variety of ways, which they are reluctant to reveal to a doctor. Their thoughts may range from a deep-seated fear on the male side of a threat to virility or plans for a second marriage in the future, to the female's fear that it may provide her partner with the opportunity for unlimited promiscuity.

More tact is required in raising the issue when the female patient has significant heart disease. Care must be taken to avoid the husband feeling any sort of pressure to have the operation for his partner's benefit. The potential for marital stress and break-up is obvious, particularly if the female partner's life expectancy is limited. The couple may well have already considered vasectomy. If not, the possibility should be mentioned and it should be left to them to discuss it and the implications, and perhaps make a joint request for the male partner to have a vasectomy. The man should at some stage be seen alone before the operation, to ensure that he has considered all the implications and it is what *he* wants!

References

1 Vessey MP, Lawless M, McPherson K, Yeates D. Fertility after stopping use of intrauterine contraceptive device. *BMJ* 1983; **286**: 106.

2 Farmer RDT, Preston TD. The risk of venous thromboembolism associated with low oestrogen oral contraceptives. *J Obstet Gynaecol* 1995; **15**: 195–200.

3 Brenner PF, Mishell DR. Contraception for the woman with significant cardiac disease. *Clin Obstet Gynecol* 1975; **18**: 155–68.

4 *Population Reports.* Lower-dose pills. 1988; series A, number 7: 1–31.

5 Rabajoli F, Aruta E, Presbitero P, Todros T. Rischi della contraccezione e della gravidanza in patienti con cardiopatie congenite. Studio retrospettivo in 108 pazienti. *G Ital Cardiol* 1992; **22**: 1133–7.

6 Elder MG. New hormone contraceptives; injectable preparations. *J Obstet Gynaecol* 1982; **3(suppl 1)**: S21–24.

7 Newton JR, d'Arcangues C, Hall PE. "Once-a-month" combined injectable contraceptives. *J Obstet Gynaecol* 1994; **14(suppl 1)**: S1–34.

8 Hawkins DF, Elder MG. *Human fertility control. Theory and practice.* London: Butterworth, 1979.

9 *Population Reports.* IUDs—a new look. 1988; series B, number **16**: 1–31.

10 Abdalla MY, Mostafa EED. Contraception after heart surgery. *Contraception*, 1992; **45**: 73–80.

11 Acker D, Boehm FH, Askew DE, Rothman H. Electrocardiogram changes with intrauterine contraceptive device insertion. *Am J Obstet Gynecol* 1973; **115**: 458–61.

12 Sherrod DB, Nicholl W. Electrocardiographic changes during intrauterine contraceptive device insertion. *Am J Obstet Gynecol* 1974; **119**: 1044–51.

13 Lehfelt H. Wilful exposure to unwanted pregnancy (WEUP). Psychological explanation for patient failures in contraception. *Am J Obstet Gynecol* 1959; **78**: 661–5.

14 *Genesis*; **38**: 8–10.

15 Centers for Disease Control. *Abortion surveillance 1975.* Atlanta: US Department of Health, Education and Welfare, Public Health Service, 1977.

16 Bennett SJ. Pregnancy following hysterectomy. *J Obstet Gynaecol* 1993; **13**: 117–25.

17 *Population Reports.* Female Sterilisation. Minilaparotomy and laparoscopy; safe, effective, and widely used. 1985; series C, number **9**: 125–67.

Index

Page numbers in **bold** type refer to figures; those in *italic* refer to tables or boxed material.